LONG-TERM RESULTS IN PLASTIC AND RECONSTRUCTIVE SURGERY

VOLUME I

*The Physician: dealing with the present but with an eye
to the past and future*

Sculpture in Wood by Jacob Goldwyn, M.D.

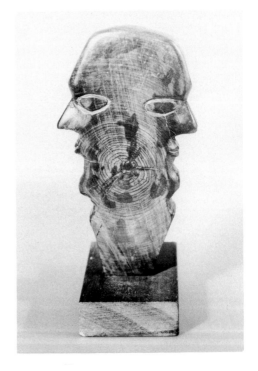

Edited by
Robert M. Goldwyn, M.D.

Clinical Professor of Surgery, Harvard
Medical School; Head, Division of Plastic Surgery,
Beth Israel Hospital; Surgeon, Beth Israel Hospital
and Peter Bent Brigham Hospital, Boston; Editor,
Plastic and Reconstructive Surgery

LONG-TERM RESULTS IN PLASTIC AND RECONSTRUCTIVE SURGERY

Little, Brown and Company, Boston

CONTENTS

PREFACE

AN unfortunate consequence of being a physician is that the crush of the present too often obscures a view of the past and a conception of the future. Daily trivia as well as demands in the office, at the bedside, and in the operating room are not conducive to gaining perspective. In their day-to-day activities, few areas of medicine are concerned with vistas; public health and psychiatry are the exceptions. It is difficult for most physicians to extricate themselves from the turnstile to get a good look backward, in order to improve their future care of patients. Moreover, the surgical residency, with its frenetic quality, is hardly a setting for contemplating and assessing long-term results. Because of the relatively short duration and frequent rotations of surgical residency, residents seldom benefit from their own observations of the eventual outcome of their treatment. In fact, the usual pattern is for the most senior resident to do the most complicated procedures in the few months or even days before departing forever from the scene.

This book was written to present the long view. That its objective serves a purpose needs no elaboration. Something, however, should be said about its shortcomings. Despite persistent efforts to keep the scope broad and the contents complete, there remain distressing lacunae. In certain areas, nobody could be found with sufficient experience and enthusiasm to review patients and to report the results. A few began the task but felt that the data would not be significant because of poor patient retrieval; in some situations, the editor and the author experienced the pain of a chapter rejected because it did not focus adequately on long-term results. If a second edition is ever justified by reader response, this type of book should be easier to produce and better to peruse because the prototype exists.

Not included in the contents by design is the large area of long-term results of cancer surgery, particularly of the head and neck. Five- to ten-year survival, for example, and death rates for neoplastic disease have been omitted. This information, though of obvious importance, is easily obtained elsewhere.

This book should help those who are younger to avoid the errors of their elders. In the words of Cicero, "Not to know what happened before one was born is to remain a child."

R. M. G.

ACKNOWLEDGMENTS

THIS book contains the life experiences of many. No professional career has the duration and breadth to encompass all aspects of plastic surgery. Whatever deficiencies this book may have, they would have been worse without the presence of my colleagues. I am extremely grateful to the contributors for their willingness not only to do hard work but to confront unyielding reality. A look backward is not always pleasant.

As in my other books, I have benefited from the complete support and wise counsel of Fred Belliveau, Vice President and General Manager of the Medical Division of Little, Brown and Company. I am very appreciative of Norma Langthorne's initial thorough evaluation of the manuscript. To Marcia Mirski and to Jane MacNeil, project editors, I am thankful for their expertise and enthusiasm, and their implacable commitment to excellence. I am indebted also to James K. Madru, copyeditor, to Phyllis Ehrlich and James Krosschell, proofreaders, and to Steve Csipke, indexer, for their singular skills.

In addition to her unusual competence, Bobbi Quigley, my secretary (who typed the entire manuscript), exhibited monumental cheerfulness despite innumerable revisions. Kay Mulcahy and Jane Sivacek, my other secretaries, also veterans (victims) of previous books, successfully and painlessly juggled me from hospital to office, to home, to library. For their equanimity, I am much beholden.

Once again I was blessed in having Marion Levine at the Francis A. Countway Library of Medicine at Harvard Medical School to verify references.

I wish to thank Richard W. St. Clair and Joan R. Warren, master photographers, for helping me with the illustrations.

I am grateful also to Dr. Joseph E. Murray for his efforts in the early stages of this book.

N. H. Antia, F.R.C.S.

Professor of Plastic Surgery, Grant Medical College, University of Bombay; Chief, Tata Department of Plastic Surgery, J. J. Group of Hospitals, Bombay, India

COMMENTS ON CHAPTER 27

Lars Avellán, M.D.

Lecturer in Plastic Surgery, University of Göteborg; Assistant Chief Surgeon, Department of Plastic Surgery, Sahlgrenska Sjukhuset, Göteborg, Sweden

CHAPTER 17

Thomas J. Baker, M.D.

Assistant Clinical Professor of Surgery (Plastic), University of Miami School of Medicine, Miami, Florida

CHAPTER 32

Arthur J. Barsky, M.D.

Professor Emeritus of Plastic Surgery, Albert Einstein College of Medicine of Yeshiva University; Consulting Surgeon, Mt. Sinai and Beth Israel Medical Centers, New York

COMMENTS ON CHAPTER 45

Norman R. Bernstein, M.D.

Professor of Psychiatry, University of Illinois College of Medicine; Medical Staff, Department of Psychiatry, University of Illinois Hospital, Chicago

CHAPTER 2

Edgar P. Berry, M.D.

Chief of Plastic Surgery, Plastic Surgical Service, Lenox Hill Hospital, New York

CHAPTER 35

G. Boering, M.D.

Professor of Oral Surgery, State University, Groningen, the Netherlands

CHAPTER 52

Raymond O. Brauer, M.D.

Clinical Professor of Plastic Surgery, Baylor College of

CONTRIBUTING AUTHORS

Medicine; Active Staff and Chief, Division of Plastic Surgery, St. Joseph Hospital, Houston, Texas
CHAPTER 45

T. Ray Broadbent, M.D.
Associate Clinical Professor, University of Utah College of Medicine; Active Staff, Latter-Day Saints Hospital and University of Utah Medical Center, Salt Lake City
CHAPTER 28

Bradford Cannon, M.D.
Clinical Professor Emeritus of Surgery, Harvard Medical School; Senior Surgeon, Plastic Surgery, Massachusetts General Hospital, Boston
CHAPTER 5

Matías Pradas Caravaca, M.D.
Resident, German Hospital, Madrid
CHAPTER 16

Salvador Castañares, M.S., M.D.
Division of Plastic Surgery, University of Southern California School of Medicine; Past Senior and Chief of Plastic Surgery, Hospital of the Good Samaritan and Hollywood Presbyterian Hospital, Los Angeles
CHAPTER 33

Thomas D. Cronin, M.D.
Clinical Professor of Plastic Surgery, Baylor College of Medicine; Active Staff and Director, Plastic Surgery Residency Program, St. Joseph Hospital, Houston, Texas
CHAPTER 45

A. Lee Dellon, M.D.
Resident in Plastic Surgery, The Johns Hopkins University School of Medicine, Baltimore
CHAPTER 44

Charles J. Devine, M.D.
Professor and Chairman, Department of Urology, Eastern Virginia Medical School; Attending Urologist and Chief, Department of Urology, Medical Center Hospitals, Norfolk
CHAPTER 18

Francisco Rodríguez Durán, M.D.
Former Assistant, San Rafael Children's Hospital, Madrid
CHAPTER 16

Isaac Eliachar, M.D.
Senior Lecturer of Otolaryngology, Technion Faculty of Medicine; Head, Department of Otolaryngology, Rambam Medical Center, Haifa, Israel
CHAPTER 12

Martin A. Entin, M.D.
Associate Professor, Department of Surgery, McGill University Faculty of Medicine; Honorary Attending Surgeon and former Chief of Plastic Surgery, Royal Victoria Hospital, Montreal
COMMENTS ON CHAPTER 46

Bromley S. Freeman, M.D.
Clinical Professor of Plastic Surgery, Baylor College of Medicine; Attending Plastic Surgeon, Methodist Hospital (Texas Medical Center), Houston
CHAPTER 22

Osamu Fukuda, M.D.
Professor of Plastic Surgery, School of Medicine, University of Tokyo; Chief, Plastic Surgery Unit, University of Tokyo Hospital, Tokyo
COMMENTS ON CHAPTER 9

Julien Glicenstein, M.D.
Professor of Plastic Surgery, Université de Paris V-René Descartes, Faculté Necker-Enfants Malades; Consulting Plastic Surgeon, Hôpital Boucicaut, Paris
CHAPTER 13

Robert M. Goldwyn, M.D.
Clinical Professor of Surgery, Harvard Medical School; Head, Division of Plastic Surgery, Beth Israel Hospital; Surgeon, Beth Israel Hospital and Peter Bent Brigham Hospital, Boston; Editor, Plastic and Reconstructive Surgery
EDITOR

Howard L. Gordon, M.D.
Assistant Clinical Professor of Surgery (Plastic), University of Miami School of Medicine, Miami, Florida
CHAPTER 32

Frederick M. Grazer, M.D.
Associate Clinical Professor of Surgery, University of California, Irvine, California College of Medicine; Active Staff, Hoag Memorial Hospital Presbyterian, Newport Beach
CHAPTER 42

Walter Guralnick, D.M.D.
Professor and Chairman, Department of Oral Surgery, Harvard School of Dental Medicine; Chief, Department of Oral Surgery, Massachusetts General Hospital, Boston
COMMENTS ON CHAPTER 26

Robert L. Harding, M.D., D.D.S.
Clinical Professor of Plastic Surgery, Pennsylvania State University College of Medicine, Hershey; Plastic Surgeon, Harrisburg General Hospital and Polyclinic Medical Center, Harrisburg
CHAPTER 7

Ulrich T. Hinderer, M.D.
Professor of Urologic Plastic Surgery, Universitas Complutensis; Head, Plastic Surgery Departments at German Hospital and St. Raphael's Children's Hospital, Madrid
CHAPTER 16

Edward C. Hinds, D.D.S., M.D.
Professor and Chairman, Department of Surgery, The University of Texas Dental Branch at Houston; Chief, Dentistry and Oral Surgery Service, The Methodist Hospital, Houston
CHAPTER 26

Bernard Hirshowitz, M.D.
Professor of Plastic Surgery, Technion Faculty of Medicine; Head, Department of Plastic Surgery, Rambam Medical Center, Haifa, Israel
CHAPTER 12

John E. Hoopes, M.D.
Professor of Surgery (Plastic Surgery), The Johns Hopkins University School of Medicine, Baltimore
CHAPTER 44

Charles E. Horton, M.D.
Professor and Chairman, Department of Plastic Surgery, Eastern Virginia Medical School; Chief, Department of Plastic Surgery, Medical Center Hospitals, Norfolk
CHAPTER 18

A. J. C. Huffstadt, M.D.
Professor of Plastic Surgery, State University, Groningen; Head, Department of Plastic Surgery, University Hospital, Groningen, the Netherlands
CHAPTER 52

Bengt Johanson, M.D.
Professor of Plastic Surgery, University of Göteborg; Director, Department of Plastic Surgery, Sahlgrenska Sjukhuset, Göteborg, Sweden
CHAPTER 17

Hugh A. Johnson, M.D., M.S. (Plastic Surgery)
Clinical Associate, Rockford School of Medicine; Plastic Surgery Consultant, Burn Unit, St. Anthony Hospital, Rockford, Illinois
CHAPTER 14

Leonard B. Kaban, D.M.D., M.D.
Assistant Professor of Oral Surgery, Harvard Medical School; Associate in Surgery, Peter Bent Brigham Hospital, Boston
COMMENTS ON CHAPTER 24

Sidney Kahn, M.D.
Clinical Professor of Surgery (Plastic), Mount Sinai School of Medicine of the City University of New York; Chief, Department of Plastic Surgery, Beth Israel Medical Center, New York
CHAPTER 37

Bernard L. Kaye, M.D.
Clinical Professor of Surgery (Plastic), University of Florida College of Medicine, Gainesville; Chief, Plastic Surgery Service, Baptist Medical Center, Jacksonville
CHAPTER 34

Lynn D. Ketchum, M.D.
Professor of Surgery, Section of Plastic Surgery, Department of Surgery, University of Kansas College of Health Sciences and Hospital, School of Medicine, Kansas City
CHAPTER 51

Jerome R. Klingbeil, M.D.

Associate Clinical Professor, Department of Surgery (Plastic), University of California, Irvine, California College of Medicine; Active Staff, Surgery Department, Memorial Hospital Medical Center of Long Beach

CHAPTER 42

Edward Lamont, M.D.

Professor of Clinical Surgery, Department of Surgery, Division of Plastic and Reconstructive Surgery, University of California, Irvine, California College of Medicine

CHAPTER 4

Xavier Latouche, M.D.

Faculté de Rennes; Chief of Clinic, Centre Hospitalier de Rennes, France

CHAPTER 13

Gordon Letterman, M.D.

Professor of Surgery (Plastic Surgery), George Washington University School of Medicine and Health Sciences, Washington, D.C.

CHAPTER 15

Michael L. Lewin, M.D.

Professor Emeritus of Plastic Surgery, Albert Einstein College of Medicine of Yeshiva University; Director of Plastic Surgery, The Hospital of the Albert Einstein College of Medicine, New York

CHAPTER 21

John R. Lewis, Jr., M.D.

Director, Institute of Aesthetic Plastic Surgery, Atlanta; Associate Clinical Professor of Surgery (Plastic), Emory University School of Medicine, Atlanta; Clinical Professor of Surgery (Plastic), University of Kentucky College of Medicine, Lexington; Chief, Department of Plastic Surgery, Doctors Memorial Hospital, Atlanta

CHAPTER 43

William K. Lindsay, M.D.

Professor of Surgery, Division of Plastic Surgery, University of Toronto Faculty of Medicine; Senior Surgeon and Head, Division of Plastic Surgery, The Hospital for Sick Children, Toronto

CHAPTER 6

Clyde Litton, M.D., D.D.S.

Chief of Plastic Surgery, Doctors Hospital, Washington, D.C.; Consultant in Plastic Surgery, Bethesda Naval Hospital, Bethesda, Maryland

COMMENTS ON CHAPTER 32

W. M. Manchester, M.B., Ch.B., F.R.C.S., F.R.A.C.S.

Professor of Plastic and Reconstructive Surgery, Auckland University Medical School; Head, Department of Plastic and Reconstructive Surgery, Middlemore Hospital, Auckland, New Zealand

CHAPTER 23

James K. Masson, M.D.

Associate Professor of Surgery, Mayo Medical School; Plastic Surgeon, Mayo Clinic, Rochester, Minnesota

CHAPTER 20

Mary Mattiello, B.S.

Patient Interviewer and Researcher, Newport Beach, California

CHAPTER 42

Frederick J. McCoy, M.D.

Clinical Professor of Surgery and Chairman, Section of Plastic Surgery, University of Missouri—Kansas City School of Medicine; Chairman, Plastic Surgery, Children's Mercy Hospital, Kansas City, Missouri

CHAPTER 25

John B. McCraw, M.D.

Associate Professor of Plastic Surgery, Eastern Virginia Medical School; Director, Plastic Surgery Residency Program, Medical Center Hospitals, Norfolk

CHAPTER 18

Jeffrey Meilman, M.D.

Fellow in Head and Neck Surgery, Roswell Park Memorial Institute, Buffalo, New York

CHAPTER 24

Bryan C. Mendelson, F.R.C.S.E., F.R.A.C.S.

Assistant Plastic Surgeon, Alfred Hospital, Melbourne, Australia

CHAPTER 20

Timothy A. Miller, M.D.
Associate Professor, Division of Plastic Surgery, University of California, Los Angeles, Center for Health Sciences; Chief, Division of Plastic Surgery, Wadsworth Veterans Hospital, Los Angeles
COMMENTS ON CHAPTER 44

Vladimir Mitz, M.D.
Chief of Clinic, Université de Paris V-René Descartes, Faculté Necker-Enfants Malades; Chief of Clinic, Hôpital Boucicaut, Paris
CHAPTER 39

Bernard L. Morgan, M.D.
Clinical Professor of Plastic Surgery, University of Florida College of Medicine, Gainesville; Program Director, Plastic Surgery Residency Training Program, Jacksonville Health Educational Programs; Chairman, Department of Surgery, Baptist Medical Center, Jacksonville
CHAPTER 36

Joseph E. Murray, M.D.
Professor of Surgery, Harvard Medical School; Chief, Divisions of Plastic Surgery at Children's Hospital Medical Center and Peter Bent Brigham Hospital, Boston
COMMENTS ON CHAPTERS 5, 12, 21, 23, 24, 50

John C. Mustardé, F.R.C.S.
Lecturer Emeritus in Plastic Surgery, Glasgow University; Consultant Emeritus in Plastic Surgery, West of Scotland Plastic Surgery Unit, Canniesburn Hospital, Glasgow
CHAPTER 10

Katsuya Namba, M.D.
Professor, Department of Plastic Surgery, Nagasaki University Medical School, Nagasaki, Japan
CHAPTER 54

Seiichi Ohmori, M.D.
Chief of Department of Plastic and Reconstructive Surgery, Tokyo Metropolitan Police Hospital, Tokyo
CHAPTER 27

Francis X. Paletta, M.D.
Clinical Professor of Surgery, St. Louis University School of Medicine; Director of Plastic Surgery, St. Louis Medical Center, St. Louis
CHAPTER 3

George C. Peck, M.D.
Associate Professor of Plastic Surgery, Temple University School of Medicine, Philadelphia
CHAPTER 30

Vincent R. Pennisi, M.D., D.D.S.
Clinical Associate Professor of Surgery (Plastic), University of California, San Francisco, School of Medicine; Director, Subcutaneous Mastectomy Data Evaluation Center, Saint Francis Memorial Hospital, San Francisco
CHAPTER 41

Alan D. Perlmutter, M.D.
Professor of Urology, Wayne State University School of Medicine; Chief, Department of Pediatric Urology, Children's Hospital of Michigan, Detroit
COMMENTS ON CHAPTERS 16, 17

Paul P. Pickering, M.D., D.D.S.
Professor of Clinical Surgery, University of California, San Diego, School of Medicine; Attending Staff (Surgery), Mercy Hospital, San Diego
CHAPTER 38

Robert Pool, M.D.
Chief, Department of Plastic and Reconstructive Surgery, William Beaumont Hospital, Royal Oak, Michigan
COMMENTS ON CHAPTER 8

Sir Benjamin Rank, C.M.G., M.S., F.R.C.S., F.R.A.C.S., F.A.C.S.
Consulting Plastic Surgeon, The Royal Melbourne Hospital, Melbourne, Australia
CHAPTERS 46, 48

Paule C.L. Regnault, M.D.
Ex Clinical Professor Agrégé, Université de Montréal
COMMENTS ON CHAPTER 42

David W. Robinson, M.D.
Vice Chancellor for Clinical Affairs, University of Kansas Medical Center; Professor of Surgery (Plastic), University of Kansas College of Health Sciences and Hospital, School of Medicine, Kansas City
CHAPTER 50, COMMENTS ON CHAPTER 22

Maurice Rousso, M.D.

Head, Service for Hand Surgery, Hebrew University; Senior Surgeon, Hand Unit, Department of Orthopedics, Hadassah—Mount Scopus Hospital, Jerusalem

CHAPTER 49

Richard Carlton Schulz, M.D.

Professor of Surgery, The Abraham Lincoln School of Medicine; Chief, Division of Plastic Surgery, University of Illinois Hospital, Chicago

CHAPTER 24

Maxine Schurter, M.D.

Associate Clinical Professor of Surgery, George Washington University School of Medicine and Health Sciences, Washington, D.C.

CHAPTER 15

Bernard E. Simon, M.D.

Clinical Professor of Surgery (Plastic), Mount Sinai School of Medicine of the City University of New York; Chief, Department of Plastic Surgery, The Mount Sinai Hospital, New York

CHAPTER 37

Richard C. Smith, M.S.

Research Director, Plastic Surgical Associates, Inc., Brookline, Massachusetts

CHAPTERS 11, 31

Wendell M. Smoot III, M.D.

Chief Resident, Plastic Surgery, St. Joseph Hospital, Houston, Texas

CHAPTER 45

Melvin Spira, M.D., D.D.S.

Professor of Surgery and Head, Division of Plastic Surgery, Baylor College of Medicine; Chief of Plastic Surgery, The Methodist Hospital, Ben Taub General Hospital, and Veterans Administration Hospital, Houston, Texas

COMMENTS ON CHAPTERS 10, 11

Richard B. Stark, M.D.

Professor of Clinical Surgery, Columbia University College of Physicians and Surgeons; Attending Surgeon, St. Luke's Hospital Center, New York

COMMENTS ON CHAPTER 6

Jan O. Strömbeck, M.D.

Docent of Plastic Surgery, Karolinska Institutet; Chief of Plastic Surgery, Sabbatsbergs Sjukhus, Stockholm

CHAPTER 40

Craig S. Sutton, D.D.S.

Senior Resident, Oral Surgery, The University of Texas Dental Branch at Houston, Houston

CHAPTER 26

Alfred B. Swanson, M.D.

Clinical Professor of Surgery, Michigan State University College of Human Medicine, Lansing; Program Director, Orthopedic Surgery Residency, Blodgett Memorial Hospital and Butterworth Hospital, Grand Rapids, Michigan

CHAPTER 47

Genevieve de Groot Swanson, M.D.

Plastic Surgeon and Coordinator of Orthopedic Research, Blodgett Memorial Hospital, Grand Rapids, Michigan

CHAPTER 47

Radford C. Tanzer, M.D.

Clinical Professor Emeritus of Plastic Surgery, Dartmouth Medical School, Hanover, New Hampshire; Consultant in Plastic Surgery, Veterans Administration Hospital, White River Junction, Vermont

CHAPTER 9

Charles P. Vallis, M.D.

Instructor in Plastic Surgery and Dermatology, Tufts University School of Medicine, Boston

CHAPTER 19

Thomas R. Vecchione, M.D.

Assistant Professor of Surgery, Division of Plastic Surgery, University of California, San Diego, School of Medicine; Attending Staff (Surgery), Mercy Hospital, San Diego

CHAPTER 38

Raymond Vilain, M.D.

Professor of Plastic Surgery, Université de Paris V-René Descartes, Faculté Necker-Enfants Malades; Head, Plastic Surgery Service, Hôpital Boucicaut, Paris

CHAPTERS 13, 39

John Watson, M.A., F.R.C.S.

Teacher Emeritus, The University of London; Consultant Plastic Surgeon and Head Emeritus, Department of Plastic Surgery, The London Hospital, London, and The Queen Victoria Hospital, East Grinstead, Sussex, England
CHAPTER 53

R. C. A. Weatherley-White, M.D.

Associate Clinical Professor in Surgery, University of Colorado School of Medicine, Denver; Adjunct Professor of Speech, University of Denver, Colorado
COMMENTS ON CHAPTER 7

George V. Webster, M.D.

Clinical Professor of Surgery (Plastic), University of California, Los Angeles, School of Medicine; Senior Attending Surgeon (Plastic), Huntington Memorial Hospital, Pasadena, California
CHAPTER 29

Richard C. Webster, M.D.

Associate Surgeon in Otolaryngology (Plastic Surgery), Massachusetts Eye and Ear Infirmary, Boston
CHAPTERS 11, 31

Menachem Ron Wexler, M.D.

Associate Professor of Plastic Surgery, Hadassah Hebrew University Medical School; Acting Chief, Department of Plastic and Maxillofacial Surgery, Hadassah University Hospital, Jerusalem
CHAPTER 49

William L. White, M.D.

Clinical Professor of Surgery, University of Pittsburgh School of Medicine; Chief, Plastic Surgery Section, University of Pittsburgh Medical Center Hospitals, Pittsburgh
COMMENTS ON CHAPTER 47

John E. Williams, M.D.

Active Medical Staff, Century City Hospital, Los Angeles, and Daniel Freeman Hospital, Inglewood, California
CHAPTER 38

Robert M. Woolf, M.D.

Associate Clinical Professor, Plastic Surgery, University of Utah College of Medicine; Active Staff, Latter-Day Saints Hospital and Primary Children's Medical Center, Salt Lake City
CHAPTER 28

Sidney K. Wynn, M.D.

Clinical Professor of Plastic Surgery, The Medical College of Wisconsin; Director, Cleft Palate Center, Milwaukee Children's Hospital; Chief, Plastic Surgery, Mt. Sinai Medical Center, Milwaukee
CHAPTER 8

The greatest friend of truth is time.
C. C. Colton, 1822

Time is the plastic surgeon's greatest ally and also his most trenchant critic.
H. W. Gillies, 1920

LONG-TERM RESULTS IN PLASTIC AND RECONSTRUCTIVE SURGERY

1 ALTHOUGH the evaluation of patients many years after treatment presumably should yield important information, these reports have been relatively scarce in the history of medicine for several reasons. Foremost is that the scientific method had to evolve before such an enquiry could be conceived and achieved. Thinking in terms of direct cause and effect and gathering and interpreting data with objectivity are recent developments in human thought. For millennia, explanations for the simplest events were sought in the unseen forces of nature ruled by myriads of deities. Slowly, in response to the challenges of the environment and the pressures of emerging civilization, the human animal, by error and design, became more adept at living on this planet. In the process, he learned more about his own body. Extraterrestrial agencies were less frequently invoked to explain biological phenomena or to cure illness. More immediate causes were considered responsible for specific events. Medicine had left its age of superstition and entered the era of empiricism.

Despite the lack of a computer to retrieve data, the physician or surrogate—shaman, apothecary, barber surgeon—did get feedback from his therapeutics. In fact, his payments or punishments frequently depended on whether the patient improved or worsened. How many surgeons today would be willing to practice under the code of King Hammurabi (about 1700 B.C.)?

If a physician performed a major operation on a seignior with a bronze lancet and has caused the seignior's death, or he opened the eye socket of a seignior and has destroyed the seignior's eye, they shall cut off his hand.

Learning from the experience of others was much more difficult in ancient times than now,

Robert M. Goldwyn

PERSPECTIVES

partly because of the absence of good records. Although the notations by the pupils of Hippocrates are one of the most remarkable examples of medical recording, they are, nevertheless, an imprecise legacy of what was then known and done. Not until the nineteenth century did European and American doctors keep even scanty records of their patients, and then primarily to collect fees.

By a statistical analysis of his records, Charles-Alexandre Louis (1787–1872), properly considered the founder of medical statistics, proved that blood-letting was valueless in the treatment of pneumonia, but unfortunately his contemporaries were blind to the virtue of his quantitative methods.

Long-term results require vital as well as medical statistics. Accurately recorded births and deaths, with the causes of the latter, are indispensable to charting the complete course of a patient. Helpful also is the census, conceived initially to levy taxes and to raise armies, but now a good source of information about who is where. Even with these aids, however, locating and communicating with patients many years after treatment is arduous. Names change with marriage, and in this country, geographical mobility is great. The average American supposedly changes residence six times during a lifetime. His whereabouts may remain unknown despite the services of the post office, the telephone company, and both public and private agencies.

Another requirement for a long-term evaluation is the survival of not only the patient but also the physician or a successor with enough interest in a follow-up. That someone other than the original physician should do a late evaluation of the patient would seem disadvantageous, yet the lack of continuity might be offset by the gain in objectivity. Ideally, the patient should be seen by both the doctor who gave the first treatment and a dispassionate, skilled medical observer. Information obtained solely from questionnaires sent to patients may be inaccurate and incomplete because of their total subjectivity. The longer the follow-up, the greater the number of variables. Both the patient and the doctor change in terms of their perceptions, expectations, and mental and physical status.

Even without the confounding factor of the passage of time, we in plastic and reconstructive surgery deal with less-defined variables than in most areas of medicine. Assessment of mortality at 5 or 10 years after colectomy for carcinoma, for example, is clear and unambiguous. In contrast, the long-term evaluation of a patient after a face lift is less straightforward, for it involves the complex process of aging and the elusive criterion of happiness. Plastic surgery shares with psychiatry the amorphous task of being concerned with human contentment. It would be hard to conclude that a rhytidectomy, no matter how well executed, was justified, or that psychotherapy, no matter how well conducted, was worthwhile if the patient stated that she was made more unhappy because of it. The legitimacy of a procedure undertaken for the removal of a cancer does not include an assessment of a patient's satisfaction with his or her life as a result of having had the cancer removed. These differences between much of plastic and reconstructive surgery and the life and death arenas of medicine may seem too basic to belabor, yet their very obviousness may obscure their importance.

A subtle, rarely articulated reason for the reluctance to do a long-term evaluation is perhaps the unconscious feeling that time and death eventually will erase all benefits of any surgery. Aesthetic surgery, for example, to reduce signs of aging is ultimately a losing battle;

so also is any type of medical or surgical treatment. The very long view can become the destructive view. It can lead to therapeutic nihilism. Why treat duodenal atresia if the baby will eventually die at age 75? All of us who are concerned with the preservation of life and the alleviation of pain are asked and required to intervene at a specific time in the life of another human being. That intervention should be appropriate, effective, and immediate. Most of us would act now to save someone's life even if we knew that 3 months later he would commit suicide.

Another problem to ponder is how long the follow-up should be. For many conditions, the answer will be found in subsequent chapters of this book, but consider an incision and drainage of an abscess. The results should be known in a few days and certainly in a couple of weeks. If it had been an infected cyst, the outcome of surgery with respect to recurrence could not be assessed in less than a few years. In essence, the follow-up should be as long as required to give the desired information. But for how long and for how much is a surgeon responsible, either directly or indirectly? Sagging of the upper lids to their preoperative appearance 10 months after an eyelidplasty would likely prompt the disappointed patient to demand an explanation. This same phenomenon, if it occurred 10 years after surgery, would not be considered the surgeon's responsibility. With some problems, time helps a surgeon's efforts and the patient's results, scar revision being a notable example. In that instance, long-term evaluation can be confusing because we do not know whether the scar would have improved to the same degree without operation. However, in other situations, long-term assessment is critical. Too often in plastic surgery we have accepted

reports on the benefits of a new lip repair with only meager follow-up of 1 or 2 years. Sometimes by choice, and frequently by necessity, we must extrapolate from the present to the future. Is it reasonable to expect that a surgeon would wait 20 years before describing a technique that seems promising? Furthermore, for some medical problems and their surgical solutions it may not be necessary to wait a decade before judging the results. This fact will become apparent from the information presented in this book. The realities of the professional marketplace encourage ambition in those with the least experience, whereas those with the most service stripes may have reached their pinnacle or plateau and are the least driven to summarize their work.

Civilization can be viewed as an accumulation of information whose validity and relevance are continually assessed by long-term follow-up. While each generation need not reinvent the wheel, it nevertheless must question the past while learning from it. Looking backward is not the same as summing up. Information derived from the experience of an individual or a nation does not have intrinsic finality. The problems of today may not exist tomorrow, or if they do, their definitions and solutions may change. The history of medicine is replete with egregious miscalculations by those who should have know better—that a specific disease can "never be cured" or "should always be treated by" a method now viewed as primitive or nonsensical.

The gathering of long-term results is a feeble anodyne to the human malady of "growing old too soon and smart too late." How relevant the Scriptures: "We are but of yesterday, and know nothing, because our days upon earth are a shadow" (Job 8:9).

2 THIS area is hemmed in between the bold publications by journalists and popular writers who stress the wonders that one can achieve by physical reworking of one's body and some popular books by plastic surgeons who write of the miracles they wreak [1, 21, 24–26, 30, 32]. Countering them are reports on the "beauty butchers" [5], who maim and injure many of their patients. Cosmetic surgical transformation has an aura of jet trendiness, tinged by tales of silicone injections for exotic dancers. Although an estimated quarter of a million people per year choose to have cosmetic surgery, there is no systematic large-scale evaluation of the effects on their lives. The explanations for this are numerous and not surprising.

Most cosmetic surgery patients have no major difficulties with their surgery or its sequelae, and they tend to disappear from medical care after routine follow-up visits to the surgeon. This phenomenon has been explained by Gifford [14], who has indicated that these people do not experience such operations as part of an illness, but rather as a way of coping actively with their lives. Therefore, the surgery produces no serious emotional reactions. There is also a diversity of specialists performing these operations—plastic surgeons; maxillofacial surgeons; ear, nose, and throat specialists—all of whom work with different segments of this patient group, frequently without communication. Add to this the varied attempts made by inexpert workers and charlatans, and the field becomes cloudier still. In addition, there are two quite widely varying factors that shape the responses of cosmetic surgery patients. First is the individual per-

6

Norman R. Bernstein

EMOTIONAL REACTIONS IN PATIENTS AFTER ELECTIVE COSMETIC SURGERY

sonality patterns of the patients operated on and the many special meaning they attribute to the operations undertaken. Second, the variety of procedures that are attempted, with different parts of the body altered, produce outcomes that are not readily comparable. Moreover, the long-term changes that come with age alter the tonus of the skin of the belly, or breast, and, in conjunction with the life situations in which they find themselves in later years, influence the ways in which patients look back on their surgery. There are also unknowable influences from the environment, such as the fate of the Vietnamese bar girls who had eyelid surgery to be more appealing to the American soldiers stationed there. The changes in the political situation after the war may have altered their lives, turning them into targets for hostility.

In a book about plastic surgery, Baker and Smith write, "Practically everyone can be more beautiful, as never before . . ." [30]. Popular books like *A New You: How Plastic Surgery Can Change Your Life* [32] and *The Miracle of Cosmetic Plastic Surgery* [1] describe a bewildering group of body-altering procedures, and the fashion magazines and newspapers continue to dramatize each procedure on navels, eyelids, hips, noses, and breasts. In spite of the early and exaggerated warning of psychiatrists about the hazards to the personalities of plastic surgery patients, it appears that only a small group of such patients decompensate and have to seek psychiatric help. Although these people do exist, they are but a tiny group within the hundreds of thousands of other patients who come for treatment. Gipson and Connolly [15] sug-

gest that for some disturbed people, cosmetic surgery can delay breakdown, but not prevent it. Dr. Palemon Rodriquez-Gomez [26], a member of the American Society of Plastic Surgeons and the Mexican Association of Plastic Surgeons, says:

We sculpt living materials. Not like working in clay or marble, perhaps, but we, too, must have artistic imagination. And our handiwork goes out into the real world with a new appearance and changed psyche, the shape and integrity of face and body restored.

Lay authors like Simona Morini also write of "body sculpture" [25] and advance an image of self-perfectability through surgery. Margaret Mead, in the introduction to MacGregor's *Transformation and Identity* [23], notes:

The fewer members of the public there are who shudder away from the reflections of their own very moderately displeasing or unfashionable faces, the easier it will be to build a climate of opinion within which those with reconstructed faces may move with a full sense of identity.

Such commentary implies that plastic and cosmetic surgery can have dividends in terms of community attitudes toward the handicapped. More and more, cosmetic and plastic surgeons are expressing interest in the psychological aspects of their work. Goldwyn [18] in particular has tried to isolate several types of psychologically unsuitable candidates for cosmetic surgery, delineating the unrealistic; the grieving; patients in psychotherapy, with an unwilling spouse or lover; the primarily schizoid, paranoid, or severly neurotic patient; or those who want a total overhaul. He cautions that the surgeon should be alert to such patients, as well as to people who seem to have the least deformity but who express the greatest concern or who are going to the surgeon to please someone else—a boss, a husband, or a lover. Kahana and Bibring [19] have attempted to delineate personality types who present problems in medical management, such as the aloof, the self-sacrificing, the querulous, and the dramatizing. Each of these efforts is valuable in terms of the short-term or intermediate care of the patient, but none yields long-term outcome data because what happens later is determined by many other factors in the social environment and future of the patient.

Few cosmetic patients come back whether satisfied or not, and the most neurotic often do not come back for psychotherapy even when they are deeply troubled. Surgery done to improve appearance, surgery of the *self-image*, should open up avenues through which we can examine the large area of unspoken but vital feelings people have about themselves and the subtle and striking ways in which their pictures of themselves may be distorted, unrealistic, or silly. However, many patients with distorted self-images are pleased and buoyed up shortly after their surgery. What happens during the long-term adjustment of these individuals? I will provide some general impressions and examples that have emerged from individual follow-up studies and psychiatric contacts over 25 years. Some of the major determinants that will be focused on are the phases of life in which the patient is operated on or from which he or she looks back on the surgery: adolescence, adulthood, or middle age. Also, the degree of personality disorder and its special relationship to the part of the body to be changed are significant. Situational and cultural aspects will be stressed.

Adolescence

Adolescence is the period of development during which there is the greatest normal concern about becoming attractive and competent. Adolescents have a poignant and persuasive need to be acceptable to people. Just as orthodonture is frequently done for middle-class adolescents, so also is cosmetic surgery. The most prominent and acceptable procedure is rhinoplasty, and such words in currency as "nose bob," "rhino," and "nose job" all indicate the way popular culture has taken this up. The overriding American optimism about fixing oneself up to face the world supports this, and the very idea of "facing" shows how imbedded cosmetic value is in our idioms. Other than for young women in show business, breast augmentations seem to be less widely performed on adolescents, with emphasis on waiting to see if the breasts will develop further.

For most adolescents the surgery is not traumatic. As one surgeon remarked, "The best result is one where your friends say how well you look, and don't seem to notice what has changed" [8]. This would be most true in the older patients who had a face lift, but numerous young people with unremarkable noses want something done about them and experience a great lift from "doing something about themselves" without a great objective alteration. The surgical intervention serves as a watershed from which the young person can often move ahead with new confidence. Goffman [16, 17, 27] and other medical sociologists have pointed out how much of our social performance is related to the way in which we bear ourselves, rather than to objective qualities. The cosmetics industry, with its enormous advertising apparatus, works relentlessly and ubiquitously to indicate that some change in hair color or coiffure, eye shadow, lipstick, or powder will transform a young person. The peculiar language of fashion—"This style really is you"—hints at the way a person needs to find equipment that will help him find a special image of himself. Plastic surgical intervention has a greater impact because it is an acute intervention, has much of the important aura of medical and surgical care, and produces a more permanent result than the easily reversible actions of ointments and eye shadows.

CASE 1

Roddy Antoon was a slender and athletic 16-year-old boy who felt his beaked nose made him ugly; he suggested that his Lebanese ancestry showed or that he might look Jewish. His family first tried to discourage him by saying that he "looked fine," but he continued for a year to complain about not being attractive to women. He had some social contacts, but was a typical, nervous, insecure adolescent, who was not scapegoated, but was not the "Big Man on Campus" he wanted to be. After much discussion, the family doctor found him a surgeon, and a rhinoplasty was performed that did not greatly alter his appearance. The surgeon had told him and his family explicitly that the change undertaken was a slight one and that the results would be a minor change. Neither the parents nor the patient could hear this, though it was carefully stated, but they all were delighted by the result. When the patient went off to college at 18, he felt he had an advantage. He felt that he looked more attractive, and his social life in college and graduate school went well. After finishing school he married. Ten years later, when he accompanied his wife for treatment of psychological troubles, he expressed himself as delighted that he had taken the step and given himself "the edge" in confidence. His wife thought he looked fine, both in his old pictures and in his present state, but the surgical intervention was experienced as a clear, positive, and useful coping effort.

CASE 2

Ernestine Putnam was a vivacious adolescent with enormous, shining eyes, a trim figure, and an unstoppable pressure of speech and flirtatiousness. She felt she was ugly because she had a large nose, and she focused all her insecurities on this. She used marijauna extensively, tried cocaine, and was dedicated to proving herself by seducing every male who came within reach. She was openly provocative in her psychiatric consultations, and was allowed to flit from one psychiatrist to another because her parents were frightened by her compulsive sexuality,

and because she had contracted a case of gonorrhea. Her school work was not given much attention, but she managed to pass. One psychiatrist she saw for treatment was supportive of her desire to have her nose altered. The surgery was performed and results were unusually satisfactory, giving her pert features that seemed charming to bystanders. What followed was a brief effort at serious and more restrained living, on the assumption that she had repaired her damaged self-esteem and no longer needed to rely exclusively on sex to attract people. However, her basic insecurities soon overflowed this restrained posture, and she resumed running around socially and taking a variety of risks, like hitchhiking and getting drunk with strangers, until she gradually settled down, finished school, and went to work several years later. She did not regret her surgery. In fact, she was pleased with her appearance to a great extent. However, her self-doubt and poor control over impulses required years to change in a slow maturational process.

Thomson, Knorr, and Edgerton [33] report from their wide experience that many psychiatric difficulties emerge in the period directly following cosmetic surgery, but are short in duration. They relate this to an upsurge of feelings that previously had been focused on the assumed physical defect. There is also some transient shame over having surgery—constant staring at and examination of the part—and a mild form of "mourning" for the old self, which gradually abates.

Adult Life

CASE 3

Pat Holden was a depressed 34-year-old, plain-looking nurse who had always been shy and jealous of her sister, a married and more comfortable and happy younger sibling. She came for psychotherapy because other nurses on the ward had been pressing her, stressing that her work was fine but that she was so grouchy and self-hating that something should be done. She had had a rhinoplasty 10 years before and felt that it had not changed her life. She underwent a period of dejected seclusion till her "black eyes" resorbed. She was embarrassed by her *visible* efforts to change her appearance, and at the same time she hoped for a great deal from the change. The change was not as great as she had hoped for, and she said that her family remarked, "It doesn't really look like you." She continued in the same role in the family—marked out as the troubled one, single, sad, lonely, and emotionally disappointed.

CASE 4

Two sisters who were trying to break out of their constricting and conventional homes each went to college, and each tried to work in nightclubs. One, Margie, sang with a band, and her sister, Donna, played jazz piano. Both dyed their hair red, dressed dramatically, and established homes away from their parents. Each ultimately married. Margie went to nursing school, obtained her degree, and continued to work part time as a nurse. She always tried very hard to be stylish. She was tense, but happy in her marriage, and showed no major signs of psychiatric disease. Donna, who had been much more disturbed from the first, flourished in a variety of different entertainment jobs, and then became a secretary and married. She had two children and a chronic mood disorder and marital strife; one of her children was disturbed. However, when interviewed 20 years after the rhinoplasties, Margie and Donna were not able to distinguish their diets, hairdos, and stylish dressing from the effect of cosmetic surgery on their life adjustments, although both were satisfied with their surgery.*

CASE 5

Barbara Ann Larson was a tall, slender woman of 40. She had never married, although she had

*Ravindra Manek [22] reported one 37-year-old woman who was married for 17 years after having a rhinoplasty and had a satisfactory marriage, but came for psychotherapy. In the course of her treatment she said that she felt that the operation had undoubtedly made her look better, but that inside she was the same. She went on to say that she did not know confidently that her husband "would have loved" her if she had retained her original aquiline nose.

had some fleeting social and sexual ventures. Her self-image was that of an unattractive woman who lacked anything a man would want. She had a habit of saying that men were interested in women only with large breasts. After several years of ruminating about this, and with the encouragement of articles in the popular press, she went to see a doctor for breast augmentation. The procedure went well initially but was followed in several weeks by a wound infection in the left breast, resulting in sloughing of tissue and the ultimate removal of the implant on that side. This left her with a horror of the asymmetry of her body, adding one more aspect to her longstanding self-dislike. Her depression was severe enough to prevent her from working for several months. Upon improving emotionally, she continued to have great difficulty functioning socially. She was pervaded by thoughts of her defect and unattractiveness, now much focused on the breast area. She did not go back for further surgery, even though a good cosmetic result seemed possible. Moreover, she was obsessed about suing the surgeon for having mutilated her, although she never took any action.

Middle Age

Middle age is another period of life in which more and more people are undergoing cosmetic surgery. In this case, surgery is frequently sought in an attempt to maintain the appearance of youth and vigor. Middle age is a time when an enormous number of divorces occur, and statistics indicate that most men who divorce after 40 remarry, while most women over 40 do not. It may be for these reasons that there is a host of women who feel economically and socially disadvantaged by their divorces and who seek to restore themselves to a more appealing condition.

CASE 6

Barbara Harding was perpetually 48 (she was actually 54), and her blond hair, regular exercise, frequent trips to Florida, and endless skin creams did not make her execrable marriage better. Her husband (age 55) was a wealthy businessman who traveled around the world, had casual affairs wherever he could, and made a special point of seducing Barbara's friends and then having them all together for lavish parties. She had had her face lifted twice in attempts to remain youthful, and while these interventions were technically successful, they never altered the worried and guilty manner she showed in trying to hold her marriage together. She was very attached to her plastic surgeon, always bringing flowers for his secretary and returning often to have any actinic ketosis examined or removed or to check on the state of her face. She saw the whole system of beautification as part of the war of attrition she was gradually losing in her marriage. She maintained all the external rituals of marriage and housekeeping and was generally known as a perfect hostess and long-suffering wife. However, her quiet unhappiness persisted. She felt that the creases that were removed from her face helped her look younger, but she knew she was not changing the relationship with her husband. Moreover, she felt she could not give up this approach to managing her life. She went for psychiatric help, but she wanted specific formulas to force her life into a new channel, and since there was no such psychoprosthesis available, her situation remained mired in the same recurring struggles. She retained a definite fear that her "lift" would shift and show her inner misery.

CASE 7

A 46-year-old married woman with two children by her first marriage and one by her second felt that she had never liked her nose. She had always been a vivacious southern charmer and was fully competent socially: "But I never liked my profile and I had to argue with John for years, before he was willing to let me go ahead. He felt that it was something superficial and that the real me was inside. I felt that too, but it still bothered me, and only when I felt more satisfied with myself, could I convince myself it was all right to do something superfi-

cial. Then I could go ahead and make this change. And I am very pleased with the result." It did not produce much reaction in her children.

Barsheid and Walster [2] have reported that people who are satisfied with their appearance are generally more well adjusted, and that neurotic people have more dissatisfaction with their looks. This is actually a cluster of ideas rather than a simple factor. For example, Schilder [28] defined the body image as the

picture of our body which we form in our mind, that is to say the way in which the body appears in our mind, that is to say the way in which the body appears to ourselves . . . we see parts of the body surface. We have tactile, thermal, pain impressions. There are sensations which come from the muscles and their sheaths . . . and sensations coming from the viscera. . . . The body schema is the tri-dimensional image everybody has about himself. . . .

He goes on to point out that just as the postural body image changes constantly, so do our perceptions about ourselves, and one part of the body image that has not been conscious can be brought into consciousness because of injury or a special attitude. We can abruptly become aware of our ears if they seem to be too large or somebody remarks on how red they have become in a social situation.

More recent psychological theorists like Erikson [12] have stressed the concept of identity in the individual and underscored that this involves a sense of continuity of one's personal history as well as an awareness of the body image and the delimitation of one's world and life. The idea of the "self" seems to involve both body-image concepts and the feelings people have, such as self-confidence and worth. Many of these qualities are tied to experiences with people around us and the ways in which we are perceived early in life.

Some investigators report that beautiful women in middle life have a particularly difficult time because the loss of this instrument for appeal to others becomes apparent, and they feel they have nothing left. However, this explanation seems too simplistic. Obviously, since the philosophers have failed to agree on a concept of beauty, and there are different types of beauty, and individual "beauties" have varied personalities, some women who have been very pretty find they have a new type of middle-aged or mature good looks that involves also a different role. Their acceptance of this role relates to what they are doing, their social environment, and the appreciation of people around them. There continues to be conflict between the idea that beauty is only skin deep and should not be consciously sought, and the obvious attitudes in society that youth and good looks are vital assets. Moreover, each organ has its special meaning to particular individuals. No area of the body has more complex social values than the female breast. Traditionally, it has been stated that breast amputation for cancer is best managed psychologically by mature women who are married, secure, and have children, so they can forgo this part of their body image and self-concept more readily. But Cope [9] has argued cogently that many women who are well established in life are still desperately shocked and feel depressed, diminished, and devalued after mastectomy. Analogously, reduction mammaplasty can have variable outcomes.

CASE 8

Ann Lattanzio felt embarrassed when she began to develop large breasts. She felt the eyes of every man were groping her, and her sisters teased her while her mother seemed rather amused (which the patient interpreted as scorn). In several relationships with men she felt herself ashamed of her pendulous breasts. So when she was in her middle twenties, she had breast reduction performed. She said that for years afterward she was unable to feel any sexual gratification from her breasts and was mortified by this. She reported being bothered by anesthesia and being "breast-conscious" for years. Nonetheless, she married when she was around 30 and has several children (which she did not nurse). Gradually, she has come to feel more confident about herself as a person and less concerned about the whole issue. When seen for psychiatric consultation about her child, she spontaneously brought up the whole matter and regretted that she had gone ahead with the operation, even though at the time of her operation she felt it had made a large difference in her appearance, confidence, and ability to move about publicly.

Other women are troubled by unnatural sensations about their breasts, noses, eyelids, or other body parts, and many experience minor symptoms of heightened attention to the cosmetically changed body part. Such patients do *not* show overall failure in adaptation.

Those women whose work is explicitly sexual are notable among candidates for breast augmentation. Stripteasers and topless dancers who had silicone injections sometimes come for psychiatric help after suicide attempts. Their self-concepts are so full of self-loathing, and their attitudes toward men and sexuality are so full of bitterness, that it is difficult to distinguish the specific attitudes toward the cosmetic surgery when they get older from their reactions to their diminished ability to compete sexually. Such people are also often the ones who received bargain-basement care surgically, with a much greater incidence of unsatisfactory outcomes and complications.

Middle-aged men are coming in increasing numbers for hair transplants and face lifts; it seems they want to wring out "a few more years" to make up for what they have missed. There is a particular feeling of envy in the middle-aged toward the so-called sexual generation and the large numbers of younger people living together without marriage. These men are especially jealous of the young and try to become "swingers" themselves. Generally, they find that it is not possible to regain their youth. After some months of experimentation, the typical male "middlescent" who is trying to make up for what he missed in college settles down. He is generally pleased with the surgical improvement in his appearance, but not greatly changed in terms of the inner feelings about advancing years and mortality. Men are no more objective about appearance than women, but their fantasies differ.

CASE 9

Bud Ryan had been a spectacular college athlete in the Southwest. He went on to a nationwide business career selling sports equipment. He had an attentive wife and three sons and two daughters. This did not keep him from philandering on business trips, but he felt his life was going well. He exercised regularly, and controlled his weight with strict dieting. He felt he was still "the same driving kid inside" until he found that he needed glasses and that his old football knee injury was causing trouble. This was a traumatic time for a man who willed everything in his life. These were changes he could not control, and they both infuriated and terrified him. A period of drinking followed, and then he developed great concern about his appearance, which led to having the bags under his eyes removed. This was followed by a short spell of self-confidence and enthusiasm, but this did not last. He became preoccupied with his appearance again and came for marital counseling, which led after a few months of therapy to a more stable acceptance of aging and a more shared parental involvement.

Traditional psychiatric formulations about personality focus on diagnostic categories. Therefore, depression, schizophrenia, phobia, and hypochondriasis are typical labels for some of these patients, but these are not the more useful formulations. They are suited to naming the reactions to a very specific aspect of psychological functioning: the investment in physical images by plastic surgery. For some patients, such labels do make the overall situation clear and help predict outcomes. Chronically depressed people are less likely to experience a positive sustained change than normal people. Anxious people, on the other hand, especially if they are young, are very likely to seem petrified of an operation, but use it as a step toward better social performance.

Vaillant [34], in a study of college students over a 30-year period, tried to list the qualities that made for the best adjustment to life. He attempted to use levels of functioning, describing *psychotic* mechanisms as the poorest, followed by *immature* mechanisms, which are found in severe depression, personality disorders, and adolescence. Then he designated a third level of *neurotic* mechanisms, and finally a level of *mature* mechanisms seen commonly in healthy adults. Unfortunately, many of the cosmetic patients who come as young people show strong *adolescent* mechanisms: fantasy, hypochondriasis, projection, masochism, and acting out are common. In fact, acting out is deeply involved in the decision to undertake plastic surgery. Yet such subjective whims lead to objective attempts at improvement of appearance and are adaptive for most. Therefore, we cannot directly utilize this type of protocol. In fact, one clear feature that Vaillant has stressed in adaptation to life is *humor*, which he acknowledges is very difficult to include as a category because there are so many types of humor: wit, sarcasm, joshing, irony, and so forth. In clinical terms, patients who can be detached enough about what they are doing to look humorously at their plastic surgery efforts are likely to do well. However, many people are too frightened by their operation to be able to see any humor in it. For example, in case 4 (the sisters who both had rhinoplasties), the one with the better adjustment could make some fun of their "fight to be gorgeous," while the less well adjusted one was always frozen when it was referred to, feeling there was an implied criticism of her as a person if any part of her was mentioned.

Loving Relations

Erikson [12], in his studies of the stages of personality development, stresses a stage of *integrity*, in which an individual can hold together and face aging, and this implies qualities of individual toughness. However, he and most other psychological theorists would agree that this feeling of self-sufficiency derives much from having loving relationships in childhood and the experience of successful relationships with others. Hence the paradox—that people who are most independent are usually people who did not have to be independent when they were young. This pattern also seems true for the long-term adjustment of cosmetic surgery patients—the ones who have had reasonably good upbringings and who continue to be both active and somewhat independent souls will be the most likely to handle the long-term adjustments to changes in appearance following cosmetic surgery. If we were to take Freud's old dictum that the ability to care for other people and the ability to do work are the qualities of normality and add to it the ability to laugh at one's self in the cosmetic situation, we would have a relatively useful indicator of long-term adjustment, and we would not need extensive psychological testing.

Random events and intercurrent diseases clearly come into the picture. For example, one woman who had lost a lot of weight (80 lb) and had undergone lipectomy for what she felt were the "awful wrinkles" on her abdomen dyed her hair blonde and set out to catch a new husband quite consciously. Unfortunately, she developed lupus erythematosus, and the illness precluded any role but that of a seriously ill invalid. On the other extreme, a man who was considering a face lift because he wanted to maintain his image at 48 as a young executive had a coronary and proceeded to seduce the intensive care nurse and run off with her to the West Coast.

Another factor in the prediction on long-term outcomes would be the determination of how much the patient is relying on the *single* procedure to transform him or her. If someone changes his or her diet, loses weight, takes up jogging, and renounces smoking, or if a woman changes her style of dress and her hair color along with the other activities, the chances are more likely that the plastic surgery is part of a program of self-improvement, which takes away some of the desperate qualities of the surgical procedure alone.

CASE 10
Tania was a 34-year-old cocktail waitress who was at the same time illegally on welfare and engaged in promiscuous sexuality with both men and women. In addition, she was strug-gling to rear her illegitimate daughter. When she came for breast augmentation she looked about 25 and seemed enormously energetic and wholesome, despite her adventures with drugs and dissipation. She felt that if her flat chest were altered, she could "get" the kind of people she wanted. Consequently, she pursued a number of surgeons until she found one willing to implant prostheses. It made little difference in her desperate, humorless, isolated, and sad quest for acceptance for herself and her child.

The Life Context

The assessment of long-term functioning of any individual depends on the situation in which he or she lives. In some cities, plastic surgery is viewed with little concern and therefore is entered into quite casually. In others, surgeons feel disinclined toward "superficial luxury surgery" and are reluctant to undertake cosmetic work—their manner makes their patients feel guilty. Another source of difficulty is the communication problem [3, 27]. Many patients are told precisely what to expect from their surgery insofar as change in appearance, and *every* patient seems to have a dream of improvement that goes beyond what they have been promised. Most adapt to this, a few sue, and some stew for a long time over what they believe to be a swindle. This difficulty is primarily psychological in origin, but there is no direct way to counter it. Time with the patient helps, but this is hard for the busy surgeon to manage. Statements by nurses must be carefully monitored. Nurses should be instructed about how and what to tell patients about their prognoses or they should be evasive and supportive when disclosure is inappropriate. It is often not feasible to develop the kind of relationship necessary to explore the sexual feelings that concern a woman contemplating a breast implant. Will her lover say it feels different? What difference will she experience? Will erotic manipulation shift the implant? Many unverbalized fantasies linger and do influence the sexual performance of patients. Written statements about results are a protection for the surgeon in terms of threats of suit, even though patients often do not read or merely scan any statement. In the longer view, efforts to improve communication enable patients to guide other patients seeking cosmetic surgery and thus have an overall beneficial influence.

Schontz [29] wrote about the problems of correlating personality patterns with the way one experiences one's body:

Body schemata, body values, and body concepts are something like cooperating partners co-managing the unified enterprise of ongoing behavior. Each makes its special contribution to the business of living. That business functions as a cohesive whole, not because its components are all alike, but because they collaborate effectively and make the most of their differences.

Or as Thomas Aquinas put it, "Beauty is what pleases me."

Final Thoughts

The problems of determining the long-term outcomes of individuals who have chosen to have cosmetic surgery are similar to the methodological problems of studies of psychiatric outcomes. In medicine the ideal patient has a specific problem and is treated for this and goes about his or her business. In elective surgery, this is often not so. Duff and Hollingshead [11] described patients with medical problems whose hospitalization was the beginning of a general life deterioration.

For the psychiatrist, the best patients are those who finish a course of therapy and then go on to lead independent lives and are not heard from again. There is some analogy here to plastic surgery; for the cosmetic surgeon, the short cross section of a patient's life that becomes apparent when a patient comes for cosmetic work does not provide much opportunity for a determination of all the social and environmental factors that will influence the future course of the patient's life. The usual cautions remain sound: to reject obviously deluded people and those whose explanations of their motives seem peculiar. Feelings on the part of the surgeon of an unusual or abrasive emotional tone between him and the patient remains a good indicator. And obviously, the surgeon should ask about previous psychiatric disease, hospitalization, and treatment as well as about thoughts of suicide and depression. Such questions do not take much time. Although formal psychiatric assessment might not be of use at all times, it can be a practical prerequisite for the many thousands of patients undergoing cosmetic surgery. Evidence continues to accumulate that the overwhelming number of patients who experience the varieties of competent cosmetic surgery absorb the experience into their lives and continue to develop in positive ways. While we would all like to see our work as pivotal in directing someone's life, we should not make this our absolute expectation. If we are successful in improving a patient's appearance, we should be content that the patient can then move ahead in life, giving less attention to appearance (although appearance remains important throughout life, be it in the cute cheerleader or the distinguished ex-professor or white-haired patriarch). Our result becomes incorporated in a complex of improved self-regard and confidence that aids the patient in facing the stresses of living.

References

1. Aronson, R.B., and Epstein, R. *The Miracle of Cosmetic Plastic Surgery.* Los Angeles: Sherbourne, 1970.
2. Barsheid, E., Walster, E., and Bohrnstedt, C. "Beauty and the Best." *Psychol. Today* 5 (10):42, 1972.
3. Bernstein, N.R. Psychological changes caused by the aging of the face: Aging and the body image. *Plastische und Wiederherstellungs-Chirurgie aus klinik und Forschung: Tagung der Vereinigung der Deutschen Plastichen Chirurgen.* Stuttgart: Schattauer, 1975. Pp. 13–19.
4. Bernstein, N.R. *Emotional Care of the Facially Burned and Disfigured.* Boston: Little, Brown, 1976.
5. Bettelheim, B. *Symbolic Wounds.* New York: Collier, 1962.
6. Boorstin, D.J. *The Image.* New York: Atheneum, 1962.

7. Bressler, B., Cohen, S.I., and Magnussen, F. The problem of phantom breast and phantom pain. *J. Nerv. Ment. Dis.* 123:181, 1956.
8. Constable, J. Personal communication, 1976.
9. Cope, O. *The Breast: Its Problem—Benign and Malignant.* New York: Oxford, 1977.
10. Dicker, R.L., and Syracuse, V.R. *A Consultation with a Plastic Surgeon.* New York: Warner, 1977.
11. Duff, R.S., and Hollingshead, A.B. *Sickness and Society.* New York: Harper & Row, 1968.
12. Erikson, E. *Childhood and Society.* (Rev. ed.). New York: Norton, 1968.
13. Fisher, S. *Body Experience in Fantasy and Behavior.* New York: Appleton-Century-Crofts, 1970.
14. Gifford, S. Cosmetic Surgery and Personality Change: A Review and Some Clinical Observations. In R.M. Goldwyn (Ed.), *The Unfavorable Result in Plastic Surgery.* Boston: Little, Brown, 1972. P. 11.
15. Gipson, M., and Connolly, F.H. The incidence of schizophrenia and severe psychological disorders in patients 10 years after cosmetic rhinoplasty. *Br. J. Plast. Surg.* 28:155, 1975.
16. Goffman, E. *The Presentation of Self in Everyday Life.* Edinburgh: Edinburgh University, 1956.
17. Goffman, E. *Stigma: Notes on the Management of Spoiled Identity.* Englewood Cliffs, N.J.: Prentice-Hall, 1963.
18. Goldwyn, R.M. Operating for the aging face. *Psychiatry Med.* 3:187, 1972.
19. Kahana, R.J., and Bibring, G.L. Personality Types in Medical Management. In N.E. Zinberg (Ed.), *Psychiatry and Medical Practice in a General Hospital.* New York: International Universities, 1965. P. 108.
20. Kane, F.J., Jr., and Simes, L. Phantom urinary phenomena in hemodialysis patients. *Psychosomatics* 18:13, 1977.
21. La Barre, H. *Plastic Surgery: Beauty You Can Buy.* New York: Holt, Rinehart and Winston, 1970.
22. Manek, R. Personal communication, 1978.
23. Mead, M. Introduction. In F.M.C. Macgregor (Ed.), *Transformation and Identity: The Face and Plastic Surgery.* New York: Quadrangle, 1974.
24. Mesinger, M *Self-Image Surgery.* New York: Bantam, 1973.
25. Morini, S. *Body Sculpture: Plastic Surgery from Head to Toe.* New York: Delacorte, 1972.
26. Rodriguez-Gomez, P. Quoted in *Chicago Tribune.* Section 2, P. 2, September 29, 1977.
27. Scheflen, A.E. *Body Language and the Social Order.* Englewood Cliffs, N.J.: Prentice-Hall, 1972.
28. Schilder, P. *The Image and Appearance of the Human Body.* New York: International Universities, 1970.
29. Shontz, F.C. *Perceptual and Cognitive Aspects of Body Experience.* New York: Academic, 1969.
30. Smith, J.W., and Baker, S.S. *Doctor, Make Me Beautiful.* New York: McKay, 1973.
31. Spitz, R. "The beauty butchers." *VIVA* 5(4):75, 1978.
32. Stallings, J.O. *A New You: How Plastic Surgery Can Change Your Life.* New York: Mason/Charter, 1977.
33. Thomson, J.A., Jr., Knorr, N.J., and Edgerton, M.T., Jr. Cosmetic surgery: The psychiatric perspective. *Psychosomatics* 19:7, January 1978.
34. Vaillant, G.E. *Adaptation to Life.* Boston: Little, Brown, 1977.

3 THERE is nothing greater than the experience of arriving at a decision to the technique most applicable in handling a major reconstructive problem. Looking back over the last three decades, I can recall some popular surgical techniques about which my impression is different today. I must say that many of the procedures used in the forties and fifties were taken from the pioneers of our profession. Although they would be considered older techniques today, I like to think of them as historically significant in the development of principles contributing to out present concept of plastic surgical reconstruction. Significant advances have been made in the last 37 years. This must be attributed to our experience in World War II, surgical postgraduate training programs, scientific meetings, and the availability of plastic surgery journals and books. We should give considerable credit to the journal *Plastic and Reconstructive Surgery.*

Taking into consideration all our newer techniques, such as microvascular and craniofacial surgery, the majority of problems in plastic reconstructive surgery are best handled by the formula: the simplest technique that has the least risk and fewest complications, that can be accomplished in the shortest time, and that produces the best functional and cosmetic result.

In our teaching program, every patient seen has a problem. All the techniques described for handling the problem are outlined either in writing or mentally. Each procedure is evaluated in terms of advantages, disadvantages, complications, and time consumed. The procedure that is the simplest, has least complica-

Francis X. Paletta

SURGICAL JUDGMENT: TWENTY-FIVE YEARS AGO COMPARED WITH TODAY

tions, is the most effective, and can be done most rapidly is chosen.

In what follows, I present examples of some problems seen 25 to 30 years ago in order to describe how I handled them then and how I would handle them now.

Reconstruction of the Eyelid

During the 1950s, major reconstruction of the eyelid associated with resection for carcinoma made use of techniques outlined by our predecessors. One procedure that I remember very well was that described by Hughes [1] (Fig. 3-1B through E), who utilized the mucous membrane and tarsal plate of the opposite eyelid. However, this method involved suturing the eyelids together for a long time before a second stage of detachment, and skin grafting on the surface of the tarsal plate (Fig. 3-1A and F). Other disadvantages were management of drainage in patients with chronic conjunctivitis, decreased vision in the elderly, interference with the opposite eyelid and loss of important tissue, and the occasional complication of entropion. The advantage was the close proximity of the donor site.

In the 1960s the concept changed to immediate reconstruction following cancer extirpation, so we began to look for other techniques. Our aim was to choose a procedure that was simple, could be performed quickly, and could use tissue of similar quality, preferably from the neighboring area. The nasolabial flap seemed to be the answer [8]. Initially, I projected the possibility of needing a mucous membrane

graft for lining, a fascial sling to maintain elevation, and the establishment of lachrymal drainage. Time has proven that these secondary procedures were seldom required (Fig. 3-2A through C). The lachrymal drainage was taken over by the opposite eyelid. No mucous membrane grafts were needed for lining since the bulbar conjunctiva shifted over nicely. Fascial slings were not necessary to cover the exposed sclera or to achieve symmetry with the opposite eyelid. Occasionally minor revisions were done in young individuals when the flap was not properly designed. It seems to me that the technique of rotating a cheek flap makes the operation a much bigger performance than is necessary. It has been my experience that reconstruction for a specific essential feature of the face is best accomplished when the transferred tissue reconstructs a specific region alone [2,3,5] (Fig. 3-3A and B). In other words, when the tissue brought in reconstructs both the nose and cheek, or both eyelids and cheek, the boundaries of the specific area being reconstructed are not clearly defined, such as the nasolabial fold. There are times in reconstruction of the upper eyelid when a switch flap from the lower eyelid may be indicated. During World War II, we used cervical neck tubes to reconstruct eyelids, but it took too long to complete the reconstruction and the eyelid was too thick (Fig. 3-4A and B).

Reconstruction of the Lip

In the early 1940s, while I was a Cancer Fellow at Barnard Skin and Cancer Hospital in St.

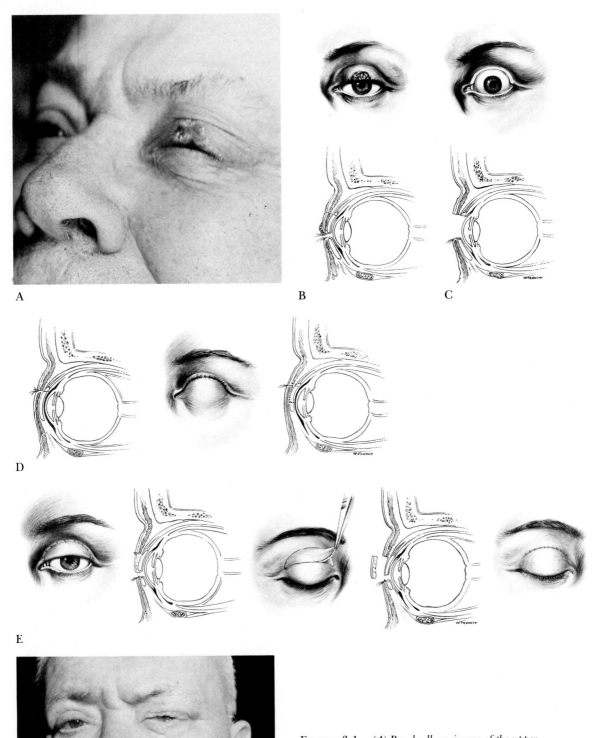

FIGURE 3-1. *(A) Basal cell carcinoma of the upper eyelid. (B) Diagram of the area excised. (C) Outline of the area excised. (D) Closure of the eyelids. (E) Detachment of the eyelids and full-thickness skin graft from the opposite eyelid. (F) Patient 2 weeks after detachment of eyelids.*

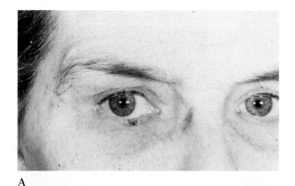

A

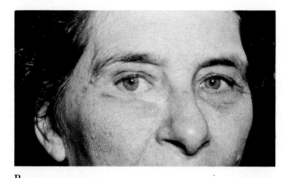

B

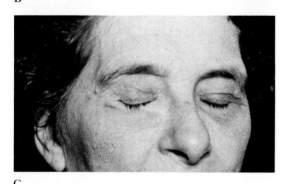

C

FIGURE 3-2. *(A) Multiple basal cell carcinoma of lower palpebral margin. (B) Reconstruction of the lower eyelid with nasolabial flap. (C) Closure of eyelids.*

Louis, there were many old techniques used to reconstruct the lower and upper lips. These procedures made use of bilateral Abbe flaps; bilateral nasolabial flaps; bilateral facial cheek flaps; rotation of composite cheek flaps, including mucous membrane, muscle, and skin; and Blair's pectoral flap (then the war-horse of facial reconstruction). Most of these facial flaps disregarded physiological principles, such as

Langer's lines, and the maintenance of muscle and nerve continuity. Although all these surgical operations got the job done, many of the niceties we think of today were overlooked. Again, my guiding formula was to use the simplest, most effective procedure—one that could be executed quickly for immediate reconstruction and that paralleled proper lines of closure without disrupting muscle and nerve continuity.

In partial resection of the upper and lower lips (Fig. 3-4C through E), the enlarged nasolabial flap works well for restoration (Fig. 3-5A through D). Mucous membrane flaps are used in the treatment of extensive neoplasms requiring excision of large areas of the oral cavity lining or for resurfacing the vermilion. Free skin grafts can also be used for lining. In patients with much larger problems, where a portion of the chin is excised, bilateral facial-cervical flaps are required to bring sufficient tissue to the area (Fig. 3-6A through C). With the present concept of immediate repair, larger margins of excision are taken, as well as frozen-section studies of the host tissue margins. Another valuable factor to consider is that resurfacing areas with skin flaps makes it possible to give additional radiation with the newer cobalt techniques.

Reconstruction of a Child's Nose

There was considerable discussion in the 1950s about when to reconstruct the nose in a child. Will one reconstruction suffice, and if it is done in early childhood, will it grow with the patient and be an acceptable nose for adulthood? If surgery is to be performed, at what age would the patient be most cooperative? It was obvious that there was limited experience in most of the discussions.

In one little girl with choanal atresia and a small amount of nasal skin (Fig. 3-7A), I elected to operate when she was 5 years old. The initial procedure was to establish an airway by removing bone in the nasopharynx and inserting tubes lined by skin grafts. Also, I chose the

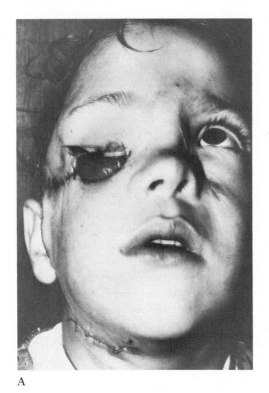

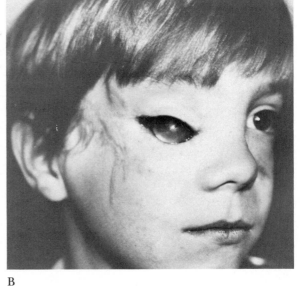

A   B

FIGURE 3-3. *(A) Gunshot wound of the eye, loss of lower eyelid. (B) Reconstruction of lower eyelid with nasolabial flap. Orbit reconstruction not completed.*

forehead for nasal skin in the belief that a larger nose would be more acceptable in adult life.

There were problems. First, the cartilage, both autogenous and homologous, was absorbed, and this prevented the attainment of a good nose contour, particularly in relation to the columella. I wanted to wait until the patient was 15 years old to insert a bone graft with the thought that this would be her final nose. One thing I have learned in nasal reconstruction is that when I tried to save a part such as the ala and interdigitate it with newly reconstructed tissue, the result never looked satisfactory (Fig. 3-7A through C). At 15 years of age, the patient was a big girl. I knew that I could never make a nose out of what was present, so I decided to start all over. The only tissue left was the arm, so I elected to use the Tagliacotian technique. I had seen Dr. J. P. Webster make a beautiful nose in a woman using this donor site. As one

can see, the operative procedures are not complete in this young girl (Fig. 3-7C).

There are two things that I would not do again. One, if I were to reconstruct a nose in a young patient, I would choose a Tagliacotian flap that would not disfigure the forehead in a growing child. If a complication does occur, as occasionally it does in a major reconstruction, or if the construction of a second nose is necessary, an untouched forehead is a singular advantage. I do not want to get into a discussion here about forehead versus arm flap and the forehead scarring. In my opinion, the forehead makes the best nose. The forehead can be well grafted to look good. Moreover, the time required for reconstruction is less with the forehead technique.

Reconstruction of the Total Columella

Most of the columellar reconstruction in the early 1950s was made from neck tubes. This required a long time for forming the tube, de-

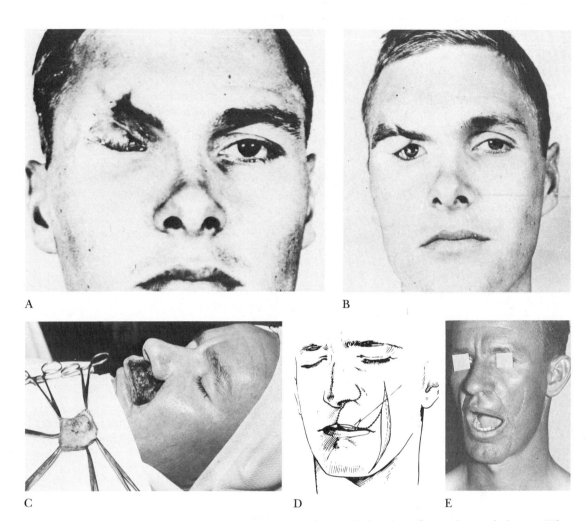

A

B

C

D

E

FIGURE 3-4. *(A) Gunshot wound of the eye. (B) Reconstruction with cervical neck tube. (C) Basal cell carcinoma of the upper lip. Resection of half the upper lip, leaving mucous membrane. (D) Diagrammatic outline of nasolabial flap for reconstruction of upper lip. (E) Upper lip resurfaced.*

laying the skin paddle, transferring the tube to the nasolabial area, delaying the opposite end of the tube, and finally transferring to the columellar region (Fig. 3-8A through C). The flap was usually too bulky and required several defatting procedures.

This technique obviously does not fit into the formula of the "simplest, quickest procedure that gets the job done." So now, reconstruction of the columella is done with an elongated nasolabial flap [8]. It can be directly applied without delay, scarring is minimal at the donor site, and the time factor is much better (Fig. 3-9A through C). A composite ear graft is satisfactory for small areas of the columella, but I do not feel that it is the best choice for columella replacement. A forehead flap is another alternative (Fig. 3-10A through C).

Large Avulsion Wound of the Hand

Shortly after starting practice in 1949, I was called to the emergency room to see a baker who had avulsed all the skin of the index, long, ring, and little fingers with the distal half of the skin on the dorsum and palm of the hand (Fig. 3-11A). In those days we were told to bury the hand in the lower abdomen. This was done, and it was a mess. There was considerable

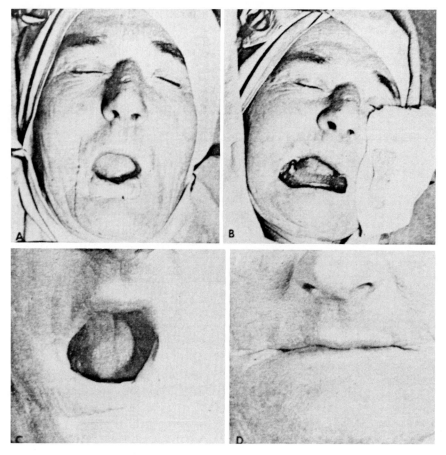

FIGURE 3-5. (A) Multiple squamous cell carcinoma of the lower lip, treated previously by radiation. (B) Excision of the lower lip with specimen. (C) Reconstruction with cer-vical facial flap (enlarged nasolabial flap folded on itself). (D) Reconstruction of lower lip following oral mucous membrane flap advancement to reconstruct vermilion.

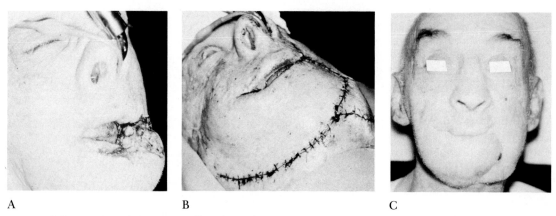

A   B   C

FIGURE 3-6. (A) Extensive squamous cell carcinoma involving anterior periosteum of the mandible. (B) Bilateral facial-cervical flaps to reconstruct the lower lip and chin. Buccal mucous membrane flaps furnished oral lining. (C) Two weeks following surgery.

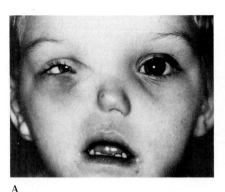
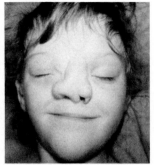
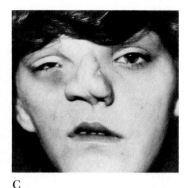

A   B   C

FIGURE 3-7. *(A) Congenital absence of right side of nose at age 5. (B) Reconstructed nose with forehead flap at age 7. (C) Nose at age 15, unsatisfactory. Reconstruction by arm flaps, not completed.*

drainage, resulting in a soupy wound and difficulty in keeping the fingers in a fixed position. Frequently the patient ended up with stiff fingers, and pedicle flaps to the digits made them look too thick in spite of repeated defatting (Fig. 3-11B). I will never bury a hand again.

Today split-thickness skin grafts are used to cover fingers wherever possible, particularly if there is paratenon present. The same treatment applies to the dorsal and palmar surfaces of the hand. If pedicle flaps are needed to cover bone or tendons with no paratenon, or if tendon, nerve, or bone-graft procedures are required, they can be patterned to the specific area. It is always advisable to have a wide-base pedicle with a patterned tip to fit the site of application. However, multiple pedicles can also be used to satisfy the position and location (Fig. 3-12A through C).

Giant Pigmented Nevi of the Forehead and Scalp

Although Ferris Smith popularized and emphasized fractional excision in the early 1940s, I did not accept the concept at the time. I

wanted to get the lesion off in a hurry, even if it required skin grafting. This was fine on the body, but was it the right procedure for the scalp?

I was impressed by early removal of giant hairy nevi in children. These nevi seemed to get larger with body growth, requiring more extensive skin grafting. I treated a little girl, 4 months of age, who had a large hairy nevus of the upper back. It was excised, and the excision was grafted with one drum of skin. Today she is in her twenties and the skin graft is approximately four times its original size (Fig. 3-13A and B).

The problem with pigmented nevi of the forehead and scalp is that if they are not excised deeply enough, pigmentation and hair will recur. However, when excision is deep, depression in the forehead results. Another problem, and one worthy of emphasis, is that skin grafting the scalp leaves an area of alopecia. The 7-month-old baby in Figure 3-14A had a hairy nevus of the forehead and scalp. The entire area was excised and skin was grafted. There was no hair on one side of the frontal-parietal area. It took a major operation to elevate the entire scalp for resurfacing the hair in the areas of alopecia (Fig. 3-14B through D). This is much more difficult in the older child and may require several procedures, particularly when the patient will not allow you to shave the entire head. I believe it is preferable to skin graft the forehead as one procedure. Pigmented nevi of the scalp should be handled by fractional excision, which produces no unsightly alopecia (Figs. 3-15 and 3-16).

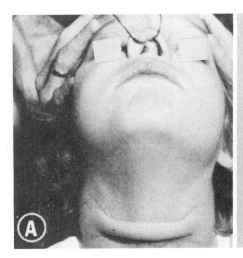
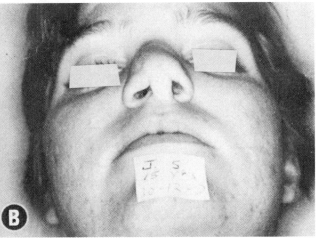

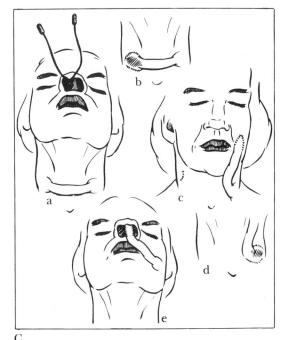

C

FIGURE 3-8. *(A) Loss of columella in a child 5 years of age; etiology: eczema and infection as a baby. (B) Reconstruction columella with a cervical neck tube. (C) Diagrammatic outline of columella reconstruction with a cervical tube.*

Reconstruction of the Chin

Twenty-seven years ago, a young boy with a burn scar on the chin was admitted with underdevelopment of the symphysis mandibulae from scar contracture. Dr. Jerome P. Webster had used a thoracoepigastric tube for major reconstruction about the face. My patient, then 12 years old, eventually would require a cartilage graft to the chin and resurfacing of the chin and neck (Fig. 3-17A).

I elected to form a thoracoepigastric tube (Fig. 3-17B). It took a long time to waltz it up to the chin, and with a teen-age male patient, there were many scars along the way. In addition, a lot of skin and fat were left over. (This reminds me of a story: Dr. J.P. Webster was visited by Sir Harold Gillies at the Presbyterian Plastic Surgery Clinic. He said, "Harold, I want to show you something." He lifted up the hospital gown of one of his patients and brought out the longest tube pedicle flap made in history. It was a thoracoepigastric tube, made in this tall woman for total reconstruction of the nose. After having completed the nasal reconstruction, he did not know what to do with the tube and the patient carried it around in her clothes.)

In my patient, after the chin and neck were resurfaced with skin and fat, an autogenous cartilage graft was attached to the periosteum

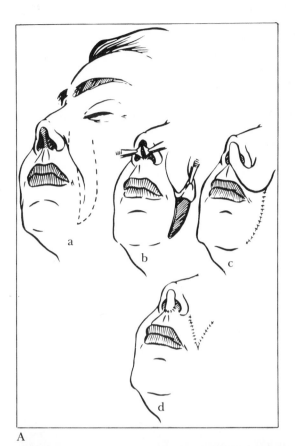

A

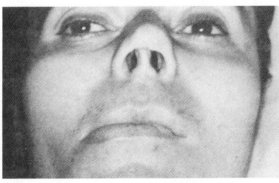

B

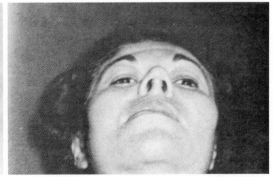

C

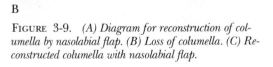

FIGURE 3-9. *(A) Diagram for reconstruction of columella by nasolabial flap. (B) Loss of columella. (C) Reconstructed columella with nasolabial flap.*

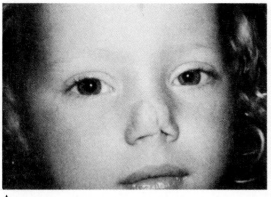

A

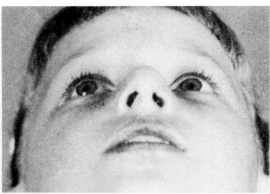

B

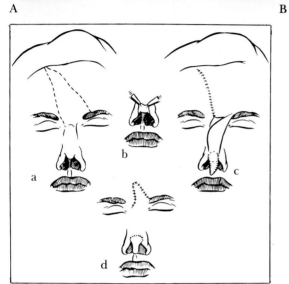

C

FIGURE 3-10. *(A) Loss of columella from treatment of hemangioma of the nose. (B) Reconstruction of columella from middle forehead flap. (C) Diagrammatic outline of forehead flap to columella.*

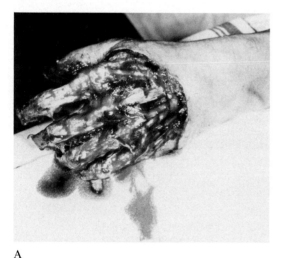

A

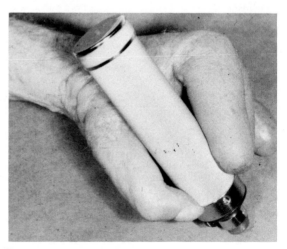

B

FIGURE 3-11. *(A) Avulsion of the fingers and hand in bakery. (B) Result following resurfacing, using the buried abdominal flap technique.*

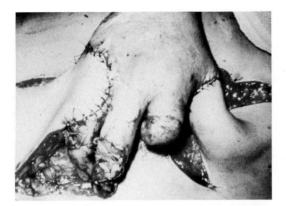

A

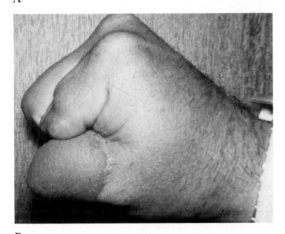

B

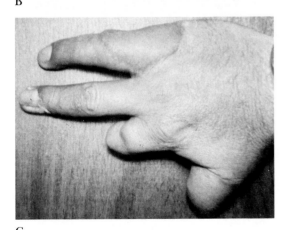

C

FIGURE 3-12. *(A) Multiple abdominal pedicle flap applied to an electric burn of the hand. (B) Resurfacing of the thumb and ulnar surface of the hand showing flexion. (C) Hand in extension.*

of the mandible, and the patient was happy with the result (Fig. 3-17C).

Today I would not use this procedure. In fact, I rarely make tube pedicle flaps except in unusual situations, e.g., for major reconstruction of the face of a woman or young girl, where I use a tube from the arm in order to spare the chest. Now most of these chin burns are resurfaced with local skin flaps or grafts. Small bone or cartilage grafts can be placed beneath the new skin under the periosteum. A graft of cartilage is preferable to one of bone, since it can be shaved easily to eliminate irregularities postoperatively.

Reconstruction Following Total Avulsion of the Ear

Again in the early 1950s, the technique of removing all the skin from the totally avulsed ear and burying the cartilage in the postauricular area or abdomen was acceptable, and may be so even today.

A policeman, age 40, came to the emergency room with total avulsion of the ear; the tissue was chewed up. I removed the skin from the auricular cartilage and kept it in saline. The postauricular area was debrided, and the skin and scalp in this region were undermined to facilitate primary closure. The auricular cartilage was placed beneath this postauricular skin flap. Attempts to reconstruct an ear with this buried cartilage were unsuccessful. The cartilage was thin and gave very little shape to the ear. This was the last patient to have this type of reconstruction. Another disadvantage of this method is the common occurrence of infection.

Until the time comes when we can replant the total ear by microvascular technique, my treatment is as follows. The totally avulsed ear (Fig. 3-18A), severely crushed and mutilated, is sent to pathology. The auricular area is cleansed, debrided, and closed primarily by skin flap advancement or skin graft (Fig. 3-18B). When the area is soft and ready for the next stage, an autologous cartilage graft taken from the rib is inserted into the postauricular

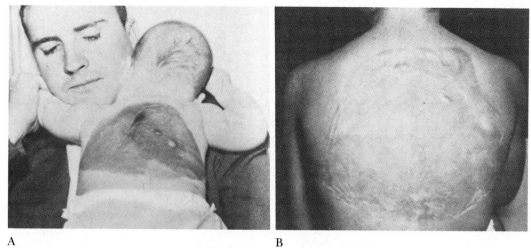

A   B

FIGURE 3-13. *(A) Baby, 4 months of age, with large hairy nevus of the back. (B) Note increased size of the one drum of skin.*

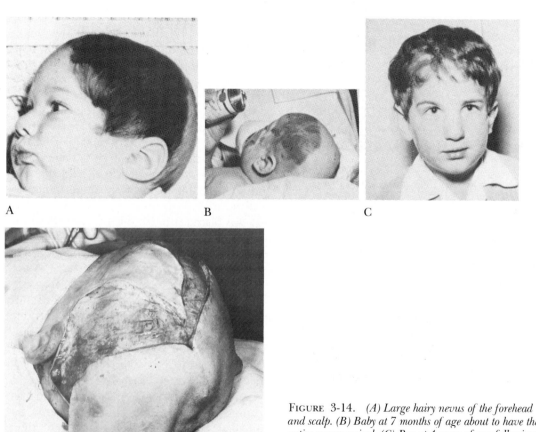

FIGURE 3-14. *(A) Large hairy nevus of the forehead and scalp. (B) Baby at 7 months of age about to have the entire nevus excised. (C) Boy at 4 years of age following excision of skin graft of scalp and rotation scalp flaps. (D) Scalp flaps elevated to resurface the nonhair-bearing skin graft of the frontal parietal area.*

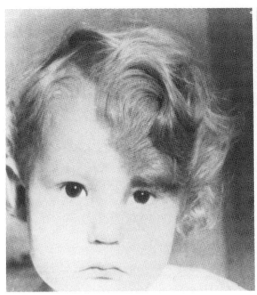
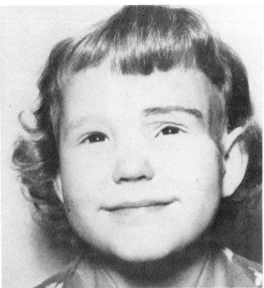

A   B

FIGURE 3-15.   *Hairy nevus of the forehead and scalp before and after excision (4 years old).*

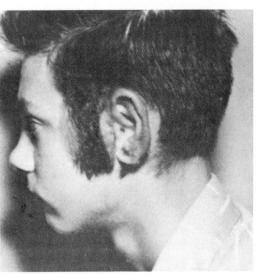
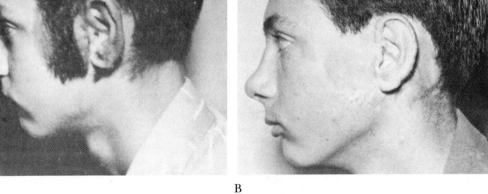

A   B

FIGURE 3-16.   *Hairy nevus of the face and scalp in 14-year-old boy before and after excision.*

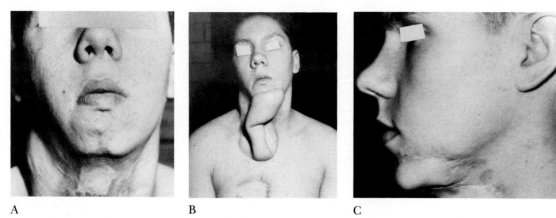

A   B   C

FIGURE 3-17. *(A) Burn-scar contracture of the chin with underdevelopment of the symphysis mandibulae. (B) Thoracoepigastric tube transferred to the chin. (C) Reconstructed chin with skin flap and cartilage graft.*

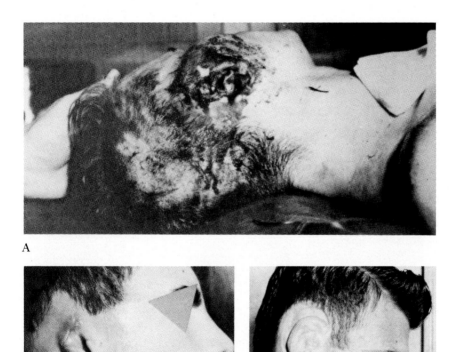

A

B   C

FIGURE 3-18. *(A) Total avulsion of ear from automobile accident. (B) Wound healed by posterior auricular skin flap advancement. (C) Reconstructed ear 1 year later.*

area. This is then followed by elevation and skin grafts 2 or 3 months later (Fig. 3-18C).

References

1. Hughes, W.L. A new method for rebuilding lower lid. *Arch. Ophthalmol.* 17:1008, 1937.
2. Paletta, F.X. Early and late repair of facial defects following treatment of malignancy. *Plast. Reconstr. Surg.* 13:95, 1954.
3. Paletta, F.X. Rehabilitation of patients with cancer of the face. *Miss. Valley Med. J.* 76:220–222, 1954.
4. Paletta, F.X. Management of carcinoma of the lip. *J. Int. Coll. Surg.* 30:162, 1958.
5. Paletta, F.X. Tumors of the Skin. In J.M. Converse (Ed.), *Reconstructive Plastic Surgery*. Philadelphia: Saunders, 1964. Vol. 1, p. 286.
6. Paletta, F.X. *Trauma*. St. Louis: Mosby, 1967.
7. Paletta, F.X. Lower eyelid reconstruction. *Plast. Reconstr. Surg.* 51:653, 1973.
8. Paletta, F.X., and Van Norman, R.T. Total reconstruction of the columella. *Plast. Reconstr. Surg.* 30:322, 1962.

4 THIS chapter is a follow-up of four decades of experience with plaster-cast models (Figs. 4-1 and 4-2). The plaster of paris cast mold has been utilized in all patients who lent themselves to the procedure (e.g., for faces, hands, and ears), and it has been used on many thousands of patients [4–7].

The plaster model is a peerless audit for clinical evaluation and follow-up of a surgical case. Its three-dimensional qualities allow opportunity for leisure study both preoperatively and during the procedure in the operating theater.

Plaster as a media for casting is easy to handle, inexpensive, long lasting, and simple to store. The plastic surgeon's records are immeasurably fortified under a litigious atmosphere. The cast model is helpful in the preoperative psychological cushioning of the patient. The surgeon who becomes acquainted with its use gains assurance, and it becomes an important diagnostic instrument.

Although photographs are mandatory and invaluable, they do not demonstrate the exactness of contour that is depicted by a three-dimensional cast model. Photographs vary with each operator, with time, with the type of film, with lighting, and with the mood of the photographer.

Cast models are especially helpful in evaluating nasal deformity. The moulage may be studied from all angles prior to surgery. Although the patient is usually operated on lying down, the surgeon rarely examines the patient in this position prior to the operation. Whether or not it is justified, postoperative rhinoplasty patients often have some minor complaint. The

34

Edward Lamont

REFINEMENTS IN THE ART OF MAKING A PLASTER-CAST MODEL

plaster-cast model proves helpful in such cases.

Few plastic surgeons have employed the cast model as routine in their practice. They have been under the impression, perhaps rightly so, that making a plaster of paris cast mold is "messy" and time consuming. Consequently, they have come to a comfortable conclusion: that "it isn't worth it anyway and is not helpful as a diagnostic or postoperative audit." After long experience it may be said that these conclusions are not valid. The introduction of the Lamont Templet (Figs. 4-3 and 4-4)* has overcome most difficulties in making a facial moulage.

Creation of the Plaster-Cast Model

PREPARATION OF THE PATIENT

The patient is prepared psychologically prior to making the plaster-cast "negative." The procedure is explained, and the patient is assured of comfort, with no obstruction to breathing. The patient is advised that within a short time after the plaster is placed on the face, there is a feeling of warmth. When a patient has breathing difficulty, a shrinking drug is used intranasally. I have had patients fall asleep during the brief time the negative is on the face.

The patient is asked to lie prone on a comfortable table, with a small pillow under the head and a pillow under the knees. The operator may place both palms gently over the face, covering the eyes and mouth and leaving

*Padgett Instruments Division, Kansas City Assemblage Co, Inc., Kansas City, Mo. 64108.

the nostrils exposed for breathing, thus demonstrating the area that will be covered by plaster. The Lamont Templet is now adjusted over the face (Fig. 4-5).

Using a cotton applicator, petroleum jelly is carefully applied to the eyebrows, the eyelashes, and mustache if one is present, and a slight amount is brushed within the nostrils (Fig. 4-6). The eyebrows and mustache are coated heavily to avoid a flattened-down appearance in the final "positive." Petroleum jelly is overlaid on the hair of the forehead and temple region. *No tubes are used in the nostrils.* The Lamont Templet is now repositioned so there is minimal leakage of plaster.

MIXING THE PLASTER OF PARIS

Rapid-setting pure white plaster of paris is used. It is available in most dental supply houses. Approximately 600 ml of cold water is poured into a shallow plastic or rubber bowl. A cup is filled with plaster, and the plaster is slowly sifted into the water. Plaster is always added to the water, never vice versa. The plaster is never poured in one mass because that procedure will cause lumpiness. Plaster is continuously added, while the bowl is gently agitated, until the surface resembles a dry, cracked desert pond. The mixture is then stirred with a light, flat ladle, which allows the plaster to combine freely with the water.

Lumps should be avoided as the mixture becomes homogenized. Experience with the mixture is the best indicator of when more plaster is needed. When more plaster is required, it is sprinkled over the surface and

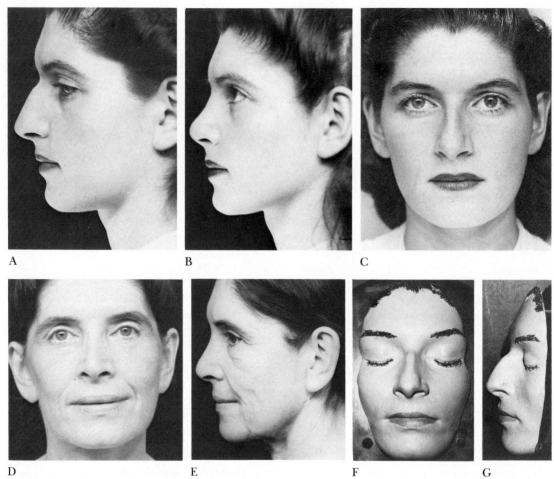

A   B   C

D   E   F   G

FIGURE 4-1. *(A) Nasal and septal deformity with block-age to breathing. (B) Postoperative rhino-osteoplasty in conjunction with septal realignment. The lower turbinates were electrofulgurated along their entire base, then frac-tured laterally. A rounded square of autogenous septal car-tilage measuring approximately 1 cm was inserted through a small incision into a superficial pocket created at the columella-philtrum angle in order to gain a gentle curve at this juncture. After 35 years, the cartilage remains intact.*

(C) Preoperative front view 35 years ago. (D) Thirty-five years following rhino-osteoplasty and septal repair. Taken several years after blepharoplasty and rhytidectomy. (E) Profile view of the patient more than 30 years after nasal surgery, taken prior to eyelid and facial surgery. (F) The plaster of paris cast moulage made of the patient 35 years ago serves as a three-dimensional record and is an ideal audit of surgical results and long-term follow-up. (G) Pro-file of the plaster-cast model prior to the initial surgery.

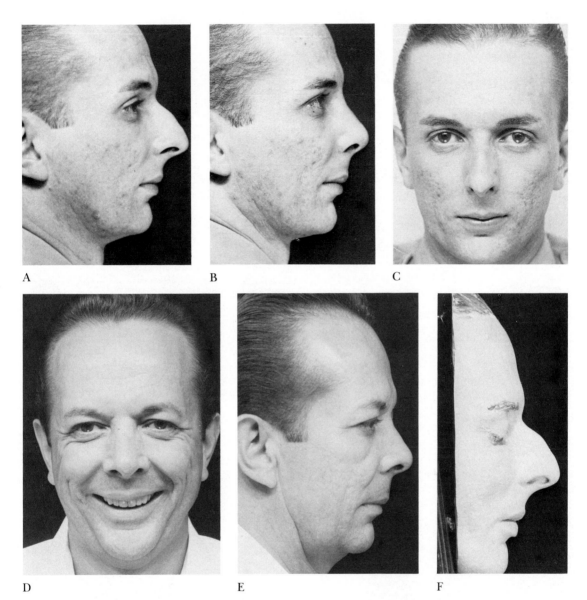

FIGURE 4-2.   *(A) Nasal deformity associated with an-*
terior septal dislocation, taken prior to surgery. (B) Rhino-
osteoplasty in combination with a swinging-door procedure,
moving the septum to the midline. The columella-philtrum
angle required recession. This was accomplished by resect-
ing the required amount of tissue, then placing a septal-
columellar-philtrum silk suture and allowing it to remain
for 3 days. (C) Front view of the patient prior to surgery,
taken 33 years ago. (D) Thirty-three years following nasal
surgery. (E) The patient profile. (F) The plaster of paris
cast moulage taken of the patient 33 years ago. It has no
peer as a comparative study for audit of results, in teach-
ing, and for long-term follow-up.

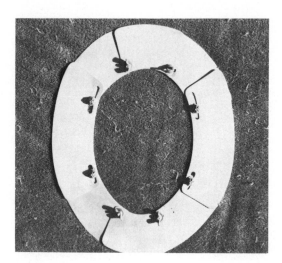

FIGURE 4-3. *The Lamont Templet: the wing screws in place allow the eight segments to form an oval. The sections may be altered to fit the size and contour of the patient's face.*

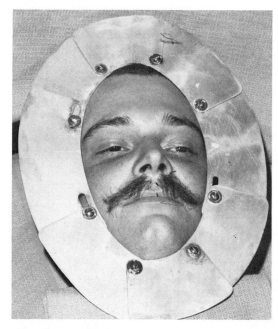

FIGURE 4-5. *The patient in a prone position on a comfortable table with a small pillow under the head and a pillow under the knees. The Lamont Templet has been fitted to the patient's face.*

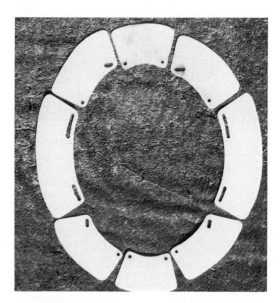

FIGURE 4-4. *The Lamont Templet shown in its eight separate sections. (Available from Padgett Instruments, Kansas City, Missouri 64108.)*

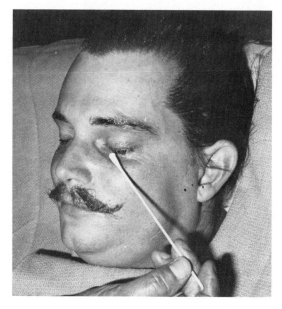

FIGURE 4-6. *Petroleum jelly is applied to the eyebrows, eyelashes, mustache, nostrils, and forehead and temple hair.*

gradually allowed to submerge; then the mixture is stirred. Until one becomes accustomed to the procedure, it is better to make a large batch than to be caught short.

If one wishes to shorten the setting time of plaster of paris, one-half teaspoonful of table salt is added to 450 ml of water, and this is used in the plaster mixture. The more salt, the more rapidly the plaster will set. Potassium sulfate, potassium alum, and other chemicals may be used to hasten the setting of the plaster [2].

To increase the time of setting, a saturated solution of borax is made. One part of this solution is mixed with ten parts of water. This will increase the setting time 25 to 30 minutes. There are a number of other chemicals that may be used to the same end [3].

APPLICATION OF PLASTER TO THE FACE

With the Lamont Templet in position, the plaster mixture, which has the consistency of thick porridge, is applied to the tip of the nose, the alae, and the columella with a camel's hair brush. The area is relayered several times (Fig. 4-7).

During this period, the plaster in the bowl has begun to set, although it is still liquid. At this point, a ladle is used to apply plaster to the face (Fig. 4-8). The remainder of the nose, the eyes, and the forehead are covered, and then the cheeks, mouth, and chin.

After the face is covered, more plaster is added as necessary. A wooden tongue depressor is used to smooth the plaster and move it into reinforcing positions (Fig. 4-9). The patient should be advised not to squint when the plaster is laid over the eyes, and not to grimace when it is placed over the mouth. The templet easily catches the plaster as it gravitates down the face, so the negative becomes a single unit.

REMOVAL OF THE MOLD

The negative is allowed to remain on the face 4 to 5 minutes. During this time, there should be minimal conversation in the room. The patient is reassured of the successful progress and advised that the plaster negative will be removed

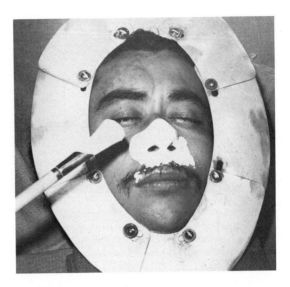

FIGURE 4-7.   *The homogenized plaster of paris mixture, the consistency of thick gruel, is initially painted onto the tip of the nose in several layers.*

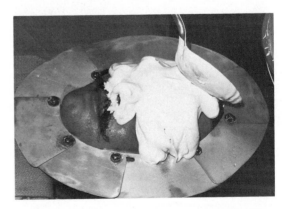

FIGURE 4-8.   *After the plaster begins to set, it is ladled over the eyes, forehead, mouth, cheeks, nose, and chin.*

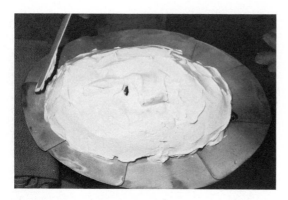

FIGURE 4-9. *While the plaster is reasonably soft, it is smoothed with a wooden tongue depressor. After allowing it to set for approximately 5 minutes, the plaster negative adhered to the templet is removed with ease.*

shortly. As soon as no plaster remains on the finger when the mold is brushed lightly, the negative may be removed.

The patient is advised not to open his or her eyes until told to do so. The templet is grasped on top, the last two fingers of each hand gain-

ing purchase on the temple regions, and the templet and negative are lifted from the face accompanied by a slight suction sound.

The face and hair are cleansed with a wet towel. Moist applicators are used to clean the eyelashes and to remove small bits of plaster on the lid margins. The patient is then led to a mirror and allowed to complete cleaning his or her face.

PREPARING THE POSITIVE

Although materials such as wax or metals can be used to create a positive, this chapter deals only with plaster of paris.

The negative is easily removed from the templet, and a coat of pure white shellac is applied to its face. It is placed in a cold-water bath for 20 minutes (Fig. 4-10). The negative is dried, and a separating mixture is applied to its face. The separating mixture consists of equal parts of pure white talc, turpentine, and castor oil (Fig. 4-11).

A new batch of plaster is mixed. However, this batch is slightly thicker than that made for

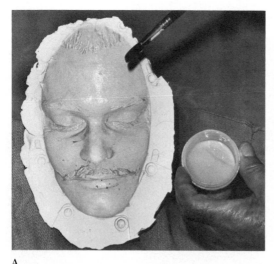

A

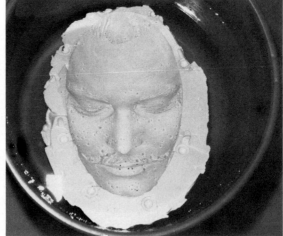

B

FIGURE 4-10. *(A) The plaster of paris negative is shellacked. The camera eye has given the negative a three-dimensional contour so that it appears as a positive. (B) The shellacked plaster negative is soaked in a cold water bath for 20 minutes.*

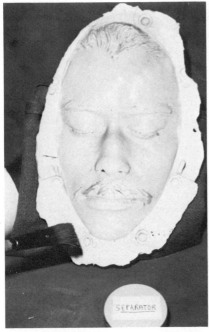

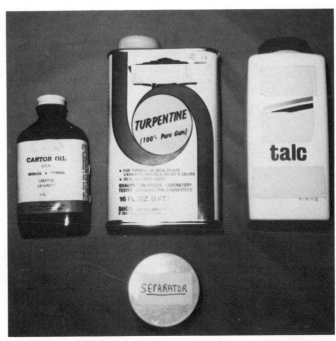

A   B

FIGURE 4-11.   *(A) The plaster of paris negative is dried, and a separating solution is painted over its face. (B) The separating solution is made up of equal parts of pure white talc, turpentine, and castor oil.*

the negative. This allows for easier separation and a longer-lasting positive. At this time, color may be added to the water if a tinted positive is desired.

The mixture is poured into the plaster negative mold with a ladle. The negative is gently agitated to allow the plaster to uniformly find its way into the crevices. Plaster is added until it reaches the edge of the negative (Fig. 4-12). It is placed in a holder for support, and before it hardens completely, a heavy-gauge wire loop is inserted into the center of the upper third, so the positive may be hung.

Separating the Positive from the Negative

After some 3 hours, the positive is broken away from the negative with a wooden mallet (Fig. 4-13). The edges of the negative are tapped along all sides, and finally it breaks away piecemeal.

The edges of the positive are smoothed with a knife and sandpaper. Any small pieces of clinging plaster are eased off. The inexperienced operator may be confronted with small artefacts created by bubbles. These are easily repaired by scraping some plaster from the back of the negative, mixing it with saliva, inserting it into the defect, and then smoothing the surface.

Finally, a submucous periosteal elevator is used to remove excess plaster from the nostrils until their exact contour is obtained (Fig. 4-14).

Storing the Cast Models

A cabinet containing slots is ideal for storage of the plaster moulages. Filed alphabetically, they are easily accessible and become part of the patient's record [8].

The more interesting models may be oil painted and hung in the laboratory and thus are available as teaching material (Figs. 4-15 through 4-21).

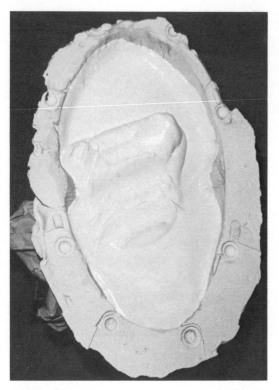

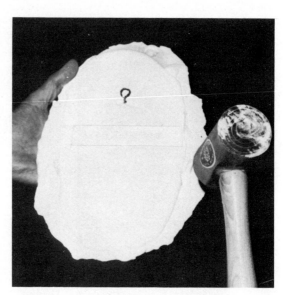

FIGURE 4-13. *The positive is allowed to set for 3 hours, then gently cracked away from the negative. The edges of the plaster moulage are now smoothed with a knife and sandpaper. The nostril openings are cleansed of plaster. The back of the moulage is labeled with an indelible pencil, and it is now part of the patient's long-term record.*

FIGURE 4-12. *A new batch of plaster is mixed, which is slightly thicker than that prepared for the negative. It is ladled onto the face of the negative while the latter is slightly agitated.*

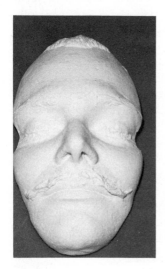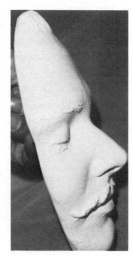

A   B

FIGURE 4-14. *(A) The plaster of paris moulage is invaluable as an adjunct in preoperative study, teaching, long-term follow-up, and auditing of surgical results. (B) The plaster-cast positive.*

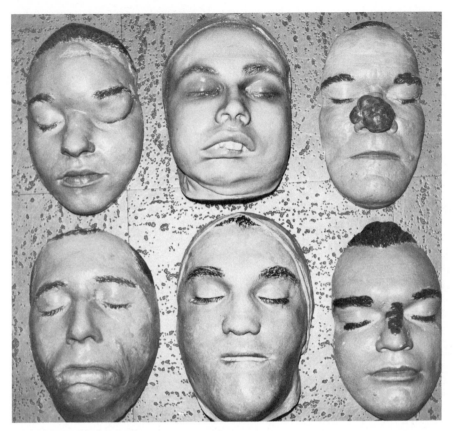

FIGURE 4-15.   *The plaster-cast model is especially valuable for teaching. Demonstrating from top left to right: giant lymphoma-hemangioma, malocclusion due to injury,* *rhinophyma, a burned face, prognathism, and hemangioma of the nose.*

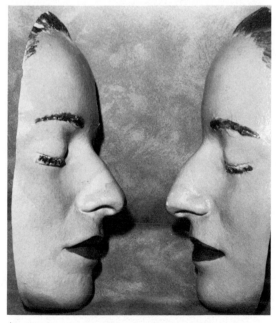

A

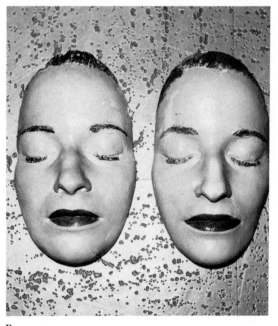

B

FIGURE 4-16.   *(A) Identical twins operated on 30 years ago. Although differences were hardly identifiable, the cast* *models reveal the dissimilarities. (B) Identical twins operated on 30 years ago.*

43

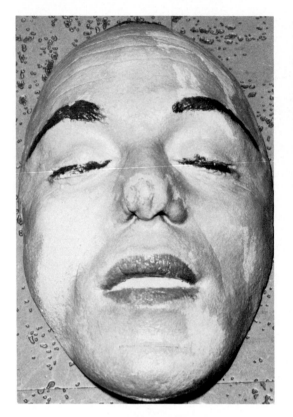

FIGURE 4-17. *Cast model: paraffinoma of the nose.*

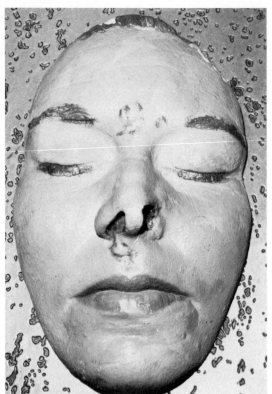

FIGURE 4-18. *Deformity due to injury. The plaster-cast model not only serves as an excellent surgical audit, but allows the surgeon to leisurely plan the operative procedure. It is ideally helpful in staged operations.*

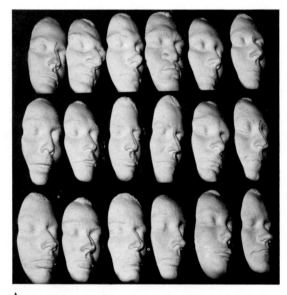

A

FIGURE 4-19. *(A) The plaster-cast moulage is easy to file in a cabinet, and available to the surgeon for studying long-term follow-up, for psychological cushioning of the patient, and as an ideal three-dimensional record. More interesting cases can be painted and hung in the laboratory. (B) Plaster-cast models of faces and hands.*

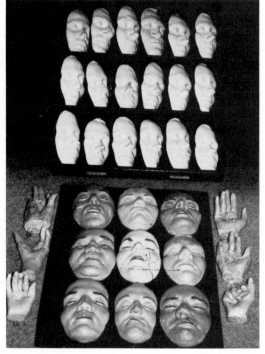

B

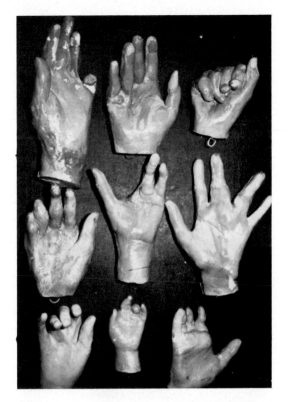

FIGURE 4-20. *Plaster-cast models of hands: injury, tumor, Dupuytrens contracture, congenital deformity. These models are helpful for long-term follow-up and teaching.*

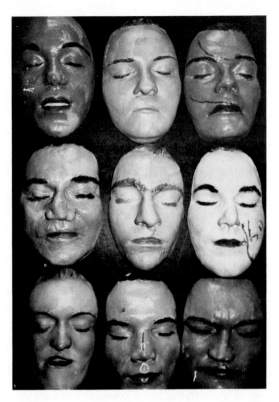

FIGURE 4-22. *Although photographs are a requirement in all plastic surgery cases, the three-dimensional plaster-cast model is a perfect partner for a true record and comparative study following plastic surgery.*

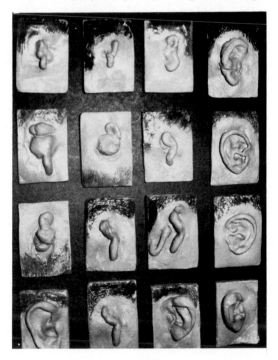

FIGURE 4-21. *Plaster-cast models of microtia in various stages of surgical reconstruction* [4].

Final Thoughts

The plaster-cast model has no substitute as an instrument for surgical planning or for auditing long-term postoperative results (Fig. 4-22). Once a routine is established, plaster models require little time to make, and when combined with photographs, black and white and color, they serve as ideal records and teaching modules.

Acknowledgment

I should like to express my indebtedness to Ms. Gertrude Hance, longtime artist non pareil with Drs. Blair, Brown, Byars, and McDowell in St. Louis, and Ms. Suzanne Postelle, R.N., equally capable in ability and experience with Drs. Updegraff and Lamont.

My thanks go also to Dr. Lynn Hilde and Dr. Conny Joy, formerly Senior Residents in Plastic and Reconstructive Surgery at the University of California Medical School, Irvine, for their help in the preparation of this chapter.

References

1. Brown, J.B., and McDowell, F. *Plastic Surgery of the Nose.* St. Louis: Mosby, 1951. P. 40.
2. Bulbulian, A.H. *Facial Prosthesis.* Philadelphia: Saunders, 1945. P. 189.
3. Clarke, C.D. *Facial and Body Prostheses.* St. Louis: Mosby, 1945.
4. Lamont, E. Reconstructive plastic surgery of the absent ear with necrocartilage. *Arch. Surg.* 48:55, 1944.
5. Lamont, E. Reconstructive surgery of the nose in congenital deformity, injury and disease. *Am. J. Surg.* 65:17, 1944.
6. Lamont. E. Reparative plastic surgery in secondary cleft lip and nasal deformities. *Surg. Gynecol. Obstet.* 80:422, 1945.
7. Lamont, E. Plastic surgery of the nose—A thirty year review. Transactions of the Asian Pacific Congress of Plastic Surgery, New Delhi, India. Vol. 1, 1970.
8. Updegraff, H. The problem of rhinoplasty. *Ann. Surg.* 90:961, 1929.

Robert M. Goldwyn

COMMENTS ON CHAPTER 4

THE use of plaster-cast models is not new; they were used in the nineteenth century, employed extensively during World War I by Kazanjian, and popularized later by the St. Louis group (Drs. Brown and McDowell). Of course, plaster-cast models are not the only way of documenting preoperative status and post-operative results. As Dr. Lamont states, photographs are also "mandatory and invaluable," but they do not give the "exactness of contour" that a three-dimensional model does. This is not the place to argue the merits and drawbacks of the various means of record keeping available to the plastic surgeon. Suffice to say that in our specialty, unlike some others in medicine, written notes are not enough; visual records are indispensable. But more important than whether one uses the camera or plaster or both for documentation is the commitment to an accurate and sufficiently long follow-up. Admittedly, such follow-up requires time and effort on the part of both the surgeon and the patient, especially if the result has been an unfavorable one.

5 WARS have always been a challenge to the surgeon, and often great medical and surgical progress and innovations emerge. World War II was certainly no exception. Just as in World War I, World War II gave a great stimulus to the efforts of surgeons concerned with reconstruction of tissue and parts damaged or destroyed by missiles, flame, or accident. Despite the military reluctance to accept specialization, it became clear by the time of the landings in North Africa that there was a compelling urgency to reorganize the medical services of the Armed Forces and prepare for the anticipated flood of injured and wounded. In order to provide the specialized care to which these men were entitled, it was necessary to designate and staff hospital centers across the country, to which, after intelligent triage, patients were assigned. Centers for vascular surgery, neurosurgery, plastic and reconstructive surgery, and hand surgery, among others, were organized.

One of the centers for plastic and reconstructive surgery was the Valley Forge General Hospital in Phoenixville, Pennsylvania. This hospital opened in 1943 under the direction of Dr. James Barrett Brown, and during the next 4 years, over 16,000 operations were carried out successfully. The purpose of this chapter is to review briefly the experience at Valley Forge General Hospital and to present a quarter-century follow-up of some of these patients.

The daily record of operations performed in the years 1943–1947 has been reviewed. The procedure performed the largest number of times was the free skin graft, totaling 2,381. This large figure is understandable since warfare inevitably involves penetration of, damage to, or loss of skin. The most frequent injury calling for skin grafting was the burn, usually

Bradford Cannon

SOME LATE RESULTS IN WORLD WAR II WOUNDED

having resulted from flaming gasoline. Burns in falling airplanes, enclosed armoured tanks, or exploding vehicles on the ground were frequent. Another large group of wounds were those involving the face and jaws. In contrast to much civilian surgery, the ramus, condyle, or coronoid processes were seldom involved. Doubtless shell fragments penetrating posteriorly would result in such massive hemorrhage or brain damage that survival would be unlikely. On the other hand, unilateral or bilateral destruction of the anterior mandible was frequent and also was frequently associated with massive skin loss.

A considerable number and variety of operative procedures were carried out during those years. They include free skin grafts, as mentioned earlier; local and remote flaps to extremities, face, nose, etc.; bone and cartilage grafts; composite grafts from the ear; ear reconstruction; fascial transplants; and revision of unsightly scars.

CASE 1

This man, who was in the 3rd Infantry Division, was struck by a shell fragment in the crossing of the Volturno River in Italy in October 1943. He had a defect in the chin and mandible as a result of this injury (Fig. 5-1A). Because of the constant drooling which he and others like him experienced, the first procedure undertaken was to mobilize the local soft tissues so that the amount of drooling from the mouth could be minimized (Fig. 5-1B). Fortunately, enough tissue remained to make this possible. Simultaneously, a chest flap was begun to provide adequate soft tissue for restoration of the chin and jaw. A rectangle of skin from the side

of the flap was inverted to provide the lining for the inner surface of the lip. After several delaying procedures, the flap was transferred to the chin, where it remained attached for several weeks. The pedicle was then severed and returned to the chest wall, and the incisions on the chin were closed (Fig. 5-1C). With the softening of the skin flap, the tissue was ready for restoration of the continuity of the mandible with a bone graft (Fig. 5-1D).

He fell in love with one of our most capable nurses who, responsible for surgical dressings, was an invaluable member of the surgical team. Thanks to her dedication and skill, all wounds were scrupulously clean and all dressings were dry. It is no exaggeration to say that the success of many operative procedures could be directly attributed to her. After their respective discharges from the army, they were married and settled on Long Island, where he was involved in an active business venture. When visited several years ago, it was clear that they had made a happy life for themselves (Fig. 5-1E). They spoke proudly of their son and several grandchildren, who were happily settled in a neighboring community.

CASE 2

This man was tank chief in Germany, and he was wounded in March 1945 when a shell struck the tank deck and exploded, causing loss of much of the middle third of the face and a segment of the mandible, and extensively injuring, but fortunately not destroying, both eyes (Fig. 5-2A and B). He was one of those so seriously deformed that one wondered whether the use of a prosthetic reconstruction, as was the practice in World War I, should be consid-

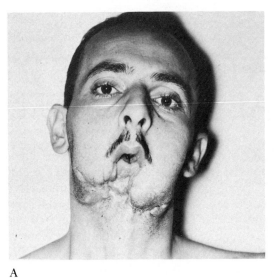

A

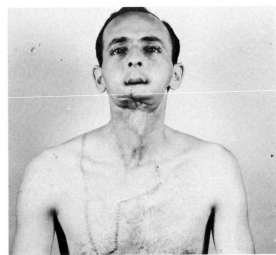

B

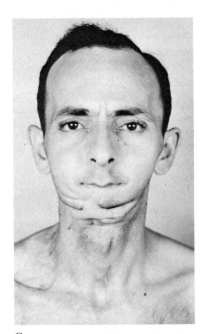

C

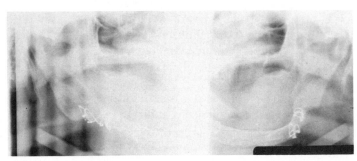

D

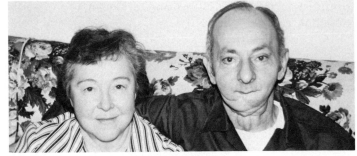

E

FIGURE 5-1.   (A) Condition after the initial wounds healed, showing massive tissue loss. (B) Remaining tissues of cheek and lip have been mobilized to control mouth drooling. Flap for ultimate repair has been delayed and is ready for transfer after turn-in of the rectangular flap needed for lining. (C) Soft tissue for restoration of chin and mandible now in place. The pedicle has been returned. (D) Recent panoramic-Zomographic radiograph of intact mandibular bone grafts. (E) Recent photograph of patient and his wife.

ered. However, the battalion surgeon responsible for the primary care wisely preserved all possible mucous membrane, suturing it to adjacent undamaged skin. Therefore, the first reconstructive procedure consisted of mobilizing the exposed mucosa for restoration of mouth lining. Despite the massive skin loss, the tissues were closed enough to minimize annoying drooling and pave the way for ultimate reconstruction of the face (Fig. 5-2C). During the same operation, preparation of a skin flap on the chest wall was started. A marginal flap of skin was later turned in to provide lining for the upper lip and the roof of the mouth. Several weeks after transfer to the face, the pedicle was divided and returned to the chest wall (Fig. 5-2D). Initially the flap covered the normal opening of the nasal passage. Eventually the passage was uncovered and the outlet lined with marginal skin flaps (Fig. 5-2E). The bony defect in the mandible was bridged with a rib graft (Fig. 5-2F). The middle of the face was supported by another bone graft crossing from zygomatic prominence to zygomatic prominence. The graft was fixed with screws to the zygoma. Of interest was the pain at the site of the screws, which promptly subsided when the screws were removed. The first bone graft was absorbed where it traversed the flap tissues. Presumably there was insufficient blood supply to ensure its viability. A second bone graft months later survived permanently and provided a foundation on which the nose and its framework were built. The nose was reconstructed with an arm flap and bone grafts were used for support. X-rays taken 25 years later revealed that the bone grafts to the mandible, the bone graft across the middle third of the face, and the struts providing a framework for the nose were intact (Fig. 5-2G).

This patient is legally blind but has travel vision and is serving as a guard in a public building in Boston. He is concerned about the color of the nose, particularly at the tip where the skin is red, a surprising finding since the usual picture of an arm flap is one of pallor (Fig. 5-2H and I). This change is said to have developed after some recent x-ray exposures. He

is able to lead a useful life and has a fine family with two children, each of whom is a college graduate.

CASE 3

This officer was a tank commander in North Africa. His tank was struck and destroyed by a German 88 shell, and he was ejected from the turret, sustaining severe burns of the face and hands and scattered burns elsewhere on the body. He also had a below-knee amputation of the leg. Captured by the Germans, he was returned on a prisoner exchange 11 months later. The destruction of skin of all four eyelids left the corneas exposed (Fig. 5-3A). Only by his frequent moving of the moist conjunctiva over each corneal surface were the eyes protected from damage. Release of ectropion of the four eyelids and repair with full-thickness supraclavicular skin grafts were of primary concern (Fig. 5-3B). Additional skin grafting of the face and total resurfacing of the nose were also performed. The residual stiffness of the hands responded to conservative treatment.

He returned to Kentucky and began raising Angus cattle. He was very active and reported that almost every year he had to have the artificial leg replaced because each soon wore out with his strenuous life. During the last dozen years he has had a political position as county clerk in his locality. His election as a state representative was reported in a recent communication. As he grew older and the farming duties became too physically arduous, he chose to seek political offices. His subsequent medical needs have been uneventful except for several basal cell carcinomata of the face (Fig. 5-3C), which have been treated surgically and appear to be unrelated to the original burns.

CASE 4

As a flight engineer on a B-24 which was shot down over Italy, this man sustained severe burns of the face, scalp, ears (Fig. 5-4A and B), and hands which required a number of skin-grafting procedures for closure of the wounds,

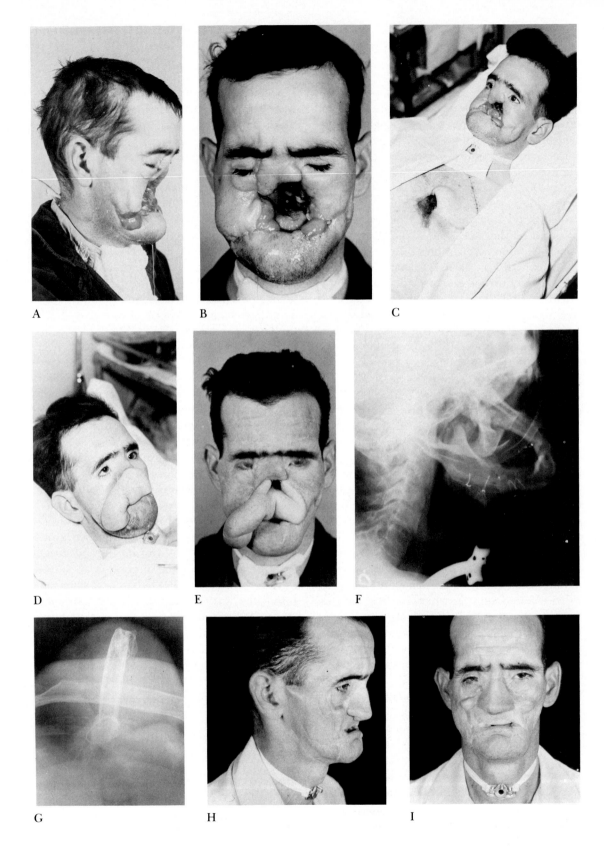

A   B   C

D   E   F

G   H   I

52

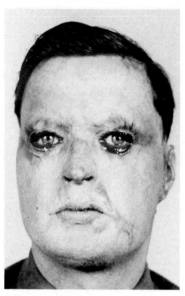
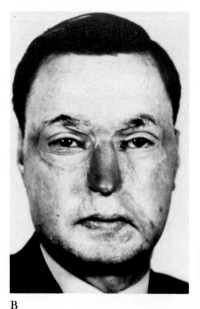
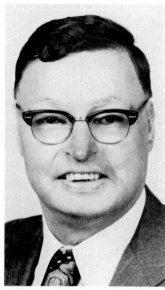

A   B   C

FIGURE 5-3. *(A) Condition on return from Germany in a prisoner exchange. (B) After multiple skin grafts to eyelids, face, and nose. Full-thickness skin grafts were used* *for eyelids. (C) Thirty years later. (From J. B. Brown and F. McDowell,* Plastic Surgery of the Nose, *1951. Courtesy Charles C Thomas, Publisher, Springfield, Ill.)*

release of contractures, and general resurfacing (Fig. 5-4C). The ears were framed with preserved cadaver cartilage (Fig. 5-4D).

Recent photographs in black and white and in color are interesting to compare. The contrasts between the various skin grafts used in resurfacing the face are minimally conspicuous in the former (Fig. 5-4E and F), but in color the contrasts are somewhat striking. However, by dint of a strong will and steadfast family support, he has been able to surmount these differences and lead a normal, active life. The preserved cartilage framework of the ears has

FIGURE 5-2. *(A) Massive loss of tissue of middle third of face. (B) After mobilization of salvaged mucous membrane. (C) Delayed transverse upper chest flap with turn-in for lining. (D) Flap in place. (E) After opening of nasal passage and shifting of a local flap for nasal floor. (F) Recent x-ray showing well-healed rib graft to mandible, the remnant of the first rib graft across the midface, and the well-healed second rib graft. (G) Recent x-ray showing the bony strut supporting the tip and dorsal ridge of the nose. (H) and (I) Recent photographs.*

been gradually absorbed, causing them to shrink but still remain recognizable.

Prior to the injury he was a boating enthusiast and used to race against Guy Lombardo, among others, on the Hudson River. On his discharge from the air force, he established and managed a boat yard in Connecticut until his recent retirement. He is the father of three children, one of whom is a law school graduate.

Final Thoughts

The preceding are examples of the types of wounds unusual in civilian practice but frequent in war times. After their discharge, each of these men made the often very difficult adjustment to his handicaps, found a place in the civilian world, and led a useful life. Others, fortunately rare, were unable to make the adjustment and have completely disappeared from follow-up. Some have died of normal causes, others have had continuing medical

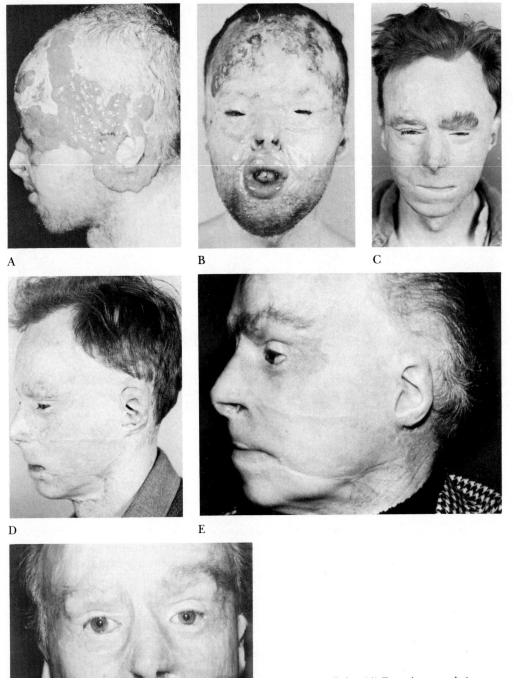

FIGURE 5-4. *(A) Extensive granulating areas of the face and scalp. (B) Massive distortion of the face after preliminary wound closure with skin grafts. (C) and (D) After resurfacing of much of the face and nose with thick-split grafts, with full-thickness supraclavicular grafts to the eyelids, with scalp grafts for the eyebrow and ear reconstruction, and with local soft tissue and a preserved cartilage framework. (E) and (F) Recent photographs revealing some of the color differences of the grafts on the face and a moderate degree of shrinkage of the cartilaginous framework of the ear.*

problems in the injured area: sensitivity to cold, dental difficulties, instability of the repair with recurrent ulcerations, color mismatch of skin grafts, etc. Many have relied on the facilities at the Veterans Administration hospitals for subsequent help. Although these hospitals have been an occasional source of follow-up information, few of these men have had to return for further significant reconstructive surgery after discharge from the military hospitals. It would appear that plastic surgeons assigned to hospital centers during World War II did an impressively adequate job in the rehabilitation of the wounded.

Joseph E. Murray

COMMENTS ON CHAPTER 5

I HAD three reactions after reading this chapter. First, the excellence of the surgical repairs; second, the long-term follow-up of the physiology of skin grafts and flaps; and finally, and most important, the psychosocial evaluation of seriously injured patients after a quarter of a century.

The surgical techniques employed were of the highest quality, but they would have been to no avail had not sound surgical principles been followed. The cases forcefully drive home the fact that sound basic surgical principles can carry the reconstructive surgery to a successful resolve. Precise refined surgical techniques are, of course, the *sine qua non* for a success story, but without solid foundation, technique alone is merely a house built on sand. In spite of the many advances of recent decades in the analysis of pedicle flaps and skin grafting, it is truly incredible that such spectacular repairs were achieved utilizing the simple principles of skin grafting and randomly based pedicle flaps.

The second unique aspect is the long-term follow-up of these skin grafts and pedicle flaps on the exposed facial surfaces. The blending of flaps and grafts over the years into a facial unit with expression and personality is an unexpected finding and illustrates that nature is truly kind in its healing process.

The final point of note is the quality of life experienced by these patients. In analyzing these lives and trying to find a common denominator, one notices the strong familial influences that ultimately lead to a stabilized society. Throughout the ages, the family unit has been the basis of a sound society, and the lives of these patients reinforce these observations. Current quests for self-identity and the trend in society toward introspectiveness are doomed to fail because selfishness is constrictive and self-defeating. The lives of these men and their families demonstrate the richness that can come from firm, giving human relationships. Truly the handicaps in these men, rather than becoming roadblocks, have been made into stepping stones.

6 THE end results of two methods of cleft palate repair will be described in this chapter. The question "What is the best method of cleft palate repair?" will be answered, adding to the active controversy that has persisted since the middle of the nineteenth century.

Aims of Cleft Palate Management

The aims and objectives of cleft palate operations have changed over the years. The earlier aims were to produce normal, or at least acceptable, speech and anatomical closure, thus stopping the undesirable transfer of air and secretions between the nose and the mouth. A relatively new objective of cleft palate repair is to foster suitable development of teeth, alveoli, and facial bones, particularly the maxillae, not only for reasons of good speech, but also for aesthetic reasons [1]. These three aims and objectives are interdependent.

Types of Cleft Palate Operations

There are so many types of cleft palate operations that it is difficult to classify them equitably. It is possible to divide them into two major groups: (1) pushback operations and (2) simple-closure operations. The pushback operations were the last to arrive on the scene. All involve complete detachment of the mucoperiosteum of the hard palate laterally and anteriorly, leaving it attached only by a posterior soft-tissue pedicle. The pushback operations fit into two main groups: the two-flap

William K. Lindsay

THE END RESULTS OF CLEFT PALATE SURGERY AND MANAGEMENT

(Figs. 6-1 through 6-3) and the four-flap procedures (Figs. 6-4 through 6-6). The four-flap procedures attempt more complete anterior anatomical closure.

Simple closure techniques (Figs. 6-7 through 6-9) are directed toward side-to-side closure and do not involve an attempt to lengthen the whole palate. They involve less dissection and detachment of the anterior mucoperiosteum than the pushback procedures do. Immediate postoperative raw areas are smaller. Modern critics of the simple-closure palatoplasty claim that it allows unnecessary fistulae or residual defects in the anterior aspects of the mouth, produces a palate of insufficient length, and is associated with inferior speech results.

Three End-Result Studies at The Hospital for Sick Children, Toronto

The initial long-term review of the results of cleft palate surgery at The Hospital for Sick Children, Toronto, was completed in 1959 [4, 5]. The patients in this first review of end results had all received a pushback palatoplasty best described as a two-flap pushback [3] (Figs. 6-1 through 6-3). This initial review of results prompted the completion of a comparable series of simple-closure operations (Figs. 6-7 through 6-9) which were reviewed in 1969 [6]. This second review of end results was completed when the patients were young. Ideal situations existed at The Hospital for Sick Children, Toronto, to follow these patients and to restudy the relative merits of pushback opera-

tions and simple-closure palatoplasties. A third review of end results was completed in 1978 [8].

SPEECH RESULTS

The speech end results following cleft palate repair have been studied three times during the author's professional lifetime at The Hospital for Sick Children, Toronto. The speech assessments have always been conducted independently by a group of experts, including a speech pathologist and a plastic surgeon who was not one of the operating plastic surgeons. Speech and numerous factors relating to speech were assessed objectively. Speech was also assessed subjectively. The subjective ratings will be reported in this chapter because, from a clinical point of view, they are more useful. Speech was assessed subjectively on either a four- or a five-point scale which ranged from normal to unintelligible. The surgeon and the speech pathologist independently assessed the speech of the children in each study. They agreed, in general, in 85 percent of their assessments. The results have been divided into two broad practical categories, especially for this chapter: those with "acceptable" and those with "unacceptable" speech. The three studies were conducted in different ways. The variables were different with respect to sample size and number of operating surgeons. Some studies were controlled more than others. It is demonstrative and reliable to compare the three studies in the following ways.

The general results of the initial study were found to be related to many variables, including the type and degree of original palatal clefting,

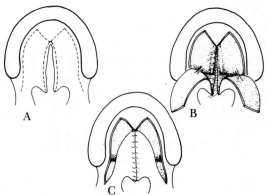

FIGURE 6-1. *Two-flap palatoplasty for isolated cleft palate. (A) The incision lines. Note that the medial and lateral incision lines are joined anteriorly by an oblique line placed to allow V-Y type closure. (B) Mucoperiosteal flaps are completely elevated and based posteriorly and on the posterior palatine arteries. The nasal mucosa and muscle were managed as in Figure 6-7D. (C) The oral mucosa has been closed. The V-Y lengthening principle is used anteriorly to gain overall palatal length or pushback.*

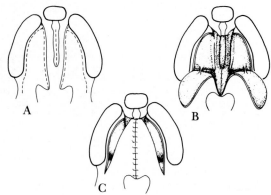

FIGURE 6-3. *Two-flap palatoplasty for bilateral cleft of the primary and secondary palates. (A) The incision lines. The oblique lines joining the medial and lateral incisions must be placed thoughtfully if significant V-Y retrodisplacement is to be obtained. (B) Elevation of mucoperiosteal flaps. Closure of mucous membrane and muscles as in Figure 6-7D. (C) Closure of oral mucosa. It will be impossible to obtain complete anterior closure unless the premaxilla has been repositioned by earlier maxillary orthopedics.*

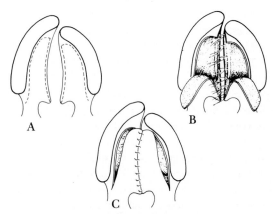

FIGURE 6-2. *Two-flap pushback palatoplasty for complete unilateral cleft of the primary and secondary palate. (A) The incision lines. Note that the medial and lateral incision lines are joined anteriorly by a line placed obliquely in a manner that will allow maximum V-Y retrodisplacement of the mucoperiosteum. (B) Mucoperiosteal flaps have been elevated with posterior palatine arteries intact, but teased out of their foramina. Soft palate lateral-release incisions have been made. The hamuli are infractured. The nasal mucosa and muscle are closed as in Figure 6-7D. (C) The oral mucosa is closed using the V-Y shift anteriorly, which shifts not only mucoperiosteum, but the whole palate posteriorly.*

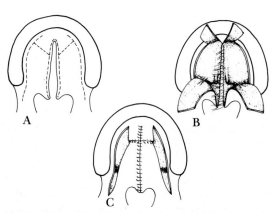

FIGURE 6-4. *Four-flap palatoplasty for isolated cleft palate. This procedure is used by some when the cleft extends forward to the incisive foramen region. It was not used in any of the studies reported in this chapter. (A) The incision lines. The oblique incision joining the medial and lateral incisions is again made in such a way to permit V-Y closure and to gain length. Care must be taken to retain a base to the anterior two flaps, yet these flaps must be mobile enough to shift them forward. (B) The four flaps are mobilized, and the nasal mucosa is closed directly. (C) Oral mucosa closure.*

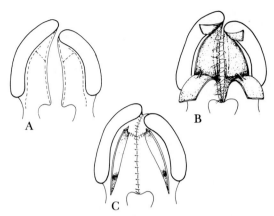

FIGURE 6-5. *Four-flap pushback palatoplasty for complete unilateral cleft of the primary and secondary palates. This operation was not used in any of the three studies. (A) The incision lines. Anteriorly, these vary considerably with the configuration of the palate. (B) Four mucoperiosteal flaps have been elevated; the two small flaps move medially and anteriorly. The nasal mucosa is closed. (C) Oral mucosa closure.*

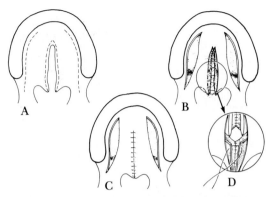

FIGURE 6-7. *Von Langenbeck (simple closure) palatoplasty for isolated cleft palate. (A) The incision lines for the margins of the soft and hard palates and for the soft and hard palate lateral release incisions. (B) Closure of the nasal mucosa. In this case, direct closure leaving the nasal mucosa intact is shown. This is possible only in the narrower and less extensive clefts. Not shown is the fact that the hamuli have been infractured, mucoperiosteal flaps have been elevated, leaving the posterior palatine artery intact, but freeing it from its foramen, and some tenuous fibers running from the region of the maxillary tuberosity to the vicinity of the posterior palatine artery have been cut. (C) Closure of the oral mucosa. Note that the anterior mucoperiosteum is still intact and there is a bipedicled mucoperiosteal flap on either side. The opportunities for pushback are not as great. The lateral open areas are not as large as with the other operations. (D) An enlarged drawing of the circled area in Figure 6-7B to illustrate one of the controversial areas. The nasal mucosa is transected and allowed to drop back with the soft palate, leaving the controversial raw nasal area. The tensor and levator muscle mass is shown, already dissected away from the posterior nasal spine and the palatal aponeurosis. These muscles are directly sutured to each other.*

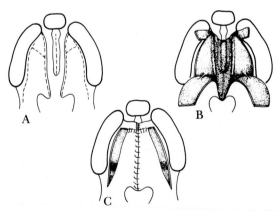

FIGURE 6-6. *Four-flap palatoplasty for bilateral complete cleft of primary and secondary palates. This operation was not used for any of the studies reported in this chapter. (A) The incision lines. It is frequently difficult to find very much mucoperiosteum for the anterior two flaps. (B) Dissection of the four mucoperiosteal flaps. Lateral soft palate release dissection, usually involving infracture of hamuli. Closure of nasal mucosa. (C) Closure of oral mucosa. The premaxilla has not been repositioned, and nothing has been done to the alveolar gap region at the time of lip closure, so complete anterior oral closure will be difficult.*

the intelligence of the patient, the presence of residual defects in the hard and soft palates, the size and shape of the velopharynx, the operating surgeon, and hearing loss (Table 6-1). No pharyngoplasty patients are included in this study. The operation was rarely done at that time. None of the patients in the initial study had the benefits of comprehensive follow-up and treatment by a "team."

In the second study, the patients were young at the time of assessment: median age 4 years. I believe that in preschool children, an experienced examiner can detect those speech defects that are likely to improve with maturation,

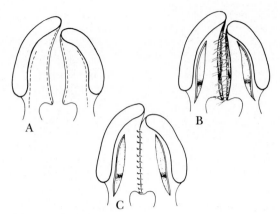

FIGURE 6-8. *Von Langenbeck (simple closure) palato-plasty for complete unilateral cleft lip–cleft palate. (A) The incision lines. (B) Mucoperiosteal flaps have been elevated, although they are not well shown in this diagram. The nasal mucosa is closed. In this anomaly, the nasal mucosa on the noncleft or medial side is continuous with the septum and vomer. More is available to manipulate. It was dealt with as described in Figure 6-7D. (C) Oral mucosa closure. Note it is impossible to obtain a two-layer closure of the alveolar portion of the cleft with this operation. Pushback is less. Lateral raw areas are smaller because the mucoperiosteum is not detached anteriorly.*

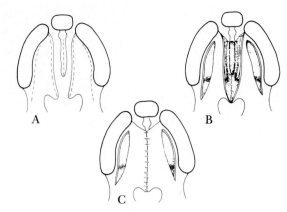

FIGURE 6-9. *Von Langenbeck (simple closure) palato-plasty for bilateral complete cleft lip–cleft palate. The configuration of this deformity varies tremendously, and line drawings can be misleading. (A) The incision lines. The inferior border of the vomer is incised and the mucous membrane is elevated from both sides of it. (B) Muco-periosteal flaps are elevated without anterior detachment, keeping the posterior palatine arteries intact. Extensive dissection is frequently necessary in the lateral release incision area for this anomaly. The cleft is usually wide, and there is usually considerable hypoplasia. The nasal mucosa is closed. Two suture lines are necessary anteriorly because of the two vomer flaps. (C) Oral mucosa closure. It is impossible to close the anterior portions of the cleft with this operation. The amount of palatal bone denuded is less, however.*

those that will respond to training, and those that will be permanent without further surgical procedures. The results in Table 6-2 are therefore a combination of the actual assessment at median age 4 years and the expected result at 8 to 10 years of age with speech maturation and speech therapy, but without revisionary surgery of any type.

Table 6-2 contains combined data from a combination of isolated cleft palate, complete unilateral cleft lip–cleft palate, and complete bilateral cleft lip–cleft palate patients repaired by one of two primary palate operations by one surgeon.

This study was designed primarily to compare two different palate operations: pushback and a simple-closure procedure. The finding (not shown in tabular form) was that the speech result would be essentially the same with the two procedures when the patients reached speech maturity at approximately 8 years of age. This study involved one operating surgeon only. No pharyngoplasties are involved in this

TABLE 6-1. *Speech Results (n = 612), Initial Study (1962) [4, 5]*

Speech	Number	Percent
Acceptable	419	68
Unacceptable	193	32

TABLE 6-2. *Speech Results (n = 111), Second Study (1969) [6]*

Speech	Number	Percent
Acceptable	91	82
Unacceptable	20	18

TABLE 6-3. *Speech Results* (n = *84*),
Third Study (1978) [8]

Speech	Number	Percent
Acceptable	58	84
Unacceptable	26	16

sample because they were not being done in the younger age group at that time.

The third study was much more controlled, but it was completed in a similar way (Table 6-3). Only isolated cleft palates were included (Figs. 6-1 and 6-7). It involved the surgery of two surgeons doing very similar procedures. Included in the unacceptable group are those patients (8 percent of the total) who were offered early secondary pharyngoplasty, this operation now being done more frequently and in a younger group.

This study involved two carefully matched samples derived from 296 isolated cleft palate patients who had isolated cleft palate repairs of either the pushback or the von Langenbeck method by two surgeons between 1963 and 1972. The pharyngoplasty rate for the 296 patients was 8 percent for the pushback group and 6 percent for the von Langenbeck group. These pharyngoplasty patients are included with the reviewed group in Table 6-3 because they must be considered to have "unacceptable" speech with respect to this primary operation.

The speech results for isolated cleft palate patients repaired by both the simple-closure and the pushback operation have been combined in Table 6-3 to make them as comparable as possible with the studies of Tables 6-1 and 6-2. The subjective speech results for the two operations were identical, although this is not shown in tabular form.

SPEECH SUMMARY

The speech results were relatively poor in the initial study for several reasons. The three speech studies are not strictly comparable. The initial study involved 612 consecutive patients with many variables, as summarized earlier.

This study, however, involved only one basic operation: a two-flap pushback procedure. The second study was designed to compare two cleft palate operations: a pushback and a simple closure. This second study involved the work of only one surgeon, but the other variables were essentially the same. The overall speech results were better in the second study: 82 percent acceptable speech versus 68 percent in the first study. The third study was again designed to compare the two cleft palate operations, but in this study, many variables were excluded to give a purer study sample, including restricting the study to isolated cleft palates. The speech results in the second and third studies were identical: 82 and 84 percent acceptable speakers, respectively. The second and third studies indicate that the speech results of the simple-closure and the pushback operation are the same.

ANATOMICAL CLOSURE—RESIDUAL DEFECTS OR FISTULAE

Most patients treated at The Hospital for Sick Children, Toronto, have had no attempt to close completely the anterior alveolar region of complete clefts of the primary and secondary palates at the time of primary lip or palate operation. All such gaps narrow spontaneously after, first, the lip surgery and, later, the palate surgery. Many abut and close completely or almost so. I have always considered it preferable to avoid extensive operating in the alveolar gap area.

The simple-closure palatoplasty (Figs. 6-7 through 6-9) does not offer the surgical satisfaction of closing the alveolar gap region. The two-flap pushback procedures (Figs. 6-1 through 6-3) likewise do not permit closure of this region unless combined with some other procedure, such as a vomerine flap. It is only the four-flap or related procedures which permit a direct anterior closure attempt (Figs. 6-4 through 6-6).

Complete closure is attempted to maximize the patient's comfort by preventing nasal escape of liquids, foods, and saliva and the oral

TABLE 6-4. *Incidence of Fistulae or Residual Defects* (n = 612), *Initial Study (1962)* [4, 5]

Site of Defect	Isolated Cleft Palate	Cleft Lip–Cleft Palate
Perialveolar	0	20%
Hard palate	0	11%
Soft palate	0	1%

escape of nasal secretions. Complete closure has a lesser, although significant, relationship to speech. The site of the fistula is important. Anterior fistulae, prealveolar, alveolar and postalveolar, affect speech less than the more posterior fistulae—those in the posterior two-thirds of the hard palate and the soft palate.

The incidence of fistulae or residual defects has been studied three times during the present generation at The Hospital for Sick Children. In the initial study, the incidence of fistulae was high at the front of the mouth, but rarely symptomatic. Fistulae farther back were less common but usually symptomatic (Table 6-4).

The second study was done to compare the simple-closure and pushback palatoplasties (Table 6-5). The incidence of perialveolar fistulae was high in the second study because only complete cleft lip and cleft palate patients were included and a considerable number were bilateral.

The comparative incidence of fistulae with the simple-closure and pushback procedures is shown in Table 6-6. Fistulae were slightly more frequent and somewhat larger in the patients repaired by simple-closure palatoplasty,

TABLE 6-5. *Incidence of Fistulae or Residual Defects* (n = 111), *Second Study (1969)* [6]

Site	Isolated Cleft Palate	Complete Cleft Lip–Cleft Palate
Perialveolar	0	31%
Hard palate	0	0
Soft palate	0	0

TABLE 6-6. *Incidence of Alveolar and Postalveolar Fistulae, Second Study* [6]

Cleft Palate Only	Simple Closure (n = 66), Complete Cleft Lip– Cleft Palate		Pushback (n = 45), Complete Cleft Lip– Cleft Palate	
	Unilateral	Bilateral	Unilateral	Bilateral
0	16%	23%	10%	21%

presumably because less collapse is produced by simple-closure methods. They were obviously more frequent in the bilateral complete cleft lip–cleft palate patients.

Summary

The incidence of fistulae was high at the front of the mouth in cleft lip–cleft palate patients. Few of these were symptomatic. Fistulae farther back were rare, but usually symptomatic. The incidence, and size, of fistulae was slightly greater with simple-closure methods when compared with pushback methods, but this difference was not enough to condemn the simple-closure methods. Fistulae in the posterior hard and soft palates should always be closed surgically. Fistulae at the front of the mouth should be closed by an interim removable plate or prosthesis and may be closed by a secondary operation when growth and orthodontia are complete, if the patient does not have to wear a removable plate bearing missing teeth.

MAXILLARY GROWTH AND DENTOALVEOLAR DEVELOPMENT

The degree to which cleft palate repair retards anteroposterior, lateral, and vertical growth of the maxilla is uncertain, although both the timing and the type of operation are important. A review by the orthodontic division of the Facial Treatment and Research Centre of The

Hospital for Sick Children, Toronto, revealed that maxillary arch contraction was much less in the patients of one particular surgeon, although the patients considered had essentially the same operations [7]. Moreover, this surgeon had produced "average collapse" in his first few years, but consistently less thereafter.

In a cleft of the maxillary complex, there is great variability in the amount of tissue present, in the relationship of the parts, and in the individual's growth potential. Moreover, there are equally important variations related to the surgical procedures.

Rapid changes occur in facial morphology following surgery. As mentioned, the degree to which cleft palate repair retards anteroposterior, lateral, and vertical maxillary growth is uncertain, although both the timing and the type of operation are important. The consensus is that the sequelae of surgical repair are the major causes of impaired maxillary growth and dentoalveolar deformities [7].

The patients in the first study all received a pushback operation. The incidence of maxillary and dentoalveolar deformities was noted to be high [4]. Data are not available to tabulate. My suspicions were raised about the possible harmful effects of surgery on lower facial bone and dental growth and development.

In the second study, the frequency of incisor crossbite in postoperative cleft lip–cleft palate patients was lower after the simpler von Langenbeck procedure than after the pushback. It is not shown in Table 6-7, but positive or normal incisors existed for 56 percent of the patients in the von Langenbeck series,

TABLE 6-7. *Comparison of Pushback and von Langenbeck Operations with Maxillary Growth and Dentoalveolar Development in Cleft Lip–Cleft Palate Patients, Second Study (1969) [6]*

Operation	Number of Cases	Buccal Segment Collapse (Percent)	Incisor Crossbite (Percent)
Pushback	71	62	50
von Langenbeck	17	12	44

TABLE 6-8. *Comparison of Pushback and von Langenbeck Operations with Crossbite Deformities in Isolated Cleft Palate Patients, Third Study (1978) [8]*

Operation	Number of Cases	Incidence of Crossbite* (Percent)
Pushback	43	56
von Langenbeck	21	19

*Chi-square, with Yates' modification, = 6.33 with 1 d.f., $p = 0.02$.

whereas this was found for only 24 percent of those in the pushback series, the remainder having an end-on relationship.

The frequency and degree of buccal segment collapse were found to be markedly less in the patients in the von Langenbeck group than in the pushback group [6].

The simpler the surgical technique, the less severe the maxillary and premaxillary deformities. These findings were for a young group of patients. However, findings and conclusions continue to be the same as these patients become older.

This aspect of cleft palate surgery was again reviewed in the third study, but for isolated cleft palate patients only (Table 6-8). Cleft lip–cleft palate patients were not included in this study. The incidence of individual tooth crossbite and buccal segment collapse was significantly higher in patients repaired by the pushback operation when compared with those repaired by the simple-closure operation. Only gross orthodontic deformities in the form of obvious crossbite were recorded. The larger raw areas left by the pushback operation, allowed to heal spontaneously, do so with scar epithelium. This must be related to the increase in the dentoalveolar deformities.

PHARYNGOPLASTY

Pharyngoplasty was carried out very infrequently during the period of the initial study, but with increasing frequency during the second and third study periods at The Hospital for Sick Children, Toronto. No frequency figures are available for the first two study periods, but pharyngoplasty was carried out on 8 percent of all cleft palate patients who had received prior treatment by primary palatoplasty in infancy during the period of the third study.

The first 96 pharyngoplasty patients treated at The Hospital for Sick Children, Toronto, during the periods of the first and (mostly) second studies were reported in 1970 [2]. The 96 patients had previous palate repair, unless they had submucous cleft palates. They all had an adequate trial of speech therapy. The average age of pharyngoplasty was 11 years, and patients were followed for periods up to 13 years from the operations. There were several operating surgeons.

Speech was rated on a five-point scale and, for this study, was converted to a percentage of normal (100 percent) figure for before- and after-pharyngoplasty comparison.

There were many variables in the sample studied. Those which proved less significant, although not always insignificant, were type of flap, cleft type, and age of operation. The significant variables in this study were type of speech defect, intelligence, hearing loss, emotional stability, age at pharyngoplasty, and experience of the surgeon.

It made no difference whether the flap was inferiorly or superiorly based or whether the flap ended up looking wide or narrow at follow-up. There was a poor correlation between preoperative type of cleft palate and the pharyngoplasty speech result. However, the type of cleft palate was more closely related to the type of speech defect, which in turn was closely related to the type of speech result following pharyngoplasty. The bilateral complete cleft lip–cleft palate patients tended to have the more serious type of speech defects, those which produced the worst results following pharyngoplasty.

Those patients who had their pharyngoplasty between 4 and 11 years of age tended to have better results than those operated on between 12 and 19 years of age, but this variable was not as strong as others.

TABLE 6-9. *Speech Improvement after Pharyngoplasty* (n = 96)

	Speech (Percent Normal)		Number of Patients
	Before	After	
Group 1: IQ 90+ No other variable*	48	98	35
Group 2: Low IQ No other variable	63	84	19
Group 3: IQ 90+ Other variables present	58	99	18
Group 4: Low IQ Other variables present	30	73	24

*Other variables include hearing loss of 20 dB or more in one or both ears and emotional instability.

Speech defects were divided into two main categories: pure nasal emission defects and the more complicated sound substitution defects. The nasal air emission group did better at all times. This was particularly true of the 20 percent who had spontaneous improvement noticeable within 10 days of pharyngoplasty.

A child with an intelligence quotient above 80, or preferably 90, is better able to discriminate between the speech sounds he or she hears and is more nearly able to reproduce them. Participation in speech therapy is always improved with a reduction of emotional and psychological problems. In addition, the data suggested that surgical experience was related to the end result.

In Table 6-9, the amount of improvement accomplished by pharyngoplasty is presented. To compact this table, nasal air emission and sound substitution defects have been combined. To delineate other variables, the patients have been divided into four groups.

Pharyngoplasty results, similar to primary palatoplasty, are related to many variables. The best results are produced in those patients with nasal air emission speech defects who have normal or better intelligence, no hearing loss, and are emotionally stable. The worst results were found in children who were substituting nonspeech sounds, whose intelligence was below 80, and who had a hearing loss.

The pushback operation with extensive lateral dissection and radical anterior mobilization of large mucoperiosteal flaps allows the soft palate to be lengthened, but leaves larger raw areas that must heal spontaneously with scar epithelium. The more limited dissection of the von Langenbeck operation permits only side-to-side closure with very little lengthening of the soft palate, and the raw areas are smaller.

It has naturally been assumed that the length of soft palate is important for velopharyngeal closure and that one may expect better velopharyngeal function with less nasal escape with the pushback closure. The findings of these studies indicate an unexplained discrepancy in this logic. The only difference between the two operations was the amount of dissection and detachment of tissue at the front of the mouth.

The end results of cleft palate patient management at The Hospital for Sick Children, Toronto, indicate that velopharyngeal function and speech are the same with both a pushback and a simple-closure palatoplasty. Maxillary growth disturbance, dentoalveolar deformity, and orthodontic deformity are less with the simple-closure (von Langenbeck) procedure.

References

1. Graber, T.M. Craniofacial morphology in cleft palate and cleft lip deformities. *Surg. Gynecol. Obstet.* 88:359, 1949.
2. Hamlen, M. Speech changes after pharyngeal flap surgery. *Plast. Reconstr. Surg.* 46:437, 1970.
3. LeMesurier, A.B. The operative treatment of cleft palate. *Am. J. Surg.* 39:458, 1938.
4. Lindsay, W.K. The Cleft Lip and Cleft Palate Research and Treatment Centre: A Five-Year Report, 1955–1959. Toronto: The Hospital for Sick Children, 1960.
5. Lindsay, W.K., LeMesurier, A.B., and Farmer, A.W. A study of the speech results of a large series of cleft palate patients. *Plast. Reconstr. Surg.* 29:273, 1962.
6. Palmer, C.R., Hamlen, M., Ross, R.B., and Lindsay, W. K. Cleft palate repair: Comparison of the results of two surgical techniques. *Can. J. Surg.* 12:32, 1969.
7. Ross, R.B., and Johnston, M.C. *Cleft Lip and Cleft Palate.* Baltimore: Williams & Wilkins, 1972. P. 159.
8. Witzel, M.A., Clarke, J.A., Lindsay, W.K., and Thomson, H.G. Comparison of results of pushback or von Langenbeck repair of isolated cleft of the hard and soft palate. *Plast. Reconstr. Surg.* 64:347, 1979.

Richard Stark

COMMENTS ON CHAPTER 6

THESE are monumental studies in the dimension of time from the Division of Plastic Surgery at the Hospital for Sick Children, Toronto. In actuality, they are the quintessence of an ongoing assay of cleft palate patients operated on as early as 1939. In all, there were three separate studies, from which one may, as has Dr. Lindsay, distill principles from data.

1. The subjective appraisal of speech by skilled speech pathologists and an external plastic surgeon bereft of patient bias by association is still one of the most meaningful methods of evaluation.
2. The earliest reliable age of speech evaluation is 4 (I would say 5).
3. Speech results are roughly equivalent for von Langenbeck and pushback palatoplasties (over 80 percent acceptable).
4. Dentoalveolar deformities are appreciably higher in pushback as opposed to von Langenbeck palatoplasties. Deformities consisted of incisor crossbite and buccal segmental collapse. Dr. Lindsay feels this is due to the large retroalveolar raw surfaces that must epithelialize.
5. More fistulae result from the simple side-to-side von Langenbeck closure. However, the reduction of fistulae in the pushback series may be the result of increased buccal segmental collapse in this group.
6. Dr. Lindsay rightfully states that anterior fistulae are rarely seriously symptomatic, while those in the velum or posterior part of the hard palate certainly may be, depending on size. He states, "I have always considered it preferable to avoid extensive operation in the alveolar gap area," to which I would agree with alacrity. The inordinate attention paid to the cleft alveolus during the past decade resulted, I feel, in overtreatment and overhospitalization of the patient.

Dr. Lindsay then discusses, in general terms, 96 patients subjected to secondary pharyngoplasties of the pharyngeal flap type. Here he says many things that coincide with the primary pharyngeal flap pharyngoplasties we have conducted at St. Luke's Hospital Center since 1955.

After pharyngoplasty, all patients (including those with a low IQ plus other problems) achieved at least 73 percent normal speech, while those with an IQ above 90 achieved 98 percent normal speech.

Although no mention is made in the discussion of primary palatoplasty (either pushback or von Langenbeck) of patient age at operation, in the secondary pharyngoplasty, Lindsay states that speech results are better in the younger group (ages 4 to 11) as opposed to those older (12 to 19). He also places importane for good speech results on the patient's IQ, the presence of hearing, the emotional stability of the patient, and the experience of the surgeon. I would agree with much of this.

For the past 24 years at St. Luke's Hospital Center, we have performed as a routine procedure for palatal clefts of all kinds, a von Langenbeck simple closure with the addition of a pharyngeal flap at the same operation. Our speech results in a continuing study have exceeded 90 percent normal speech. Results are consistently better if the operation is performed before the onset of speech. We prefer 1 year of age. Results are poorer in patients who are mentally retarded. Hearing loss at 1 year of age is usually due to serous otitis, which is ephemeral.

Contrary to Dr. Lindsay's finding that the experience of the surgeon is most important when performing a secondary pharyngoplasty in an older child whose scarred velum obscures part of the pharyngoplastic operation, our series of simple-closure palatoplasties cum primary pharyngeal flap has been performed largely with the preceding result by plastic surgical residents via unexcelled exposure of the pharynx through the open palatal cleft. This is a distinct advantage that primary pharyngeal flap has over the secondary pharyngoplasty operation.

I agree that it matters not whether the pharyngeal flap is based superiorly or inferiorly, nor how wide it remains in the dimension of time. Performed early, the flap-tethered velum tends to grow in length as the result of this traction force.

7 THE number of operations available for repair of a cleft of the palate is in itself an admission that no single one is ideal or universally acceptable. The choice and timing of the surgical intervention, therefore, can be said to depend in part on the operator's surgical philosophy and, indeed, on his or her own personality. The decision represents a summation of one's training, experience, clinical astuteness, and technical skill. It may be influenced also by the mutual respect and restraint existing among members of a coordinated interdisciplinary cleft palate team, who offer a breadth of knowledge and experience greater than that possessed by one person. The surgeon's natural desire to correct a congenital malformation early and thus to allay the anxieties of the parents must be tempered by wisdom based on the fund of knowledge derived from clinical and basic research, including retrospective studies.

A working familiarity with the various cleft palate operations gives the surgeon a number of options for different clinical situations and alternative techniques to be applied during the course of a palate repair. Decision making is an important part of a sophisticated service, but the suitability and long-term effects of a particular procedure are not always readily apparent at the outset. Many cleft palate repairs produce results that appear quite satisfactory during the early postoperative course. Unfortunately, however, some are accompanied by complications affecting growth and development, and related functions, and the full impact of these complications may not be evident for several years (Fig. 7-1).

Bone grafting of the alveolar process and hard palate during the first year of life illustrates this point well. When it was first proposed, early primary bone grafting to correct a deficiency and provide stability and contour appeared to be a good concept. The graft itself

Robert L. Harding

CLEFT PALATE

probably had no ill effects on growth and development. The widespread mobilization of mucoperiosteal flaps to cover the bone grafts did, however, have an undesirable effect on biological growth processes in many young patients. After this gradually became clinically evident, many of the surgeons who had had long experience with this surgical plan abandoned early primary bone grafting and became more selective in the timing of the operation.

Because of the concern about violating the oral mucoperiosteum, the members of our Cleft Palate Clinic did not accept early primary bone grafting as a logical procedure in a rapidly growing infant. We do not, therefore, have a long-term experience with that operative plant. A few surgeons in the United States still use early primary bone grafting, but the number of advocates is dwindling. During the past decade, the debate on bone grafting revolved about the matter of timing, not about the concept of the operation. There is a place for bone grafting in cleft palate surgery, but we believe it should be delayed until at least 12 years of age. An increase in the breadth of the maxillary ridge takes place at about 11 years. This growth change may be only 2 or 3 mm, but it would seem prudent to defer bone grafting until after all the important growth changes are complete and the teeth are in a normal occlusion for the patient. Any time thereafter, we will use autogenous iliac bone grafts as a fashioned block and/or cancellous chips for the late closure of alveolar and anterior palatal clefts, the stabilization of maxillary segments, the restoration of contour, and the repair of large palatal fistulae. This service is frequently designed to satisfy the requirements of the orthodontist. Lessons gained through experiences such as early bone grafting should serve as a guide in future surgical protocols.

Normal craniofacial growth follows an or-

derly and discernible pattern. It is a time-linked change with differential growth velocities along different planes. At birth, 60 percent of the facial breadth, 45 percent of the height, and 30 percent of the depth are complete. During the postnatal period, 70 percent of the growth takes place in the anteroposterior dimension or sagittal plane. Therefore, the sagittal plane becomes the one most affected by a midline growth failure, and the dental expansion and holding prostheses which are designed to correct deficiencies in width will be of little benefit in the anteroposterior plane.

The goal in cleft lip and palate surgery is the attainment of an aesthetic and functional reconstruction that will enhance the patient's ability to participate in society. Aesthetics cannot be divorced from growth, structural relations, and function, nor function from structural relations and aesthetics—all are interdependent. Patients with velopharyngeal insufficiency, or with deafness, or with structural malrelations or other deviations from a normal range lose something in aesthetic qualities. It is essential to keep these important interrelationships in mind during the planning and closing of a cleft of the palate. Growth is a multifactorial phenomenon with many variables and unanswered questions. We do not know the real stimulus to growth, but we are aware of many factors that can affect the basic genetic pattern, including surgical intervention. Ortiz-Monasterio et al. [26, 27] and other groups [30] have illustrated that normal midfacial development takes place when there is no treatment of a facial cleft (Fig. 7-2). In our society, surgical intervention is a social necessity, however, and that introduces variables into a complex system. The only thing that we, as surgeons, can decide is what operation to do and when to intervene.

Time tends to made a surgeon more conser-

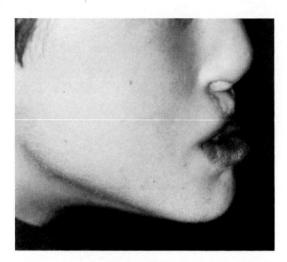

FIGURE 7-1. *Midface retrusion resulting from midline growth failure secondary to lip or palate surgery or both. Maxillary retrusion can be part of the genetic heritage and is made worse by surgical intervention and restrictive fibrous tissue. There was no tendency for midface retrusion in this patient's family.*

vative. A surgeon who is inquisitive enough to review the results of his or her surgical efforts will eventually find a way to alter or improve techniques to accomplish goals more easily. It will become obvious that surgery is a traumatic episode that stimulates a differential biological response. Retrospective studies and familiarity

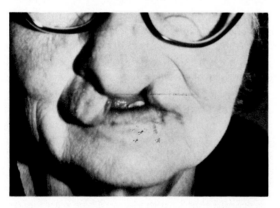

FIGURE 7-2. *A 65-year-old female with an unoperated cleft lip and cleft palate. There is normal development of the bony framework. (Reproduced, with permission, from H. K. Cooper et al.,* Cleft Palate and Cleft Lip. *Philadelphia: W. B. Saunders, 1979.)*

with the related biological information invariably has an effect on one's surgical protocol. There is presently available a body of knowledge which helps us make a judgment in our surgical approach to cleft palate habilitation.

Growth morphologists, supported by longitudinal data and several surgeons (Dingman [6], Rehrmann [29], Johanson [14], and others [28, 30]) through retrospective studies, have warned of the risk to growth and development of extensive surgery at an early age, particularly over the bony parts. This hazard was even recognized in the last century when Dieffenbach [4, 5] first introduced a "bone-flap operation" to avoid some of the structural malrelations that occurred following surgery. His surgical recommendation has been an accepted method of cleft palate repair by several surgeons [13] in the United States. Slaughter and Pruzansky [33] in this country and Schweckendiek [24] in Germany recommended primary closure of the velum with a delayed closure of the hard palate to preserve the integrity of the oral mucoperiosteum and the growth potential of the maxilla. In addition, one should be aware of the studies performed on primates by Kremenak [16–18], Atherton [1], and others, who have demonstrated that mucoperiosteum is one factor related to growth and the direction of bone modeling. It is apparent that growth is a gentle force that can be altered by an opposing force or restricted by scar tissue. It takes only a Simonart's band to retain a premaxilla in a good position. The form and function of craniofacial structures are related to the integrity of all related structures and systems, and the deformity or dysfunction of one structure will have repercussions in all related structures. This is a craniofacial biological concept.

These consensuses, as well as retrospective studies on our patients, have caused us to pursue a more conservative surgical protocol in primary cleft palate repairs performed at an early age. When possible, clefts of the palate have always been repaired in patients at approximately 1 year of age. I believe there is a functional advantage associated with early surgery on the palate, but the operative procedure must be so planned that it will interfere as little as possible with normal biological growth processes and thus avoid acquired malformations with their associated malfunctions. If it is logical to repair a nerve under magnification, and it is a fact that scar tissue will limit the gliding of a tendon, then it should also be logical to develop a surgical protocol that will limit restrictive scar tissue on young, growing palatal segments.

Cleft Palate Surgery

Most residents, after completing their formal training and finding themselves in a new and unsupervised medical environment, will and should use the techniques in which they have been trained and with which they are familiar. As they gain experience, they will probably try other operations or modifications. It is always stimulating to employ new methods or to alter one's technique, especially if it should lead to an improved result. As one acquires familiarity with a procedure, modifications become easier. Unfortunately, we are today witnessing a period in which residents and surgeons in private practice and academic centers are performing fewer and fewer operations for cleft lip and palate. This universal development is the result of the leveling off or even decrease in the number of patients born with a facial cleft and the increasing number of plastic surgeons interested in cleft surgery. When surgical opportunities decrease, so does technical competence. Until one gains more experience, therefore, the young surgeon establishing a practice would be wise to adhere to basic procedures. These are more likely to lead to a good result with fewer complications than some of the more sophisticated and extensive approaches.

It is unfortunate that the surgeon must wait until a patient's growth is essentially complete before it is possible to make a final evaluation of the effects of the surgical intervention for cleft lip and palate. An acquired deformity induced by a surgical procedure, however, may become evident before an individual's growth is complete. It is also difficult to compare on opera-

tion performed today with a similar approach carried out 15 or more years ago because of changes that have taken place in supporting and related fields and the continual flow of new information. For example, anesthetic agents and technology have improved such that the surgeon can work in a more relaxed manner. In addition, new and improved instruments and materials make it possible for the surgeon to perform operations more easily today than similar procedures 15 or 20 years ago. It therefore has become possible to devote more attention to fine technical details, which is a nice surgical dividend.

In evaluating the long-term results of surgery on the palate, most of this chapter is devoted to the operative procedures that we have used for several years in our clinic and which have gradually led to improved results. For approximately 15 years, we have been keeping accurate longitudinal data on our patients as a means of evaluating our surgical experience. A review of these data has persuaded us to alter our surgical protocol from time to time. Good clinical records and a periodic recall of patients with a cleft can lead to sound surgical impressions similar to those gained from the detailed data essential for investigative work.

It is not necessary to review the historical "forced compression" cleft palate procedure of Brophy because it has not been in general use for many years. It is one example of an operation that was abandoned following retrospective clinical reviews. Nevertheless, the surgeon should be aware of the risks to the facial structure associated with forced compression, because some methods recently proposed to reposition a protruding premaxilla have a compression effect, and others may be proposed in the future.

One of the common operations has been the von Langenbeck procedure [35] and it is still a basic method for cleft palate repair, even though it has declined in popularity for surgery performed at an early age. After employing his operation for many years, we finally abandoned it for clefts involving most of the hard palate. Many of the palates repaired by the von

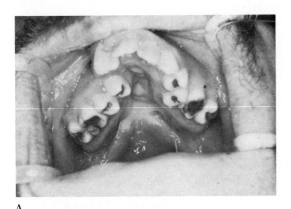

A

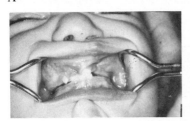
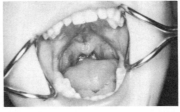
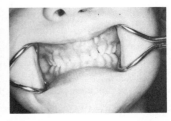

B

FIGURE 7-3. *(A) Apparently this palate was closed by the Von Langenbeck method, after which scar contracture created the maxillary arch and dental malrelations. This acquired deformity will require surgical intervention and orthodontia for correction. (B) This palate was repaired* *with sliding mucoperiosteal flaps similar to those of the von Langenbeck operation, but the closure of the alveolar cleft was deferred. The patient acquired a good structural and functional result through the period of eruption of the deciduous dentition, and this probably will persist.*

Langenbeck technique turned out well, but others did not. Some patients developed postoperative structural malrelations that did not lend themselves to orthodontic correction (Fig. 7-3 A and B). We were not able to determine with accuracy which patients would or would not develop scar contracture and structural deformities, and that may mean our selection of cases was not sophisticated enough. It appeared that those patients who had a wide cleft of the palate, and in whom mucoperiosteal flaps were lowered from the palatal vault to close the cleft, developed a greater deposition of fibrous tissue and a higher incidence of maxillary arch constriction. The extensive elevation of mucoperiosteal flaps followed by the proliferation of fibrous tissue may lead to contracture and a deleterious effect on growth and the direction of bone modeling, as demonstrated in primates and in retrospective human studies [6, 12, 20, 22, 23, 30]. The amount of fibrous tissue

formation and the extent of contracture following a cleft palate repair were not always directly related to the width of the cleft, because such tissue formation and contracture also occurred following the repair of narrow clefts. Scar tissue has a three-dimensional contracture, and on the palate the most obvious manifestation is the medial movement of posterior maxillary teeth by cicatricial orthodontia. This creates the so-called hour-glass deformity (Fig. 7-4A and B). In addition, scar tissue can lead to a false ankylosis in the region of the pterygoid plates or create a restrictive lip and retard the forward drift of the maxilla and reduce the length of the soft palate, which is already deficient. There may also be some effect on the vertical height. For these reasons, therefore, we no longer consider the von Langenbeck repair as a routinely desirable operative procedure for the closure of a cleft which involves the hard palate, as Dieffenbach [4] recognized in the last

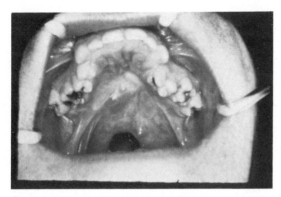

A

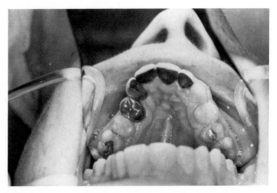

B

FIGURE 7-4. *(A) "Hourglass" deformity due to scar contracture following a cleft palate repair. Note raised scar extending across the hard palate at the level of the bicuspid teeth. Evidently this palate was closed by the von Langenbeck method. (B) An hourglass deformity producing a* *canine-shaped maxillary arch. Such acquired deformities are not readily apparent in the early postoperative period but only after months or years. This palate also was closed by the von Langenbeck method.*

century. When the cleft involves not more than one-third of the posterior hard palate, the oral mucoperiosteum adjacent to the cleft can be raised through a relaxation incision posterior to the tuberosity to permit closure along with the cleft of the soft palate. This will avoid extensive elevation of hard palate flaps, but still will not eliminate the risk of scar contracture. It is the sliding oral mucoperiosteal flaps that lead to scar contracture and structural malrelations in an unpredictable number of patients. When scar hypertrophy and contracture can be controlled medically, that important step in medical progress will be reflected in surgical philosophy.

The opinions we have developed to guide our surgical judgments are based on data that fall into several categories. First, we have longitudinal data on about 400 patients varying in age up to approximately 15 years. Second, for a larger number of patients, the hard and soft data are incomplete, but it is available for limited studies. And for many other patients, we have only a clinical evaluation with no hard data. There are many patients in this later category that had operative procedures we no longer employ, and some were done by us and some by other surgeons. We have also given weight to our judgment from information on biological growth processes, including research

on primates [16–18], and retrospective studies of our own, as well as those of other professionals as reported in the literature [12, 20, 22, 23, 30].

The cleft palate operations we were performing about 15 years ago were considered to be conservative and included many of the popular procedures of the day. Our protocol has been revised from time to time based on our experiences, but the original list on which we have pure data includes the following:

1. Cleft of the soft palate only:
   a. The soft palate was repaired at 12 months of age.
   b. The soft palate was closed in three layers.
   c. About one-half the patients had a two-flap lengthening or pushback operation based on the V-Y principle similar to the Veau-Wardill-Kilner palatal flaps.
2. Clefts of the hard and soft palate only:
   a. The median cleft of the hard palate was closed at 12 months of age, with a bilateral vomer flap when feasible.
   b. The hard palate was closed with sliding mucoperiosteal flaps in another group of patients. This method, which was based on the von Langenbeck repair, was later abandoned.
   c. A primary veloplasty was performed at

12 months of age in a group of patients in whom a vomer flap was not feasible, and the repair of the hard palate was deferred until there was less risk of structural impairment. This plan was started later in the longitudinal study program.

3. Clefts of the lip and palate:
   a. At 12 months, the hard palate was closed with a unilateral or bilateral vomer flap which extended anteriorly only to the incisive foramen. This was not feasible in all patients.
   b. At 16 months, the soft palate was then repaired by a three-layer closure.
   c. Half the patients had an associated two-flap pushback procedure in conjunction with repair of the soft palate.
   d. The vomer flap, soft palate repair, and two-flap lengthening procedure were all carried out in a single operation in a few instances.
   e. Sliding mucoperiosteal flaps were used to close the hard palate when the vomer flap was not feasible. This operation was later abandoned.
   f. A primary veloplasty was introduced later in the longitudinal program instead of sliding mucoperiosteal flaps when a vomer flap was not feasible. Repair of the hard palate was then deferred.

4. Primary veloplasty:
   a. At 12 months, a primary veloplasty was done in a group of patients in addition to those in whom a vomer flap was not technically feasible.

Preoperative maxillary orthopedic appliances are advocated by some clinicians prior to or in conjunction with cleft lip and palate surgery. It is true that such prostheses can improve the relationship of structures that are free to move, and the new position may be retained with a holding prosthesis. We have gradually given up nearly all preoperative maxillary orthopedic appliances. We have learned that the arch and segmental relationships will undergo favorable change through the influence of growth and the eruption of the deciduous dentition, pro-

vided the repaired lip is not restrictive and the maxillary arches or segments are not "locked in" as a result of surgical intervention (Figs. 7-5 and 7-6). A retrospective study of our cleft lip and palate patients who were not treated with a preoperative maxillary orthopedic appliance revealed that when the lip was supple and the alveolar cleft had been left open to be repaired at a later age, and there had been minimal or no violation of the oral mucoperiosteum, 89 percent had no crossbite, or one limited to the canines, or a buccal crossbite (Fig. 7-7). Such limited crossbites can usually be corrected with an expansion prosthesis by 4 or 5 years of age, provided the maxillary segments are not restricted by scar tissue.

REPAIR OF CLEFTS OF THE SOFT
PALATE ONLY

The cleft involvement of the soft palate was described as being minimal, one-third, two-thirds, or complete. The width of the cleft, tissue deficiency, neuromuscular function, and other pertinent observations were recorded. All reparable clefts of the soft palate were closed in three layers (Fig. 7-8 A and B). An incision was made first along the margins of the cleft to permit the oral and nasal mucosa to retract and to create a raw surface without the sacrifice of any tissue. A modified S-shaped relaxing incision was then made which extended medially around the tuberosity to the posterior border of the hard palate. The hamular process was frequently finger fractured when the soft palate flaps were being mobilized for approximation at the midline. But this fracture was carried out only when necessary to assist in relaxation of the palatal flaps. There is no anatomical reason to expect the fracture of the hamular process of the pterygoid plate to have any ill effect on eustachian tube function, and this proved to be true in clinical studies. About half the patients had a two-flap, V-Y lengthening operation in conjunction with the soft palate closure. In all clefts involving two-thirds or more of the soft palate, the levator muscle was detached from the posterior border of the hard palate. Ana-

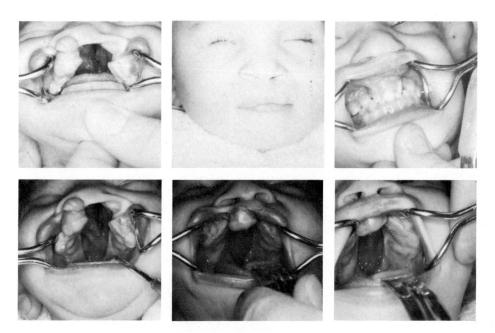

FIGURE 7-5. *Satisfactory maxillary segmental relations enhanced by not "locking in" the alveolar ridges surgically at an early age. This encourages molding and dentoalveolar adaptation under the influence of a supple lip matrix and biological growth processes.*

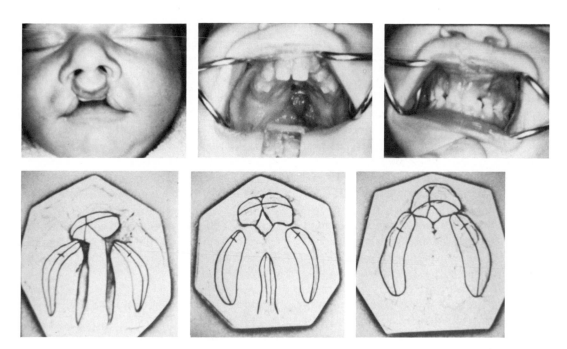

FIGURE 7-6. *A supple lip, a nonrestrictive palate, and a delayed repair of the alveolar clefts have encouraged dentoalveolar adaptation and a satisfactory arch alignment for this patient. There is a crossbite limited to the maxillary left cuspid tooth. The patient had a two-staged palatal repair without an associated pushback procedure. (Photocopies of casts from Lancaster Cleft Palate Clinic.)*

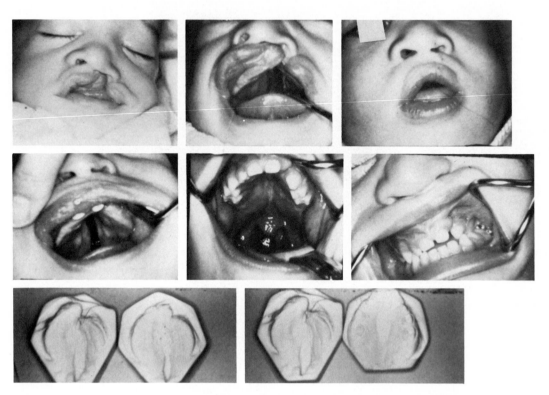

FIGURE 7-7. *Following a unilateral cleft lip repair, this baby had a supple lip and narrowing of the palatal cleft. A two-staged palatal repair with a two-flap pushback was* *carried out with a delay of the alveolar cleft. The patient has a left buccal crossbite which is easily correctable by orthodontia because the segment is not restricted.*

tomically, in the absence of a cleft, the levator muscles of the soft palate are not attached to the posterior border of the hard palate. The muscle layer was well approximated in each cleft repair, but the levator muscles were dissected and realigned only in some of the patients. We could not determine any particular advantage among those patients who had realignment of the levator muscles compared with those in whom the muscles were detached and simply well approximated. In both instances, the palate seemed to function well so far as elevation and traction were concerned. We did not determine if any gain in length of the palate was realized by realignment of the levator sling. However, we did do a retrospective study on the increase in length of the soft palate in those patients who eventually needed a pharyngeal flap, and we compared them to a group that did not require a pharyngeal flap.

We found little difference in the velocity of growth in length among both groups of patients up to 3 years of age who had had a repair of the palate without an associated pushback operation. After the age of 3, there was a decreased velocity of growth in the length of the palate among those patients who eventually developed a velopharyngeal incompetence. The reason for this decreased rate, which appeared over a year following the repair, could not be determined.

REPAIR OF CLEFTS OF THE HARD AND SOFT PALATE ONLY

Clefts of the palate can be designated as involving one-third, two-thirds, or the complete soft palate and one-third, two-thirds, or the complete hard palate, and the complete cleft terminates anteriorly at the incisive foramen.

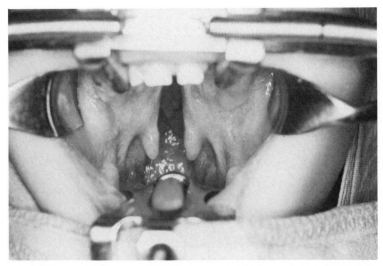

A

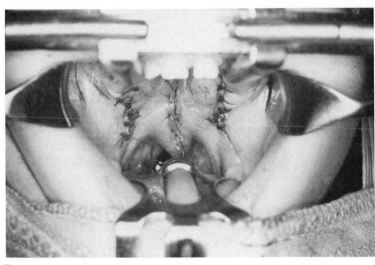

B

FIGURE 7-8. *(A) A preoperative cleft of the soft palate. (B) Repair of the cleft of the soft palate without an associated Veau-Wardill-Kilner two-flap retropositioning oper-* *ation. The levator muscles of the soft palate were detached from the posterior border of the hard palate, and the soft palate was repaired in three layers.*

Clefts that involve the alveolar process are considered with the lip embryologically, but from a practical point of view, they are considered part of the cleft of the palate. When possible, the cleft of the hard palate was closed with a bilateral vomer turnover flap. This would convert the complete cleft into a cleft of the soft palate only, which would then be repaired 4 months later. The majority of clefts involving the soft

and hard palates do not lend themselves to a vomer flap repair of the hard palate because either the cleft is too wide or the nasal septum is well above the palatal shelves. In one group of patients in whom the vomer flap was not a suitable procedure, we elected to close the hard palate with sliding mucoperiosteal flaps of the von Langenbeck type and to close the soft palate 4 months later (Fig. 7-9). An attempt was

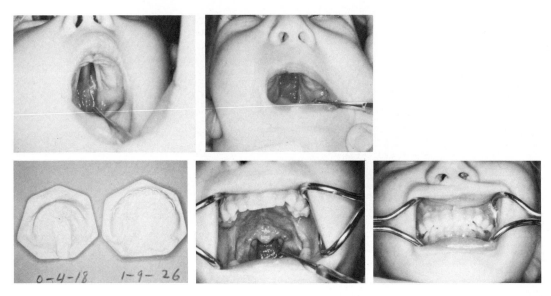

FIGURE 7-9. *A complete cleft palate repaired in two stages. The hard palate was closed with sliding mucoperiosteal flaps of the von Langenbeck type. The soft palate was closed 4 months later without an associated pushback procedure. This patient has a good palate with no cicatricial orthodontic deformity, and it is unlikely that any unfavorable structural alignment will develop.*

made to retain some of the attachments at the posterior border of the hard palate to resist shortening of the soft palate secondary to postoperative contracture in the hard palate. However, contracture also takes place in other directions. Even though we may have preserved some length with this two-staged operation, we observed that in some patients we produced dentoalveolar malrelations through cicatricial orthodontia. Because of the risk of structural malrelations associated with the sliding mucoperiosteal flaps, this method of closing the hard palate was gradually abandoned. Our interest was then turned toward a primary repair of the velum with a delay in the repair of the hard palate. This approach will be discussed in the section on primary veloplasty.

REPAIR OF CLEFTS OF THE LIP AND PALATE

In accordance with our protocol, a cleft of the palate associated with a cleft of the lip, whether unilateral or bilateral, was repaired in two stages. These palates can easily be closed in a single operation, but we adopted the two-staged approach in the hope of reducing structural malrelations to a minimum. Many clefts involving both the lip and palate are amenable to a vomer flap repair of the hard palate. This was usually carried out at 1 year of age, and the vomer flap was extended anteriorly only to the incisive foramen. The vomer flap was raised and then turned over and placed beneath the margin of the oral mucoperiosteum. In this way, there was minimal violation of the integrity of the oral mucoperiosteum (Fig. 7-10 A and B).

Four months following the vomer flap palatoplasty, the soft palate was repaired with the usual three-layered closure following detachment of the levator muscles from the posterior border of the hard palate. Some of the patients had a combined two-flap pushback procedure of the Veau-Wardill-Kilner type associated with the soft palate repair. For a small group of patients, the vomer flap, the soft palate repair, and the two-flap lengthening procedure were combined into a single operation for comparative studies. The posterior palatal

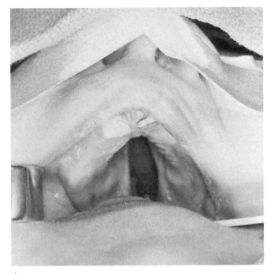

A

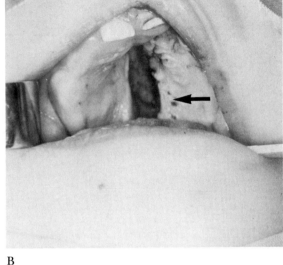

B

FIGURE 7-10. *(A) A cleft palate suitable for repair of the hard palate by a vomer flap that will extend anteriorly only to the incisive foramen. The alveolar cleft is left open to encourage dentoalveolar adaptation. (B) Vomer flap turned over beneath the edge of the left palatal mucoperiosteum. The cleft of the hard palate will then close by second intention. Even this comparatively simple palate operation is associated with a lag in the growth curve for 6 months, and this is followed by a period of recovery, so the curve approximates the normal in 1 year. Following some extensive operations, recovery may not be complete.*

neurovascular bundle was preserved, and length was gained in the two-flap pushback by stretching the bundle out of its canal, then dissecting it from the undersurface of the mucoperiosteal flaps, and finally removing the posterior bony rim of the posterior palatal foramen on each side. The raw nasal surface created by the retropositioning operation was covered with posterior nasal mucosa as described by Cronin [3] in some of the patients. In other patients it was left raw to heal by second intention. It was our impression that the patients gained very little by lining the nasal surface, but this cannot be scientifically validated from our data. Of the patients who had their palate procedures performed in a single operation, some turned out well and others developed structural malformations. The elevation and retropositioning of the mucoperiosteal flaps with subsequent scar contracture seemed to be the factor that caused the structural malformations.

THE PRIMARY VELOPLASTY

Our surgical protocol has changed with time. Out of respect for the integrity of the oral mucoperiosteum, we gradually adopted the primary veloplasty for some cases in which the vomer flap repair of the hard palate was not technically suitable. Restoration of the posterior soft palate matrix enhanced the narrowing of the cleft of the hard palate if there was an associated cleft of the lip and alveolar process. The molding is similar to that following a lip repair. The cleft may narrow to the point where the palatal shelves are in close proximity. Then the hard palate cleft can be repaired by raising the edges of the oral mucoperiosteum and suturing the flaps together (Fig. 7-11). This requires very little elevation of the mucoperiosteum. If the alveolar ridge is intact, the primary repair of the soft palate will have less effect on the width of the hard palate cleft. Some narrowing may take place through growth of the palatal shelves, but there is also an increasing width of the arch

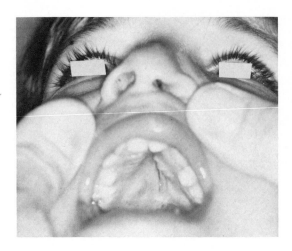

FIGURE 7-11. *Reduction in width of the hard palate cleft following a primary veloplasty. The patient had a cleft of the lip, alveolar process, and palate.*

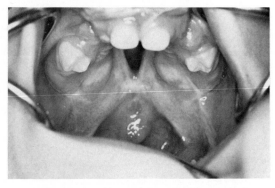

FIGURE 7-13. *A primary veloplasty with a persistent large anterior fistula or hard palate cleft and a deficient soft palate with velopharyngeal incompetence. This patient cannot acquire oral-nasal balance and acceptable speech without additional physical restoration. The goal must be socially acceptable speech and structural relations that will enhance facial balance.*

which may affect cleft width. As soon as the patient is cooperative, a dental prosthesis can be used to cover the cleft of the hard palate until a decision is made concerning repair of the cleft. The repair of the hard palate is usually delayed until 6 years of age or even older, depending largely on the width of the cleft. Occasionally a cleft is wide enough to consider a permanent prosthesis (Fig. 7-12). One disadvantage with a primary repair of the velum is that there is

some sacrifice in length of the soft palate, and this is particularly evident in the wider cleft (Fig. 7-13). This contributes to velopharyngeal incompetence, which together with the anterior palatal cleft leads to a deficient quality of speech. The primary repair of the velum is a good operation, but not for all cleft palates. The surgeon must use surgical judgment in selecting an operative plan for repair of a cleft of the palate. Whatever the plan, the goal is ac-

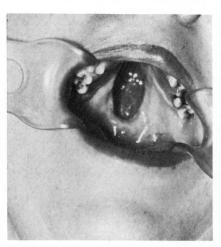
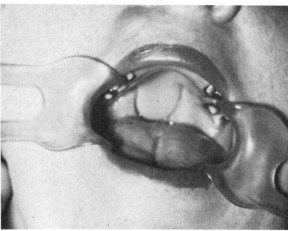

FIGURE 7-12. *A persistent wide cleft of the hard palate following a primary veloplasty. This was closed with a prosthesis, after which the patient was in oral-nasal balance. (Prosthesis by William Harkins, D.D.S.)*

ceptable speech and normal structural relations. A primary veloplasty is a good operation for the average complete cleft of the lip and palate because of the tendency for the hard palate cleft to narrow substantially. The patient may then be able to build up a fairly good oral pressure, provided there is velopharyngeal competence, with little risk of structural impairment. The hard palate cleft repair can then be delayed.

Results and Discussion

Our surgical philosophy, like that of most surgeons, has undergone continual change based on our past experience and a review of our data. We feel there is both a structural and functional advantage to be gained with early restoration of a facial cleft, particularly the soft tissue matrices. The type and timing of all operative procedures should be planned so as to interfere as little as possible with biological growth processes in an infant. It has already been stated that our experience has taught us to respect the integrity of the oral mucoperiosteum and the hazards associated with fibrosis and scar contracture, particularly over the bony parts. A tight, scarred lip, as well as scar tissue in the region of the pterygoid plates, and a primary pharyngeal flap can limit the normal forward drift of the maxilla (see Fig. 7-1). Scar contracture in the palate may dislocate teeth and the alveolar process or limit expansion in all directions. Unfortunately, one cannot predict with accuracy which patients will develop a scar contracture that will create structural malrelations. We have substantially reduced the incidence of structural malrelations with our present surgical plan, in which we strive to obtain a supple lip that will gently mold the underlying maxillary segments. We further strive to limit the surgery on the hard palate to a vomer flap that extends anteriorly only to the incisive foramen when the repair is performed at an early age. Whenever a vomer flap is not feasible, we will consider a primary veloplasty, particularly for the patient with a complete cleft of the lip and palate, and we will then delay the

repair of the hard palate. When neither a vomer flap nor primary repair of the velum seems appropriate, we may consider a delay of the palate repair for 5 or 6 years. At that time, considerable development has taken place, reducing but not eliminating the risk of structural deformation following surgical intervention. A temporary prosthesis can be used during the delay, and these have been worn as early as 3 years of age. We gradually curtailed the sliding mucoperiosteal flaps of the von Langenbeck type and those operations which transfer oral mucoperiosteum and leave denuded bone to heal by second intention. This includes island flaps and the two-flap pushback procedure. In addition to the risk of scar contracture following an island flap transfer, there is loss of suppleness and mobility of the soft palate, which affects velopharyngeal competence. Skoog [32] modified the two-flap pushback operation and transposed bilateral buccal flaps raised lateral to the tuberosity and alveolar ridge to cover the raw donor areas of the mucoperiosteal flaps. He believed that this aided healing and reduced the amount of scar tissue. This technology may have merit, but I do not have enough experience with it to comment. We have become more selective in our use of the two-flap pushback and still use it occasionally to help close the wider clefts and those with a substantial deficiency of the soft palate. The advantage to be gained must be balanced against the risk encountered from raising oral mucoperiosteal flaps. The decision making might best be made in an interdisciplinary conference where all facts and modalities can be weighed. Undoubtedly, many patients have had sliding mucoperiosteal flaps and pushback operations with good results. Nevertheless, structural malrelations do occur, and they are not always predictable. Some are difficult to treat and costly in terms of time and money.

In our experience, the pushback or lengthening type of operation, particularly the two-flap design which we generally used, has not contributed substantially to our functional results. Speech is one measure of function and is one indication of a satisfactory cleft palate repair. In a group of our patients who had two-staged palate repairs with the hard palate closed by a vomer flap at 1 year of age and the soft palate 4 months later without an associated pushback operation, an analysis revealed that 73 to 76 percent have acceptable speech. The range in percentages arises from the fact that some patients did not always perform at the same level on successive visits. Those who did not probably had a borderline velopharyngeal competence. Since this percentage is about the same as the national average of acceptable speech following palatal repair, we did not feel that retropositioning procedures would contribute that much more to our results and might add to the risk of structural impairment.

We do not ordinarily use a primary pharyngeal flap in conjunction with a soft palate repair. An exception to this opinion is the patient with a wide cleft of the soft palate that requires additional tissue to facilitate a repair. In this situation, the pharyngeal flap will compensate for a deficiency in the length of the soft palate and enhance velopharyngeal competence. A pharyngeal flap is not a normal anatomical structure, and about 75 percent of the patients will not need a pharyngeal flap because they will not develop velopharyngeal incompetence following the usual cleft palate repair. Our other objection to the routine use of a primary pharyngeal flap at an early age is the risk of interfering with the forward positioning of the maxilla. In general, we elected to use superior-based pharyngeal flaps as a secondary procedure for the surgical management of velopharyngeal incompetence. The pharyngeal flap is a good rehabilitative operation when used secondarily, and the interference with the forward drift of the maxilla is then measured in a very few millimeters, which alone does not impair facial balance. Usually we do the pharyngeal flap operation at between 3½ and 6 years of age. If the velopharyngeal gap is large at 3 or 3½ years of age with signs suggesting velopharyngeal incompetence, and if the speech scientist believes that there may be little to be gained from therapy, the pharyngeal flap operation is not delayed any longer. For other patients, a decision is made at no later than 4 years of age on the need for a pharyngeal flap. This decision again is based on the size of the velopharyngeal gap and other factors such as hypernasality, facial grimaces, the presence of glottal stops, and poor articulation. There is another group of postoperative cleft palate patients who will demonstrate a gradual improvement in oral-nasal balance with intelligible speech and a decreasing nasality up to 5½ to 6 years of age. If we perceive this improvement taking place, we delay the pharyngeal flap operation until that age when the need for a pharyngeal flap can be substantiated. Many in this group will so improve that a flap will be unnecessary. An investigative study on our pharyngeal flap patients revealed no ill effect on hearing sensitivity and no particular auditory disadvantage compared with controls. We were also unable to determine any alteration in the bony architecture as a result of performing the flaps as a secondary procedure.

All surgery on the palate is a traumatic episode, and some procedures are more injurious than others. There is no such thing as elevating the oral mucoperiosteum in an atraumatic fashion. It is only a matter of degree. We observed a lag in the growth curve following all surgery on the palate, including a procedure as comparatively simple as a vomer flap carried forward only to the incisive foramen. This lag lasted approximately 6 months, after which there was an accelerated rate of growth such that the curve approximated the normal in about 1 year. In some of the more extensive operations, recovery was not complete.

At one period of time in our surgical management, we routinely closed the cleft in the alveolar ridge along with the vomer flap. We were aware that these patients develop fibrous tissue in the alveolar cleft and that occasionally bone is formed. We then decided there might be some advantage in not "locking in" the alveolar ridges at an early age so that the segments would be free to undergo molding and dentoalveolar adaptation under the influence of a restored lip matrix and biological growth processes (see Figs. 7-5 through 7-7). Therefore, we decided to carry the vomer flap anteriorly only to the incisive foramen. The closure of the lip has a significant effect on the reduction of the alveolar and palatal cleft and on maxillary segmental relationships and positioning. Since we have deferred closure of the alveolar cleft, we have observed the development of a more favorable relationship between the maxillary segments during the early stages of arch development. We noted that the segmental relationships began to change prior to 3 years of age, and improvement continued through the period of eruption of the deciduous dentition. Many patients with a unilateral or bilateral cleft lip and palate will develop an end-to-end arch relationship (Figs. 7-3B, 7-5 through 7-7). This will frequently take place without the aid of maxillary orthopedic appliances. With freedom of the maxillary segments and the absence of a heavily scarred palate, the orthodontist will find it much easier to correct any crossbite that develops. Skoog [32] indicated that he had satisfactory structural relations on a 5-year follow-up evaluation of patients who had a primary periosteoplasty. He also recognized that one must wait until the postpuberal stage to make a final assessment.

Few of our patients complained about leakage of liquids into the nose at the site of the unrepaired alveolar cleft, particularly after the palate was closed and the segments assumed a reasonably good relationship. A substantial part of maxillary growth has taken place by 6 years of age, so that closure of the alveolar process could be considered at that time if structural relations are satisfactory. At approximately 11 years of age, there is an increase of about 2.5 mm in the width of the maxillary arch. Because of this late growth change, we prefer to delay repair of the alveolar cleft for most patients until the twelfth year.

We have routinely resisted early primary bone grafting in the alveolar ridge and palate, as previously mentioned. But the concept of a bone graft at a later age is good, and we frequently use bone in conjunction with a delayed alveolar cleft repair to provide stability and contour. We also find bone grafts very helpful

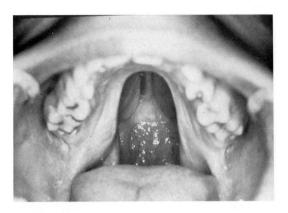

FIGURE 7-14. *A "horseshoe" type cleft palate with inadequate soft tissue available for a repair.*

in closing large palatal fistulae in the hard palate. The majority of surgeons would now agree with the delayed timing of bone grafts in cleft surgery, but that would not have been true in the 1960s.

We have not studied a group of patients who had a restoration of the levator sling compared with a group in whom the levator muscles of the soft palate were separated from the posterior border of the hard palate and merely well approximated. The levator muscles are routinely detached from the posterior border of the hard palate in all clefts involving more than two-thirds of the soft palate. Elevation and traction of the velum apparently seems to be good in either case, provided the muscle layers are well approximated.

Some clefts, such as a horseshoe cleft, are just too wide to permit a reasonable surgical repair (Fig. 7-14). We feel that these patients are best treated with a speech-aid prosthesis. We do not believe that a cutaneous, skin-covered pedicle flap is a logical means of restoring these wide clefts (Fig. 7-15). The skin-lined flap does not contribute ciliated epithelium or a mucous blanket to the nasal surface. Instead, sebaceous material accumulates on the superior surface creating a foul odor. This becomes an objectionable social problem which is impossible to correct by nasal irrigations. Skin on the oral surface is not associated with this problem because it is mechanically cleansed. The problem

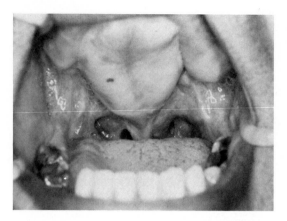

FIGURE 7-15. *A skin flap with a skin lining on both the oral and nasal surfaces used to repair an extensive palatal cleft. Part of the skin flap was used as a pharyngeal flap. The patient has an edentulous maxilla. A skin flap is not a wise choice in this situation.*

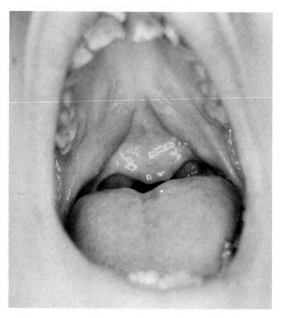

FIGURE 7-16. *Submucous cleft palate with a submucosal nonunion of the soft palate muscles, a palpable notch in the posterior border of the hard palate, and usually a small and/or partially cleft uvula. Patient is saying "ah" to demonstrate the notch in the posterior hard palate.*

arises only when there is full thickness skin on the nasal surface. We have found it necessary to take down some of these skin-lined pedicle flaps in order to eliminate the constant foul odor. These flaps are only an adynamic mass of tissue which requires an associated pharyngeal flap in order to develop any velopharyngeal competence.

SUBMUCOUS CLEFT PALATE AND CONGENITAL VELOPHARYNGEAL INCOMPETENCE

Submucous cleft palate and congenital velopharyngeal incompetence in the absence of a submucous cleft are now quite common diagnoses. At one time they were considered to be relatively rare. It is not definite whether these deformities are actually more common today or whether there is just an increasing awareness of these malformations. The presence of a submucous cleft palate is not an indication for an operation (Fig. 7-16). We have learned that some of these patients will develop good quality speech without surgical intervention. They should have a sophisticated speech evaluation and appropriate therapy before they are operated on. The surgical correction of velopharyngeal incompetence is directed toward the reduction in the size of the velopharyngeal port. Simply restoring soft palatal muscle con-

tinuity in a submucous cleft palate is inadequate. Palatal lengthening operations as an isolated procedure have also been disappointing. For many years we have used the superior-based pharyngeal flap exclusively, which has given our patients a good service. Other surgeons have different preferences for the management of velopharyngeal incompetence. If there is evidence of limited mobility or fatigability, we will frequently use a palatal lift prosthesis for several months. This may help to improve muscle function such that an operation may be unnecessary, or it may enhance the level of velopharyngeal competence along with the pharyngeal flap.

Congenital velopharyngeal incompetence occurs in the absence of a submucous cleft palate and is another diagnosis being made with increasing frequency (Fig. 7-17). The diagnosis is most often made after removal of the tonsils and adenoids. There is no submucosal separation of soft palate musculature and no palpable notch in the posterior border of the hard palate. There is a discrepancy in the relative size

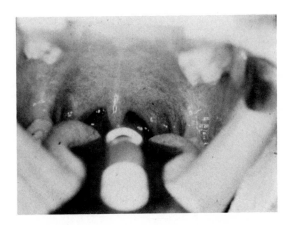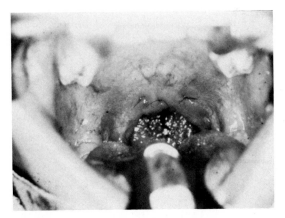

FIGURE 7-17. *Congenital velopharyngeal incompetence without the physical findings associated with the submucous cleft palate. Velopharyngeal competence was acquired with a superior-based pharyngeal flap and an opposing rectangular nasal palatal flap based posteriorly.*

or function of the soft palate and pharynx, and the patient is not in oral-nasal balance. The palate may be normal and the pharynx large, or the pharynx normal and the palate short. Or there may be a neuromuscular deficit. If velopharyngeal incompetence persists after a trial on speech therapy, the patients are treated in the same manner as those with a submucous cleft palate. With experience and a good clinical evaluation, candidates for surgical intervention can be identified before a prolonged course in speech therapy is undertaken.

Late Complications

The two most common prolonged and late complications following cleft palate surgery are the persistence of rhinolalia aperta or cleft palate–type speech and acquired structural malrelations. We have reduced the incidence of structural malrelations on our service by respecting the integrity of the oral mucoperiosteum at an early age and planning a surgical program that in our experience is associated with the least risk of scar contracture and structural impairment. If hypernasal speech persists, then attention must be directed toward the velopharyngeal incompetence. Sur-

gical preferences vary considerably in the management of velopharyngeal incompetence. Our own preference for many years has been to use the superior-based pharyngeal flap, together with a rectangular nasal palatal flap, to reduce the size of the velopharyngeal gap, provided muscle function is good. The two flaps are sutured together to essentially create a closed wound.

Arch malrelations vary most often in accordance with the breadth or width dimension. Anteroposterior or depth dimension can be affected, whereby the patient may have a midface retrusion and a false mandibular prognathism with a Class III malocclusion (see Fig. 7-1). A patient may have a genetic tendency for such a retrusion, and this may be accentuated by surgery. Many of these malformations cannot be managed by orthodontia alone, and the best planning is an interdisciplinary setting. Some patients will need combined surgery and orthodontia. Others will require a high degree of planning and technology with facial osteotomies, structural realignment and bone grafts, and additional aesthetic and dental procedures to acquire a maximum benefit. Many of these malformations are most difficult to treat and more costly in terms of time and money than the initial malformation. The consumer is becoming more knowledgeable and raises more questions about surgically induced malrelations. The dissatisfied patient tends to wander from clinic to clinic and is frequently lost to follow-up. We still like to repair palates at an early age, but we believe that we have reduced our number of acquired deformities by pursuing a conservative surgical protocol with respect for biological growth processes.

Final Thoughts

The best way to provide service to a cleft palate patient is through the concerted effort of an interdisciplinary team in which mutual respect and restraint prevails. Although it is not an easy task, it is essential to maintain good records so that one's surgical experience can be reviewed from time to time and the surgical protocol altered accordingly. The key words in cleft palate surgery are *type* and *timing*. Through a review of our own patients, we have learned that the type and timing of surgical intervention are critical to the reconstructive program. In a surgical challenge as complicated as cleft lip and palate, it is unlikely that there will ever be a single, universal operative plan. Surgeons will disagree, and this is healthy.

It was a critical review of a large group of our patients that stimulated us to adopt a conservative surgical protocol, particularly when surgical intervention is performed at an early age. There is no single surgical plan that can claim to be conservative. Our surgical philosophy developed not only through a retrospective study of our patients, but from knowledge available on biological growth processes, wound healing, and the effects of scar contracture on young, actively growing structures. We were also influenced by clinical research and retrospective studies that have become generally available information. Some knowledge of medical history and the experience of former surgeons will help to prevent the repetition of mistakes. We have tried many cleft palate procedures, but our experience has persuaded us to curtail most of the operations that extensively violate the integrity of the oral mucoperiosteum at an early age. These include the von Langenbeck repair, retropositioning operations, and island flaps. Not that these operative proposals are bad, but again the issue is a matter of type and timing. The quality of speech is one important

guideline in the successful management of a cleft of the palate. Our present surgical protocol can be summarized as follows:

1. Repair the lip when the infant weighs 10 pounds. Preserve tissue and develop a supple, nonrestrictive lip.
2. Start palate repair at 1 year. For a cleft of the soft palate, do a three-layer closure without a two-flap lengthening. For a complete cleft palate, repair the hard palate with a vomer flap if feasible, and close the soft palate 4 months later. Otherwise, consider a primary veloplasty. If neither a vomer flap nor a primary veloplasty seems appropriate, consider a delayed repair and a temporary prosthesis.
3. For those patients with velopharyngeal incompetence, consider a pharyngeal flap and/or prosthesis, depending on the physical findings.

Our goal in cleft palate surgery should be the restoration of oral-nasal balance with acceptable and intelligible speech without jeopardizing the patient's genetically determined facial relations. With our present plan, we are able to obtain acceptable speech in a percentage of patients equal to national averages and with less interference with structural relations than we formerly witnessed. The surgical procedures are less exciting, but the results are more gratifying and our structural complications are fewer in number. Cleft palate patients will not become a simple problem. Whatever is planned for these patients surgically should be so designed that it will not create a malformation more difficult and costly to treat than the original anomaly.

References

1. Atherton, J.D., Lovius, B.B.J., and Maisels, D.O. Growth of bony palate of pig consequent to transpositioning oral and nasal mucoperiosteum. *Plast. Reconstr. Surg.* 56:110, 1975.
2. Converse, J.M. *Plastic and Reconstructive Surgery.* Philadelphia: Saunders, 1977. Vol. 4.

3. Cronin, T.D. Method of preventing raw area on the nasal surface of the soft palate in pushback surgery. *Plast. Reconstr. Surg.* 20:474, 1957.

4. Dieffenbach, J.F. Über das Gaumensegel des Menschen und der Saeugenthiere. *Litt. Ann. Heilkd.* 4:298, 1826.

5. Dieffenbach, J.F. *Die operative Chirurgie.* Leipsig: Bockhaus, 1845. Vol. 1.

6. Dingman, R.O. Long term results of cleft palate surgery. Lecture given at the annual meeting of the American Society of Plastic and Reconstructive Surgery, Los Angeles, 1970 (unpublished).

7. Dorrance, G.M. Congenital insufficiency of the palate. *Arch. Surg.* 21:185, 1930.

8. Downs, W. Craniofacial morphology in cleft palate and cleft lip deformities. *Surg. Gynecol. Obstet.*, 88:359, 1948.

9. Fara, M., Hrivnáková, J., and Sedláčková, E. Submucous cleft palates. *Acta Chir. Plast.* (Praha) 13:221, 1971.

10. Friede, H., and Johanson, B. A follow-up study of cleft children treated with primary bone grafting. *Scand. J. Plast. Reconstr. Surg.* 8:88, 1974.

11. Grabb, W.C., Rosenstein, S.W., and Bzoch, K.R. *Cleft Lip and Palate: Surgical, Dental, and Speech Aspects.* Boston: Little, Brown, 1971.

12. Harding, R.L., and Mazaheri, M. Growth and spatial changes in the arch form in bilateral cleft lip and palate patients. *Plast. Reconstr. Surg.* 50:591, 1972.

13. Hyslop, V.B., and Wynn, S.K. Bone flap technique in cleft palate surgery. *Plast. Reconstr. Surg.* 9:97, 1952.

14. Johanson, B. Early treatment of cleft lip and palate. In R.M. Cole (Ed.), *Proceedings of the Second International Symposium of Cleft Lip and Palate.* Chicago: Cleft Lip and Cleft Palate Institute of Northwestern University, 1970.

15. Kilner, T.P. Cleft lip and palate technique. *St. Thomas Hosp. Rep.* 2:127, 1937.

16. Kremenak, C.R., Huffman, W.C., and Olin, W.H. I. Growth of the maxillae in dogs after palatal surgery. *Cleft Palate J.* 4:6, 1967.

17. Kremenak, C.R., Huffman, W.C., and Olin, W.H. II. Growth of the maxillae in dogs after palatal surgery. *Cleft Palate J.* 7:719, 1970.

18. Kremenak, C.R., Huffman, W.C., and Olin, W.H. Maxillary growth inhibition by mucoperiosteal denudation of palatal shelf bone in non-cleft beagles. *Cleft Palate J.* 7:817, 1970.

19. Krogman, W.M. *Tabulae Biologicae.* The Hague, Netherlands: Junk, 1941.

20. Krogman, W.M., Mazaheri, M., Harding, R.L., Ishiguro, K., Bariana, G., Meier, J., Canter, H., and Ross, P. A longitudinal study of the craniofacial growth pattern in children with clefts as compared to normal, birth to six years. *Cleft Palate J.* 12:59, 1975.

21. Limberg, A. Nerve Wege in der radikolen Uranoplastik bei angeborenen Spaltendeformationen: Osteotomia Interlaminaria and Pterygomaxillaris, resectio marginis foraminis Palatini und neve Plattchennaht, fissura ossea occulta und ihre Behandlung. *Zentralbl. Chir.* 54:1745, 1927.

22. Maples, A.H., Mazaheri, M., Harding, R.L., Meier, J.A., and Canter, H.E. A longitudinal analysis of the maxillary growth increments of cleft lip and palate patients. *Cleft Palate J.* 11:450, 1974.

23. Mazaheri, M., Harding, R.L., and Nanda, S. The effect of surgery on maxillary growth and cleft width. *Plast. Reconstr. Surg.* 40:22, 1967.

24. Millard, D.R. Jr. Wide and/or short cleft palate. *Plast. Reconstr. Surg.* 29:40, 1962.

25. Millard, D.R., Jr. A new use of the island flap in wide palate clefts. *Plast. Reconstr. Surg.* 38:330, 1966.

26. Ortiz-Monasterio, F., Rebeil, A.S., Valderama, M., and Crus, R. Cephalometric measurements on adult patients with non-operated clefts. *Plast. Reconstr. Surg.* 24:53, 1959.

27. Ortiz-Monasterio, F., Serrano, R.A., Barrera, P.G., Rodriguez-Hoffman, H., and Vinegeras, E. A study of untreated adult cleft palate patients. *Plast. Reconstr. Surg.* 38:36, 1966.

28. Pruzansky, S. Factors determining arch form in clefts of the lip and palate. *Am. J. Orthod.* 41:827, 1955.

29. Rehrmann, A.H. Effect of early bone grafting on the growth of upper jaw in cleft lip and palate children: A computer evaluation *Minerva Chir.* 26:874, 1971.

30. Ross, R.B., and Johnston, M.C. *Cleft Lip and Palate.* Baltimore: Williams & Wilkins, 1972.

31. Schweckendiek, W. Die Ergebnisse der Kieferbildung und die Sprache nack der primäen Veloplastik. *Arch. Hals Ohr-Nas-Hehlk-Hk.* 180:541, 1962

32. Skoog, T. *Plastic Surgery,* Stockholm, Sweden, 1974 (Distributed by W.B. Saunders Co., Philadelphia).

33. Slaughter, W.B., and Pruzansky, S. The rationale for velar closure as a primary procedure in the repair of cleft palate defects. *Plast. Reconstr. Surg.* 13:341, 1954.

34. Veau, V., and Bord, S. *Division Palatine, Anatomie, Chirurgil, Phonetique.* Paris: Masson, 1931.

35. von Langenbeck, B. Further experiences of repair of the hard palate by freeing the mucoperiosteal covering of the palate. *Arch. Klin. Chir.* 5:1, 1864.

R. C. A. Weatherley-White

COMMENTS ON CHAPTER 7

DR. ROBERT Harding was an inspired choice on the part of the editor of this book to write a chapter on the long-range results of cleft palate surgery. For over two decades he has been the principal plastic surgeon for the Lancaster Cleft Palate Clinic, the first and probably most important interdisciplinary unit in the United States devoted to both rehabilitation and research into the cleft anomaly. His contribution reflects this wide experience as well as his ability to analyze his results, retaining what he and his colleagues find useful, avoiding fads, and yet being constantly prepared to modify his approach when a change in surgical technique seemed appropriate, based on hard data provided, in part, by his nonsurgical colleagues. This conservative and yet self-critical philosophy should serve as a model for all surgeons involved in cleft palate repair.

The past few decades have seen a steady and rather undramatic improvement in the standard of care afforded the cleft child. The principal influences responsible for this rewarding change have been, ironically, nonsurgical. Foremost of these was the introduction by Sir Ivan Magill of controlled endotracheal anesthesia, which affords a precise level of anesthesia and ensures adequate ventilation and prevention of aspiration of blood during the procedure. This technique is safer by a quantum degree than either insufflation or local infiltration. Consequently, the surgeon is more relaxed and can devote his full attention to the fine points of the operation itself. It is a foolhardy surgeon who will today, except under very rare circumstances, expose his cleft lip or cleft palate patient to the risks of surgery without competent endotracheal anesthesia.

A second major influence has been the growth of interdisciplinary cleft palate clinics, of which there are now over 200 in North America. The rehabilitation of a cleft palate child is too complex to be left entirely in the hands of one individual. Even though the surgeon will be making the ultimate surgical decision, he should give great weight to the opinions of the other members of the cleft palate team. Speech therapists, orthodontists, pediatricians interested in growth and development, and otolaryngologists all have a disciplined body of information arising from their training which can greatly benefit the integrated care of the child. In addition, by moving the evaluation of surgical results from the surgeon alone into the sphere of an objective group, a far more honest and realistic appraisal ensues, unfettered by emotional involvement. The surgeon whose results are consistently poorer than those of his colleagues will hopefully be shamed into either improving his techniques or dropping cleft lip and palate work in favor of some less demanding aspect of plastic surgery.

It will be noted that I have said little about the influences of surgical techniques on the changing standards of cleft palate surgery. The side-to-side mucoperiosteal flap repair (von Langenbeck) was introduced in the nineteenth century, and the retroposition procedure (Veau-Wardill-Kilner) was introduced over 50 years ago. Since then, several new surgical concepts have been proposed by thoughtful and innovative surgeons, such as the primary pharyngeal flap of Stark, the island flap of Millard, and the levator sling reconstruction of Edgerton. None of these has made any significant impression on the dominance of procedures standardized 150 years ago. This is probably less a commentary on the innate conservatism of plastic surgeons than on the almost total inability of the state of the art to provide a statistically valid comparison, in terms of functional speech results, between different types of surgical procedures.

In addition, the recommended timing for surgical repair varies greatly. Dr. Harding feels strongly, as do I, that palatoplasty should take place at about 1 year of age. Correction of a grossly abnormal anatomical mechanism before the onset of connected speech will theoretically prevent many of the secondary compensatory mechanisms from developing—abnormal tongue movements, grimacing to prevent nasal escape of air, and the use of the glottal stop—which are so hard to reverse in therapy. Yet protocols have been advocated, varying from closing the velum in early infancy along with the cleft lip to a totally nonsurgical approach until the midteens, thus avoiding *any* trauma to the maxillary complex during its growing period. Again, no long-range studies involving hard objective data substantiate these dramatic claims, leaving them as yet unproven.

The evaluation of the relative success of cleft palate surgery falls ultimately into two broad categories: speech and skeletal growth. From a functional standpoint, the repaired mechanism should not only be able to occlude the velopharyngeal valve, thus allowing the impounding of an intraoral breath pressure adequate for the production of "high pressure" consonant sounds and precluding nasal escape, but also should provide a supple palate which will move briskly to open and close the valve when appropriate phonetically. A scarred and immobile palate, even when of adequate length, will be unable to produce this precise activity, and the voice quality will be unsatisfactory. This is clearly demonstrated in Dr. Harding's chapter, and it cannot be too strongly emphasized.

The growth aspects of cleft palate surgery, and in particular the need to avoid procedures which, although initially attractive, are found in the long run to retard facial growth, are so well described that commentary is redundant. Dr. Harding points out with great clarity how, by drawing on the experience and hard data of his colleagues in facial growth morphology, he has modified his surgical techniques over the years to arrive at a protocol that is individualized rather than applied wholesale to all patients. This protocol yields consistently good functional results without harming the normal growth processes of the face.

It is relevant at this point to mention some of the significant variables that affect the repaired cleft palate population as a statistical unit and can drastically alter, to the point of invalidation, any broad-ranged study designed to assess the effects of surgical procedures on the cleft.

1. The skill of the individual surgeon, rather than the type or timing of a particular procedure, will probably have the greatest influence on the outcome of surgery from the standpoint of both facial growth and eventual speech. Any study which ignores this variable, for example, comparing procedure A as performed by Surgeon A with procedure B by Surgeon B, is patently invalid no matter what sophisticated methods are used to attain the outward appearance of statistical validity.

2. The availability and quality of speech therapy for the individual patient are of at least equal importance as the technical ability of the surgeon. Assuming a competent operation, the speech production of a child to whom excellent rehabilitative facilities are available on a twice-weekly basis is almost always going to exceed that of a child in a distant rural area whose parents can barely afford six-monthly evaluations. This geographic factor is ignored in most cross-sectional studies.

Dr. Harding has been able to avoid these significant variables which weaken the thrust of so many otherwise excellent papers, and he has made use of his fortunate position, that of being the principal surgeon in a high-volume clinic with superb investigative facilities, working closely with respected professionals in allied fields (and obviously in an atmosphere of high mutual regard between these often-fractious disciplines) to synthesize a lifetime of experience into a logical plan for the surgery and rehabilitation of the patient with cleft palate. This chapter is a remarkable contribution to the plastic surgery literature.

8 A PAUCITY of properly evaluated long-term results in cleft palate surgery was found in perusing the literature. Brodie [6] in 1941 confirmed the fact that lateral width of the maxilla is attained early in life; however, downward and forward growth is not complete until past the age of puberty.

Graber [19] in 1950 reached the conclusion that patients with closure of cleft palates early in life by the mucoperiosteal technique exhibit deficient patterns in maxillary growth laterally, anteroposteriorly, and vertically, early surgical trauma being the greatest cause of these deformities.

Farkas and Lindsay [14, 15] have reported on the morphology of adult faces following repair in both unilateral and bilateral cleft lip–cleft palate in childhood. They felt that the long-term narrow faces some of these patients exhibit may be the result of the combined effect of embryonal damage of the tissues and surgery, and they cited references to previous work of Pruzansky [41], Ross [42], Subtelny and Sakuda [44], Maisels [29], and Handleman and Pruzansky [20]. Farkas and Lindsay found the same general features of the face in adults with repaired unilateral cleft lips–cleft palates as in adults with the bilateral and isolated cleft palates, i.e., longer facial profile, a horizontally narrower face, and a narrower labial fissure. This finding could suggest that prenatal and postnatal development of the middle third of the face is similar in all patients with cleft lips and/or cleft palates of whatever form. Long-term studies of other methods besides mucoperiosteal elevation techniques may or may not disprove this theory.

Birch and Lindsay [2] reported in 1971 that anterior and alveolar palatal fistulae were frequent and unimportant in their repaired bilateral cleft lip–cleft palate cases. They stated that had these early treated patients been fitted with

Sidney K. Wynn

CLEFT PALATE SURGERY

fixed bridges (as is done at the present time), anterior palatal fistulae would have required closure. If the premaxilla was in good condition, the fistula was large; if it was small or displaced posteriorly, the fistula was small. They classified their speech results of the 59 adult cases studied as follows: only 19 percent had normal speech, 69 percent had intelligible speech with minor defects, 10 percent had intelligible speech with gross defects, and 2 percent had unintelligible speech. It was found that the best overall appearance was often found in patients who had few operations.

Farkas and Lindsay [16, 17] in 1972 and 1973 reported a study on 145 adult cleft lip–cleft palate patients operated on in childhood, comparing similar data on 100 normal Caucasian Canadians. The interorbital distance in both male and female patients with isolated cleft palate was the same as that in controls. They felt that in cleft lip–cleft palate patients, the defect in lip and jaw together with a compensatory growth in the nasal-frontal process contributes to the creation of this wider interorbital space. They suggest that clefts in the palate only, surrounded by a firm bony frame, do not influence the formation of the upper third of the face. Since their data did not differ significantly from that obtained by cephalometric studies, they believed the facial surface measurement was accurate for morphological study.

Pickrell [39] in 1972 reported that he had maxillary collapse in all instances where the cleft involved the alveolus and the maxilla in an adult group of patients. The Veau-Wardill-Kilner operation was used at the time surgery was done on these 100 cleft lip–cleft palate patients 22 to 27 years ago. In his group of 19 cleft palate only patients, 7 had clefts extending halfway through the palatal bone, and in 12 the defect was extremely wide and extended almost to the alveolar border. In the speech evaluation, only 28 percent had complete velopharyngeal closure (as assessed by cinefluorography) with good speech; none had perfect speech. This study also showed that 39 percent had fair speech and 33 percent had marked nasality with poor speech. Apparently, then, the cleft only group had the poorest overall speech results.

In Pickrell's cleft lip–cleft palate group of 51 patients evaluated by Dr. Massengill, 71 percent had complete velopharyngeal closure with a speech rating of good (but none perfect). The remaining 29 percent were rated as having poor speech.

Farkas and Lindsay [17], in a study in 1973, reported on 74 patients, 49 men and 25 women between the ages of 16 and 20, who had had surgical repair of complete (57 cases) and incomplete (17 cases) forms of unilateral cleft lip–cleft palate before the age of 2 years. The lip operation was mainly by the LeMesurier quadrangular flap technique, and the palate was repaired by modified Dorrance pushback operation at about 2 years of age. Seventy-three of the 74 patients had orthodontic treatment. They found the same general features of the face in adults with repaired unilateral cleft lips and cleft palates as in adults with repaired bilateral cleft lips and cleft palates and those with isolated cleft palates, that is, a longer facial profile, a horizontally narrower face, and a narrower labial fissure. These findings suggested that prenatal and postnatal development of the middle third of the face is similar in all patients with cleft lips and/or cleft palates in whatever form. They were surprised to find that the so-called normal side of the face in patients with unilateral cleft lips and cleft palates was always

Research supported by a private grant from Miss Ida Soref, without whose financial support this chapter would not have been possible.

narrower, in many cases abnormally narrow. The extent of the cleft did not seem to influence this fact in males. The different finding in females possibly could be explained by the small number of females with incomplete clefts in comparison with females with complete clefts in their study. They suggested that the abnormally developed noncleft side of the patient with a unilateral cleft lip–cleft palate was influenced by an anomaly of the development of the face equally on both sides. The labial fissure in their study has always been symmetrical in proportion with the size of the face. The smaller labial fissure length seems to be a logical consequence of narrowing the face.

Bishara [3] in 1973 studied the influence of palatoplasty on cleft length and facial development. He reported in his conclusions that the V-Y palatoplasty and the extent of the cleft in the palate did not produce consistently significant changes in the dentofacial relationship of those individuals with isolated clefts in the palate.

Ortiz-Monasterio et al. [35] in 1974 stated that the careful evaluation of late treatment of patients with clefts of lip and palate is not very encouraging. Labial clefts alone had excellent cosmetic results surgically, but they required elaborate orthodontic and sometimes segmental osteotomies. All unoperated patients have good facial growth and collapse is rare, but the maxillary segments are outwardly rotated. He felt that early aggressive surgery resulted in serious collapse. The incidence of ear, nose, and throat (ENT) and hearing problems is the same in unoperated adults and children operated on in infancy. This suggests that there is room for improvement in the methods of handling palatal fissures in order to achieve good nasal and pharyngeal function. Not only is late closure of the palate difficult, but results are disappointing. Even with good anatomical repair producing a long, soft, and mobile palate, speech results are poor. Phoniatric training was found to be very helpful for the group operated on between 6 and 12 years of age, but it had little effect on teenagers and none on adults with a well-established speech pattern.

The reasons for the delayed treatment in his study were both socioeconomic and cultural.

Caldarelli [10] in 1975 reported on a group of cleft lip–cleft palate patients 16 years and older who were selected at random in order to study the type and frequency of middle ear disease. He concluded that at best this would have to be a pilot study. Caldarelli suggested that in the absence of uniform prophylactic otologic care, a significant number of patients seem to be immune to the presumed handicap of cleft-related middle ear pathology. He felt that this study reemphasized the need for long-term otologic surveillance of the patient with a cleft. It also supported the emerging recognition that cleft palate is not purely a congenital disruption of the velar morphology, but rather a constant, complex interrelationship between velar and otic pathology. Prudent therapy, then, would imply recognition and comprehension of these variations in cleft form and their specific otic pathologic sequelae.

Moller [34] in 1975 reported on long-term results in 113 patients, 58 with both cleft lip and cleft palate and 55 with cleft palate only. Chronic otitis media was found in only 3 percent of the ears, and cholesteatoma was found in only 1 percent. A hearing loss of more than 30 dB was found in 6 percent of 6-year-old patients, but the frequency was reduced to 2 percent in 15-year-old patients.

Honjo et al. [21] reported in 1975 that in order to reevaluate the role of Passavant's ridge, 10 adult cleft palate patients with a marked ridge were examined by a radiographic and cineradiographic method. The following results were obtained: (1) height of the ridge varies with the vowels, (2) height of the ridge in consonant syllable phonation is related not to velopharyngeal closure required for each consonant but to the succeeding vowels, and (3) tongue position for vowel phonation has a great effect on the appearance of the ridge. In conclusion, formation of Passavant's ridge is not associated with the degree of velopharyngeal closure necessary for the specific speech sound, but it is closely related to the tongue position for vowel production. Thus the significance of

Passavant's ridge in cleft palate speech remains quite doubtful.

Yules [50] reported in 1975 that the incidence of conductive hearing loss in adults who have had cleft palates approximates 50 percent. That their ear disease arises during infancy had been previously well documented. The serous otitis media which develops in infancy and persists through adolescence is presently best treated by tympanic aeration tubes. Whether or not a limited adenoidectomy is a useful adjunct to treatment remains to be conclusively demonstrated. The eventual outcome of ear disease would seem to suggest so. The end product of recurrent serous effusions and/or ear infections can be a chronic draining ear and/or cholesteatoma which, following the attainment of adolescence, is best treated by mastoid tympanoplasty with ossicular reconstruction.

Pannbacker [36] in 1975 reported the investigation of selected oral language skills and their relationship to speech intelligibility in 40 cleft palate and normal adult speakers. Connected speech samples were analyzed to determine spoken language status, which included response length, grammar or syntax, and vocabulary size. The subjects were judged for intelligibility by two groups of listeners: sophisticated and unsophisticated. It was concluded that (1) cleft palate speakers used shorter responses and were more consistent in their language usage, (2) there were no significant differences in syntax and vocabulary, (3) for cleft palate speakers there was a relationship between intelligibility and language measures, (4) unsophisticated listeners were more consistent in judging intelligibility, and (5) sophisticated listeners rated cleft palate speakers poorer than unsophisticated listeners.*

A study by Blocksma et al. [5] in February 1975 reported that a large percentage of postoperative cleft palate cases require pharyngeal flap or pharyngeal implant secondary surgical procedures to improve speech. Indeed they reported that this was necessary in as many pa-

*I believe the key to good speech investigation is to have sophisticated listeners, rather than the surgeon, rate speech.

tients after radical lengthening procedures as after conservative closures. Their conservative approach named (1) the modified von Langenbeck (no pushback), 49 percent; (2) the Veau-Wardill-Kilner V-Y pushback, 79 percent; (3) the island flap, 51 percent; (4) the Dorrance method, 63 percent; and (5) the von Langenbeck method, 40 percent. This seems to be a great number of secondary procedures.

Bishara et al. [4] in 1976 concluded in their study of the effects of palatoplasties on facial growth that the different palatoplasties investigated do not produce significantly different results in anteroposterior and vertical skeletal and dental relationships as examined from lateral cephalograms. These were the results in the Veau-Wardill-Kilner and von Langenbeck palatoplasties. Therefore, the addition of speech results and the details of dental occlusion become more critical factors in the evaluation of the effects of these palatoplasties.

Coerdt [11] reported in 1977 that of a total of 3,681 operations for hare lip and cleft palate, 139 patients operated on between 1951 and 1975 were compared with the aid of exact measurements and the impressions to ascertain whether early orthodontic treatment had an influence on the growing maxilla. Forty-nine percent of 200 patients who were followed up had normal speech, 39 percent had minimal disturbances of articulation, and 12 percent had poor speech. In 13 out of 16 of these patients, pharyngoplasty improved the speech. The palate repairs were of mucoperiosteal elevation techniques.

The general consensus now is that mucoperiosteal elevation cleft palate techniques may account for late-growth maxillary retardation. Kremenak et al. [25, 26] demonstrated that when strips of mucoperiosteum are removed from the growing palate in dogs, narrowing of the maxilla results. This may partially account for some of the poor speech and developmental long-term results seen in mucoperiosteal-type cases.

The musculature of the soft palate is of prime importance in speech. Techniques that describe separation of the soft palate from the hard palate at the aponeurosis are certain to cut some innervation in that area, as described by Broomhead [7]. This could account for some of the problems in the Veau-Wardill-Kilner V-Y pushback cases and the island flap techniques.

Simple closure of only the posterior soft palate (modified von Langenbeck procedure) is being proposed by some surgeons at this time [5]. Their theory is that the anterior palate bony defect will narrow enough that they can perform a simple closure as a later procedure. Objective measurement data confirming this theory have not been forthcoming to this author's satisfaction. Thirty years of observation reveal that the wide cleft palate defects will not narrow sufficiently to be closed without secondary wide mucoperiosteal elevation for the anterior closure. These are the patients that could be identified in our long-term study [48] as having greater maxillary problems. The modified von Langenbeck technique with the simple soft palate closures still requires 49 percent of the cases to have secondary operative procedures such as pharyngeal flaps or implants to improve speech. Some of the cases require the use of prosthetic palate plates for the anterior palate closure until anterior surgical palate closure can be done, if ever. This may be feasible in areas where orthodontists and prosthodontists are readily available; however, in many areas this is not possible. With all these facts in mind, I believe a restatement of the osteotomy procedure is now pertinent.

Long-term results were reported by this author in 1976 [48] after cleft palate closure by the bilateral osteotomy technique. Our completed study included cephalometric examinations, dental study casts, profile photographic studies, audiologic exams, and speech evaluations of patients aged 16 to 24. In determining what is actually the result of cleft palate surgery, we come to the realization that we are speaking of multiple deformities. Figures 8-1 through 8-12, showing variations of cleft palate osteotomies as done at the Milwaukee Children's Hospital, adequately illustrate practically every type of cleft palate deformity encountered. Accurate evaluation can be done by

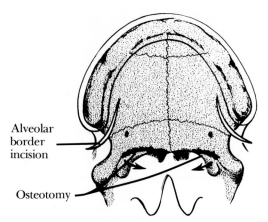

Alveolar border incision

Osteotomy

FIGURE 8-1. *Minor soft palate defect or submucous cleft palate, hamulus osteotomy only.*

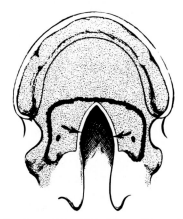

FIGURE 8-2. *Incomplete cleft palate small bone defect, osteotomy into notch.*

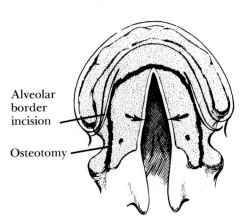

Alveolar border incision

Osteotomy

FIGURE 8-3. *Incomplete V-shaped cleft palate, osteotomy to anterior notch.*

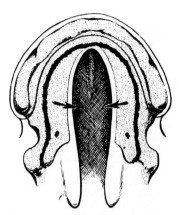

FIGURE 8-4. *Incomplete horseshoe cleft palate, osteotomy to tip of notch.*

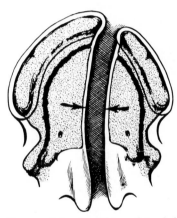

FIGURE 8-5. *Complete unilateral cleft palate, osteotomy hamulus to anterior.*

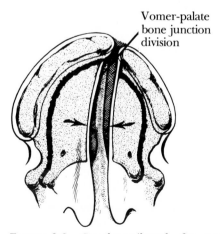

Vomer-palate bone junction division

FIGURE 8-6. *Complete unilateral—firm vomer attachment, divided vomer—palate junction prior to osteotomy.*

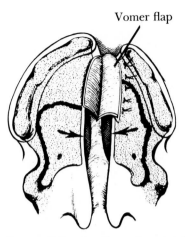

Vomer flap

FIGURE 8-7. *Complete unilateral cleft, wide type cleft vomer flap prior to osteotomy. Osteotomy on attached side to posterior vomer.*

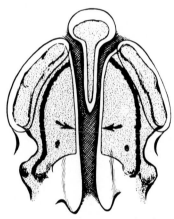

FIGURE 8-8. *Bilateral cleft palate, narrow with free vomer, osteotomy hamulus to anterior.*

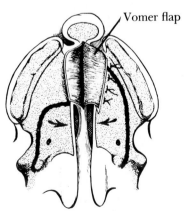

Vomer flap

FIGURE 8-9. *Bilateral cleft palate, unilateral vomer attachment, vomer flap prior to osteotomy.*

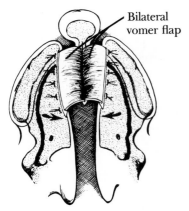

FIGURE 8-10. *Bilateral wide complete cleft palate, free floating vomer, bilateral vomer flap prior to complete osteotomy.*

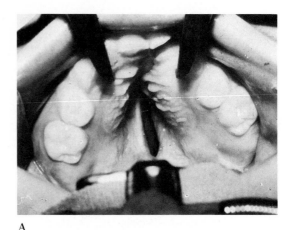

A

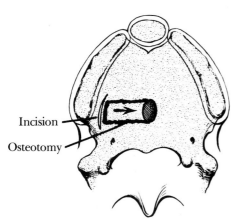

FIGURE 8-11. *Central palate fistula. Use localized osteotomy. Avoid wide mucoperiosteal elevation.*

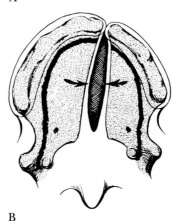

B

FIGURE 8-12. *(A) Osteotomy location used secondarily only when soft palate is closed by a modified von Langenbeck procedure. (B) Demonstrates open anterior cleft often found several years after simple soft palate closure by modified von Langenbeck technique.*

recall of postoperative cleft palate patients in their teens and early twenties. Their developmental shortcomings become apparent and give insight into future surgery. There are many other factors that must be considered; that is, variations in culture, ethnic derivation, intelligence of the patient, cooperation of the parents, motivation, personality, and financial background all eventually count toward a long-term result. Therapy such as orthodontia can vary in long-term results. An individual who has a child at a medical center where multiple facilities are available and money is no object is indeed very fortunate; however, those in rural

areas or financially wanting and having no available orthodontist may have further problems. Interested speech pathologists, dentists, orthodontists, audiologists, and a plastic surgeon willing to see the patient develop past the age of puberty are essential.

The osteology of the palate bone and, consequently, the arterial anatomy (especially the location of the egress of the greater palatine artery) changes between early infancy (Fig. 8-13A and B) and the age of 5 years (Fig. 8-14). The bony structure of the medial and lateral pterygoid plates is considerably more posterior to the alveolar ridge in the 1-year-old than in a

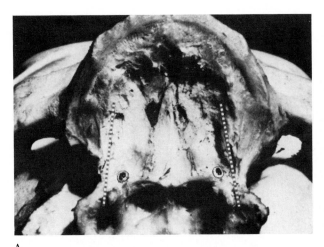

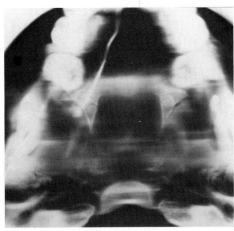

A

B

FIGURE 8-13. *(A) Base of skull, 1-year-old infant. Note the posterior opening of the greater palatine foramen and the more posterior position of pterygoid plates (O marks the* *foramen). (B) X-ray tomogram with wire in greater palatine foramen extending anteriorly to approximate position of the greater palatine artery.*

child who is already 5 years of age. This has been determined by our own specimen studies, and these differences of the palate osteology have not heretofore been emphasized in anatomical texts. The bony structures begin to get more ossified and thus harder to move by the age of 2 and older. The greater palatal foramen is also located more posteriorly and medially in the 1-year-old infant. In this author's article of 1976 [48] and in previous publications and

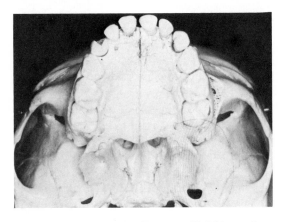

FIGURE 8-14. *Base of skull, 5-year-old child. Note how the pterygoid plates are now closer to the posterior alveolus. Note also the decrease in area between the greater palatine foramen and the alveolar area.*

movies [23,24,45,47,49], the location of the greater palatal foramen has been placed too forward on the palate. Thus, when placing the initial chisel in these cases, it is a simple matter to feel the notch between the medial and lateral pterygoid plates and move up anteriorly with the chisel series and still avoid cutting through the greater palatine artery. The pterygoid plates and the greater palatal foramen migrate gradually to just behind and medial to the posterior alveolar border by the age of 5. The maxillary sinus is a small structure before the age of 1 (Fig. 8-15) as compared with age 5. Consequently, the osteotomy going only into bone is much easier at a younger age. Calcium is continually being laid down to make harder bone. Comparison of each and every surgical technique over a long term is an impossibility on a completely accurate basis. This type of research outline would require the following parameters: surgeons with similar abilities, patients with similar ages, and similar techniques of speech evaluation and hearing and cephalometric comparisons. True humility should rapidly surface in the plastic surgeon who reevaluates his 15- to 20-year postoperative cleft palate patients. An apparent good result immediately or within a few years post-

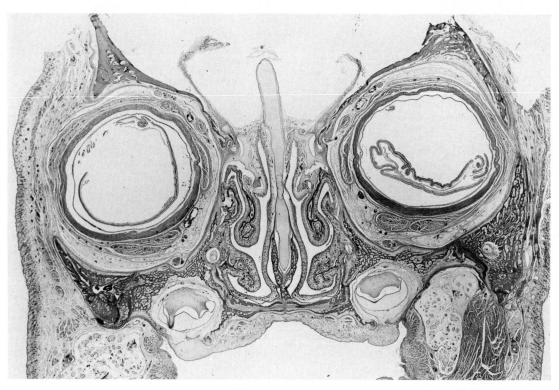

FIGURE 8-15. *Coronal cross section of infant palate. Note the small maxillary sinus in comparison with tooth bud. Note also the large area of bone readily available for osteotomy to but not through the maxillary sinus.*

operatively may prove to be a poor result on reevaluation.

It stands to reason that waiting for osteotomy until this older age is not as safe and is much more difficult to perform. The younger the infant (we start at age 9 months), the more expedient is the surgical procedure. Thus there is a more rapid osteoblastic activity with reconstruction of a bony palate. Histologic sections taken at the palatal shelf–nasal junction revealed a considerable number of osteoblasts lined up on each side of the bony palate shelf in the palate (Fig. 8-16). Maher [27] in 1977 reported on the circulation of the palate. He demonstrated multiple perforating vessels and connections through the bony palate shelves. He also states that there is circulation coming through the superior alveolar artery to the inci-

sive foramen that connects up with the greater palatine arterial system. In a personal conference, Dr. Maher [28] stated to this author that "the osteotomy procedure would cut off less circulation to the palate shelves than mucoperiosteal palate closure techniques previously described."

The surgical technique, because of editorial cutting with strict space limitations, has been described inadequately in previous publications. Hopefully these few additional comments will help to clarify previous writings [46,47,49]. Initial incisions are made just inside the alveolar area (Fig. 8-17A through E). They start behind the tuberosity of the superior maxilla on each side and come forward about three-fourths of the length of the hard palate. This is actually a combination relaxing incision and the incision into which the chisels are placed. The initial chisel used is ordinarily a straight chisel. The one we use first is 13.5 cm in length and 7 mm in width, and it is placed by feeling the notch between the hamulus process medially and the

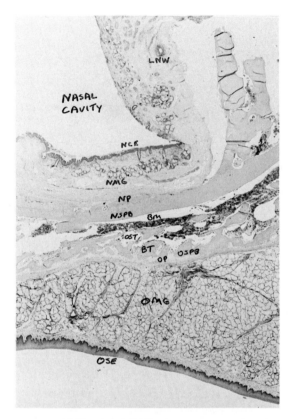

FIGURE 8-16. *Photomicrograph of the coronal section of hard palate depicts from top to bottom, nasal cavity, lateral nasal wall (LNW), nasal columnar epithelium (NCE), nasal mucous glands (NMG), nasal periosteum (NP), nasal surface of palatine bone (NSPB), bone marrow (BM), bony trabeculae (BT), with osteoblasts (OST), oral surface of palatine bone (OSPB), oral periosteum (OP), oral mucous glands (OMG), and oral squamous epithelium (OSE). Original magnification, 100×.*

the greater palatine foramen (medially) and the alveolus (laterally). The bone is divided and then moved with a medial wedging action with the one to three chisels in place. The number of chisels depends on the severity of the palate defect. This will usually produce a fracture into the anterior area of the palate cleft. The length of defect present actually dictates the linear osteotomy. The chiseling is done straight down into the bone itself without any mucoperiosteal elevation. It is known from our previous studies that the osteotomized bones of infant palates regenerate new bone at the osteotomy margins. If the palate shelf does not move over easily by the wedging action, additional chiseling may have to be done anteriorly with the use of a 15-mm length, 2-mm width small curved chisel. This can be introduced into the anterior portion of the incision at the front of the osteotomy area in a tangential fashion to produce a guided fracture in the proper location, depending on the type of palate with which one is dealing. The circumference of the palate vault is diminished as the levering action of the chisel brings the palatal shelf toward the midline. This simultaneously shortens the radius within the arch of the palate. When this is done, the opportunity to approximate the palatal shelves is improved.

In a complete cleft palate, as one wedges the palatal shelves toward the midline, it is very possible that the anterior fracture itself will extend in some cases into the anterior location of the incisive suture line in the infant. This may explain why the wedging action so simply moves the palate shelf over in the complete cleft palate in a 9- to 12-month-old baby. It could be speculated from a practical standpoint that this suture line is still not solid in these infants. In those palates in which there is a very firm vomer attachment and a narrow cleft, it is advisable to take a 15-cm length, 7-mm width straight osteotome and split the vomer-palate junction. This will help the palatal shelf come down below the level of the vomer. The wedging action of the osteotome is performed to reduce the radius of the vault of the palate for easier closure.

lateral pterygoid plate. One chisels into this area to a depth of approximately 1 cm, dividing the plate in a perpendicular fashion between the lateral and medial pterygoid plates. This chisel should be left in place as the adjacent series of chisel cuts is made anterior to this. The second chisel used ordinarily is approximately 13.5 cm in length also and 5 mm in width. A third chisel of the same type is then used, still further forward on the palate, just inside the alveolus to about the canine region. Each chisel is maintained in place, allowing the next to go adjacent to it. Thus the chisels are kept between

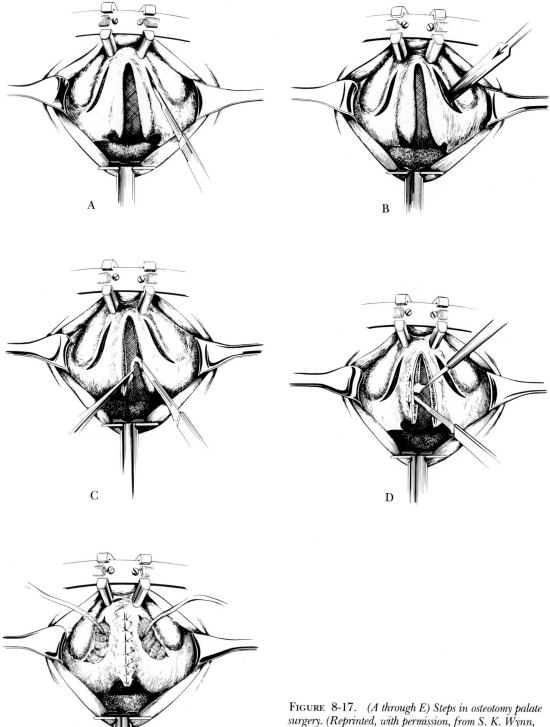

FIGURE 8-17. *(A through E) Steps in osteotomy palate surgery. (Reprinted, with permission, from S. K. Wynn, Long-term results after cleft palate closure by bilateral osteotomy technique. Plast. Reconstr. Surg. 58:71–79, 1976.)*

In cases in which the medial palate shelves are acutely angled above the level of the lower border of the vomer, an additional technique is utilized. The 1-cm right-angle Padgett elevator can be introduced through the cleft on the nasal side of the nasal mucosa in conjunction with the osteotome wedging action. An assistant pulls firmly on the right-angle elevator to help move the palate shelf in an oral direction as the wedging by the lateral osteotome is being activated. This helps reposition the palate shelf in its proper position on the vomer. If the cleft palate is very wide with a vomer attachment, it is advisable to do a vomer flap procedure preliminary to the osteotomy operation (Figs. 8-18 through 8-20). On the side on which the vomer is attached, make a guided fracture with the 2-mm chisel to the posterior area of the vomer attachment after the initial osteotomy.

When moving the palate shelves toward the midline, the leverage should not be applied against the alveolar ridge. In this way, injury to erupted or unerupted teeth is avoided.

Following the completion of the osteotomy procedure, the edges of the entire palate cleft are stripped and pared. The entire palate is closed with the 3-0 nylon suture, and gauze packs are placed in the osteotome wedge areas. The packs are removed in 5 days. The void fills in rapidly with granulation tissue within a few days. Mucous membrane usually covers this area within 2 weeks.It has been demonstrated by later x-ray reviews that this area fills in with bone (Fig. 8-21A and B).

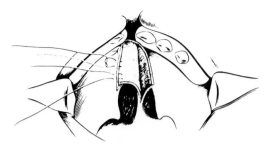

FIGURE 8-19. *Vomer flap booked.*

If a central opening must be left between the vomer flap area of closure and the posterior osteotomy closure in the soft palate, this opening can be closed easily at a later date with a localized type of osteotomy by making a small incision inside the alveolar border. Using the 2-mm chisel tangentially, form a guided fracture above and below the area of the fistula so that tension is completely removed. Then with a minimal elevation of the mucoperiosteum on each side of the fistula, the fistula can be sutured together with a 3-0 or 4-0 nylon on a half-circle small needle (PR-2 Davis and Geck). The usual packing is placed in the area of the osteotomy and removed in 3 to 5 days. Anatomically, the musculature of the soft palate is brought into optimum functioning position when osteotomy techniques are used to bring the palate edges into approximation. This obviates the necessity of separate muscle dissection, which could lead to further scar formation. It is my opinion that detaching the levator musculature from the palate bone and turning

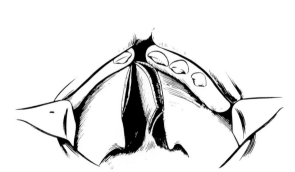

FIGURE 8-18. *Vomer and palate incisions for vomer flap.*

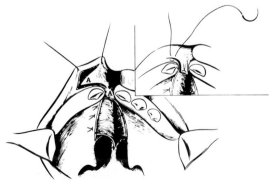

FIGURE 8-20. *Anterior alveolar area closed with labial rotation flap.*

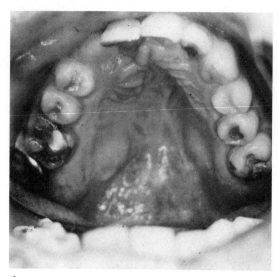

A

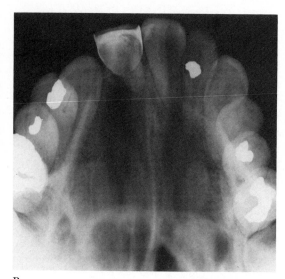

B

FIGURE 8-21. *(A) Healing obtained in complete uni-lateral cleft of the palate, after bilateral osteotomy technique. (B) Postoperative occlusal x-ray film of the same patient. Note complete lateral bone fill-in and reconstruction* *of bony palate. (Reprinted, with permission, from S. K. Wynn, Long-term results after cleft palate closure by bilateral osteotomy technique.* Plast. Reconstr. Surg. *58:71–79, 1976.)*

its direction is not necessary in the osteotomy-type procedures, as evidenced by the excellent postoperative elevation of the soft palate on phonation. This has been witnessed by both clinical examination and cinephonation studies.

Dr. Donald Babbitt, chief radiologist at the Milwaukee Children's Hospital, verifies the fact that cinefluoroscopy studies of these children postoperatively have revealed excellent palate motion with good velopharyngeal closure [1]. A complete file of these cinefluorography tapes has been kept at Milwaukee Children's Hospital Radiology Department.

The osteotomy method in surgery has been studied in depth from the long-term standpoint. The proportional measurement tables were taken from cephalometric measurements of 41 operated cleft palate patients aged 16 to 24. These were compared with a study by Mestre [32] of unoperated clefts. Both the incomplete and complete types revealed no undue superior maxillary developmental problem according to Dr. Thomas McGowan, the orthodontist who performed this study at the Milwaukee Children's Hospital Cleft Palate Center. Here reproduced in part is Dr.

McGowan's orthodontic portion [31] of the long-term cleft palate research project done by the Milwaukee Children's Hospital Cleft Palate Team (Fig. 8-22, Table 8-1).

Complete orthodontic records were taken on 41 cleft lip–cleft palate patients. The records included

1. Intraoral photographs
2. Extraoral portrait photographs
3. Orthodontic study models
4. Panoramic dental radiographs
5. Lateral cephalometric radiographs

The sample includes 17 posterior (second-degree) cleft palate subjects, 17 unilateral (third-degree) cleft palate subjects, and 7 bilateral cleft palate patients. The age of this population varied from 16 to 24 years.

The lateral cephalometric headplates were traced on a 0.003 matte acetate tracing paper. A 4-H tracing pencil was used, and all measurements were recorded to the nearest ½ mm or degree.

Angular and linear measurements were used to study facial development. The absolute

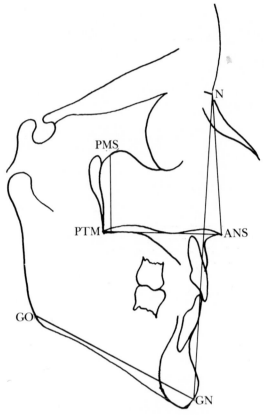

FIGURE 8-22. *Cephalometric measurement diagram.*
N-Nasion.   The intersection of the internasal suture with
the nasofrontal suture in midsagittal plane.
ANS-Anterior nasal spine.   This point is the tip of the
anterior nasal spine seen on the x-ray film from the
norma lateralis.
GN-Gnathion.   The most inferior point in the contour of
the chin.
GO-Gonion.   The point that is the most inferiorly, poste-
riorly, and outwardly directed on the jaw angle.
PTM.   The point of intersection of the palatal plane as it
crossed the tuberosity of the maxilla.
PMS.   The point midway between the most superior and
posterior points of the ascending maxilla drawn perpen-
dicular to PTM-ANS. (Reprinted, with permission,
from S. K. Wynn, Long-term results after cleft palate
closure by bilateral osteotomy technique. Plast. Reconstr.
Surg. 58:71–79, 1976.)

linear size of parts was not considered, but rather a proportional percentage of investigated areas was utilized. This was described by Mestre [32] as follows:

Proportional and angular measurements are particularly suitable, if not preferable, in a cross-sectional study of this type. In comparing cross-sectional samples, individual variation in the dimensions of the head must be considered. For example, a large individual may reveal larger linear measurements than a smaller individual. Yet both may be comparable in age and development. The inequity can be partially overcome by utilizing angular and proportional measurements.

The results of anteroposterior position of the chin in this study indicate that in the posterior cleft palate patients, there was no significant difference with the unoperated sample at the 0.05 level of confidence. The position of chin point (pagonion) relative to cranial base was sella-nasion.

This angle SNPOG relates the chin point horizontally to the cranial base.

The position of chin point in the operated complete unilateral cleft palate sample did have a significant difference (79.75 mm unoperated, 75.44 mm for operated) when compared with the unoperated unilateral patients. As described by Pionek [40], the linear distance S-N is greater in the complete unilateral cleft patient than in the posterior cleft patient. This may account for the more acute angle in complete unilateral cleft patients. The length of the mandible from gonion to gnathion in both second- and third-degree cleft patients was for all practical purposes the same (75.79 to 75.88 mm).

The vertical position of chin point is indicated by (N-S-GN). The more obtuse the angle, the more vertical is height to the total face, with the endpoints being nasion and gnathion. The vertical position of the chin in the operated and unoperated posterior cleft samples showed no significant difference at the 0.05 level of confidence. The height in the complete unilateral samples did show a significant difference. The linear difference in the operated second- and third-degree samples was 124.56 mm (sec-

Table 8-1. *Cephalometric Proportional Measurements*

	Second-Degree Clefts		Third-Degree Clefts	
	Mean	S.D.	Mean	S.D.
From Mestre [32]:				
1. $\dfrac{\text{N-ANS}}{\text{N-GN}}$	43.62	3.04	43.24	8.51
2. $\dfrac{\text{PMS-(PTM-ANS)}}{\text{N-ANS}}$	50.43	5.81	47.21	6.53
3. $\dfrac{\text{CO-GO}}{\text{GO-GN}}$	80.38	7.80	82.61	9.24
4. $\dfrac{\text{ANS-PTM}}{\text{GO-GN}}$	67.37	5.51	66.27	6.10
From our osteotomy procedure [48]:				
1. $\dfrac{\text{N-ANS}}{\text{N-GN}}$	43.20	1.72	42.52	2.02
2. $\dfrac{\text{PMS-(PTM-ANS)}}{\text{N-ANS}}$	52.40	6.40	51.40	4.30
3. $\dfrac{\text{CO-GO}}{\text{GO-GN}}$	77.60	7.83	81.13	6.57
4. $\dfrac{\text{ANS-PTM}}{\text{GO-GN}}$	72.56	6.26	72.22	5.94

Reprinted with permission from S.K. Wynn, Long-term results after cleft palate closure by bilateral osteotomy technique. *Plast. Reconstr. Surg.* 58:71–79, 1976.

ond degree) to 130.12 mm (third degree). This difference may account for the more obtuse angle in the operated third-degree sample.

The percentage of ramal height to mandibular body length showed no significant difference in the second-degree unoperated and operated groups at 0.05 level of confidence. The same was true for the third-degree groups.

The anteroposterior position of the maxilla is determined by S-N-ANS. The complete posterior cleft and complete unilateral cleft groups showed no statistical difference in the unoperated and operated samples. The difference in the complete unilateral cleft samples did, however, approach significance at the 0.05 level.

The vertical height of the total face was measured and compared with the Mestre [32] sample. Nasion to anterior nasal spine was measured proportionately to total facial height (nasion-gnathion). The percentage in the second-degree unoperated sample is 43.62

compared with the operated sample at 43.20. There is no significant difference at the 0.05 level of confidence. The third-degree samples showed similar results, with the unoperated at 43.24 percent and the operated at 42.52 percent. This again was not significant at the 0.05 level of confidence.

Posterior maxillary vertical dimension was compared with the height of the middle part of the anterior face measured nasion to anterior nasal spine (ANS). The posterior vertical height was measured from posterior maxillary summit (PMS) to the palatal plane (PTM-ANS). This measurement was described as follows:

In preparation for measuring posterior maxillary height, the tuberosity of the maxilla as it ascends to form the anterior outline of the pterygomaxillary fissure was traced from the lateral headplate. This surface continues upward and then curves sharply forward to become the superior surface of the maxilla as it progresses forward to form part of the floor of the orbit. On this curved posterior-superior outline of the maxilla, the most superior and most posterior points were selected. A point midway between these two points was designated as the posterior maxillary summit (PMS). From this point the vertical distance to the palatal plane was measured and recorded as the posterior maxillary height.

The second-degree unoperated cleft showed a 50.43 percent PMS-(PTM-ANS)/N-ANS, while the operated posterior cleft showed a 52.40 percent reading. This difference was not significant at the 0.05 level of confidence.

The third-degree unoperated sample had a 47.21 percent (PMS-PTM-ANS)/N-ANS, while the operated sample was 51.40 percent. This difference was significant at the 0.05 level of confidence.

N-ANS in a noncleft sample reported by McGowan [30] was 55.23 mm. The same distance in the operated complete unilateral cleft sample is 55.47 mm. This would seem to indicate that PMS to PTM-ANS is larger than previously reported. The degree of difficulty in locating PMS may also be the reason for this difference.

The total maxillary length (ANS-PTM) was measured proportionate to mandibular body length (GO-GN). The second-degree unoperated and operated samples showed a significant difference at the 0.05 level of confidence. The percentage readings respectively were 67.37 and 72.56. The same is true of the third-degree samples, with the unoperated at 66.26 percent and the operated at 72.23 percent. The difference could be attributed to mandibular body length, which in the surgical second-degree sample was 75.79 mm and 75.89 mm in the third-degree sample. This compares with 81.69 mm in a noncleft sample reported by McGowan [30].

The data gathered were statistically analyzed at the Marquette University Computing Center. The null hypothesis was used to study the unoperated and operated groups.

The lack of raw data in the published article of Mestre [32] made it difficult to locate the exact area of variance when the difference in data was significant at the 0.05 level. It was necessary to compare the operated sample with the noncleft sample when information was not available to explain the variation.

I am principally concerned with the maxilla or primary area of surgical intervention in this chapter. The discussion will be directed to midfacial development.

The position of ANS relative to cranial base SN is comparable to that of the unoperated sample. If cranial base length is comparable to that of noncleft patients, then the most anterior limit of the maxilla would have to be considered near normal.

The posterior limit of the maxilla is described by N-S-PTM. The location of the posterior limit of the palate was not easily discernible. The position of PTM in the second-degree operated group was not significantly different from that in the unoperated cleft. In the third-degree operated sample there was a significant difference compared with the unoperated group. The operated mean was 75.5°, while the unoperated was 70.57°. This measurement had the greatest variation in the second-degree (72.48°) and third-degree (70.57°) unoperated samples of Mestre [32], lending some credence to the difficulty of picking up the landmark PTM.

Anterior facial height was comparable in the groups studied. Total facial height was larger in the cleft sample, 124.56 mm for the second-degree group and 130.11 mm for the third-degree group, when compared with a noncleft sample, 122.30 mm. But the percentage of middle facial height (N-GN) was comparable.

Posterior midfacial height indicates that PMS to (PTM-ANS) appears to be larger in the operated sample than in the unoperated sample. N-ANS in the surgical sample was 53.85 in the second-degree and 55.47 in the third-degree groups. This distance, N-ANS, in a noncleft sample was 55.25. The higher percentages in the surgical sample studied would then seem to be the result of a larger PMS to PTM-ANS distance. The reason for this could be investigator error in picking up PMS, or it may be due to increased growth potential in the posterior face. As previously reported by Pionek [40], there is a decreased gonial angle in the osteotomy group.

The distance from the anterior nasal spine to the pterygomaxillary point compared with the mandibular corpus length in the operated sample appears to be nearly the same as in the unoperated group. The percentages of the unoperated samples are 67.37 for the second-degree and 66.26 for the third-degree groups. In the surgical sample the percentage is 72.56 for the posterior clefts and 72.22 for the complete unilateral clefts. This variation could be due to increased maxillary length or diminished mandibular length. The GO-GN length in this sample (76.09 mm) was less than that reported in a noncleft sample (81.69 mm). This may be the reason for the higher percentages in the surgical group leaving the alternative that maxillary length is greater than that reported in the unoperated group. The former is more likely, still leaving maxillary length comparable to the unoperated sample.

The medical artists in the audiographics department of the Medical College of Wisconsin evaluated the facial profiles of the 41 surgical subjects. Being a subjective evaluation, the results could always be contested (Figs. 8-23, 8-24, and 8-25).

The patients were classified as (1) ideal profile, (2) acceptable profile, and (3) concave profile. The posterior clefts had ideal profiles in all 17 patients. The complete unilateral clefts had 8 patients with ideal profiles, 7 with acceptable profiles, and 2 with concave profiles. The bilaterals, which were included in the sample, but not reported on, had 4 as acceptable, while 3 were considered concave.

After careful study of McGowan's results [31] and the profile studies [48], it was concluded that in the complete cleft lip–cleft palate cases, the only unacceptable profiles were those in which secondary wide mucoperiosteal elevations were done to close the anterior palate.

In view of the fact that there is no way of knowing which palates will narrow enough anteriorly after just soft palate closure, it is felt best to commence originally with a more anterior type of osteotomy for immediate com-

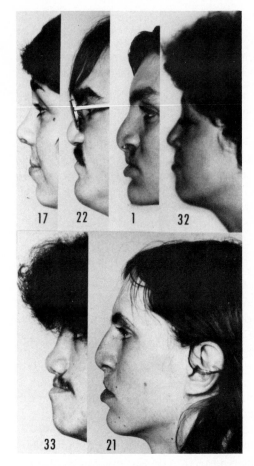

FIGURE 8-23. *Profile views, bilateral complete cleft palate cases. (Reprinted, with permission, from S. K. Wynn, Long-term results after cleft palate closure by bilateral osteotomy technique.* Plast. Reconstr. Surg. *58:71–79, 1976.)*

plete closure. However, if it is a very wide cleft, do the vomer flap as a preliminary procedure. These cases do not show the postpuberal superior maxillary developmental problems. This fact was emphasized by Dunn [13] in 1952 and reiterated by Stenström and Thilander [43] in 1974.

Some pure-tone hearing sensitivity measurements in 200 cleft palate cases repaired by the bilateral osteotomy technique were conducted in children from 3 to 13 years of age. This group of bilateral osteotomy cases had an average of 10.6 dB better hearing for 500, 1000,

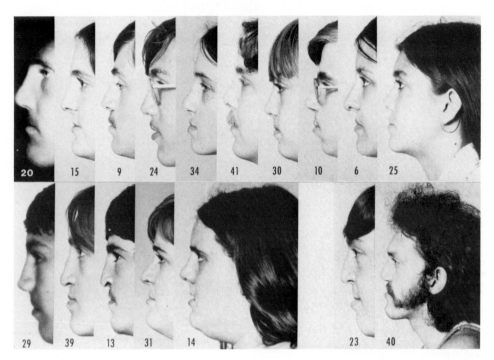

FIGURE 8-24. *Profile views, unilateral complete cleft palate cases. (Reprinted, with permission, from S. K. Wynn, Long-term results after cleft palate closure by bilateral osteotomy technique. Plast. Reconstr. Surg. 58:71–79, 1976.)*

and 2000 Hz than a group with palates repaired by the mucoperiosteal elevation operative procedures. The study was conducted by Miller and Wynn [48,33] (see Table 8-2).

This difference in sensitivity was fairly constant upon repeated pure-tone evaluations conducted periodically in later years. The actual long-term difference was 9.5 dB better pure-tone sensitivity for 500, 1000, and 2000 Hz for the cleft palates repaired by the bilateral osteotomy technique.

As stated previously, there is a marked paucity of published long-term research on cleft palate closures by techniques other than the bilateral osteotomy, with the combination of cephalometric measurements for superior maxillary development, hearing, and speech on the same patients. Thus it is impossible to compare methods accurately. Nevertheless, there is

enough conglomerate evidence in the literature today regarding results with the Dorrance, V-Y, von Langenbeck, and Veau-Wardill-Kilner procedures to be convinced that these mucoperiosteal techniques do not reproduce the speech results demonstrated by the osteotomy operation.

In the previously published study by this author [48] of long-term osteotomy results in 93 patients, 88.2 percent showed adequate velopharyngeal functioning for speech and vocal quality. The speech and voice evaluations were done by four qualified speech pathologists: Susan Marks, M.S., Kathleen Miner, M.S., Ralph Leutenegger, Ph.D., and Robert Beecher, M.S. The remaining 11.8 percent of the patients required secondary management (see Table 8-3).

In a recent and as yet unpublished study, files of 74 primary bilateral osteotomy surgery cases performed by this author and 46 primary closures by mucoperiosteal techniques (Dorrance, V-Y, von Langenbeck, etc.) were reviewed. These were all consecutive cases pulled from the files of the Milwaukee Children's Hospital

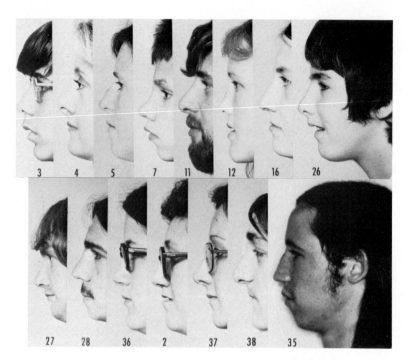

FIGURE 8-25. *Profile views, incomplete cleft palate cases. (Reprinted, with permission, from S. K. Wynn, Long-term results after cleft palate closure by bilateral osteotomy technique.* Plast. Reconstr. Surg. *58:71–79, 1976.)*

TABLE 8-2. *Hearing Table*

Cleft Palate Bilateral Osteotomy Repair Technique	Other Cleft Palate Repair Technique	Difference
18.0 dB	28.6 dB	10.6 dB

Note: Mean pure-tone air conduction thresholds at 500, 1000, and 2000 Hz (speech frequencies) for cleft palates repaired by the osteotomy technique (N = 200) and cleft palates repaired by other techniques (N = 140). Age range 3 to 13 years. Thresholds in decibels according to ANSI.
Reprinted with permission from S. K. Wynn, Long-term results after cleft palate closure by bilateral osteotomy technique. *Plast. Reconstr. Surg.* 58:71–79, 1976.

TABLE 8-3. *Speech Table*

Type of Cleft	Number of Cases	Voice Quality 1*	2†
Bilateral complete	20	17	3
Single complete	28	25	3
Incomplete	45	40	5
Total number of cases	93	82	11
Percentages	100%	88.2%	11.8%

*Normal quality or quality deviation unrelated to palatal function. In all but one of these cases, cinephonation study was normal; and in all cases, speech stimulability testing demonstrated the ability to achieve velopharyngeal closure and normal vocal quality.
†Abnormal quality related to palatal function requiring secondary management.
Reprinted with permission from S. K. Wynn, Long-term results after cleft palate closure by bilateral osteotomy technique. *Plast. Reconstr. Surg.* 58:71–79, 1976.

Cleft Palate Center by speech pathologist Amy Papador, M.S., and reviewed by our speech department chief Susan Marks, M.S. All cases had been referred for evaluation because of various problems and were previously reviewed by the entire Cleft Palate Team at Milwaukee Children's Hospital in the past 6 years (1971–1977). There was no attempt made at sifting out children with intellectual, emotional, and/or motor deficits, so the total figures must take this into account. Table 8-4 reveals that at least a 30 percent greater number of children required secondary surgical management for speech if they had a mucoperiosteal-type surgical procedure as compared with an osteotomy procedure. It also should be pointed out that these figures do not include many children who underwent osteotomy procedures and never came through the center for evaluation because there were no speech problems. The percentage difference, therefore, could possibly be even greater. All patients in our mobile society are difficult to follow if they have no loyalty to the team members because addresses and phone numbers change so frequently and are extremely difficult to track down.

Another interesting fact brought out in this study was that 82 percent successful speech and quality results were obtained with the initial superior-based pharyngeal flap procedures performed on 16 of the 74 patients seen by this author. Six percent of this flap group required secondary augmentation procedures to produce successful speech results. Twelve percent of the 16 patients never returned for official speech evaluation because of various reasons, e.g., financial, poor parental control, distance required to return, etc. However, all these patients were seen after surgery, and their operations were considered successful (in spite of the fact that many surgeons must be considered unsophisticated listeners). One can assume, therefore, considering that one surgeon (i.e., S. K. Wynn) did the pharyngeal flaps on both the postosteotomy and postmucoperiosteal cleft cases, that the chances for overall successful speech in the former are at least 98 percent as compared with a highest possible figure of 87

TABLE 8-4. *Unpublished Speech Table*

	Percentage
Primary bilateral osteotomy surgery and secondary management (n = 74):*	
Number not requiring secondary management of any type: 55	75
Flap being considered: 1	1
Number requiring secondary management	
a. Surgery: 16	22
1. 82 percent successful speech and quality results postflap.	
2. 6 percent successful speech results after augmentation procedure.	
3. 12 percent of patients never returned for reevaluation postflap.	
b. Prosthesis: 2	2
Secondary management subsequent to primary closures by other surgical techniques (Dorrance, V-Y, von Langenbeck, etc.; n = 46)	
Number not requiring secondary management of any type: 17	37
Flap being considered: 4	9
Number requiring secondary management	
a. Surgery: 24	52
1. 79 percent successful speech and quality results postflap.	
2. 4 percent also needed an appliance.	
3. 8 percent of patients never returned for reevaluation.	
4. 8 percent poor speech results.	
b. Prosthetic appliance: 1	2

*Includes children with intellectual, emotional, and motor deficits.

percent in the latter (assuming that the 8 percent of postmucoperiosteal cases who never returned were added in as successful speech results with the 79 percent of the evaluated group).

Jolleys [24] in 1954 concluded that the speech function was found to be better following operations performed before 2 years of age than following operations after 3 years of age. He also noted that there was a significant reduction in length of the soft palate in patients who had late operations. I go along with this thinking and start closure of the cleft palate, or indeed sometimes do a complete closure, at the age of 9 months.

To further confuse the picture, much emphasis was placed on, and a great deal of "jumping on the bandwagon" occurred concerning, primary bone grafting in clefts. This has simmered down now that adequate follow-up has been done, with the conclusions by Friede and Johanson [18] in 1974:

The bone graft of the anterior maxilla healed in every instance, but it resulted in an abnormal maxillary development with increased frequency of both lateral and anterior cross bites. The local and general maxillary growth retardation gave our cleft patients a pronounced maxillary retrognathia which increased with age. When fully grown, the facial profile of our patients will frequently be concave, in many cases to such an extent that we cannot recommend primary bone grafting.

The time has come to make some sense out of the confusion. Unfortunately, when first presenting the osteotomy operation, I used the term *bone-flap operation*. This term should not have been used, since it was confused with the original bone-flap procedures in which the chiseling was often actually done right into the nasal cavity. In some instances, such as in the earlier writings of Peer [37,38], Davis [12], and Brown [8,9], use of banding around the entire palate, through the nasal cavity and oral side, was noted. This is not done in this author's described osteotomy procedure. The osteotomy should be done just lateral to the nasal wall, since in this procedure the nasal cavity is not entered and the nasal tissues are stretched toward the midline. This is important in maintaining good circulation of the palate and good long-term results.

Recently I had the opportunity to see some of the simple (modified von Langenbeck) relaxing incision cases with closures of just the soft pal-

ate performed at another hospital when the patients were 1 year of age. The anterior palate had remained open. When I saw them, these children were over 4 years old (unfortunately poor speech habits had already become firmly established). In view of this fact, a bilateral osteotomy procedure was performed in order to close the posterior palate without wide mucoperiosteal elevation (Fig. 8-12). These patients actually had vocal quality that was not good enough even following the anterior osteotomy procedure. It was still necessary to do pharyngeal flaps in these patients to improve speech. Thus, in this type of case, the opportunity for early primary osteotomy with possible immediate palate lengthening and complete closure and better speech was lost.

It has actually been demonstrated at the surgical table by wire measurements from between the central incisor dental area on the alveolus and the tip of the uvula that a 1- to 1.5-cm gain in length can be obtained in a primary osteotomy operation in an infant. These actual measurements of length, which were just recently instituted, merely confirm that which has been observed at the operating table by the naked eye for over 30 years. Some recent typical examples in complete cleft patients aged 9 to 12 months follow:

Case I.   Immediate preop, 4.5 cm; postop, 5.5 cm
Case II.   Immediate preop, 3.8 cm; postop, 5.9 cm
Case III.   Immediate preop, 4.4 cm; postop, 5.9 cm
Case IV.   Immediate preop, 4.8 cm; postop, 5.8 cm
Case V.   Immediate preop, 4.0 cm; postop, 5.5 cm

It is true that the method of wire-length measurement can have some degree of error because of the increase in convexity of the palate postoperatively. However, the lengthening actually may be even more than indicated, since there is a higher arch present in the preoperative cleft palate with a consequent greater cur-

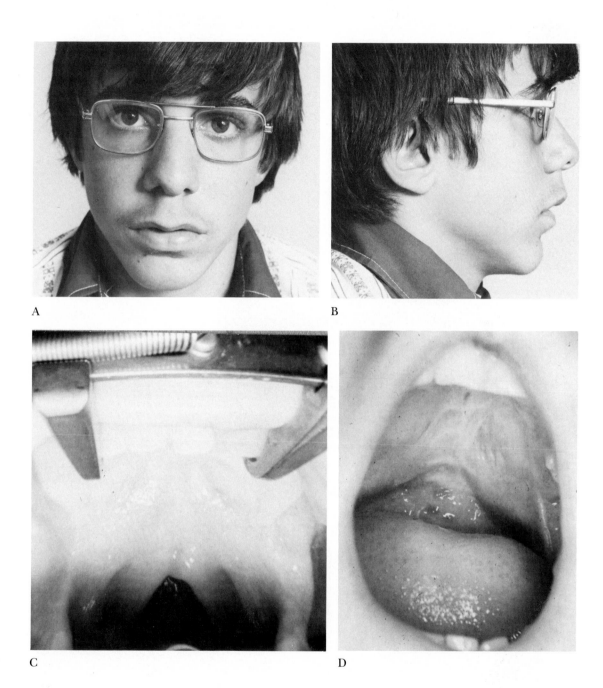

A

B

C

D

FIGURE 8-26. *(A through D) Incomplete cleft palate case, front view, side view, preoperative and postoperative views.*

vature of the wire in this preoperative measurement.

With all these facts in mind, the conclusion has been reached that early osteotomy procedures are here to stay for the best long-term demonstrable results until something still better comes along. I believe that reverting to only

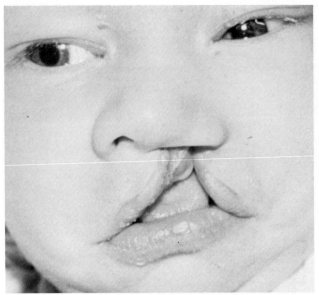

A

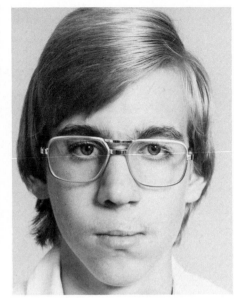

B

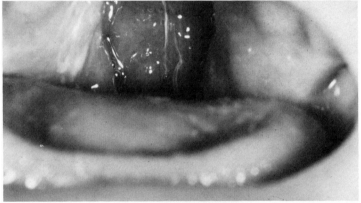

C

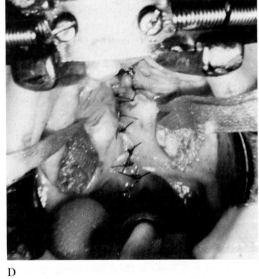

D

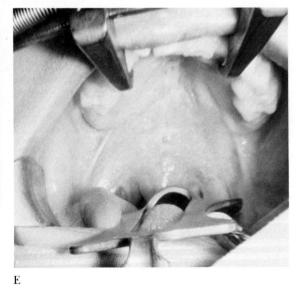

E

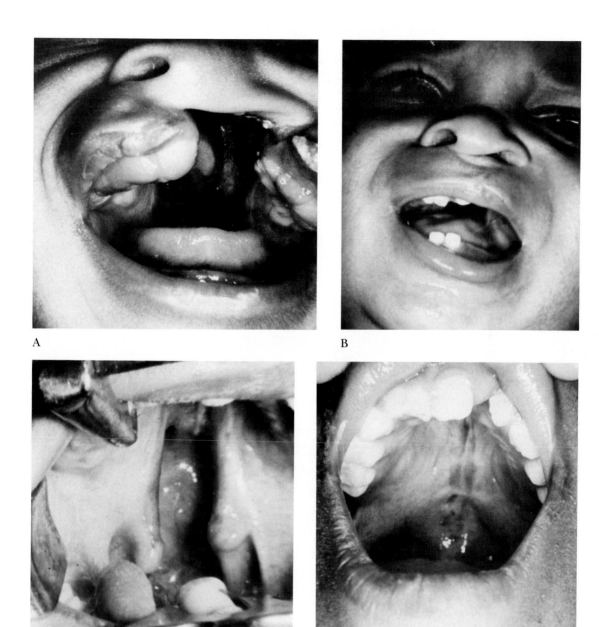

A

B

C

D

FIGURE 8-28.   (A and B) Wide complete cleft lip–cleft palate case. (C) Primary vomer flap procedure for anterior palate. (D) Osteotomy closure to complete posterior palate closure 6 months later.

FIGURE 8-27.   (A through E) Unilateral complete cleft lip–cleft palate case.

simple soft palate closures is again repetitive pioneering.

To give the anterior palates to the prosthodontic dentist is not always possible from the standpoint of location, willingness of the patient, and financial considerations. Why bow to this when an over 30-year proven technique is presently available for the learning?

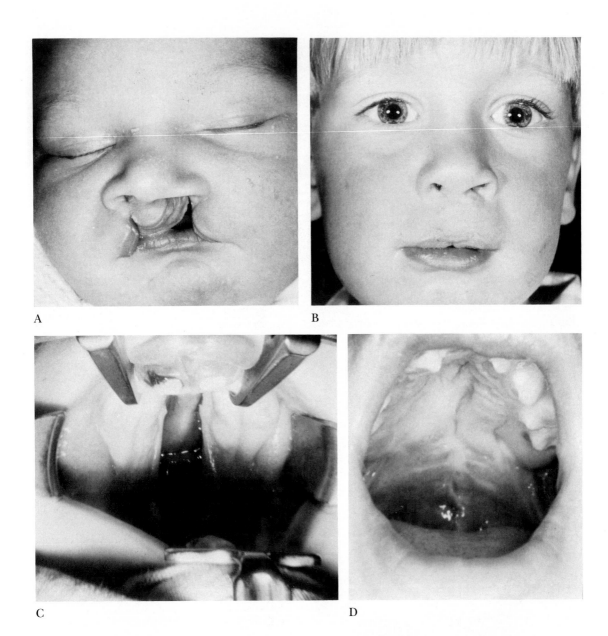

A   B

C   D

FIGURE 8-29. *(A through D) Bilateral cleft lip–cleft palate, primary closure effected by osteotomy technique.*

The following are five case examples:

Case I. Simple closure of isolated incomplete cleft palate by osteotomy. Here no superior maxillary developmental problems present themselves in osteotomy techniques (Fig. 8-26A through D).

Case II. Unilateral complete cleft lip–cleft palate case (Fig. 8-27 A through E).

Case III. Vomer flap surgery primarily, then lateral osteotomy palate closure. This procedure can readily be done as early as 9 months of age and does not cause retardation in growth of the superior maxilla, as proven by our cephalometric case studies. It is used immediately before or 6 months prior to a bilateral osteotomy closure in the

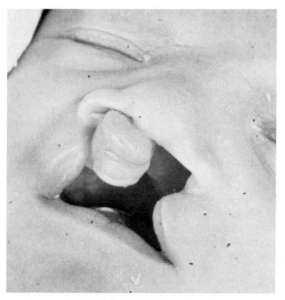

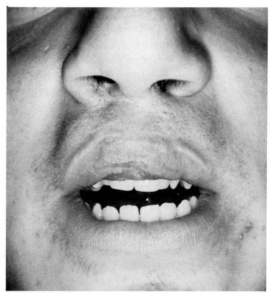

A

B

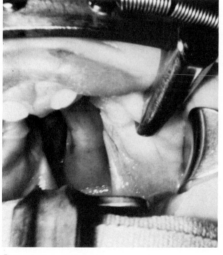

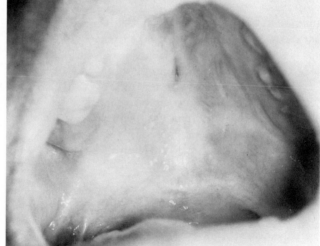

C   D

FIGURE 8-30.   *(A through D) Wide bilateral cleft lip–cleft palate case: vomer flap anterior closure, osteotomy posterior closure. Split-thickness upper labial sulcus skin graft reconstruction, whistle lip operation, and addition of fixed dental bridge.*

very wide, complete cleft palate cases only (Fig. 8-28A through D).

Case IV. Bilateral cleft lip–cleft palate case (Fig. 8-29A through D).

Case V. Vomer flap closure primarily, followed by osteotomy closure, superior labial sulcus

skin graft deepening, whistle lip operation, and later, dentures (Fig. 8-30A through D).

This chapter brings out long-term results in cleft palate surgery with different techniques. It details an efficient, basic surgical technique called *palatal osteotomy*. It is applicable to several classes of gnatho-urano-staphyloschises. There are minor variations as to the extent of the osteotomy, but nonetheless the principle is essentially the same in all instances of repair regardless of cleft form differences.

The completed work on the bilateral osteotomy procedure demonstrates that (1) it reconstructs the bony vault of the cleft palate; (2) it provides a soft, flexible, and mobile soft palate; (3) it provides maximum function of the eustachian tube in order to prevent socially significant hearing problems (audiology research has demonstrated that hearing is 10.6 dB better than hearing levels in children who have had closure of the cleft palate by other techniques, e.g., mucoperiosteal types); (4) it allows adequate maxillary mandibular posterior occlusal dental relationship; (5) vertical and horizontal development of the maxilla is comparable with an unoperated cleft sample; and (6) speech and voice research data have reflected successful communication results on 88.2 percent of the cases studied. Skeletal development and speech and hearing data will continue to be accumulated because it is agreed that the success of any primary cleft palate repair is contingent upon the results achieved in each of these areas over a long period.

In view of these facts gleaned from over 30 years of experience and ongoing research, it is felt that the bilateral osteotomy procedure in cleft palate surgery is a conservative and successful method of repair of the cleft palate.

Acknowledgment

I wish to acknowledge the aid and encouragement extended to me in the preparation of this chapter by the Milwaukee Children's Hospital Cleft Palate Team: Susan M. Marks, M.S., C.C.C., Kathleen Miner, M.S., C.C.C., Robert Beecher, M.S., Amy Papador, M.S., Thomas J. McGowan, D.D.S., M.S., Harvey Kleiner, M.D., Jerry E. Friedman, M.D., Earl G. Rosen, D.D.S., Ralph R. Leutenegger, Ph.D., Alfred L. Miller, Ph.D., Wilbert W. Wiviott, M.D., Marta M. Muller, M.D., Donald P. Babbitt, M.D., Byoung W. Kim, Ph.D., Michael S. Levine, M.D., Paul L. Lurenz, D.D.S., and Wendy Puza.

References

1. Babbitt, D.P. Personal communication, 1978. Experiences gleaned at the Milwaukee Children's Hospital from over ten years of cinefluorographic studies of bilateral osteotomy palate closures as compared to mucoperiosteal techniques.
2. Birch, J.R., and Lindsay, W.K. An evaluation of adults with repaired bilateral cleft lips and palates. *Plast. Reconstr. Surg.* 48: 457, 1971.
3. Bishara, S.E. The influence of palatoplasty and cleft length on facial development. *Cleft Palate J.* 10: 390, 1973.
4. Bishara, S.E., Ortho, D., Enemark, H., and Tharp, R.F. Cephalometric comparisons of the results of the Wardill-Kilner and von Langenbeck palatoplasties. *Cleft Palate J.* 13:319, 1976.
5. Blocksma, R., Leuz, C., and Mellenstig, K. A constructive program for managing cleft palates without the use of mucoperiosteal flaps. *Plast. Reconstr. Surg.* 55:160, 1975.
6. Brodie, A.G. On the growth patterns of the human head. *Am. J. Anat.* 68:209, 1941.
7. Broomhead, I.W. The nerve supply of the muscles of the soft palate. *Br. J. Plast. Surg.* 4: 1, 1952.
8. Brown, G.V.I. The surgical treatment of cleft palate. *J.A.M.A.* 87: 1379, 1926.
9. Brown, G.V.I. *The Surgery of Oral and Facial Diseases and Malformations* (4th ed.). Philadelphia:Lea & Febiger, 1938.
10. Caldarelli, D.D. Incidence and type of otologic disease in the older cleft palate patient. *Cleft Palate J.* 12: 311, 1975.
11. Coerdt, I., Full-Scharrer, G., and Hosl, E. Long-term results in surgical treatment of cleft lips and palates. *Prog. Pediatr. Surg.* 10: 1, 1977.
12. Davis, W.B. Harelip and cleft palate. *Ann. Surg* 87: 536, 1928.
13. Dunn, F.S. Management of cleft palate cases involving the hard palate so as not to interfere with the growth of the maxilla. *Plast. Reconstr. Surg.* 9: 108, 1952.
14. Farkas, L.G., and Lindsay, W.K. Morphology of the adult face following repair of bilateral cleft lip and palate in childhood. *Plast. Reconstr. Surg.* 47: 25, 1971.
15. Farkas, L.G., and Lindsay, W.K. Morphology of the orbital region in adults following the cleft lip–palate repair in childhood. *Am. J. Phys. Anthropol.* 37: 65, 1972.
16. Farkas, L.G., and Lindsay, W.K. Morphology of adult face after repair of isolated cleft palate in childhood. *Cleft Palate J.* 9: 132, 1972.
17. Farkas, L.G., and Lindsay, W.K. Morphology of the adult face following repair of unilateral cleft lip and palate in childhood. *Plast. Reconstr. Surg.* 52:652, 1973.
18. Friede, H., and Johanson, B. A follow-up

study of cleft children treated with primary bone grafting. *Scand. J. Plast. Reconstr. Surg.* 8: 88, 1974.

19. Graber, T.M.   Changing philosophies in cleft palate management. *J. Pediatr.* 37: 400, 1950.

20. Handelman, C.S., and Pruzansky, S.   Occlusion and dental profile with complete bilateral cleft lip and palate. *Angle Orthod.* 38: 185, 1968.

21. Honjo, I., Kojima, M., and Kumazawa, T.   Role of Passavant's ridge in cleft palate speech. *Arch. Otorhinolaryngol.* (N.Y.) 211: 203, 1975.

22. Hyslop, V.B., and Wynn, S.K.   Bone flap technique in cleft palate surgery. *Plast. Reconstr. Surg.* 9: 97, 1952.

23. Hyslop, V.B., Wynn, S.K., and Zwemer, T.   Bone flap technique in surgery of the cleft palate. *Am. J. Surg.* 92: 833, 1956.

24. Jolleys, A.   A review of the results of operations on cleft palates with reference to maxillary growth and speech function. *Br. J. Plast. Surg.* 7: 229, 1955.

25. Kremenak, C.R., Jr., Huffman, W.C., and Olin, W.H.   Maxillary growth inhibition by mucoperiosteal denudation of palatal shelf bone in non-cleft beagles. *Cleft Palate J.* 7: 817, 1970.

26. Kremenak, C.R., Jr., and Searls, J.C.   Experimental manipulation of midfacial growth: A synthesis of five years of research at the Iowa Maxillofacial Growth Laboratory. *J. Dent. Res.* 50: 1488, 1971.

27. Maher, W.   Distribution of palatal and other arteries in cleft and non-cleft human palates. *Cleft Palate J.* 14: 1, 1977.

28. Maher, W.   Personal communication, 1978.

29. Maisels, D.O.   The timing of the various operations required for complete alveolar clefts and their influence on facial growth. *Br. J. Plast. Surg.* 20: 230, 1967.

30. McGowan, T. J.   A study of the development of a multiple regression equation used in predicting the position of incisor teeth from certain roentgenographic cephalometric criteria in subjects with excellent occlusions. Marquette University M. S. thesis, 1967.

31. McGowan, T.J.   Mature, surgically repaired osteotomy cleft patients compared to unoperated oral clefts at maturation. Presented as part of research project of Cleft Palate Team, Milwaukee Children's Hospital, Milwaukee, Wisconsin, 1977.

32. Mestre, J., DeJesus, J., and Subtelny, J.D.   Unoperated oral clefts at maturation. *Angle Orthod.* 30: 78, 1960.

33. Miller, A.C., and Wynn, S.K.   Better hearing results in cleft palates. Read at the 32nd Annual Meeting of the American Cleft Palate Association, April 1974.

34. Moller, P.   Long-term otologic features of cleft palate patients. *Arch. Otolaryngol.* 101: 605, 1975.

35. Ortiz-Monasterio, F., Olmedo, A., Trigos, I., Yudovich, M., Velasquez, M., and Fuente-Del-Campo, A.   Final results from the delayed treatment of patients with clefts of the lip and palate. *Scand. J. Plast. Reconstr. Surg.* 8: 109, 1974.

36. Pannbacker, M.   Oral language skills of adult cleft palate speakers. *Cleft Palate J.* 12: 95, 1975.

37. Peer, L.A.   Cleft palate deformity and the bone-flap method of repair. *Surg. Clin. North Am.* 39: 313, 1959.

38. Peer, L.A., Hagerty, R., Hoffmeister, F.S., and Collito, M. B.   Repair of cleft palate by bone flap method. *J. Int. Coll. Surg.* 22: 463, 1954.

39. Pickrell, K.L., Clifford, E., Quinn, G., and Massengill, R.   Study of 100 cleft lip-palate patients operated upon 22 to 27 years ago by one surgeon. *Plast. Reconstr. Surg.* 49: 149, 1972.

40. Pionek, G.D.   A cephalometric roentgenographic study of cleft palate individuals surgically treated by the bone flap method. Marquette University M. S. thesis, 1970.

41. Pruzansky, S.   Pre-surgical orthopedics and bone grafting for infants with cleft lip and palate: A dissent. *Cleft Palate J.* 1: 164, 1964.

42. Ross, R.B.   Cleft lip and palate. *Appl. Ther.* 8:694, 1966.

43. Stenström, S., and Thilander, B.   Management of cleft palate cases using a modified Dunn procedure with skin graft to vomer flaps. *Scand. J. Plast. Reconstr. Surg.* 8: 67, 1974.

44. Subtelny, J.D., and Sakuda, M.   Muscle function, oral malformation and growth changes. *Am. J. Orthod.* 52: 495, 1966.

45. Wynn, S.K.   Bilateral osteotomy cleft palate surgery. From Davis & Geck Surgical Film Catalog; a 16-mm sound movie available through A.C.S., and also available through Plastic and Reconstructive Surgery Film Catalogue, 1977.

46. Wynn, S.K.   Technical clarification of the bone-flap method in surgery for cleft palate. *Am. J. Surg.* 98: 811, 1959.

47. Wynn, S.K.   In N.G. Georgiade and R.F. Hagerty (Eds.), *Symposium on Management of Cleft Lip and Palate and Associated Deformities.* St. Louis: Mosby, 1974. Pp. 153–160.

48. Wynn, S.K.   Long term results after cleft palate closure by bilateral osteotomy technique. *Plast. Reconstr. Surg.* 58: 71, 1976.

49. Wynn, S.K., and Miller, A.   Better hearing results in cleft palate repaired by the bone-flap technique. *Cleft Palate J.* 7: 455, 1970.

50. Yules, R.B.   Current concepts of treatment of ear disease in cleft palate children and adults. *Cleft Palate J.* 12: 315, 1975.

Robert Pool

COMMENTS ON CHAPTER 8

WYNN presents the broad thesis that the bilateral osteoplastic palate repair he espouses is superior to surgical repairs using mucoperiosteal flaps. If this is true, then everyone should be using the osteoplasty repair and abandoning procedures that use mucoperiosteal flaps in their various forms. I will leave it to the reader to distill from Wynn's exuberant advocacy whether this thesis is true on the whole or in some of its parts.

A remarkable biological fact which emerges from this study is that the palate heals with normal appearing bone after the osteoplasty repair even when that surgical defect consists of bone, periosteum, and mucous membrane. Does this mean that a bony defect of the palate is better repaired by the body than a defect of similar size which consists of periosteum and mucous membrane? At this point it is necessary to make an important distinction. There is a substantial difference between elevating a mucoperiosteal flap and leaving a defect of periosteum and mucous membrane. I think that the two are not the same. There is clinical and experimental evidence which demonstrates that when the defect of periosteum and mucous membrane is adjacent to the alveolar ridge, then alveolar collapse will be precipitated. I refer the reader to animal research by Kremenak and Searls [1], which demonstrates this effect. The postoperative hour-glass deformity after the Veau-Wardill-Kilner repair is adequate clinical evidence of that fact. In that same regard, it is worth examining one significant short series to which Wynn refers. He quotes Stenström's work, where the vomer flap was used as a preliminary procedure in closure of wide clefts. The major thrust of Stenström's report, however, was that he did not leave a raw area, but covered the void with split-thickness grafts under the vomer flap. He demonstrated, to my satisfaction at least, remarkable long-term results both in maxillary arch form and mucous membrane replacement, and I have used split grafts in 10 similar cases with excellent results.

The speech results that were achieved in this series are certainly better than reported with some of the mucoperiosteal flap procedures, but they are approximately equal to Stark's series, where a conservative von Langenbech palatoplasty was performed with a primary pharyngeal flap. Stark reports that 83 percent of his patients had normal speech and required no secondary procedures.

I agree with Wynn wholeheartedly in condemning palatal procedures that use intravelar muscle dissection. He states accurately that palatal scar, decreased vascularity, and risk of denervation are hazards. Whether or not separation of the soft palate from the posterior margin of the hard palate gives denervation is an interesting hypothesis and is possible but as yet unproven.

I am impressed that Wynn's series demonstrated that hearing was 10 dB better than in a comparable series using mucoperiosteal flaps. This could be due to more appropriate preservation of tensor and levator velopalatal muscles. This chapter is certainly the best presentation of the osteoplasty repair to date and gives an excellent long-term follow-up on this fascinating and provocative series of techniques.

Reference

1. Kremenak, C.R., Jr., and Searls, J.C. Experimental manipulation of midfacial growth: A synthesis of five years of research at Iowa Maxillofacial Growth Laboratory. *J. Dent Res.* 50: 1488, 1971.

9   RECONSTRUCTION of the auricle is a knotty problem which has baffled plastic surgeons for many years. The frustrations encountered are epitomized in the words of Bouisson, a French surgeon, who consoled his colleagues in the following manner: "The accolades for Tagliacozzi who, in the sixteenth century, pretended to make ears, should no longer trouble the sleep of surgeons. Their creations would be so dissimilar to those of nature that patients would have to hide them under their hair with more care than they would the amputation site itself." Nevertheless, the struggle has continued. The efforts of surgeons such as J. F. Dieffenbach, Sir Harold Gillies, George Pierce, Jerome Webster, Barrett Brown, and Lyndon Peer testify to the many ingenious and sometimes fanciful attempts designed to produce an inconspicuous ear.

During the past 20 years or so, a rekindling of interest in the subject has resulted in the development of several procedures which are capable of producing an acceptable auricle. The author, using autogenous costal cartilage [22], has advocated a method which Furnas [12] and Brent [2,3] have modified, using an open framework which requires less material. Gorney [13] and Davis [6,7] have extended the use of conchal cartilage to create an entire auricular framework. Using a very different concept, Cronin [4,5] has succeeded in building nicely contoured auricles with an inorganic framework of silicone rubber, a technique which has been pursued most enthusiastically by Ohmori [15,16]. Yarchuk [30] has even fashioned acceptable ears by the injection of preserved homografts of diced cartilage, based on the original experiments of Limberg [14], but the incidence of absorption early in the

Radford C. Tanzer

RECONSTRUCTION OF MICROTIA

postoperative course has rendered the method unacceptable.

Most plastic surgeons feel that although conchal cartilage is an excellent material for constructing partial losses of the auricle, the available cartilage is insufficient for a complete reconstruction. So the principal decision involves the selection of either autogenous rib cartilage or an inorganic material such as silicone rubber for construction of the auricular framework.

Throughout the rather extensive series of articles describing these varied methods, one is struck by the scarcity of long-term follow-up reports. Techniques are discarded in favor of later modifications, with no information on the fate of the older methods. So it is with the hope of encouraging more frequent long-term reports that this opportunity is taken to present an extended follow-up of all but one of the cases of complete microtia treated and followed over a 19-year period.

Personal Experience with Microtia

CASES STUDIED

I operated on 44 patients with complete microtia between 1957 and 1971. For the most part, these patients were characterized by a deformity composed of a diminutive lobule surmounted by a nubbin of rolled-up cartilage representing the elements of the auricle. Two had a diminutive concha and ear canal; the others had atresia of the ear canal and absence of the concha. Only one patient required complete reconstruction of both ears, although several had significant bilateral deformities requiring less than complete reconstruction on the second side. In the patients with unilateral deformities, 23 occurred on the right, 20 on the left. The sex ratio was 34 male and 10 female. Thirty-six patients reside in the United States or Canada, 5 in Brazil, and 1 each in Mexico, South Africa, and Pakistan. Twelve had had previous operations on the auricle, ranging from 1 to 17 procedures, and 2 had had reconstructions of the middle ear.

Every case required the fabrication of a complete framework. A number of patients with other congenital deformities, including 21 patients with constricted (cup and lop) ears, were omitted from the study in order to reduce the number of variables.

METHODS OF RECONSTRUCTION

Autogenous costal cartilage was used exclusively for the fabrication of the framework, although conchal cartilage from the same or opposite side is favored for the reconstruction of less severe defects.

Variables in technique were kept at a minimum to make the postoperative follow-up more meaningful. The original procedure and two minor variations were used throughout the series. The variations were designed to shorten the length of time required to complete the reconstruction and did not deviate from the original concept. The method of removing rib cartilage and fabricating the framework, the use of suture material, and the postoperative care remained constant during the entire series. Twelve of the cases had had previous operative procedures, so it was sometimes necessary to do a preliminary revision in order to improve the quality and vascularity of skin to be used as cover. In several instances this entailed the replacement of scarred integument by free, full-thickness grafts.

The *temporary-tunnel technique*, also referred to as the valise-handle technique, was used in the first 19 patients with microtia [22,23,28]. After a preliminary rotation of the diminutive lobule into a transverse position, a cartilage framework was fashioned from the sixth, seventh, and eighth rib cartilages of the opposite chest wall and was embedded subcutaneously in the mastoid area. Four months later the framework was elevated from the side of the head by creating a large aperture beneath it which served to place the auricle at a satisfactory angle to the head and which developed at the same time a well-defined posterior conchal wall. Finally, the conchal cavity was deepened, the tragus was constructed, and the temporary tunnel, which had contracted in the meantime to a smaller size, was completely closed (Figs. 9-1 and 9-2).

The *four-stage procedure* was used on the next 22 patients. One patient required bilateral correction. The reconstruction consisted of (1) rotation of the lobule, (2) fabrication and embedment of the framework, (3) elevation of the auricle without the creation of a valise handle, and (4) construction of the tragus and conchal cavity [24]. This method produced an auricle that lay closer to the side of the head than the previous method. However, it had the advantage of simplicity, while still producing an acceptable reconstruction (Fig. 9-3).

The *three-stage procedure* was used on the last three patients. This method combined rotation of the lobule and fabrication and embedment of the cartilage framework in one operative procedure [25,28]. This not only reduced the number of stages, but also permitted more accurate placement of the lobule. It is the method of choice, provided the lobule does not require extensive mobilization in order to place it at its proper level.

Thirteen-Year Review

The first cartilage framework was embedded in 1957, and 13 years later the first comprehensive review of all cases was completed. Forty-four reconstructions in 43 patients were included in the review, which was based on a perusal of all records, direct interviews and examinations in 17 cases, and the results of a questionnaire in 26 cases.

OPERATIVE COMPLICATIONS DURING THE RECONSTRUCTION

No complications caused permanent marring of the appearance of the reconstructed ears. An exposure of the cartilage transplant occurred in five instances. Three of these appeared as small losses of free skin graft on the medial surface of the ear, and all healed under conservative management within 30 days. On two occasions, small areas of exposed cartilage occurred on the free margin of the reconstructed helix several days after the embedment of the cartilage transplant. These losses were due presumably to undue tightness of the compression sutures used to snug the skin into the helical sulcus. Both were treated by first excising an ellipse of compromised skin surrounding the defect and then undermining and advancing the medial skin margin to permit closure without tension. Both areas remained stable thereafter. One factitious ulcer, resulting from persistent scratching of the skin graft lining the auriculocephalic sulcus, required regrafting. One cartilage framework seemed too large after its embedment and was removed, trimmed down to suitable size, and reimplanted.

Five pleural tears, incurred during the course of removal of donor cartilage, caused no sequelae. Three seromas of the abdominal wall at the site of embedment of surplus cartilage required aspiration.

POSTRECONSTRUCTION COMPLICATIONS

Several abnormalities of form required correction. A shallow helical sulcus was revised in

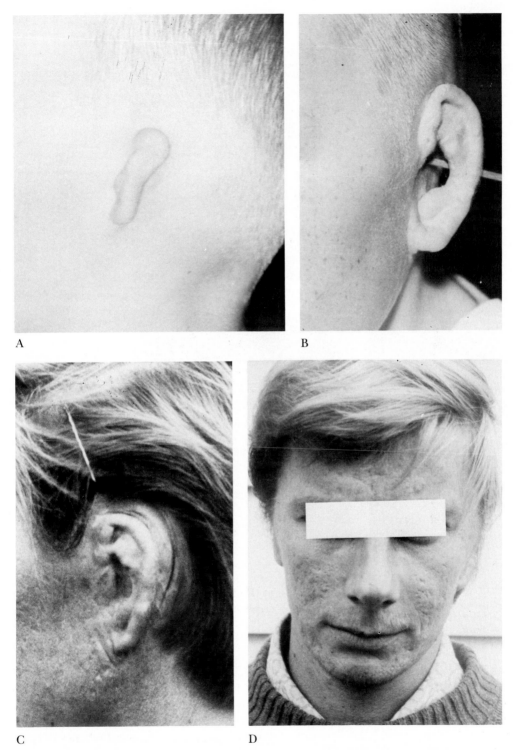

A

B

C

D

FIGURE 9-1. *(A) Six-year-old boy with microtia and atresia of the ear canal. (B) Reconstructed auricle, using the temporary tunnel technique, which gives access for middle* *ear exploration. Later, the tragus will be constructed and the tunnel closed. (C and D) Fifteen years after reconstruction.*

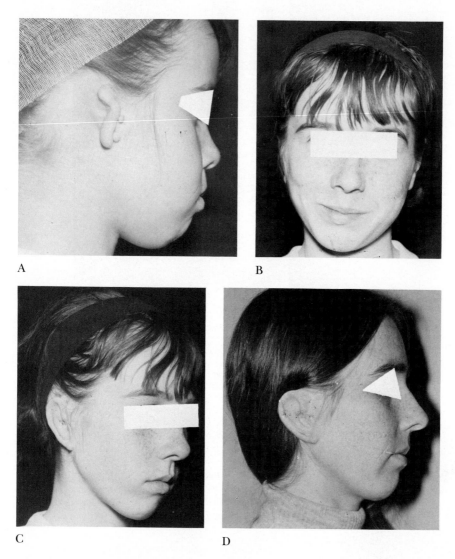

FIGURE 9-2. *(A) Six-year-old girl with microtia and atresia of the ear canal. (B and C) Four years after reconstruction by the temporary tunnel technique. (D) Fourteen years after reconstruction.*

three instances. One contracture of the conchal cavity required excision of cartilage and the addition of more skin graft. In two instances, resuturing was required when the anterior arm of the helical cartilage became displaced forward as a result of loosening of the fixation sutures. Three patients reconstructed by the valise-handle technique developed small perforations in the free skin graft closing the aperture that required secondary closure.

Long-Term Follow-up

In 1976 a long-term study of this same group of patients, together with one additional patient subjected to the three-stage method, was undertaken [26,27]. All but 1 of the 44 cases (including one bilateral reconstruction) were surveyed, 4 by direct interview and 39 by questionnaire. The length of time after reconstruc-

128

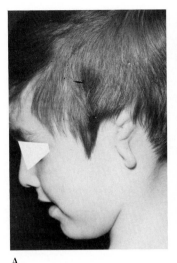
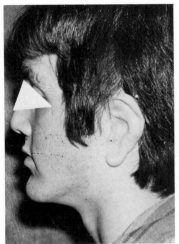
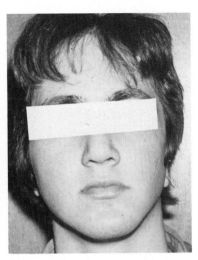

A   B   C

FIGURE 9-3. *(A) Six-year-old boy with typical microtia and atresia of the ear canal. (B and C) Nine years after a four-stage reconstruction of the auricle.*

tion ranged from 6 to 19 years (Table 9-1). The study was undertaken with three principal objectives in mind: (1) to determine the growth potential of the reconstructed auricle, (2) to discover any late changes not apparent in the earlier survey, and (3) to make a rough evaluation of the effect of the congenital deformity on the social life of the patients.

METHOD OF STUDY

The material was gathered by questionnaire, except for four patients interviewed directly. The heights of both normal and reconstructed

TABLE 9-1. *Length of Follow-Up*

Number of Years from Cartilage Embedment to 1976 Review	Number of Auricles
6 to 9	26
10 to 14	13
15 to 19	5

Reproduced, with permission, from R.C. Tanzer, Microtia —A long-term follow-up of forty-four reconstructed auricles. *Plast. Reconstr. Surg.* 61:161, 1978.

auricles were recorded twice by relatives, one by measurement and another by tracing the auricular contours on transparent film. The tracings were measured when the questionnaire was returned, and the measurements supplied by the families were averaged with our measurements of the tracings to give the figures which were used in the study. The records of 37 patients were sufficiently well documented to compare measurements taken at the completion of the reconstruction with those taken in 1976.

In addition, information was obtained concerning the chest incision, lack of definition of the auricular concavities, softening and exposure of the framework, and extrusion of the wire sutures used in the construction of the framework. Also, the patients were asked to evaluate the effects of the deformity on their daily social contacts, and the families were requested to comment if their opinion varied from that of the patient.

RESULTS

The height of the reconstructed ears, measured at the time of completion of surgery, varied from 4.9 to 6.6 cm, compared with 5.1 to 6.8 cm on the normal side. The bar graph (Fig. 9-4) compares the increase in height of the 37 pairs

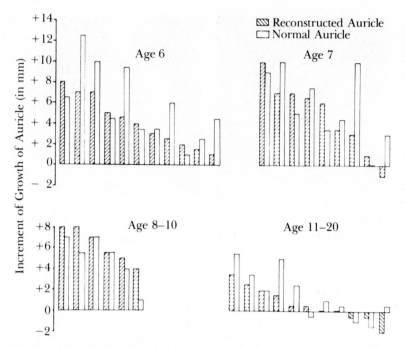

FIGURE 9-4. *Comparative increments of growth in 37 pairs of reconstructed and normal auricles, with patients grouped by age at start of reconstruction. Growth is measured from the time of completion of the reconstruction to 1976. (From R. C. Tanzer, Microtia—A long-term follow-up of forty-four reconstructed auricles. Plast. Reconstr. Surg. 61:161, 1978.)*

of auricles on which data are complete. An increase in height is noted in 31 reconstructed ears and in 33 normal ears, while 6 reconstructed and 4 normal ears are recorded as showing no growth or an actual decrease in height, the maximum decrease being 2 mm. The average increase in height of the reconstructed ears is 3.6 mm; that of the normal ears, 4.4 mm.

Table 9-2 shows a breakdown of the patients according to age group. The average increment of growth of both reconstructed and normal auricles is virtually the same in patients operated on during the first decade of life. Almost one-third of the patients were treated during the second decade of life, and as one might expect, even though the follow-up period is longest in this group, the growth factor is negli-

TABLE 9-2. *Increments of Growth in Reconstructed and Normal Auricles*

Age at Start of Reconstruction	Number of Cases	Average Number of Years, Follow-Up	Average Increase in Height (in millimeters)	
			Reconstructed Ear	Normal Ear
6	11	8.0	+4.1	+5.8
7	9	8.2	+4.8	+5.8
8 to 10	6	8.2	+6.2	+5.0
11 to 20	11	9.8	+0.7	+1.5

Reproduced, with permission, from R.C. Tanzer, Microtia—A long-term follow-up of forty-four reconstructed auricles. *Plast. Reconstr. Surg.* 61:161, 1978.

gible. Only two reconstructed ears and four normal ears in this group show more than a 2-mm increase in height (Fig. 9-4).

LATE COMPLICATIONS

Shallowness of contours, especially loss of depth of the helical sulcus, had been corrected three times in the early postoperative period and was noted again by five patients during this survey. Three of these patients had had surgery prior to our reconstruction, indicating the significance of the scar in the production of this deformity.

Exposure of the cartilage framework had taken place five times during the course of the reconstruction, as noted earlier. The integument had remained stable in the three patients who evidenced spontaneous healing and in the two auricles that had been closed surgically. None of the remaining 38 patients had sustained any exposure of cartilage, although no special restriction had been imposed, other than the avoidance of contact sports such as football and wrestling unless proper headgear was used.

Eleven patients recalled the removal of extruding metal sutures used during the fabrication of the framework. In fact, the extraction of 20 sutures was recorded in the 1970 survey, several patients having experienced this on two or more occasions.

The knot of the metal suture is usually found at the base of a small tract within the free skin graft on the medial surface of the reconstructed auricle. Because of a lack of symptoms, patients are advised to inspect the back of the ear with a mirror, or have it inspected by a family member, every 2 weeks during the first year after surgery. Once a tract is detected, the suture is very simply removed in toto by picking up the knot with a hemostat, cutting one side of the loop, and gently extracting the suture. In no instance has the sinus persisted following suture removal. The tolerance of cartilage for the prolonged presence of an extruding suture was made evident in a patient who had had a reconstruction of the auricle to correct a post-traumatic deformity. He was aware of a small

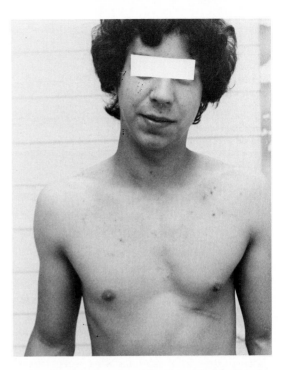

FIGURE 9-5. *Depression of the chest wall, 10 years after the removal of the left sixth, seventh, and eighth rib cartilages.*

area of chronic inflammation for almost a year, at which time a suture presumably extruded itself completely and the lesion healed. When we saw him later in follow-up, a small indentation on the helical rim was the only residual.

A depression of the chest wall in the region of the operative incision was reported by seven patients (Fig. 9-5). All but one of these were male, and all were in the 6- and 7-year age group except one, an 11-year-old child with a poorly developed skeletal framework. The usual description was a "hollowness" or "depression" of the chest. One described a protrusion of the ribs superior to the site of cartilage removal. Another noted a "twisted" chest wall which became less noticeable as growth proceeded. The follow-up period in this group of seven patients averaged almost 10 years. In addition, three of the chest scars were hypersensitive and one was hypertrophic.

Only one of the group of 43 patients had had a subsequent operation on the reconstructed

TABLE 9-3. *Patient's Estimate of Effects of Deformity on Daily Social Contacts*

None*	23
Minor	15
Moderate	4
Severe	0

*One patient replied "Satisfied."
Reproduced, with permission, from R.C. Tanzer, Microtia —A long-term follow-up of forty-four reconstructed auricles. *Plast. Reconstr. Surg.* 61:161, 1978.

auricle after release from our care. It consisted of a secondary release of the ear from the side of the head and a reduction of the lobule's prominence.

PSYCHOLOGICAL EFFECTS

An attempt was made to gain some impression of the psychological status of the patients by asking for comments on the effects of the microtia on social contacts and activities. In the cases of the four patients who were directly interviewed, all are completely adjusted and feel that the microtia plays no significant role in their lives. Two are happily married, and one has just finished medical school. The response of the entire group is tabulated in Table 9-3. Of 10 parents who added comments of their own, 9 echoed their children's favorable opinions. In one case, the patient expressed dissatisfaction with the result and the mother likewise felt disappointment, stating that her child suffers from self-consciousness. Of the 14 patients over 21 years of age, 6 are married.

Discussion

How large should one make a reconstructed ear? Since no valid answer to this question has been offered in the past, this constituted one of our principal objectives in carrying out this late postoperative study. Symmetry between the reconstructed and normal ear, particularly when the reconstruction is done in young children, will depend on two factors: the growth potential of the normal ear and the growth potential of the rib cartilage transplant.

GROWTH POTENTIALS

Farkas [10] has noted that after the rapid growth spurt in the first year of life, ear growth in males slows down. In fact, it undergoes periods of almost complete cessation between years 1 and 2, 3½ and 4, 7 and 9, and 11½ and 13½. After 9 years of age, the ear grows only about 5 mm up to the time of maturity. In females, the growth pattern is more regular. Since the reconstruction is usually postponed until 6 years of age, one might assume that growth of the normal ear up to the time of maturity would not be substantially more than 5 or 6 mm.

Rib cartilage, on the other hand, has a much greater potential for growth after age 6. The viability of autogenous rib cartilage transplants has been documented by numerous authors. Farkas notes that the maximum growth of hyaline rib cartilage occurs during the first 4 years of life, but that the thickness of the cartilage increases during the first 30 years of life, the sharpest growth spurt taking place between 12 and 18 years of age.

EXPERIMENTAL EVIDENCE OF
CARTILAGE GROWTH

In 1941 Dupertuis [8] demonstrated definite growth of auricular cartilage in young rabbits, a finding that was confirmed by Stoll and Furnas [21] and by Allison, Achauer, and Furnas [1]. Growth occurred in cartilage that was removed both extraperichondrially and subperichondrially. Peer's group [18,29] also repeated Dupertuis's experiments but failed to note any growth in the transplants. Young [31] also failed to observe, over a period of 18 months, any growth of rib cartilage implanted subcutaneously in dogs.

CLINICAL EVIDENCE OF
CARTILAGE GROWTH

Clinical evidence of growth of cartilage transplants is meager. Padgett and Stephenson [17] examined two autogenous cartilage grafts buried in the abdominal wall 8 and 13 years after embedment, noting that the cartilage appeared viable and without evidence of absorption. Dupertuis [9] transplanted costal cartilage grafts denuded of perichondrium to reconstruct the nasal bridges of two children and found 6 mm of growth in each instance when measured through the skin several years later. A third patient displaying the Treacher-Collins syndrome received costal cartilage grafts to both malar regions. When measured 4 years later at the time of reimplantation of more cartilage, both grafts had increased 6 mm in length.

Conclusions

1. Based on studies of 37 patients with reconstructed microtia 6 to 19 years after operation, one may conclude that an auricle reconstructed with autogenous rib cartilage grows, except for minor variations, at roughly the same rate as the normal auricle up to the time of maturity. The conclusion is based on measurements of the height of auricles at the completion of surgery and again in 1976. The relative importance of the cartilage graft and the soft tissues in this increased height has not been determined, although it can be assumed that since most of the patients had a substantial amount of lobule present, at least part of the growth is attributable to enlargement of this structure. Farkas found that the height of the lobule increases from 5 mm at 5 months of age to 10 mm at puberty.

A breakdown of patients into four age groups shows that growth of the reconstructed auricle is active and roughly parallels growth of the normal auricle up to age 10. During the second decade of life, growth of both reconstructed and normal ears declines abruptly, confirming the growth pattern outlined by Figalova and Farkas [11].

2. Auricles constructed with autogenous rib cartilage in patients ranging from 8 years of age to maturity should be made the same size as the normal auricle, with the expectation that growth of the auricles will be comparable on each side. In children 6 or 7 years of age, since

growth of the normal ear exceeded that of the reconstructed ear by 3 mm or more in almost half the cases, it seems reasonable to make the reconstructed ear about 2-mm longer than the opposite ear.

3. This long-term study of 43 patients with reconstructed microtia indicates that softenning, shrinkage, and extrusion of the auricular framework can be avoided by using the surgical procedures described.

4. A postoperative depression of the chest wall at the operative site has been noted as a late complication in 16 percent of the cases. Throughout the series, a single technique has been used, consisting of the removal of the sixth, seventh, and eighth rib cartilages, together with their perichondrium, leaving the synchondrosis between the sixth and seventh ribs intact. In view of this late complication, it is suggested that a subperichondrial dissection of the rib cartilages is preferable in order to promote the postoperative deposition of a rigid, plate-like rib substitute which will minimize deformation of the chest wall [19,20].

An expeditious method of removal of the sixth, seventh, and eighth rib cartilages is illustrated in Figure 9-6. A T-incision of the perichondrium of the eighth rib (shown in dotted lines) is made, and the rib cartilage is separated and removed. The pattern of the proposed framework (A) is placed over the sixth and seventh ribs and the synchondrosis. The required amount of cartilage is marked out (vertical dotted lines). The perichondrium of the sixth and seventh ribs is then incised (horizontal dotted lines) and is peeled away from the anterior surfaces and sides of the two ribs in the direction indicated by the arrows, leaving the synchondrosis intact (crosshatched area). After dividing the two ribs laterally, they can be partially lifted, and the separation of the perichondrium from the visceral rib surfaces can be done under direct vision. The perichondrium should be reconstituted as well as possible by suturing, and any unattached strips should be replaced as free grafts.

5. Loss of definition of the auricular contours, noted by 11 percent of our patients, can

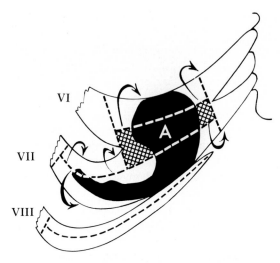

FIGURE 9-6. *A suggested method of subperichondrial removal of rib cartilage designed to avoid late distortion of the chest wall (see text for details). (From R. C. Tanzer, Microtia. In D. W. Furnas (Ed.),* Clinics in Plastic Surgery *(Vol. 5). Philadelphia: Saunders, 1978.)*

be minimized by taking precautions during the fabrication and embedment of the framework. The helical sulcus should be kept as deep as possible, and a strip of cartilage should be added to the helix if necessary to emphasize the depth. When the pocket in the mastoid region is prepared for reception of the framework, the skin cover should be kept as thin as possible without endangering the subdermal plexus of vessels. After the framework has been embedded in the pocket through a conchal incision, the skin cover should be allowed to slide centrifugally into the concavities of the scapha. This maneuver creates a circular skin defect on the conchal floor which should be closed by a full-thickness skin graft rather than a primary closure, which is likely to cause undue tension on the skin cover.

6. Metal sutures have been used in construction of the framework since they lend stability during construction and embedment. Extrusion must be expected occasionally, particularly on the back of the ear where the free skin graft creates a vulnerable site. The sutures are easily removed, and no complications have been experienced in our series. The incidence of extru-

sion can be lessened by embedding the knot below the surface of the cartilage at the time of placement of the suture.

7. Of forty-three patients with microtia corrected by autogenous rib cartilage graft, 88 percent have been relieved of serious emotional burdens, judging from responses obtained during this study. In most instances, they also have been spared the need for further operative revisions.

References

1. Allison, G.R., Achauer, B.M., and Furnas, D.W. Growth of homotransplanted ear cartilage in baby rabbits. *Plast. Reconstr. Surg.* 55:479, 1975.
2. Brent, B. Discussion of Microtia: A Panel Presentation. In R.C. Tanzer and M.T. Edgerton (Eds.), *Symposium on Reconstruction of the Auricle.* St. Louis: Mosby, 1974. P. 89.
3. Brent, B. Ear reconstruction with an expansile framework of autogenous rib cartilage. *Plast. Reconstr. Surg.* 53:619, 1974.
4. Cronin, T.D. Use of a Silastic frame for total and subtotal reconstruction of the external ear: Preliminary report. *Plast. Reconstr. Surg.* 37:399, 1966.
5. Cronin, T.D. Use of a Silastic Frame for Construction of the Auricle. In R.C. Tanzer and M.T. Edgerton (Eds.), *Symposium on Reconstruction of the Auricle.* St. Louis: Mosby, 1974. P. 33.
6. Davis, J.E. On auricular construction. *The International Microform Journal of Aesthetic Plastic Surgery,* Otoplasty, 1972-C.
7. Davis, J. Auricle Reconstruction. In M.N. Saad and P. Lichtveld (Eds.), *Reviews in Plastic Surgery.* Amsterdam: Excerpta Medica, 1974. Pp. 109–140.
8. Dupertuis, S.M. Actual growth of young cartilage grafts in rabbits. *Arch. Surg.* 43:32, 1941.
9. Dupertuis, S.M. Growth of young human autogenous cartilage grafts. *Plast. Reconstr. Surg.* 5:486, 1950.
10. Farkas, L.G. Growth of Normal and Reconstructed Auricles. In R.C. Tanzer and M.T. Edgerton (Eds.), *Symposium on Reconstruction of the Auricle.* St. Louis: Mosby, 1974.
11. Figalová, P., and Farkas, L.G. Localisation of auricle by means of anthropometric methods. *Acta Chir. Plast.* (Praha) 10:7, 1968.
12. Furnas, D.W. Problems in Planning Reconstruction in Microtia. In R.C. Tanzer and M.T. Edgerton (Eds.), *Symposium on Reconstruction of the Auricle.* St. Louis: Mosby, 1974. P. 93.

13. Gorney, M., Murphy, S., and Falces, E. Spliced autogenous conchal cartilage in secondary ear reconstruction. *Plast. Reconstr. Surg.* 47:432, 1971.
14. Limberg. A.A. Late results of homotransplantation with chopped cartilage. *Acta Chir. Plast.* (Praha) 4:59, 1962.
15. Ohmori, S., Matsumoto, K., and Nakai, H. Follow-up study on reconstruction of microtia with a silicone framework. *Plast. Reconstr. Surg.* 53:555, 1974.
16. Ohmori, S., Nakai, H., and Matsumoto, K. Unfavorable Results of External Ear Reconstruction Using Silicone Frame—Their Avoidance and Treatment. In D. Marchac and J.T. Hueston (Eds.), *Transactions of the Sixth International Congress of Plastic and Reconstructive Surgery.* Paris: Masson, 1976.
17. Padgett, E.C., and Stephenson, K.L. *Plastic and Reconstructive Surgery.* Springfield, Ill.: Thomas, 1948. P. 98.
18. Peer. L.A., Walia, I.S., and Bernhard, W.G. Further studies of the growth of rabbit ear cartilage grafts. *Br. J. Plast. Surg.* 19:105, 1966.
19. Ravitch, M.M. Disorders of the Chest Wall. In D.C. Sabiston (Ed.), *Textbook of Surgery: The Biological Basis of Modern Practice* (11th ed.). Philadelphia: Saunders, 1977. Pp. 2143–2152.
20. Robiscek, F., Mullen, D.C., Hall, D.G., and Masters, T.N. Technical considerations in the surgical management of pectus excavatum and carinatum. *Ann. Thorac. Surg.* 18:549, 1974.
21. Stoll, D.A., and Furnas, D.W. The growth of cartilage transplants in baby rabbits. *Plast. Reconstr. Surg.* 45:356, 1970.
22. Tanzer, R.C. Total reconstruction of the external ear. *Plast. Reconstr. Surg.* 23:1, 1959.
23. Tanzer, R.C. An analysis of ear reconstruction. *Plast. Reconstr. Surg.* 31:16, 1963.
24. Tanzer, R.C. Total reconstruction of the auricle: The evolution of a plan of treatment. *Plast. Reconstr. Surg.* 47:523, 1971.
25. Tanzer, R.C. Correction of Microtia with Autogenous Costal Cartilage. In R.C. Tanzer and M.T. Edgerton (Eds.), *Symposium on Reconstruction of the Auricle.* St. Louis: Mosby, 1974. P. 46.
26. Tanzer, R.C. Microtia—A long-term follow-up of forty-four reconstructed auricles. *Plast. Reconstr. Surg.* 61:161, 1978.
27. Tanzer, R.C. Microtia. In D.W. Furnas (Ed.), *Clinics in Plastic Surgery.* Philadelphia: Saunders, 1978.
28. Tanzer, R.C., Belluci, R.J., Converse, J.M., and Brent, B. Deformities of the Auricle. In J.M. Converse (Ed.), *Reconstructive Plastic Surgery* (2nd ed.). Philadelphia: Saunders, 1977. Vol. 3, p. 1671.
29. Walia, I., Peer, L.A., Bernhard, W.G., and Gordon, H.W. Does growth occur in young rabbit ear cartilage grafts transplanted in young rabbits? *Plast. Reconstr. Surg.* 29:259, 1962.
30. Yarchuk, N.I., Limberg, A.A., and Nekachalov, V.V. Clinical and histological characteristics of late results of otoplasty using diced cadaver cartilage. *Acta Chir. Plast.* (Praha) 17:188, 1975.
31. Young, F.A. Autogenous cartilage grafts. *Surgery* 10:7, 1941.

Osamu Fukuda

COMMENTS ON CHAPTER 9

THIS chapter by Dr. Tanzer is extremely interesting and noteworthy because his data show that the reconstructed ear does grow fairly well although less so than the normal ear. The information presented by Dr. Tanzer on the basis of his systematic study should contribute to our understanding of the suitable age for ear reconstruction. Although follow-up records on growth of the auricle in my series of patients are insufficient for evaluation, and although it is difficult to ascertain the rates of growth for operations done at various ages and with different types of remnants, I nevertheless was able to determine that up to 8 mm of growth occurred between 4 and 11 years after cartilage grafting in 30 children who had ear rebuilding. The average growth in height of the ear was 4.4 mm. If one breaks down these data to patients operated on between the ages of 5 and 7, the growth was 4.2 mm, and in patients who had their surgery between the ages of 8 and 12, the increment in height was 4.7 mm. Therefore, I completely agree with Dr. Tanzer's findings that the reconstructed ear grows, although I do not know yet which part grows the most—the grafted cartilage or the lobule. When two pictures at the same magnification are superimposed, it seems that the lobule grows a great deal and the contour of the cartilage is also larger, but less significantly. In two patients who had a very undeveloped lobule, there was only 1 and 2 mm of growth, respectively, after 6 and 8 years.

Another factor to take into account is that the growth pattern of the normal ear seems a little different in the Japanese. In my study, height of the ear in most children around 5 or 6 years of age is 5.5 cm for the male and the female. Although the adult female has a fairly small ear, generally 6.0 cm or slightly longer, the adult male usually has a larger ear, more than 6.5 cm and frequently greater than 7.0 cm. I believe the average size of the auricle differs in various races, and I have observed that many people in Africa have comparatively small ears.

Concerning complications after using a costal cartilage graft, I have reported in detail in a forthcoming publication. My thoughts are essentially those of Dr. Tanzer. On the deformity of the thorax, my associate, Dr. A. Yamada, recently presented a follow-up study in which he said the occurrence of the projection at the rib superior to the site of cartilage removal was seen frequently when the donor area comprised the sixth, seventh, and eighth ribs, but less commonly when the seventh, eighth, and ninth ribs were used. He presumed that the differences were due to the direct attachment of ribs one to seven to the sternum and the relative lack of attachment to the sternum of ribs eight and nine. He also mentioned that this deformity was seen more often and more severely in the group operated on at ages 5 and 6, but was less frequent and milder in the older age group. The deformity became more apparent 1 year after the operation and then showed little change. This protrusion is not noticeable in females because it is hidden by the developing breast.

10

Basis of Technique

For the past 20 years, it has been the author's contention that auricular cartilage itself, stripped completely bare of all connective tissue and muscle, is sufficiently pliable to permit bending into a gentle fold in order to produce an anthelical ridge at whatever site desired, and that the position of this fold can be permanently maintained by the insertion of three or four side-to-side mattress sutures of nonabsorbable material which are left in situ indefinitely [2–4].

Where no anthelical fold already exists (Fig. 10-1A) and the ears are sticking straight out, the stripping away of subcutaneous tissue and muscle must be carried out on the posterior surface of the auricular cartilage to the extent that it is necessary to free the postauricular skin from the whole of the surface of the auricular cartilage. In patients with ears of this type, the site of the proposed anthelical fold is marked with ink on the anterior surface of the ear skin when it is held in the desired shape with the fingers. The site of the mattress sutures is marked on either side of the proposed anthelical summit (about 8 mm on either side of the summit line), and these marks are tattooed through the cartilage with some biological ink. Once the sutures have been inserted so that they lie on the anterior perichondrium but do not pierce the anterior skin, they are then tightened sufficiently to produce the desired anthelical fold, and the ends of the sutures are cut off short, close to the knot. This point of technique is extremely important, for if suture ends of even a few millimeters are left protruding from the knots, they may lead to the postoperative development of sinuses and to com-

John C. Mustardé

RESULTS OF OTOPLASTY BY THE AUTHOR'S METHOD

plications which may vitiate the whole procedure. The author has found that none of the present-day synthetics can be tied sufficiently tightly to allow the suture ends to be cut off immediately at the knot. White silk, 3-0 or 4-0, therefore, is still used and produces excellent results. Silk can be cut off immediately beyond the knot without fear that any untying of the suture will result.

A wedge of skin about 1 cm wide having been removed from the posterior surface of the ear at the time the skin was reflected over the whole extent of the auricular cartilage on the posterior surface, the continuous pullout suture inserted to close the wound will lie in a position slightly posterior to the bridging permanent sutures without producing significant reduction of the postauricular sulcus. Packing of the ear with damp cotton and light compression bandages for 10-12 days completes the procedure. However, after the bandages are removed, patients, or their parents, are told that some form of protection of the ears, such as a ski cap, must be worn while the patient is sleeping for at least a month. This last precaution is to prevent inadvertent rolling onto the ear and tearing of the sutures through the cartilage. By about 6 weeks following surgery, sufficient scar tissue will have been laid down to form an added strengthening against such an eventuality unless undue force is applied (Fig. 10-1B through D).

Where an anthelical fold already exists (Fig. 10-2A), the technique must be modified in order to obliterate the existing fold before a new fold can be created at the desired site. The site of the new fold and the position of the mattress sutures are marked as before, with the ear being rolled into position by means of the fingers. Once the posterior skin of the ear has been completely dissected free, all connective tissue and muscle on the posterior surface of the auricular cartilage in the region of the anthelix are carefully dissected away, leaving bare perichondrium exposed. The cartilage of the tail of the helix is freed with blunt scissors from the cartilage of the antitragus right up to the point at which the cartilages join. Insertion of the sutures and the subsequent steps of the operation are carried out as before. It is quite easy to roll the cartilage into a new position, despite there having been a previous anthelical fold, provided that dissection of all existing subcutaneous tissue and muscle is carried out meticulously so as to remove as much as possible of the prestressing factors that would tend to pull the ear back into its original shape (Fig. 10-2B).

Postoperative Results

In more than 600 ears operated on during some 20 years, only 10 again became so prominent that they had to be reoperated by the author. All these became prominent within the first year (except one, which will be discussed later). At the secondary operation it was found that in four ears the sutures had either sliced through the cartilage or had been pulled through as a result of force applied to the ear. In the other six ears, no evidence of the sutures cutting through was found, and it would appear that either the sutures had not been tied tightly enough or they had slackened, or there had been some further growth of the concha of the ear which tended to throw the ear forward. It is interesting to note at this point that before the author had begun to operate on ears using the

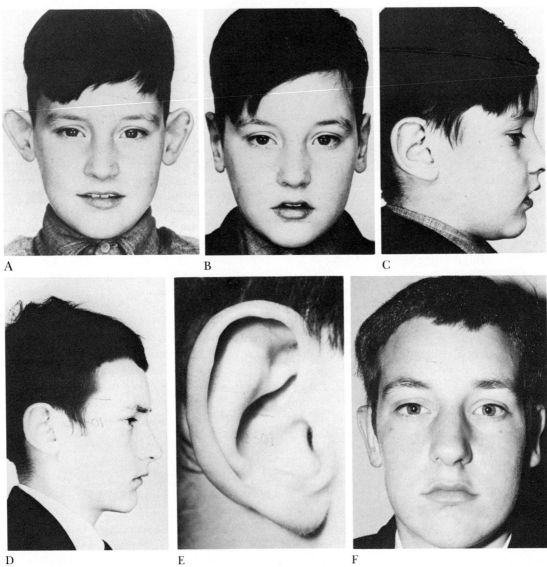

A   B   C

D   E   F

FIGURE 10-1. *Prominent ears with no anthelical folds present. (A) Preoperative. (B) Postoperative, full-face (after 4 months). (C) Postoperative, lateral (after 4 months). (Reproduced, with permission, from J. C. Mustardé, The correction of prominent ears with buried mat-* *tress sutures. In T. Gibson (Ed.),* Modern Trends in Plastic Surgery. *London: Butterworth, 1964. Pp. 233–236.) (D) Postoperative, lateral (after 4 years). (E) Postoperative, lateral (after 10 years). (F) Postoperative, full-face (after 10 years).*

regimen just described (which is never carried out before the age of 4, i.e., before the child goes to school but after the main growth of the ear has taken place), children with prominent ears had been operated on at ages as young as 2 years. Moreover, in a number of children operated on at this early age, it was found that with continued growth of the ear, and particularly of the concha, some recurrence of prominence took place.

Complications in the postoperative phase have been few in the author's hands, and although he has seen, in consultation, a number of children in whom a small sinus had occurred

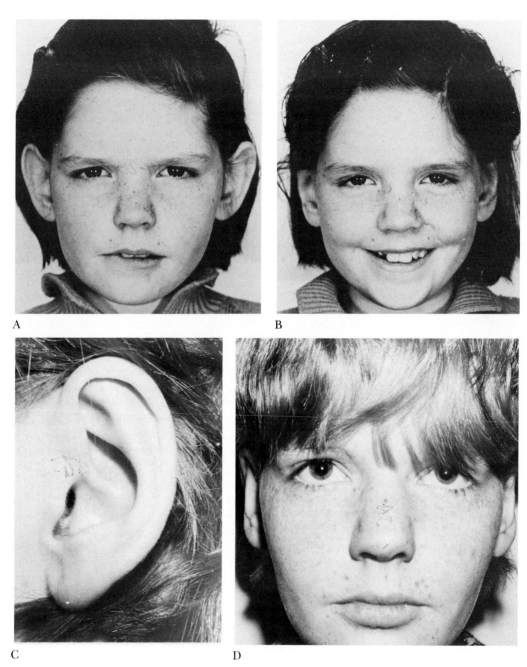

FIGURE 10-2. *Prominent ears with anthelical fold present. (A) Preoperative. (B) Postoperative (after 1 year). (C) Postoperative, lateral (after 1 year). (D) Postoperative, full-face (after 10 years).*

over a buried suture, in the author's own experience there have been only six such patients. It is felt that this is largely due to meticulous tying of the knots in such a manner, and with such material, that they will not become untied with the passage of time and, even more important, the ends of the sutures will not protrude more than 1 mm beyond the knot itself. Extrusion of the silk sutures per se does not seem to occur, and although sinuses have occurred as late as 3 years after surgery in a number of patients referred to the author for secondary opinion, the majority have appeared within 2 or 3 months after surgery. The infection can generally be controlled with the use of topical antibiotic creams until about 6 months after the operation, when the affected suture or sutures can be removed. After this length of time, about half the patients referred to the author for this complication have not required further surgery, but in the other half it was deemed advisable to reoperate a few months after removal of the suture or sutures and reposition the ear with fresh sutures. In none of these cases has there been any further complications.

Dr. Charles Horton [1] has told the author of one patient in which a postoperative sinus appeared behind the ear and led eventually to widespread infection with destruction of the auricular cartilage. This is the only instance of which the author is aware of this most alarming complication.

Long-Term Results

In an attempt to assess long-term results in patients who had prominent ear correction carried out by the preceding technique, letters were sent to 97 patients who had been operated on 10 years or more before. The patients were asked whether they were satisfied with the results of their surgery, and whether their ears had shown any signs of recurrence of the prominence. They were asked also if they were prepared to come in to be examined and photographed. Thirty-eight patients wrote back stating that they were satisfied with the operation, and four said that they thought there had been some tendency toward recurrence of the prominence, but they were still happy with the result. Three patients wrote saying that their ears had again become promi-

nent, but they did not wish further surgery. Twenty-three patients appeared for a clinical assessment, and the remainder did not reply. Of the 23 patients examined, there was an almost uniformly satisfactory permanence of the retropositioning of the ears (Figs. 10-1E and F, 10-2C and D, and 10-3A and B), but in 5 of the patients, one ear had come slightly forward compared with the other. All 5 of these patients had had preexisting prominent anthelical folds with deep conchas, and it was difficult to say whether the slight prominence was due to growth of the concha subsequent to the operation or to one of the possible faults mentioned. Two patients had obvious bilateral recurrence of some degree of prominence but seemed unconcerned by it, and one patient had a recurrence of prominence that had necessitated a repeat operation carried out by another surgeon, using the author's technique, about 2 years after the first surgery. The final result was satisfactory.

In almost all the patients, the upper half of the ears had lost the slightly overcorrected, flattened look which tends to be evident for the first year or so following surgery, and with the minimal change described, the ears looked very natural. However, where the upper half of the ear remained too flat, the lower anthelical fold appeared sometimes a little too prominent.

Closer questioning of the patient who had had a second operation revealed that he had been teased at school *because* he had had an operation to correct his prominent ears, and on a number of occasions other boys had pulled on his ears deliberately. It is difficult to assess just how much this type of handling may have influenced the postoperative course, but the author has been told by other surgeons of a number of children whose ears have again become rapidly prominent after surgery, following teasing trauma by their companions.

It is of interest that in the author's series there have been no instances of late rejection of the silk sutures, although in one patient the silk sutures could be seen and felt, ridging underneath the skin and the scar on the postauricular

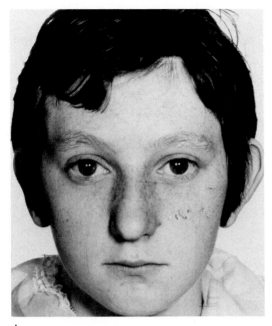
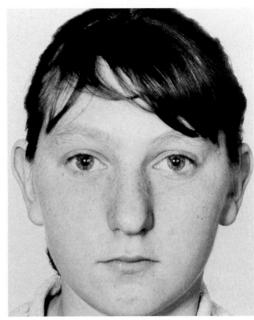

A   B

FIGURE 10-3.   *Prominence of one ear only. (A) Pre-operative. (B) Postoperative (after 10 years).*

sulcus. The skin was very mobile over the sutures, and until the patient was lost to follow-up 5 years later, it was deemed unnecessary to interfere with them in any way.

Final Thoughts

The technique of correction of prominent ears described originally by the author would seem to be a satisfactory one, and producing as it does a perfectly normal, rounded anthelix without evidence of injury to the auricular cartilage, it compares very favorably with alternative procedures. From cases referred because of postoperative complications and from discussion with other surgeons, it is obvious that meticulous attention to detail must be carried out, particularly with a view to avoiding formation of a fistula or fistulae leading to the buried

nonabsorbable sutures. The two points which the author considers of most importance are, first, that material should be used which will allow the suture to be cut off as close to the knot as possible, and second, closure of the postauricular skin wound must be carried out with great care so as to avoid any possibility of epithelial edges turning inward and coming into contact with the buried suture material.

One patient on whom the author operated several years ago was a prisoner in an American penitentiary. Although the cartilages of his ears were somewhat thickened and very resilient, it was still possible to construct folds without any great difficulty, so the operation was carried out in the usual manner. It has lately been reported to the author that this patient's ears subsequently became as prominent as they had been before surgery, which prompts the thought that it may well be that the correction of cosmetic deformities in a prison environment leads to its own complications. Certainly the possibility of fellow inmates being tempted to prove the worth of the cosmetic correction enters one's mind.

References

1. Horton, C. Personal communication, 1978.
2. Mustardé, J. C. Prominent Ears: Effective Formation of Anti-helix Fold Without Incising Cartilage. Paper presented at the Second Congress of the Transactions of the International Society of Plastic Surgeons, London, 1959.
3. Mustardé, J. C. The Correction of Prominent Ears with Buried Mattress Sutures. In T. Gibson (Ed.), *Modern Trends in Plastic Surgery*. London: Butterworth, 1964. Pp. 233–236.
4. Mustardé, J. C. Correction of Prominent Ears Using Buried Mattress Sutures. In J. C. Mustardé (Ed.), *Plastic Surgery in Infancy and Childhood*. Edinburgh: Churchill/Livingstone, 1971. Pp. 306–312.

11

THE outstanding ear has been a challenge to those interested in aesthetic surgery from the very beginnings of our specialty, and it remains so. Gross correction of ludicrous protrusion may satisfy patient and parent alike, but it is only when our field can provide an almost perfect imitation of pleasing normalcy that we can justify "interfering with nature" and ease the goad that drives us on in our quest for perfection. The purpose of this chapter is to show long-term results. In order to make these understandable, it is necessary to mention the techniques employed. Because differing combinations of methods were used, it is important that the reader understand some details of the techniques so that he may evaluate how well they worked, as revealed by the results. Therefore, in the first part of this chapter we shall discuss techniques and how they relate to what we conceive to be the surgical dynamics of otoplasty. The latter part of the chapter will concentrate on long-term results so that the reader may judge for himself the procedures involved.

Otoplasty for correction of prominent ears or improvement of unduly protruding portions of ears consists almost entirely of efforts to modify the skeleton of the ear itself. Because results of anthelical incising (Fig. 11-7C) were so imperfect, even though Luckett's [5] teachings were accepted almost universally in the mid-1940s, we began a systematic investigation of every approach that seemed to allow alteration of the elements of the ear to more closely approximate aesthetic normalcy. Obviously, anatomy and the dynamics of cartilage springs and soft tissue coverage were involved. Like every plastic surgeon, we would press the helix and lobule with our fingers to see how the ear

Richard C. Webster
Richard C. Smith

OTOPLASTY FOR PROMINENT EARS

would look when it no longer protruded abnormally. In doing so, we produced a normal-appearing anthelical fold and superior crus, or from the front, we hid the helix behind an outstanding conchal rim. It seemed to us that two fundamentally different problems, (1) the lack of development of normal anthelical and superior crural folds and (2) the protruding conchal rims, caused the differing observations under these circumstances. Moreover, these existed in isolation or in combination to produce abnormal prominence. Because we could think of no convenient way to provide the patient with 24-hour-a-day pushing forces that would give results as aesthetically satisfying as those provided by our fingers, we wondered whether appropriate pulling forces might not be used instead. Immediately, this led logically to the concepts (1) that if what attached the ear in its protruding position to the head could be severed, (2) that if the structures thrusting the lateral portions of the ear away from the head could be excised or flattened, and (3) that if the cartilaginous spring could be weakened or curved short of incising completely through it, then these pulling forces could be lessened. We felt that we would have to analyze the anatomy, learn how to diagnose the variations of the deformity, and then test with long-term observation the various techniques devised to learn the answers to the questions that logical reasoning imposed.

We shall show a few short-term results to make certain points that long-term results are not needed to demonstrate. We apologize in advance for some of the photography. Unfortunately, not all the photographs taken many years ago exactly match those taken in recent years. We also wish to make it plain that lack of emphasis in this chapter on cartilage weakening and suture techniques does not mean that we condemn these. The fact is that we have used them throughout our careers and continue to use them. However, they have been more fully documented in recent years than have the particular pull-in techniques that we will show in more detail here. This chapter is not meant to be a treatise on how to do otoplasty. For that purpose, the student is referred to videotapes [15] which show the actual dynamics of the surgical approaches in the fresh cadaver, and for more detail on the various studies performed, the student is referred to a microfiche monograph [16] which discusses otoplasty at greater length. Photographs in this chapter, originally reproduced in that microfiche, appear here with the permission of the copyright owners.

We must admit that after over 30 years we still have no absolute answers, but we do believe that some verifiable conclusions can be drawn from certain short- and long-term results studied. The interested reader is invited to look further into what we originally thought was going to be a relatively simple project. Perhaps he too will want to answer the questions that this work and that of others in the last 30 years leave unsolved.

Pertinent Anatomy

In this chapter, *superior* means toward the top of the head; *posterior*, toward the back of the head; *lateral* or *outward*, away from the middle of the head; *medial, cranial,* or *inward,* toward the middle of the head.

Figures 11-1 and 11-2 show the structures of the external ear. Elevations or eminences on

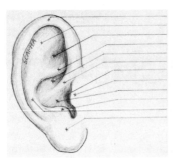

Helix
Superior crus
Fossa triangularis
Inferior crus
Cymba conchae
Crus of helix
External auditory canal
Tragus
Cavum conchae
Antitragus
Anthelix
Lobule

FIGURE 11-1. *Right auricle, lateral surface.*

the cranial surface of the cartilage correspond to concavities in the lateral surface. The helical crus partially divides the conchal cavity into the cymba conchae and the cavum conchae. The anterior extrinsic ligament extends from the root of the zygomatic process to the tragus and spina helicis. The posterior extrinsic ligament runs from the mastoid process to the posterior surface of the concha. These ligaments and other fibrous tissue attach the cartilage to the head, with envelopes of soft tissue and skin providing further attachments. Severance of the anterior ligament or excision of the spina helicis allows the auricle to wobble about. If the posterior auricular muscle is disconnected from its attachment to the ponticulus, and if the posterior ligament is severed, the auricle becomes "floppy" (can be moved in many directions). The conchal cup, shaped roughly like half a globe, can be slid or rotated forward to the extent that the external auditory canal is impinged upon or occluded. In animals, where survival dictates highly developed stereoacous-

tical function, ligaments allow and muscles cause rapid sliding of the bowl on the underlying tissues so that the concha can rotate toward the sound source. In human beings, this mobility is limited unless undermining and severance free up the concha so that it can be rotated easily. Sercer [10] believed that a short anterior ligament was the cause of prominent ears. We do not agree that it is even an important cause, but it is true that its severance will allow the ear to be flattened to the head with greater ease than when it is intact.

Blood and nerve supply to the external ear are so good that we have not yet observed vascular or permanent neural problems with any of the techniques to be mentioned in this chapter. Of course, with extremely radical undermining it would be possible to jeopardize blood supply, but to date, we have not seen slough with any of these otoplastic maneuvers personally performed.

An appreciable portion of the conchal cartilage rests against the mastoid process as the latter slopes medially toward the canal. The eminentia triangularis, resting against soft tissue overlying the temporal bone, and the more medial parts of the conchal cartilage provide the main buttresses thrusting the rest of the external ear away from the skull. A rocker effect is produced when the auricular cartilage just posterior to the eminentia triangularis is pushed closer to the head. The anterior part of the helix and the spina helicis rock outward to produce a fullness just anterior to the ear. The cauda helicis separates from the conchal and antitragal cartilage, is fastened to them by an intrinsic ligament or band of fibrous tissue, and, to a large extent, dictates much of the position of the lobule.

Diagnosis

Diagnosis takes into account such factors as age, sex, tendency toward keloid, strength of cartilaginous spring, and the positions and sizes of the parts of the ear relative to each other, the

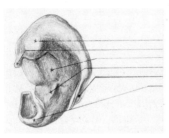

Eminentia triangularis
Spina helicis
Eminentia conchae
Ponticulus
Cauda helicis
Cartilage of external
   acoustic meatus

FIGURE 11-2. *Right auricular cartilage, cranial surface.*

face, the head itself, and the hair. Physical diagnosis relates to the tissues themselves, and aesthetic diagnosis is required to tell us what is disharmonious about the appearance of the ear. Many authors [1,9,17] have discussed aesthetic goals. These sum up to a harmonious balance, with the ear showing gentle folds and smooth contours and not overcorrected or looking like an "operated ear."

Many normal or "unoperated" ears have helices hidden from the front by parts of the anthelix, but most surgeons agree that one should not try to hide the helix. Most normal ears seem to have the helix protruding from the scalp about 1.5 to a little over 2 cm. Wright [17] states that 1.5 cm "seems best." The upper and lower poles of the ear should not be unduly prominent in relation to the middle portion of the ear. The lobule should be positioned harmoniously with the rest of the ear. The ears should be bilaterally symmetrical, particularly with regard to the lateral margins of the helices when viewed from the front. Slight asymmetries of the anthelical portions and lobules are less noticeable than those involving the helices.

In general, the anthelical fold or conchal rim should be about 2 to 5 mm medial to the outer protrusion of the helix. It should be sharp only in its inferior crus. The anthelical fold and its superior crus should be shaped like the side of a cone, with the sharper curve located inferiorly near the antitragus. The superior portion should angle forward. The superior crural convexity should fan out gently into the fossa triangularis and scapha. The scaphal plane should sit about 60 to 90 degrees to that of the outer concha, and it should not be too broad. The fossa triangularis should face more laterally than anteriorly. There should be no excessive tubercle of Woolner (Darwin himself credited Woolner with the original description), and neither the trague nor the antitragus should be unduly prominent.

After the cosmetic surgeon has studied many normal ears, he will develop the sense of proportion required in diagnosing aesthetic disharmonies. He then will take into account what

the correction of one factor may do to make something else aesthetically too prominent. When he can decide with wisdom what concavities, convexities, planes, and angles need to be changed in relation to others, he then will have the aesthetic diagnosis. With this he knows the goals of surgery and can analyze the anatomical factors requiring alteration. Only then can he select the technical modalities most likely to produce the anatomical and aesthetic modifications desired.

Operative Techniques

We have classified as *pull-in techniques* those in which laterally prominent cartilage is moved medially by pulls transmitted to it through soft tissue and/or skin left attached to it, this soft tissue or skin being sutured under tension to cartilage, soft tissue, and/or skin located medially. We have classified as *suture techniques* those in which laterally located cartilage is moved medially by sutures running from it to medially situated cartilage or soft tissue. Of course, almost all procedures correcting protrusion, even *incising techniques* where cuts are made completely through cartilage at or near the anthelix, involve application of pulling forces to move protruding parts medially. Therefore, our use of the term *pull-in* does not imply that other approaches do not employ pulling mechanisms. While there may be certain important differences between pull-in techniques and suture techniques, as we have just defined them, many of the remarks made in some detail about pull-in techniques apply equally to suture techniques, particularly those dealing with directions of pulls. A better functional classification of techniques based on surgical dynamics and goal oriented will be used in the section discussing results.

It will be noted that where technical points can be made in legends close to diagrams or photographs, we have elected to place them there rather than in the text. The reader will not be required to search back and forth from text to illustration so much under these circumstances.

CONCHAL AND ANTHELICAL CARTILAGE INCISING TECHNIQUES

In our experiments in the 1940s, we tried many cartilage incising and excising techniques. Ely [2], in 1881, excised a roughly elliptical piece of cartilage with attached anterior and posterior skin from the triangular fossa and concha where the auricle separated from the head (Fig. 11-3B and C). Conchal protrusion also can be corrected by the excision shown in Figure 11-3D and E, with or without excision of the attached skin. If anthelical curvature is present, the recurving rim can be placed to cover the lateral edge of the remaining cartilage of the conchal cup, preventing some of its sharp edge from showing (Fig. 11-7C). However, we found it difficult to get symmetrical and controlled

correction of protrusions of the helical margins, and even with careful suturing or appropriately wide undermining, a ridge and a depression frequently developed at the overlapped lateral conchal area. This approach did nothing to help with production of normal-appearing superior crural curvatures.

Luckett [5], in 1910, recommended incising through the cartilage to break its spring and to produce an anthelical fold. He removed an ellipse of conchal cartilage adjacent to the anthelix for correction of conchal protrusion. We tried every described modification of his techniques, and we evolved some others, including dicing, beveled incisions, and multiple incisions, and found none that gave what we considered satisfactory results. Essentially, the only places where we found that we could incise completely through cartilage in the anthelical region without producing abnormally sharp edges were in the most inferior parts of the fold and in the

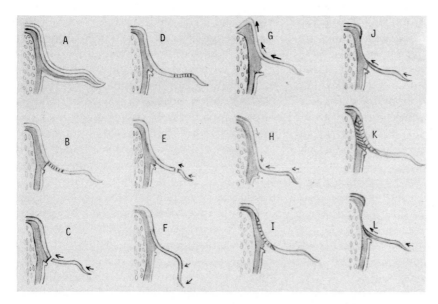

FIGURE 11-3. *Section of the right ear from above. Small circles indicate the mastoid; the gray area indicates soft tissue. Skin and soft tissue removed from the auricle in all except (A) so that cartilage shows clearly. (A) Prominent concha. (B) Crosshatching shows conchal cartilage to be excised close to the floor. (C) Arrows demonstrate effect. (D) Excision near anthelix. (E) Effect. (F) Diminishing conchal prominence by rolling part of the conchal cartilage into scapha and producing a new conchal rim or anthelix closer to the conchal floor and farther from the helical edge. (G) Anterior rotation of the conchal cup from anterior placement of the mastoid end of the mastoid-auricle suture or anterior placement of the cranial edge of skin excision followed by defect closure. Canal impingement. (H) Opposite effect with posterior placement. (I) Cartilage to be excised from conchal wall and floor. (J) Result. (K) Excision of mastoid soft tissue to be performed. (L) Effect.*

inferior crus. These incisions allowed a little more bending in of unincised portions with a given application of pull-in force. Long-term results of our efforts (occupying much of the forties) often showed hidden helices, helical asymmetries, abnormal widths of the scapha, and sharp edges (Fig. 11-7A through C). No technique evolved or worked with since is as certain to correct helical prominence, but none so frequently produces such irreversible departures from normalcy.

PULL-IN TECHNIQUES

Skin Excision Alone. Although it was claimed almost routinely that excision of postauricular or mastoid skin alone would not correct auricular prominence, we noted as early as 1943 that use of the postauricular area as a donor site for full-thickness skin grafts at times led to auricular asymmetry, with the donor ear being pulled closer to the head than its counterpart. While waiting for long-term results of the cartilage incising techniques, we began varying the amounts and shapes of skin removed for skin grafts from the postauricular and mastoid areas. On 1- to 5-year follow-up, the skin excision, even without undermining, produced a pulling-in of the auricle if the defect was made large enough. If the excision extended far enough posteriorly in the mastoid area, the ear could be plastered against the head with almost no retroauricular sulcus reappearing, even with long follow-up. Unpleasant flattening and, at times, crumpling of parts of the conchal cup occurred, and the great tension of closure with large defects led to a fair number of hypertrophied and somewhat unstable scars.

Pull-in forces exerted on the auricle differed in their effects on the canal, conchal floor, conchal wall, anthelical fold, scapha, and helix depending on the strengths of the cartilage spring, the elasticity of the skin and soft tissues, their sites of attachment, the shape of the mastoid, the slope of the conchal floor and wall, the amount of skin removed, and the relative positions and amounts of undermining of the edges of the defect on the auricle and mastoid. With skin excision and no undermining, the conchal attachments to the head tended to prevent conchal-floor cartilage from sliding forward or backward. Since the conchal floor was limited in its excursion, tension of closure was greater than when the concha could slide out of the way unhindered. Pull-in forces then tended to concentrate their effects where cartilage bent most easily. In almost all prominent ears we noted that the major bending effects occurred in the anthelical area. Beyond certain extremes, anthelical bending was followed by a flattening and increase in the area of the conchal floor at the expense of the medial part of the conchal wall (Figs. 11-3H and 11-10A through D) and the more the lateral part of the conchal wall transformed into the anthelical fold. The scapha began to increase in size and face posteriorly, and the helix became more and more hidden. Beyond this point, the conchal wall began to buckle, with bulges and concavities appearing.

Closure of skin defects on the mastoid had almost no effect on the ear. Closure of those on the back of the auricle produced differing effects depending largely on the size of the defect, the position of the defect edges, and the location of the attachments of soft tissue and skin when these were undermined and separated from cartilage immediately adjacent to the defect. Soft tissue, except for perichondrium, tends to slide much more on the posteromedial surface of the ear than on its anterolateral surface. Therefore, even without undermining, a strong enough pull on the lateral edge of the defect produced some bending of the anthelix and thus moved the helix medially somewhat. If the lateral edge was undermined so that the skin or skin and soft tissue were attached only at the scapha or back of the helix, then the pull was transmitted directly to these areas (Fig. 11-10E through G). The farther back on the scaphal area or the closer to the helical edge the pull was transmitted, the more bending effect there was on the anthelix. The closer the lateral edge of the defect was to the retroauricular sulcus and the less the lateral undermining was, the less we noted the bending effect to be on the anthelix. When the medial edge of the skin excision was very close to or in the retroauricular sulcus, or when the medial edge was undermined to the mastoid, closure produced external pulls on the skin and soft tissue of the mastoid close to the sulcus. However, this tissue would only move laterally to the limit of its capacity to stretch. Some flattening of the conchal cup with increase of the conchal floor area would occur, but whether the cup rotated forward or not depended largely on the effective directions of pulls established. With no undermining of the conchal floor, anterior rotation was limited in any event. The more anteriorly on the mastoid the medial pull on the lateral cartilage came from, the more tendency there was to anterior rotation (Fig. 11-10A and B). The more posteriorly on the mastoid, the more the conchalfloor flattening effect was likely to be (Figs. 11-3H and 11-10C and D).

Skin Excision and Undermining of Cartilage Floor. With no undermining of the floor of the concha and fossa triangularis, pull-in forces resulting from closure of retroauricular skin excisional defects produced their main effects on the auricle lateral to the sulcus. As the floors were undermined farther and farther forward, the attachments of the ear to the head were severed and the concha and fossa triangularis rotated more and more easily. As they did so, more and more of the walls of these parts came in contact with the head and were added to the original area of the floors. When the rotation occurred, the forces bending the cartilage, mainly in the anthelical areas, lessened, and curvatures produced by the pull-in forces diminished. It was found that undermining as far forward as the canal allowed cartilage and skin to impinge on the canal to the point of occlusion. Excision of impinging cartilage, leaving skin intact, sufficed to prevent functional impediment ordinarily. However, rarely it was necessary to excise skin and/or perform a Z-plasty (Fig. 11-13A through D). If 5 to 10 mm of soft tissue just behind the canal was left un-

severed, undermining farther forward than the canal above and just below it did not produce significant functional impairment. However, undermining anteriorly inferior to the canal has dangers and did little to help correct prominence in most cases.

Undermining superiorly can go far enough forward to sever the anterior extrinsic ligament. The rocker effect mentioned before, producing an unnatural fullness just anterior to the helix, could be minimized by removing part of the rocker or the floor of the fossa triangularis itself, or the bulge produced by it could be diminished by excision of the spina helicis (Figs. 11-21D and 11-22B).

The plane of undermining was found to be most convenient between the soft tissue of mastoid and perichondrium. However, it could be between perichondrium and cartilage. Wright (personal communication) reported that the latter helps prevent sharp edges from showing in the floor when large excisions of cartilage take place there. He deliberately allows some hematoma to form in this space.

The extent of undermining was determined by pressing the fingers on the lateral structures or by pulling medially on the lateral skin or perichondrial flap edge at each stage of the undermining process. If undermining is excessive enough to allow too much rotation of concha and triangularis at the expense of the desired bending in the anthelical and/or superior crural folds, concha-mastoid or triangularis-mastoid sutures could be used to prevent the undue rotation. Concha-mastoid sutures also have been found helpful in correcting overenthusiastic undermining just behind the canal.

In general, the combination of skin excision and undermining was most useful in cases with well-developed anthelical and superior crural folds and with moderate prominence of the conchal rim. However, in patients with thin, flexible cartilage that bends easily at the anthelical folds, it also could be used to produce or increase the folds themselves (Figs. 11-4 and 11-5) if enough medial pull was placed on the helix and scapha and if undermining was appropriately limited.

Skin Excision, Undermining of Floor, and Excision of Mastoid Soft Tissue and/or Cartilage from Eminences. Between the helical and conchal rims and the skull are mastoid soft tissue and the cartilage of the eminences (Fig. 11-2) and the walls of the fossa triangularis and concha. These tissues were compressed when pull-in forces were applied to the lateral components. Removal of parts of these tissues (Figs.11-3I through L and 11-10E) allowed the same pull-in forces to move the lateral structures closer to the head or permitted lesser pull-in forces to move the lateral components the same distance medially (Fig. 11-9). However, if a given skin excision produced desired bending effects in the anthelical fold areas, these bending effects were diminished as the conchal and triangular fossa floors and medial walls were more and more trimmed and as mastoid soft tissue was excised. The undermining required to expose these structures allowed more and more anterior rotation of the cartilage, and the physical removal of structures holding the conchal rim away from the head permitted this rim to move medially, both effects acting to diminish the bending effect of the pull-in forces.

Incisions made through cartilage at right angles to the anterior surface of the cartilage left a junction of undersurface of anterior skin at right angles to the cartilage remaining. These sharp angulations revealed themselves between 2 weeks and 6 months postoperatively by step-like depressions in the floors (as the skin draped over the incised edges of cartilage and anchored to the mastoid soft tissue or periosteum). These sharp edges were found to be prevented easily with a slight increase in the curvatures of the eminences by draping the fossae over the fingertip of the surgeon while paring or incising discs from the eminences with a long, straight (not bent) cutting edge such as that on a No. 11, No. 10, or No. 20 scalpel blade (Figs. 11-6 and 11-9A and B).

Amounts and locations of cartilage to be excised were determined by repetitively testing with finger pressure on the helix and lobule or conchal rim or by pulling medially on the flap of skin and/or perichondrium left attached laterally (Fig. 11-9E and F). Today we still know no better way. The same remark applies to excision of mastoid soft tissue (Fig. 11-9C). We do not excise periosteum of the mastoid, and we have not violated the attachments of the 5- to 10-mm band of soft tissue behind the canal in many years. An extremely important aesthetic landmark in the anterior half of the conchal floor and cavity is the crus of the helix. This should be left intact. If too much cartilage is excised and ridges show from buckling of cartilage left in the floor when pull-in forces are applied, we found that this buckled cartilage should be pared away or the conchal wall should be sutured to mastoid to prevent it from moving far enough anteriorly to produce the buckling.

Perichondrial and/or Soft Tissue Flaps. Pull-in forces can be exerted on laterally prominent cartilage by elevating perichondrium and/or soft tissue to the cartilaginous site where one wishes to have pull-in forces applied and then suturing the ends of the flaps to cartilage or soft tissue located medially (Fig. 11-10F and G). Except for skin suturing, we found that sutures used to provide long-lasting pulls should be permanent ones. When these flaps were used, we observed that the extent of skin excision could be lessened quite appreciably. The remarks made so far regarding undermining, excisions of mastoid soft tissue and/or excisions of cartilage from eminences, and directions of pulls in conjunction with skin excision apply also to use of flaps in conjunction with these techniques.

Cartilage Weakening or Abrading. Abrading, scoring (partial thickness incising) (Figs. 11-21C through F and 11-22A and B), or thinning of the cartilage in the anthelical and superior crural fold regions may be employed singly or in combination to provide easier bending from medial pulls applied to laterally prominent parts by skin excisions, by soft tissue and perichondrial excisional edges or flaps sutured medially under tension, or by sutures running

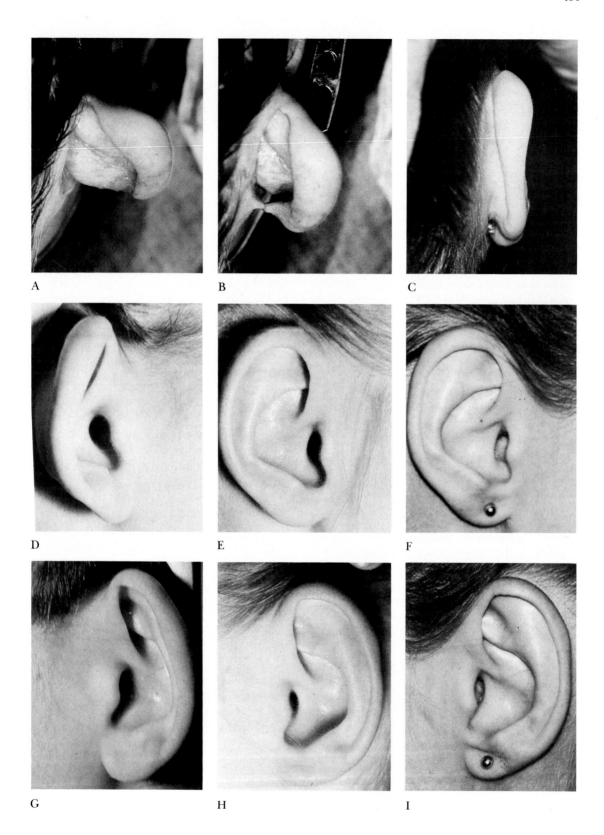

A

B

C

D

E

F

G

H

I

from the lateral structures to anchorage points situated medially.

Thinning auricular cartilage to weaken it from the posterior approach was found to be possible by bending it over the finger on the anterior surface to produce a posterior convexity that could be curetted, pared, or abraded by rasping or, later, by use of motor-driven equipment [12]. However, even with great care, it was difficult to get such smoothly graduated thinning that when the pull-in forces were applied, the subtle and differing curvatures of normal folds were well imitated (Figs. 11-7B and 11-23A).

We had hoarded septal cartilage in the scalp and used it for grafts in facial areas and had noted that scoring or abrading it on one side caused it to develop curvatures away from the treated surface. To apply these observations to auricular cartilage in making desired curvatures in otoplasty, it was necessary to get to the anterior surface. This we did by (1) undermining the upper edge of the posterior skin excision defect to the helical edge and then beyond it on the anterior surface to provide an anterior tunnel, (2) dissecting through the space between the cauda and the concha to then tunnel superiorly on the anterior surface, (3) dissecting anteriorly and superiorly through the upper

end of a through-and-through incision made in the anthelical fold proper, and (4) making incisions on the anterior skin. We tried four of these: (1) a short one hidden by the helix at the anterosuperior end of the superior crural fold that we were trying to produce, (2) a long one hidden by the helix at the junction of the scapha with the helix (Figs. 11-21C through F and 11-22A and B), (3) a short one just inside the edge of the inferior crus, and (4) a longer one made just inside the undeveloped conchal rim that we were about to make into an anthelical fold. Although we did cut through (from behind) the cartilage at the upper anterior end of the superior crus to make tunnels, it never occurred to us to incise extensively the junction between the helix and scapha, as so brilliantly performed by Stenström [13, 14].

In some cases of thinning or weakening of cartilage or when we wanted it to develop new curvatures of its own, we used no sutures, relying on dressings and the pull-in forces to maintain the curvatures produced. In others, removable sutures over bolsters or permanent buried sutures were employed. Kaye [4] described a clever technique for applying permanent sutures from the anterior surface. We like his approach when we are trying to make an ear with an underdeveloped anthelix and without appreciable conchal protrusions imitate a normal ear on the other side (Fig. 11-25A). It was found to be more convenient to put the knots in the scaphal area rather than down in the conchal cavity. However, the suture bulk may show more under these circumstances.

Whatever is used for scratching or abrading the anterior surface, we learned early that only a few months are needed to reveal any gross ridges or irregularities produced. Loose particles must be put back in their original sites or removed. Even so, ridges from partial-thickness incisions or scoring, "pebbling" from "fish-scaling" (multiple crescentic, beveled, partial-thickness incisions), and "cobblestoning" from morselization [1,8] (Fig. 11-24D) or dicing partial-thickness incisions ultimately show all too often. As one uses these techniques more

FIGURE 11-4.   (A) Adult right ear from above. Undermining already performed. Cranial edge of skin excision was in the retroauricular sulcus. Note the eminentia triangularis and conchae contacting the soft tissue covering the skull. 52/9/8 (this means that the photograph was taken on September 8, 1952). (B) Effect of one skin suture. Pull rotates the conchal cup forward slightly and bends anthelix, both effects lessening helical prominence. Floors of concha and fossa triangularis are flattened and enlarged. 59/9/8. (C) From above and behind. 74/1/22, 21 y, 4 m (this means that this photograph was taken on January 22, 1974, 21 years and 4 months after the first photographs; similar notations will be used where the follow-up period is important to an interpretation of the result). (D) Right lateral. 59/9/8. (E) Normal anthelix and superior crus. (F) 74/1/22, 21 y, 4 m. Very little change from the 1-year result. (G) Left lateral. 52/9/8. (H) 53/9/23, 1 y. Anthelical and superior crural curvatures increased. Part of former conchal wall now flattened into conchal floor, the area of which has increased. (I) 74/1/22, 21 y, 4 m. Very little change from the 1-year result.

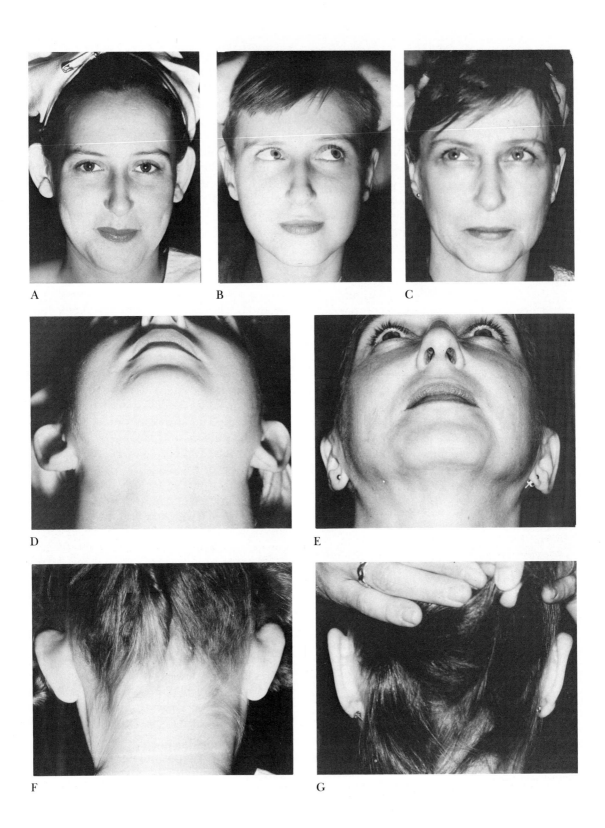

A B C

D E

F G

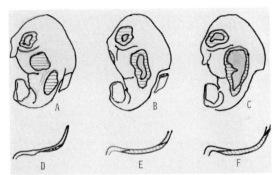

FIGURE 11-6.   *Cartilage excisions and incisions. Cranial surfaces of right ear in (A) through (C). Cross sections of floor of concha of right ear from above shown in (D) through (F). Parings or full-thickness beveled disc excisions from eminences allow ear to sit closer to head. Cross-hatching shows excisions. Gray areas represent undersurface of anterior skin exposed by disc excisions. (A) Cauda and inferior crus incised, one full-thickness and two partial-thickness excisions. (B) Spina helicis and attachment of cauda excised. Cross-hatching surrounding gray areas shows beveling. (C) Cauda and floor and part of conchal wall removed. (D) through (F) Compare with diagrams just above these cross sections.*

FIGURE 11-5.   *(A) 52/9/8. Lack or underdevelopment of anthelical folds and superior crural curvatures. Helical, conchal, and lobular prominences present. Right ear: skin excision, undermining, and cauda resection. Left ear: skin excision, scapha to concha suturing, and undermining. (B) 53/9/25, 1 y. Good prominence correction. Relatively good symmetry. Excellent formation of folds of anthelices and superior crura. Lower right helix hidden by conchal rim. (C) 74/1/22, 21 y, 4 m. Less skin excised on left. Scapha-concha suturing used instead. (D) View from below. 52/9/8. Observe cuplike auricles with underdevelopment of folds of anthelices and superior crura. (E) 74/1/22, 21 y, 4 m. Lobular prominence well corrected, but on the patient's left a slight extra bulge is present just posterior to the antitragus in this view. The cauda was not removed on this left side. (F) Back view. 52/9/8. Sulci are at junctions of eminentia triangularis and concha with the head. (G) 74/1/22, 21 y, 4 m. Sulci go to same junctions, but these now are in slightly different positions. Lower right helix where cauda was excised is pulled in more than one on left side. Scapha-concha suture ridging is apparent on left side in otherwise excellent long-term result of suture technique.*

and more, the better one gets at eliminating grosser abnormalities. However, making a truly normal-appearing superior crus by weakening, abrading, or scoring, and/or suturing (without some undue sharpening or concentration of curvature [Figs. 11-22B, 11-24D, and 11-25A], rippling, and/or slightly apparent depressions and elevations) remains one of the most difficult feats in cosmetic surgery.

SUTURE TECHNIQUES

Pull-in forces can be applied to laterally prominent structures by sutures that draw them medially. By the extent to which these work, certain other technical aids are needed less or eliminated. We have used sutures for many years, but they have their drawbacks too and should be put in context with alternatives available. We have not used the more recently introduced, slowly disappearing suture materials in otoplasty. Our comments apply to permanent suture materials such as monofilament nylon and polypropylene, white silk and siliconized silk, and braided and coated multiple-filament material such as polyester or nylon. In recent years we have been using white Tevdek.

Suture techniques can and really almost always should be used with one or more of the other techniques mentioned. We learned early that sutures tend to cut through both cartilage and soft tissue (Figs. 11-23B through F and 11-24A and B). To prevent this as much as possible, we found it necessary to (1) use at least 4-0 sutures applied in sufficient numbers, (2) include perichondrium on the anterior surface of the cartilage and, if applied to mastoid soft tissue, include mastoid periosteum, (3) take large enough bites to resist cutting through, and (4) place them far enough away from the center of the curve or bend being constructed to provide a long enough lever arm to "get the bend" with less pull than when applied close to the center of the curvature.

Unfortunately, this attempt to get a long enough lever arm forced us to situate the su-

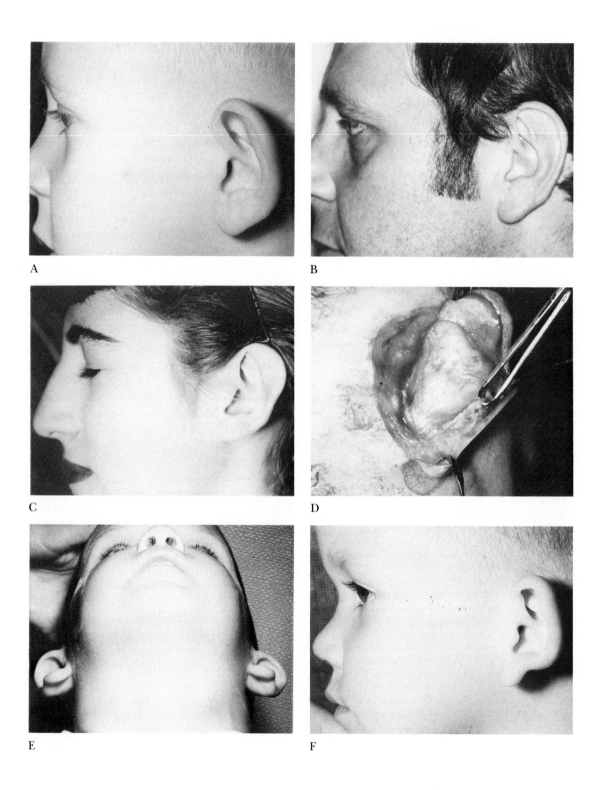

A

B

C

D

E

F

tures far enough out in the scapha that we observed bowstringing, ridging, or suture tenting (Figs. 11-5G, 11-21, and 11-23B through F) in the posterior views in many patients. Occasionally, the suture eroded through the skin or scar to become exposed. It then had to be removed–not always an easy task. While on the subject of discomfort, we and Wright (personal communication) both observed "moderate to severe pain, particularly on manipulation of the auricle, and visibility of the mattress suture when the ear is pulled."

The actual permanent buried sutures tested were (1) scapha to fossa triangularis, (2) scapha to concha, (3) scapha to mastoid, (4) fossa triangularis to concha (with inferior crus intact), (5) fossa triangularis to concha (advancing lateral cartilage of incised inferior crus anteroinferiorly on medial cartilage), (6) fossa triangularis to mastoid, (7) anthelical incised edge to concha (to cover incised conchal edge with anthelical rim), (8) concha to mastoid, (9) cauda to concha, (10) anterolateral part of lobule to concha, and (11) anterolateral part of lobule to posteromedial portion of lobule. The directions of provided pulls described earlier applied to sutures as well as to skin excisions and peri-

chondrial flaps. Certain sutures were found more valuable or safer than others. Those buried deeply enough to produce no bowstringing, such as sutures 4, 5, 6, 7, 9, 10, and 11 from the preceding list, extruded less than those in which suture tenting was observed. Concha-mastoid sutures rarely produced posterior ridging unless too few were used to pull the conchal wall too far back on the mastoid. They could produce some anterior buckling if used to rotate and flatten too much conchal wall into floor in patients with insufficient underming and insufficient excision of discs and/or mastoid soft tissue. With enough undermining, they could cause impingement on the canal. Scapha-mastoid sutures caused the worst bowstringing, with scapha-concha sutures in second place. These last two "spit" most often.

The main technical points in using permanent sutures were found to be (1) use enough of them to create the effect desired, (2) consider the directions of pulls required and take into account the adverse effects of each possible placement of both ends of the suture, (3) use as nonreactive a suture as possible, (4) take a large enough bite into tissues resisting cutting through of the suture, (5) use a large suture but one that still will be hidden by skin, (6) overcorrect a small amount to allow for some "cutting in," and (7) share the pulls with the other modalities mentioned. Wright [17] has provided a concise and superb guide to help the surgeon interested in technical aspects.

TECHNIQUES FOR CORRECTION OF A PROMINENT LOBULE

There are several causes of prominent lobules. The position of the lower part of the cauda helicis (Fig. 11-2) is one governing factor. If this portion sits laterally, the lobule almost always sits laterally. If, in addition, the lower part of the cauda is thrust forward, then the lobule hangs down from its distal end and faces forward. In most of our cases, detachment of the cauda (Fig. 11-6A and B) from the rest of the auricular cartilage or excision of it (Figs. 11-6C, 11-7D through F and 11-8A through D) was

FIGURE 11-7. *(A) Conchal protrusion with underdeveloped anthelical and superior crural folds. (B) Twenty-five-year result. Cauda excised. Curetting and scalpel shaving of cartilage to thin and weaken it was excessive and allowed acute angulation of superior crus to occur. Note excessive width of scapha. (C) Three-year result of excision of lateral conchal cartilage, coverage of the incised edge of conchal cartilage by the curved anthelix fold, and a through-and-through incision of cartilage in area of superior crus. Compare with (B). This kind of result of the 1940s led to the search for better methods. (D) 52/9/8. Posterior surface of right ear. Same patient as that in Figures 11-4 and 11-5. Observe the eminences. Cauda grasped by clamp. On this right side it was excised. It is also a simple matter to transect its attachment to the rest of the auricular cartilage by a scissor or scalpel cut made just above where the clamp is holding the cauda. (E) A not uncommon lobular prominence viewed from below. 55/5/24. There is also a conchal and helical prominence. Cauda is situated laterally and thrusts forward. Lobule hangs vertically and faces downward. (F) 55/5/24. Lobule drops downward from distal end of caudal cartilage (see also Fig. 11-8A and B).*

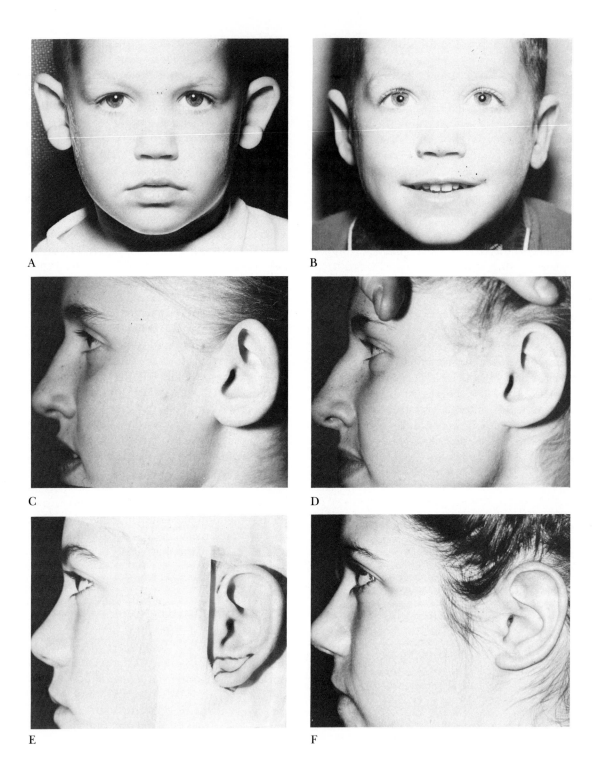

A

B

C

D

E

F

found to allow the lobule to rotate medially, with closure of the postauricular skin defect continuing downward on the back of the lobule to its lowest attachment to the head (Figs. 11-9 and 11-10H through L). Sutures from cauda to concha pulled the lobule in somewhat, but the excess of skin and soft tissue in the posteromedial half of the lobule relative to that in the anterolateral half became compressed and resisted some of the desired lobular prominence correction. It was found necessary to remove this compressed and "bunched" excess at the medial part of the back of the lobe. If this was not done, the lower and posterior border tended to protrude around a dimple where the suture "tacked" the cauda to the concha. The same observation was made on suturing the undersurface of the anterolateral skin and soft tissue either to the posteromedial skin and soft tissue or to the concha. In fact, we found that practically never were these sutures needed if the cauda was detached, if the helical and conchal prominence was corrected, and if the postauricular skin excision was continued down to the lowest attachment of the lobule to the head.

Cauda was detached by several kinds of cuts and by excising a small amount of it (Fig. 11-6A and B). The most convenient way to detach it was to punch one blade of a small scissors through the highest part of the cleft between the cauda and concha, bluntly elevate the an-terior skin to the helical margin while aiming obliquely lateral and upward, and then snip across the attachment.

Occasionally the lobule was both prominent and enlarged. Subcutaneous separation into an inner and an outer half allowed the peripheral parts of the latter to be rolled around to the posterior surface. When the best correction of prominence and enlargement was achieved by this rolling and sliding of the two halves, the excess appearing medially and superiorly was trimmed away. Although a permanent buried stitch between the halves was used in a few cases, it was found that a through-and-through stitch over bolsters or a meticulously applied bandage sufficed. Rarely, the protrusion and enlargement were excessive enough to require the technique shown in Figure 11-8E and F.

TECHNIQUES FOR CORRECTION OF AN UNDULY PROMINENT TRAGUS AND/OR ANTITRAGUS

In our practice it was rare to find grossly abnormal protrusion of these structures in isolation. However, correction of other parts of prominent ears at times revealed an unpleasant prominence of one or both of these landmarks relative to the corrected parts. An incision just inside the tragal edge allowed access for direct trimming of the protruding edge of the tragal cartilage. Redraping the skin permitted precise trimming of the skin excess. The prominent antitragal cartilage could be exposed by an incision on the conchal side just inside the rim or, better (except where skin had to be excised), through incisions already made. Sharp or blunt dissection laterally on the inferior part of the conchal cup exposed the antitragal cartilage edge well, so that it could be trimmed appropriately (Fig. 11-9I).

GENERAL REMARKS ON THE TECHNIQUES STUDIED

Very early in our careers we found it unnecessary to shave the hair. Draping was done only to keep hair from interfering with the operation.

FIGURE 11-8. *Lobular problems. (A) 55/5/24. See also Figure 11-7E and F. Observe cupping with deficient anthelices. (B) 57/1/23, 1 y, 8 m. Skin excision pull-in to produce anthelix; skin and disc excision for conchal prominence correction. Cauda excised. (C) 55/3/7. Prominence of concha, helix, and lobule. Ridge between antitragus and helix. (D) 58/2/25, 3(−) y. Prominences corrected by skin and disc excision. Ridge mentioned still present, although cauda excised. (E) 70/12/28. Conchal and helical prominence. Prominent and enlarged lobule here requires more than transection or excision of cauda because there is an excess of skin and soft tissue, particularly on the posteromedial side of the lobule. Marking indicates the full-thickness wedge with larger surface posteromedially to be excised. (F) 73/11/5, 2 y, 10 m. Skin and disc excision for pull-in correction of helical and conchal prominence. Even longer flaps than this survive well.*

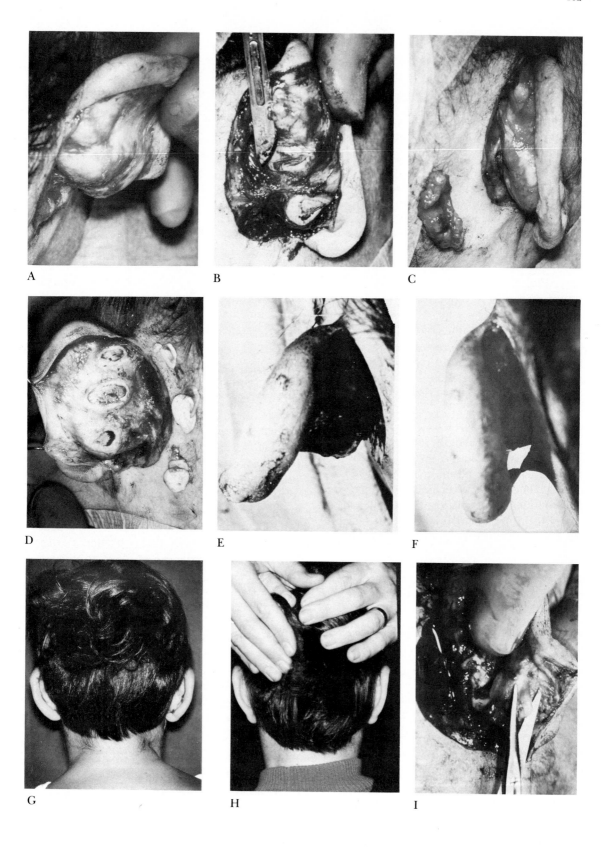

A

B

C

D

E

F

G

H

I

Attempts to get good hemostasis should be made, but well-molded compression dressings were even more important. We found it helpful in attempts to get symmetry to have both ears and as much of the head and face showing as possible. Because most of our retroauricular wounds were closed under some to much tension, we did get varying degrees of scar widening. From 6 months on, we found little difference between the sides closed with meticulously applied, very fine sutures and those closed with larger material and less time devoted to detail. For many years now we have

---

FIGURE 11-9. *Disc and skin excision and antitragal trimming. (A) Conchal and lobular prominence present. Good anthelix in this patient. Right ear from above. It is draped over the surgeon's fingers. Observe the three eminences. Between the conchal ones is a band of soft tissue still attached to the conchal cartilage and still protecting the canal from impingement. Undermining above and below this band went farther forward but did not encroach on the 5- to 8-mm-thick band left intact behind canal. (B) Surgeon's finger in fossa triangularis drapes cartilage over fingertip and protects the skin, while straight scalpel cut produces a beveled incision to remove cartilaginous disc from the eminentia triangularis. Discs have already been excised from the conchal eminences. (C) Mastoid soft tissue excised sits on mastoid skin. Obviously helix and conchal rim of ear with soft tissue and discs removed will sit closer to head than when these tissue masses were interposed between them and the skull. (D) Left ear showing beveled excisional defects, the anterolateral skin of the conchal and fossa triangularis walls and floors, and the cartilaginous discs themselves sitting on the mastoid. (E) Another patient at this stage. Left ear from above. Observe wedge-shaped defect between ear and mastoid. This defect was formerly occupied by cartilage of the eminences and wall. (F) Closure of skin defect pulls skin attached to scapha and helix medially and mastoid skin laterally. First effect of medial pull on auricle depends on strength of cartilage and its attachments to the head. The wedge-shaped defect may close with little bending at the anthelix or the anthelix may bend a fair amount before the defect is closed. When the defect is eliminated by contact of conchal wall or floor with the head, then the anthelix bends more until the conchal wall begins to crumple or slide forward. Increased bending at the anthelix is shown here. Scar contraction eventually eliminates dead space observed here between skin and cartilage. (G) Preoperative view of this patient. Good case for lenticular or elliptical skin excision, because midportion of ear most prominent. (H) 6 m. Prominence corrected and depth of sulcus restored. (I) Pointed and prominent antitragus exposed and about to be trimmed (right ear from behind).*

used Davis and Geck 4-0 mild chromic on the posterior skin and 6-0 on the anterolateral skin. These are used in a continuous fashion. The advantage of these over most other materials is that no suture removal is needed.

Results

To a large extent, the photographs and legends should speak for themselves. We have endeavored to supply the reader with precise dating and postoperative intervals so that he may make his own interpretations and judgments of the results. Here and there, the reader may have to refer to the section on techniques to get a fuller understanding of what was done. Where we found it necessary to explain certain technical choices by mentioning observed results, we did so. Therefore, some material on results appears in the section on technique. Much of that will not be repeated in this part of the chapter.

We mentioned earlier that we would use a more goal-oriented classification based on surgical dynamics in this section. Here we will list most suture techniques with the rest of the pull-in methods, not as something special and separate. Dynamically, a technique may be used for several purposes; another also may be employed for several purposes, and some are the same as those of the first technique and some differ. It is the satisfaction of as many goals as possible with the creation of as few impediments or adversities as possible that the selection of techniques is all about. Some examples from the results shown will be referred to by figure number to make certain points clear.

GENERAL OBSERVATIONS
ABOUT LONG-TERM RESULTS

In all cases, we found no significant retardation of growth of the ear as a result of surgery done often as early as 4 or 5 years of age (Figs. 11-11, 11-12, 11-13 and 11-14). Aside from growth at essentially normal rates, very few changes occurred in the ears themselves after 2 years, ex-

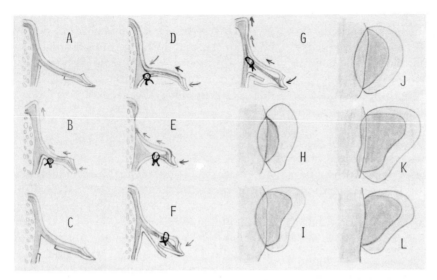

FIGURE 11-10. *Pull-in techniques. (A through G) Right ear from above. Anterior skin not present except for that in scaphal and helical areas. Gray represents soft tissue other than skin. (H through L) Right ear from behind. Darker gray represents skin excision from auricle and/or mastoid region. (A) Anterior placement of cranial edge of post-auricular skin excision. (B) Closure rotates conchal cup anteriorly, tending to impinge on canal. Tendency increases with increased undermining separating concha from mastoid. (C) Skin excision from ear and mastoid near sulcus with cranial edge of defect situated posterior to the auricular edge of the defect. (D) Leaving skin and soft tissue attached to cartilage helps here in closure's exerting pull on the conchal wall medially and posteriorly to increase the conchal floor area. Tendency to rotate the conchal cup anteriorly is diminished. In both parts B and D conchal rim and helix prominence are lessened. The closer the auricular edge of the skin defect is to the scapha and helix edge, the more bending effect there is on the anthelix. (E) Perichondrium, soft tissue, and skin undermined producing a flap attached to the scaphal area. Soft tissue and cartilage removed from conchal floor. Closure bends anthelix and slides conchal wall forward into floor. Anthelix bending would be greater if floor undermining and excisions had not been performed. (F) Flap of soft tissue and perichondrium attached to scapha is sutured to conchal cartilage. Note overlapping of posterior auricular skin and bending of anthelix. Helical prominence lessened. No effect on conchal floor. (G) Perichondrial and soft-tissue flap based on scapha near helix sutured to mastoid soft tissue. Conchal cup rotates forward because of direction of pull shown here. Anthelix bends, conchal rim and helical prominence diminish, and overlapping of postauricular skin occurs. (A through G) Many of the same effects will occur with sutures running from cartilage to cartilage or from cartilage to soft tissue if the sutures are positioned as are the skin edges or soft tissue flaps demonstrated here. (H) Closure of mastoid and auricular defect here will produce little bending effect on anthelix. (I through L) The contour of the helix edge dictates largely the shape of the excision. (L) The final sulcus tends to be most anteriorly situated when the cranial edge of the skin defect is placed originally in the preoperative sulcus at the junction of the auricle with the mastoid.*

cept for late complications of suture techniques. Among these were spitting due to exposure or late infection (Fig. 11-25B) and cutting or tearing through of one or more sutures. Keloids (Fig. 11-25I) were uncommon and were never seen on the anterior surface of the ear above the lobule. We could find no definite relationship between the incidence of keloids and the methods used. In a few cases, deepening of the sulcus and loss of scar hypertrophy continued beyond 2 years. More widening and hypertrophy of scars occurred in cases where skin was closed under great tension than in those where tension was minimal. However, by the end of 6 months, most of this widening and hypertrophy had occurred.

In fact, we found that the most significant shortcomings or failures of otoplasty had manifested themselves partially or entirely within the first 6 months. Many shortcomings were

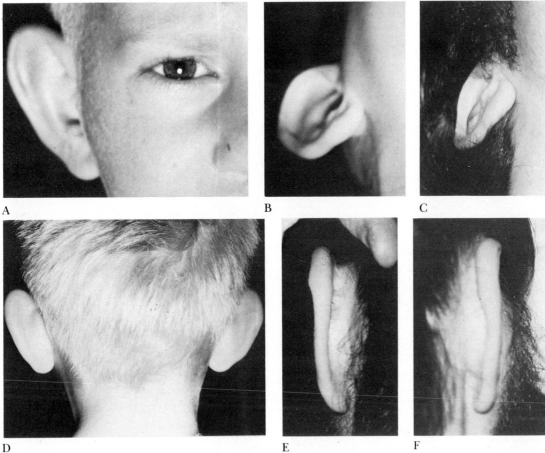

FIGURE 11-11.   *(A) 53/6/22, 5 years old. Should have increase of anthelical curvatures and some lessening of conchal prominence. (B) 53/6/22. Note underdevelopment of anthelix. (C) 76/2/17, 22 y, 8 m. Skin excision without undermining. Note bending of anthelix and diminution of helical prominence. Moderate lessening of conchal prominence. (D) 53/6/22. (E) 76/2/17, 22 y, 8 m. Mastoid skin* *has stretched out to cover part of conchal wall. No sutures from scapha to concha used, but scar ridges imitating those often seen with scapha-concha suturing show tension of closure and explain bending effect on anthelix. (F) 76/ 2/17, 22 y, 8 m. Good sulcus. Scar line just behind anthelix.*

noted as early as 2 to 4 weeks after surgery. Most inadequate or excessive corrections, asymmetries, and canal impingements could be diagnosed by then. Conchal-floor irregularities; scaphal grooving from sutures; and ridging, grooving, pebbling, cobblestoning, and rippling from cartilage thinning, scoring, abrading, morselizing, and suturing took up to 6 months or occasionally 1 year to reveal themselves in full glory. Suture bowstringing and

scar ridging could increase for more than 2 years.

Occasionally, we noted that degrees of prominence changed, particularly in adolescence. Almost always this was found to be the result not of changes in the relationships of certain parts to other parts of the ear, but of changes in the contour of the face or head or changes in the slope of the mastoid process. Of course, the hair-style changes of recent years

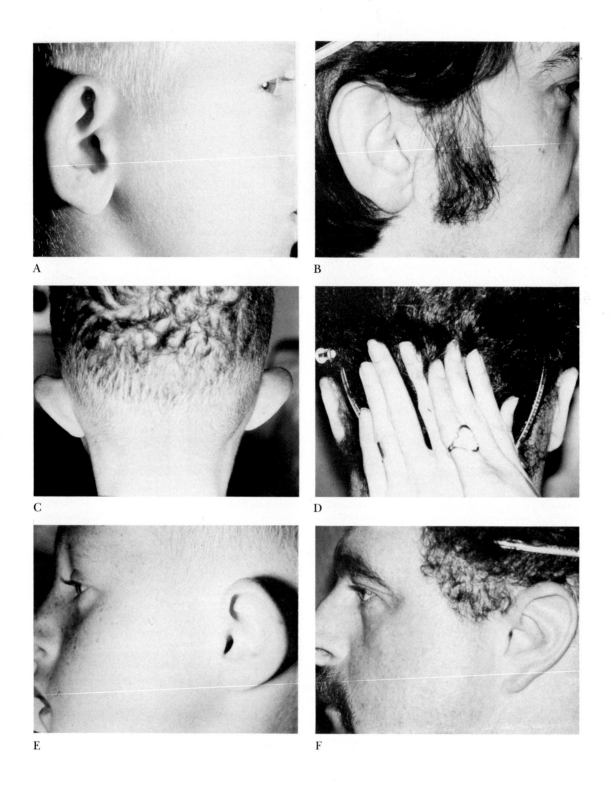

A

B

C

D

E

F

have had a profound effect on judging degrees of prominence, but I am speaking here about prominence in relation to head and face.

RESULTS OF TECHNIQUES MOVING THE AURICLE CLOSER TO THE HEAD WITHOUT BENDING THE ANTHELIX

This goal is dictated by conchal prominence and/or excessive height of the posterolateral wall of the fossa triangularis in the presence of a good anthelical and superior crural fold. Between the lateral aspects of the ear and the skull are the mastoid soft tissues and the floors and walls of the concha and fossa triangularis. Procedures allowing desired changes in the positions, shapes, or amounts of these tissues may allow the lateral edges or rims to move medially.

Anterior Rotation of Conchal Cup and Fossa Triangularis. This change in position allows lateral components to move medially. Almost all pull-in forces applied to the walls or tissues lateral to the walls tended to rotate the floors of the fossae anteriorly, unless these pulling forces were applied at such an angle to the cartilage that backward pulling on the cartilage medial to the point of application was greater than medial and anterior compressing of this cartilage. These forces were applied by pulls on skin or soft tissue or perichondrium attached to the cartilage at that site, or they were applied by sutures anchored to the cartilage. Thus all the basic pull-in techniques were used. In order to prevent as much bending of the anthelix as possible, it was learned that skin or soft tissue and/or perichondrial edges or their effective

---

FIGURE 11-12. *(A) 53/6/22. Same patient as in Figure 11-11. (B) 76/2/17, 22 y, 8 m. Normal side view. (C) 52/7/9. Upper part of ear prominent. (D) 76/2/24, 23 y, 5 m. Prominence correction with skin excision and undermining. (E) 52/7/9. No superior crus. (F) 76/2/24, 23 y, 5 m. Undermining of eminentia triangularis and upper conchal areas so extensive that these areas rotated forward and did not allow pull-in forces to be strong enough on scaphal area to bend cartilage in superior crural region.*

attachment sites to cartilage should be as far medial to the anthelix as possible. Furnas [3] has written an excellent article on conchamastoid suturing. Our concha-mastoid suturing was similar to his, and our fossa triangularis–mastoid suturing produced much the same effect on the upper pole and helix as that described by Spira [11]. For the case in which no pull should be transmitted to the scapha to produce even the slightest bending effect on the anthelix, conchally based perichondrial flap–mastoid or concha-mastoid suturing techniques were found to be preferable to those in which the pulls were produced mainly be skin excisions (Figs. 11-15B,11-18F,11-19B and 11-22C and D). Those medial parts of the walls rotated into contact with the mastoid in effect became parts of the floors of the fossae, thus adding to the total area of the floors.

Of course, without undermining the floors, thereby severing their attachments to the mastoid, anterior rotation was limited by the capacity of the attachments to stretch. To get more anterior rotation, undermining was required. It should be done in most cases (Figs. 11-4 and 11-9), but with the safeguards already listed (Fig. 11-13A through D). We found slight canal impingement to cause no significant problems, but it can be overdone. At primary surgery or in revisions, if it is recognized that undermining has been excessive, concha-mastoid suturing can anchor the cartilage so that its anterior rotation is limited or so that the floor is pulled posteriorly.

Flattening of Floors and Conversion of Medial Walls into Floors. These shape changes allow lateral components of the auricle to move medially. Pull-in forces applied from behind to the walls of the fossa triangularis and concha tended to flatten them into the floors as well as to make them slide or rotate anteriorly unless the backward component of pull was made great enough to overcome the more usual anterior rotating component. For a given pull, the more rotation allowed by undermining, the less com-

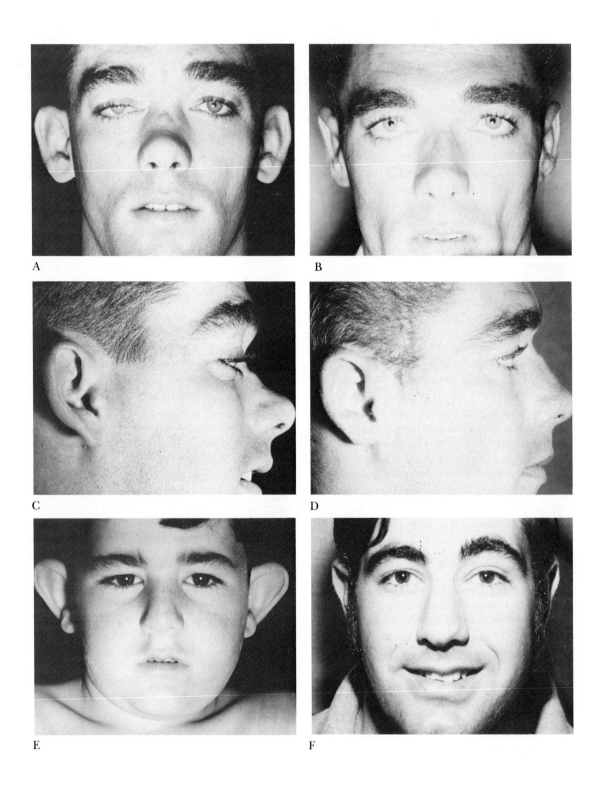

A

B

C

D

E

F

pression there was of the mastoid soft tissue deep to the floors and the less flattening there was of the medial parts of the walls to convert them into additional parts of the floors. Because the conchal wall in particular is curved in at least two dimensions, it resisted conversion into a flat shape. Rapidly increasing forces were required to flatten each additional millimeter of conchal wall into floor. In addition, compressions in the cartilage built up rapidly and were relieved by buckling at some point. The greater the pulling forces required, the more likely was the stretching and parting of tissues and the cutting through of sutures. However, within limitations, conchal and fossa triangularis wall flattening into floor was found to be a helpful part of bringing lateral structures of the ear closer to the head (Figs. 11-12A and B, 11-14C and D, and 11-15E and F).

Excisions of Interposed Tissues. The third main way to move lateral auricular parts medially is to remove tissues between these parts and the skull (Figs. 11-16 through 11-21). Several methods have been discussed. Segments of lateral conchal wall (Figs. 11-3D and E and 11-7C), medial conchal wall (Fig. 11-3B and C), medial conchal wall and conchal floor (Figs. 11-3I and J,11-7B,C,E, and F, 11-9D through F, and 11-10E), conchal and fossa triangularis floors (Figs. 11-6A and D and 11-9A through

---

FIGURE 11-13. *(A) 52/10/27. Preoperative. Observe contour of upper part of eminentia triangularis medial to helix on patient's right. (B) 54/8/6, 1 y, 9 m. Skin excision, undermining, and cartilage removal from outer part of fossa triangularis. Excessive undermining behind canal allowed impingement on canal. Therefore, this impinging cartilage excised. Note buckling of helix near fossa excision. No discs from eminentia excised. Skin excision from left lobule excessive. Mastoid soft tissue excised on right side. (C) 52/10/27. Preoperative. (D) 54/8/6, 1 y, 9 m. Needed secondary Z-plasty to skin of canal (performed on 53/9/14). (E) 53/6/8. Deficient anthelices. Protrusion more severe in upper half of ears. (F) 70/1/2, 16 y, 7 m. Good, symmetrical correction with skin excision, mastoid soft-tissue excision, and undermining only. Undermining of concha limited in order to ensure that main effect of pull would be anthelical bending, not anterior rotation of conchal cup.*

C), and mastoid soft tissue (Figs. 11-3K and L, 11-9C, and 11-10E) were removed in our series. Obviously, removal of these tissues made it possible for lesser pulls to draw the lateral parts of the ear toward the head. Also undermining required to get to these tissues added to the ease of rotation just described.

RESULTS OF TECHNIQUES THAT BEND THE ANTHELIX

This goal is dictated by helical prominence resulting from lack or underdevelopment of normal curvatures of folds in the anthelical area (Figs. 11-21 through 11-24). As mentioned, only rarely have we seen a patient with prominence due solely to lacking or underdeveloped anthelical folds. Almost always there is some conchal prominence as well. However, the otoplastic surgeon should know how to produce controlled bending of the anthelix, for he or she will see cases in which helical prominence is caused mainly by lacking or diminished curvature of these folds.

Focusing on fundamentals, the cartilage of the ear that lacks normal anthelical folds has its own structural integrity. Medial pressure on the helix will cause the cartilage to bend into shapes resembling the normal folds, but the cartilaginous spring restores the lack of curvature as soon as the pushing force is released. We employed medial pulling forces to the scapha to produce similar curvatures (Figs. 11-4, 11-5, and 11-10A through G). The variables included (1) site of pull, (2) pulling agent, (3) strength of pull, (4) direction of pull, and (5) site of medial fixation of pulling agent. We also tested various methods of changing the cartilage spring itself to lower its resistance to the bending forces. The techniques employed were (1) incising completely through the spring with single and multiple incisions, beveled incisions, oblique multiple incisions, through-and-through dicing incisions and morselization, etc.; (2) weakening by abrading, scoring, thinning, and morselizing the posterior surface; and (3) weakening and building new intrinsic curvatures by abrading,

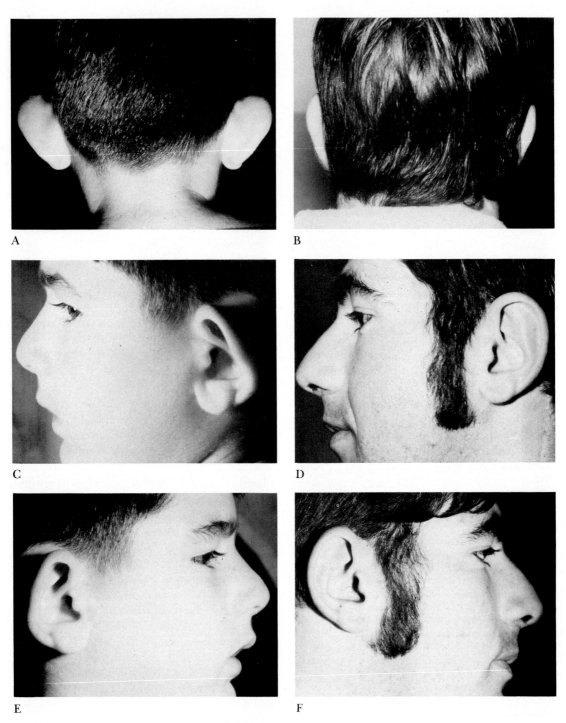

FIGURE 11-14. *(A) 53/6/8. Same patient as in Figure 11-13E and F. (B) 70/1/2, 16 y, 7 m. Good sulci present but hidden by hair. (C) 53/6/8. (D) 70/1/2, 16 y, 7 m. No discernible retardation of growth of ear caused by surgery in childhood. Good curvatures of anthelix and superior crus. (E) 53/6/8. Preoperative. (F) 70/1/2. Normal appearance postoperatively.*

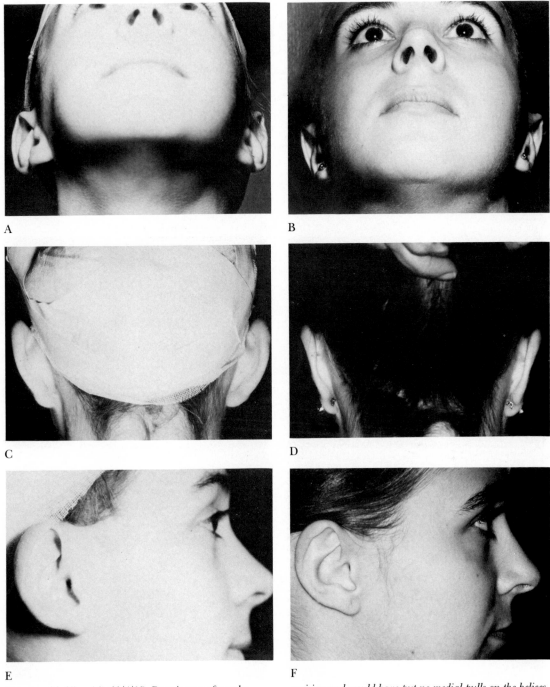

E

F

FIGURE 11-15. *(A) 61/4/15. Prominence of concha, helix, antitragus, and lobule. Underdevelopment of anthelix. (B) 72/1/2, 10 y, 7 m. Skin excision, limited undermining, excision of discs and cauda. Lower portions of helices hidden slightly but were almost hidden before surgery. Concha-mastoid sutures would have allowed less skin excision and would have put no medial pulls on the helices themselves. (C) 61/4/15. Skin markings shown. (D) 73/10/2, 12 y, 5 m. Sulci shown. Less skin excision at lower level of helices would have been wise. (E) 61/4/15. (F) 73/10/2, 12 y, 5 m. Conchal floor normal. Curvatures of anthelix and superior crus increased.*

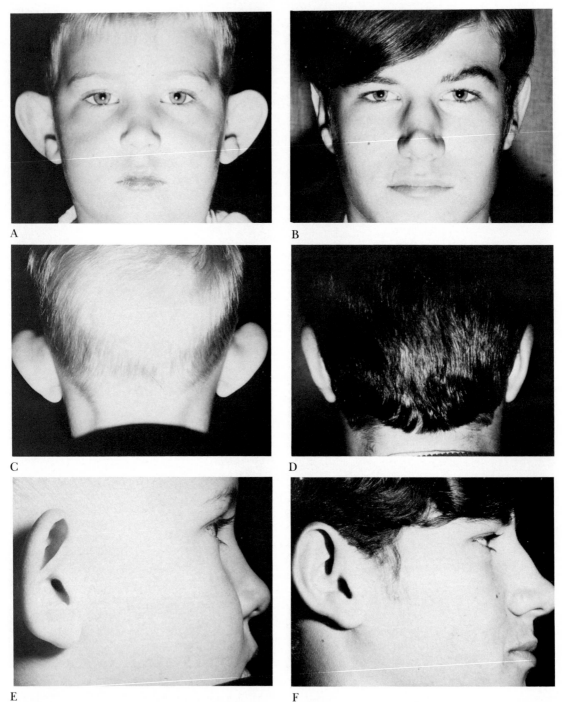

A

B

C

D

E

F

FIGURE 11-16. *(A) 57/5/9. Prominence of antitragus, helix, lobule, and concha. Anthelix folds undeveloped or missing. (B) 69/7/1, 12 y, 2 m. Skin excision. Undermining limited to that allowing cartilage disc excision from eminences. Cauda excised. (C) 57/5/9. Contours of emi-* *nences can be observed. (D) 69/7/1, 12 y, 2 m. Good sulci. (E) 57/5/9. Fossa triangularis facing forward. (F) 69/7/1, 12 y, 2 m. Normal appearance of folds and floor. Fossa triangularis now facing anterolaterally.*

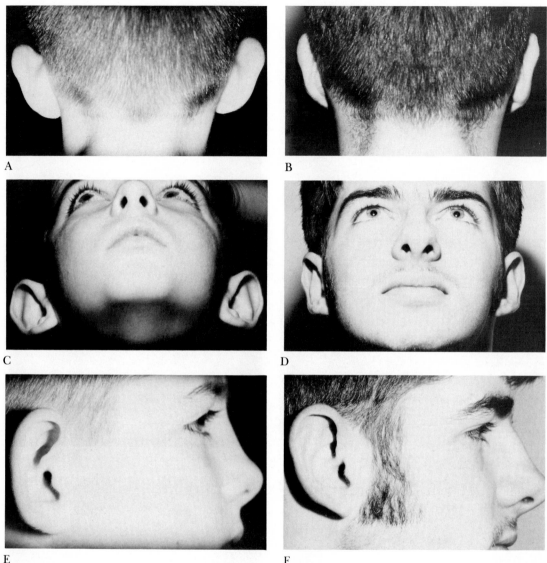

FIGURE 11-17.   *(A) 59/12/24. (B) 70/1/5, 10 y. Skin excision, wider undermining, disc excisions, and excisions of attachments of cauda to rest of cartilage. Good sulci. (C) 59/12/24. Marked conchal protrusion apparent. Anthelix folds present but slightly undeveloped. (D) 70/1/5, 10 y. More curvature to folds. Good symmetry. (E) 59/12/24. (F) 70/1/5, 10 y. Normal appearance. Superior crus gently curved.*

scoring, thinning, and morselizing the anterior surface.

Pulling Variables.   The factors tested were as follows:

1.   SITE OF PULL.   The farther away from the center of the anthelical curvature the effective center of the pulling forces was placed, the greater the bending effect on the hinge-like area was found to be (Fig. 11-10D through G).

2.   PULLING AGENT.   The pulls on the scapha were exerted by (a) sutures, (b) skin and soft tissue (nonundermined), (c) skin and soft tissue (undermined), (d) perichondrium (nonundermined), and (e) perichondrium (undermined).

174

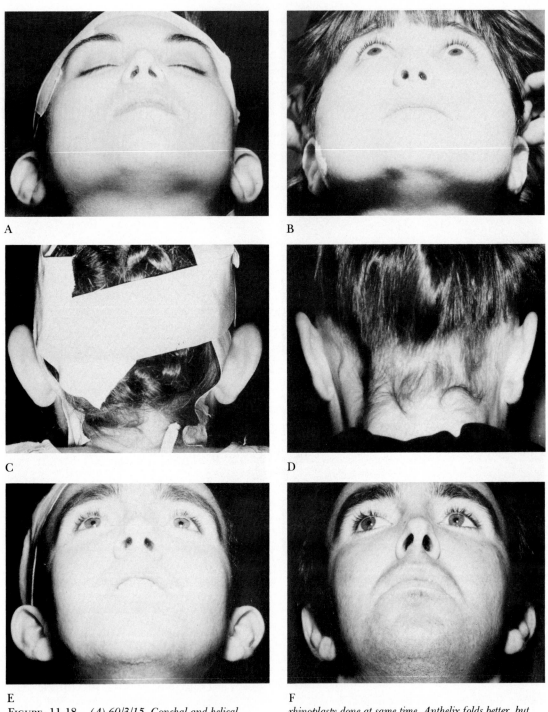

E

F

FIGURE 11-18. *(A) 60/3/15. Conchal and helical prominence. Underdevelopment of anthelical fold. Missing superior crural fold. (B) 68/3/30, 8 y. Skin excision, undermining, and disc excision. Cauda excision performed as well, mainly to get additional cartilage to use in revisional*

rhinoplasty done at same time. Anthelix folds better, but undermining and disc excisions performed to get cartilage for nose did not allow skin excisional pulls to apply enough to scaphal or helical areas to produce normal superior crural folds. (C) 60/6/22. Prominence of lobule, helix, and

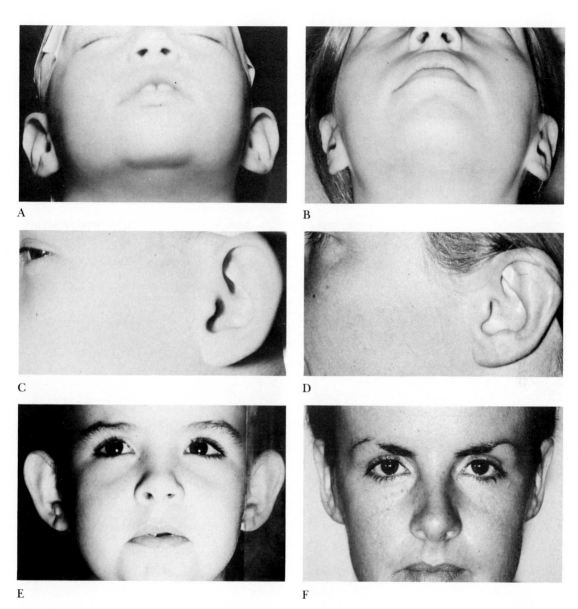

FIGURE 11-19.   *(A) 61/2/16. Asymmetric prominence.*
(B) 66/2/3, 5 y. Asymmetrical correction. Inadequate im-
provement of lobular prominences. Skin excision, under-
mining, and excision of discs and cauda. Concha-mastoid
suture would have provided less medial pull on helix just

concha. (D) 63/11/25, 3 y, 5 m. Prominences well and
symmetrically corrected. Good sulci. Skin excision, under-
mining, disc and cauda removals performed. (E) 62/3/26.
Protrusions of helix, conchal rim, and lobule. Anthelix
folds present. (F) 70/10/5, 8 y, 6 m. All areas symmetri-
cally improved with skin excision, undermining, and disc
and cauda excisions.

above lobule. Where helix is hidden or almost hidden be-
hind conchal rim preoperatively, suture should be substi-
tuted for skin excision or larger disc excision with very little
skin excision should be considered for correction of the
conchal prominence at that level. (C) 61/2/16. (D) 77/9/6,
16 y, 6 m. Conchal floor and anthelical folds normal in
appearance. (E) 54/8/17. This last example of skin excision
and disc removal for conchal setback has prominent conchal
rims with deficient anthelix folds. Helical protrusion
is marked, and the ears are large in the vertical dimen-
sion. (F) 77/8/30, 23 y. With prominence corrected, the
ears no longer seem so large. There is good symmetry and
no undue protrusion of any auricular parts.

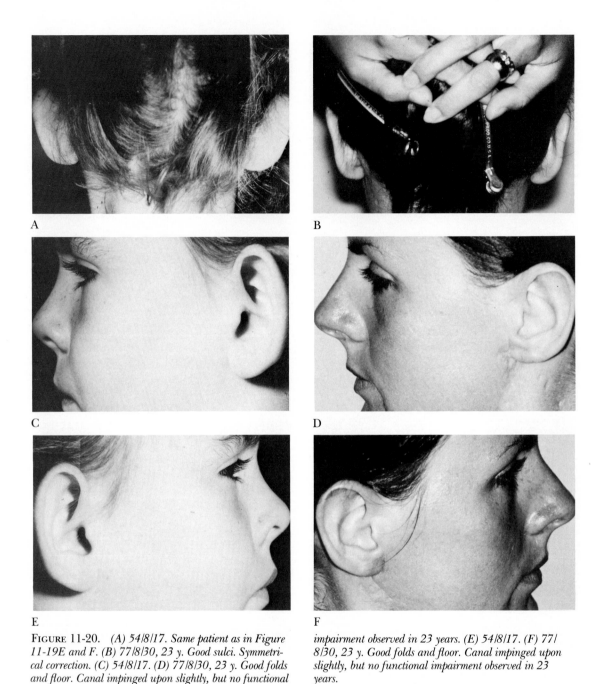

FIGURE 11-20. *(A) 54/8/17. Same patient as in Figure 11-19E and F. (B) 77/8/30, 23 y. Good sulci. Symmetrical correction. (C) 54/8/17. (D) 77/8/30, 23 y. Good folds and floor. Canal impinged upon slightly, but no functional* *impairment observed in 23 years. (E) 54/8/17. (F) 77/ 8/30, 23 y. Good folds and floor. Canal impinged upon slightly, but no functional impairment observed in 23 years.*

As mentioned, Wright [17] and Kaye [4] have written excellent articles on sutures applied to the scapha. The monumental work in this regard is that of Mustardé [6,7]. As far as the scaphal ends of the sutures are concerned, we found that it was wise, in addition to observations already mentioned, to make the bites paralleling the fold, to make the bites large, to tighten the knot to just begin to curve the cartilage grasped between the upper and lower strands of the mattress suture, and to overcorrect by just a tiny amount, except in through-

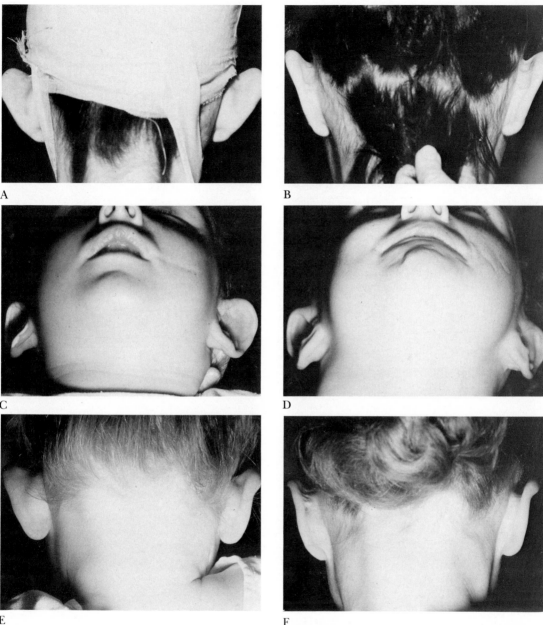

FIGURE 11-21.   *(A) 67/6/2. Scapha-mastoid suture technique to be used. (B) 67/12/28, 6 m. Ridging or tenting from scapha-mastoid sutures easily apparent. Some recurrence of prominence of upper portions of ears. (C) 52/1/14. Asymmetrical prominence. Lack of superior crural fold, left side. (D) 53/6/13, 1 y, 5 m. Scapha-mastoid sutures, skin excision, undermining limited to that needed to perform slight mastoid soft-tissue excisions carried out on both sides and to that needed to excise the spina helicis performed on left side. Anterior skin flap with edges* at scapha-helix junction elevated and anterior surface in anthelix fold area weakened by scoring and abrading with rasp. Helical spine excised on left. Presence of anthelix fold on right made these last maneuvers unnecessary there. Observe suture ridging or tenting produced by scapha-mastoid sutures. (E) 52/1/14. Groove where anthelical fold present should be noted on right side. (F) 53/6/13, 1 y, 5 m. Slight ridging noted on right, more on left. Skin excision minimal on both sides but a little greater on left than on right.*

178

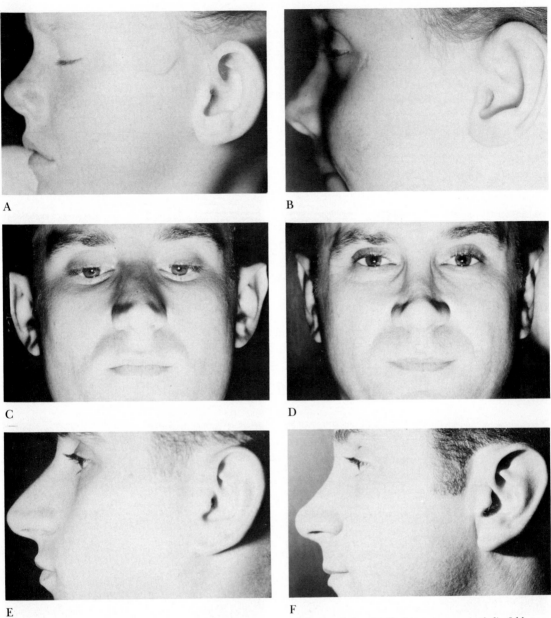

A

B

C

D

E

F

FIGURE 11-22. *(A) 52/6/13. Same patient as in Figure 11-21C through F. (B) 53/6/13, 1 y, 5 m. Scar at helix-scapha junction slightly visible still. Superior crural fold where cartilage was weakened by scoring and abrading is slightly sharper than normal. The right ear had no weakening, and its fold is normal in appearance. (C) 59/*

6/10. Conchal and helical prominence. Anthelix folds present. (D) 71/10/26, 12 y, 4 m. Concha-mastoid and triangular fossa wall–mastoid white silk sutures. Limited undermining and skin excision. Actual overcorrection achieved. (E) 59/6/10. (F) 71/10/26, 12 y, 4 m. Practically no change observed in the folds.

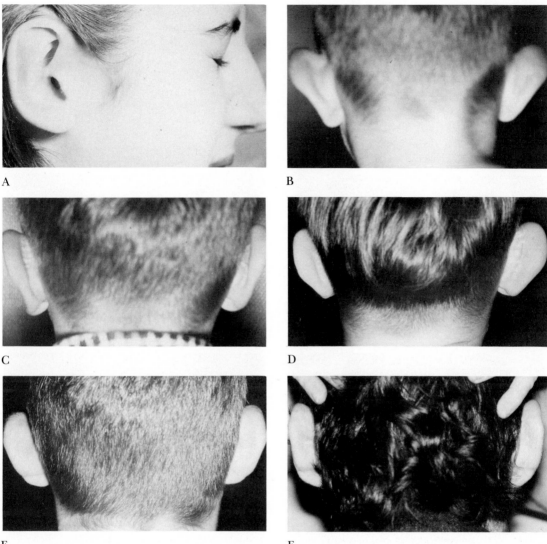

A

B

C

D

E

F

FIGURE 11-23.   *(A) 52/2/29, 3 y, 2 m. Result of excision of cartilage from conchal wall area, weakening of cartilage in superior crural region, and suturing in the latter area. Superior crus became too sharp and imitates the one on the left ear made by incising completely through the cartilage (see Fig. 11-7C). Scapha appears too broad. (B)*

54/7/30. (C) 54/11/26, 4 m. Scapha-concha sutures used. Ridging beginning to show. (D) 56/2/15, 1 y, 6 m. Secondary surgery will be required to correct this recurrence of original problem. (E) 65/9/17. (F) 76/4/5, 11 y, 6 m. Scapha-concha siliconized white silk sutures combined with slight skin excision and excision of discs and cauda.

and-through incising or morselizing procedures. The less that was done to weaken the spring, the more need there was for sharing the suture pulls with other pulls, such as those provided by skin excisions in excess of those required just to get rid of overlaps produced by the sutures to scaphal cartilage itself. When

working from the posterior surface, we placed the knots there. On the anterior surface, we found it more convenient to place the knots in the scaphal groove than in the concha, but results showed that knots with larger, stiffer suture material became visible. When scaphal-mastoid sutures were used with anterior expo-

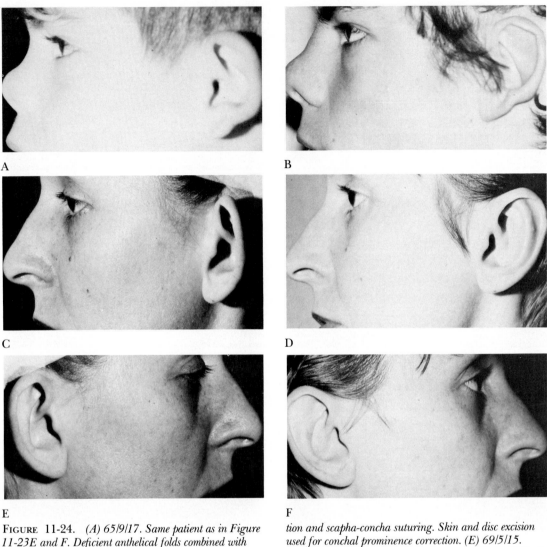

A

B

C

D

E

F

FIGURE 11-24. *(A) 65/9/17. Same patient as in Figure 11-23E and F. Deficient anthelical folds combined with conchal prominence. (B) 76/4/5, 11 y, 6 m. The sutures cut through and the folds disappeared. (C) 69/5/15. Superior crus missing. (D) 69/9/23, 4 m. Excessive curvature of superior crus from weakening with morseliza-* *tion and scapha-concha suturing. Skin and disc excision used for conchal prominence correction. (E) 69/5/15. Superior crus present but underdeveloped. (F) 69/9/23, 4 m. Discs and skin excised. Concha-mastoid suturing. No morselization. Good correction. Normal superior crural curvature.*

sure, posterior wounds had also been made, and the knots were placed at the mastoid end (Fig. 11-21D and F). If the knots were placed on the scaphal surface, we tried to flatten the knots by crushing them into the cartilage, but we found this maneuver unnecessary in most cases with the softer suture materials available in recent years.

If the skin and soft tissue excision extended to the scapha, and if the edge was not undermined, sutures applied to this edge that closed the excisional defect were found to exert pulling forces on the scapha. Actually, because the skin and soft tissue slid somewhat even without undermining, the lateral skin excision edge could even be over slightly on the conchal side of the anthelix with effective application to the scapha of pulling forces set up by sutures closing this edge to the other edge of the skin excisional defect. More precise concentration of the pulling forces could be provided by undermining the skin and soft tissue laterally to some predetermined line on the back of the scapha.

Suture bites taken in the perichondrium and soft tissue on the posterior surface of the scapha were tried. However, pulling forces applied through these bites were found to be of a temporary nature for the most part because the sutures gradually cut through these soft tissues. Undermined perichondrium and soft tissue or perichondrium, soft tissue, and skin in the form of flaps based out at some predetermined line on the scapha were found to distribute pulls nicely to the scapha, resist stretching, and hold well with enough sutures used at their medial ends (Fig. 11-10E through G).

We found it difficult with sutures applied to the anterior scaphal surface to avoid the occurrence of a somewhat concentrated scaphal groove at the site of the sutures (Figs. 11-24D and 11-25A). Also observed was a tendency toward too concentrated a superior crural fold or curvature, particularly when weakening or spring-changing techniques on the cartilage itself also were used (Figs. 11-22B, 11-24D, and 11-25A). All too often we ended with a somewhat "bunched," too tightly rolled superior crus, with the wall of the fossa triangularis facing too far forward rather than laterally (Figs. 11-22B, 11-24D, and 11-25A), or with varying degrees of loss of the crural curvature and/or failure of correction of the helical prominence (Figs. 11-22F, 11-23B through F, and 11-24A through D). Of course, with the number of cases in the series, we had some good results (Figs. 11-4G through I and Fig. 11-5), but we never developed the feeling that suturing alone should be used to solve the problem of the lack of superior crus on a routine basis. For the lower part of the anthelix, the tight rolling just mentioned was not bad, and at this level, we found sutures to be more useful. However, their use to roll lateral conchal wall into anthelix

in correcting conchal prominence was an aesthetic mistake in most cases. The scapha was made too broad, and the site of the lower end of the superior crus was moved too far forward.

Application of pulling forces by suturing the edges of skin defects or scaphal-based perichondrial flaps (Fig. 11-25C through H) gave more normal (less concentrated) curvatures than did the use of sutures to cartilage. Apparently the forces were better and more diffusely distributed to the areas being pulled on. The cutting in and grooving from sutures that applied their pressure intensely to very limited areas was not observed with these techniques. However, one can damage cartilage in elevating perichondrial flaps, and their use was found to be followed by thickening of the area enclosed by the flap posteriorly and the cartilage anteriorly. Skin excision alone with closure of the defect was found to produce normal-appearing folds, but the medial edge had to be so far medial that some medial displacement of the conchal rim almost always had to take place. Also, without use of cartilage weakening or cartilage or flap suturing, skin excision alone had its failures. When combined with any of the techniques producing or allowing medial displacement of the conchal rim, the failure rate in the production of anthelical curvatures was higher (Figs. 11-12E and F and 11-18A and B).

3. STRENGTH OF PULL. In most cases it was found wise to apply the pulls strongly enough to get the folds desired and then to slightly overcorrect. The greatest overcorrection had to be used when skin alone was the pulling agent. However, no overcorrection could be used where the areas had had through-and-through morselization or cartilaginous incisions. These patients would remain in the overcorrected state (Figs. 11-23A and 11-24C and D). We have commented on the need for enough sutures.

4. DIRECTION OF PULL. A pull at a right angle to the plane of the scapha, where the pulling force was being applied, exerted the greatest bending effect. The greater the departure from a right angle, the less bending ef-

182

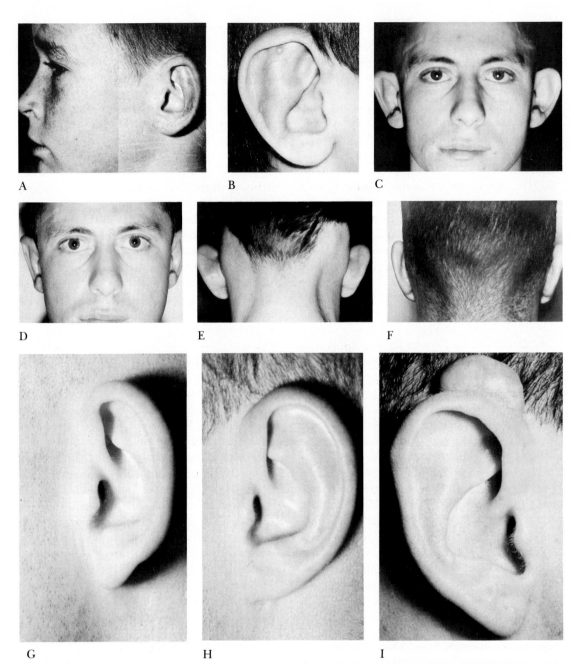

FIGURE 11-25. (A) 68/11/26, 1 y. Kaye technique.
Superior crus curvature slightly excessive. (B) 77/8/9, 3 y.
Acute perichondritis from scapha-concha and scapha-fossa
triangularis sutures. Suture removal, drainage, and
antibiotic-cured patient. (C) 53/1/31. Bilateral conchal
prominence. Left anthelix more deficient than right. (D)
54/3/29, 1 y, 2 m. Pull-in with skin excision, helix-based

perichondrial and soft-tissue flaps, and undermining. (E)
53/1/31. Ridiculously overdone "prep." (F) 54/3/29, 1 y,
2 m. Sulcus deeper on left. Perichondrial flap sutured to
concha on left, to mastoid on right. (G) 53/1/21. (H) 54/
3/29, 1 y, 2 m. Good curvatures and floor. (I) 56/12/6, 3
y, 9 m. Keloid in another patient.

fect there was. However, the farther medially on the concha that we attached the ends of perichondrial flaps, the more thickening we observed; and the farther medially on the concha that we placed the medial ends of scapha-concha sutures, the more bowstringing became apparent. The worst thickening was seen in patients where the flaps were sutured to mastoid tissues (Fig. 11-25F), and the most visible bowstringing was in those where scapha-mastoid sutures were employed (Fig. 11-21B and D).

5. SITE OF MEDIAL FIXATION OF PULLING AGENT. Comments have already been made about this variable. With flap and suture techniques, we finally settled in most cases on siting the medial fixation points or lines in the fossa triangularis or concha about the same distance from the center of the curvature of the fold (produced by finger pressure on the helix) as the distance between the center of the fold and the site of the pull being applied at that level to the scapha. When the scaphal distance was shortened and the conchal distance increased, sutures tended to pull out more or the scapha tended to be too wide. When the opposite arrangement was used, the sutures tended to pull out more or the scapha tended to face backward too much.

Changing the Anthelical Cartilaginous Spring to Diminish Resistance to Bending Forces. The variables studied were as follows:

1. INCISING COMPLETELY THROUGH THE SPRING. Incisions completely through the cartilage have been mentioned (Fig. 11-7C). For a short while, we tried morselizing with the morselizing teeth on both sides of the cartilage. The results were not good enough to make us wish to continue with that approach (Fig. 11-24C and D).

2. WEAKENING BY ABRADING, SCORING, THINNING, AND/OR MORSELIZING THE POSTERIOR SURFACE. Work done on the posterior surface had two advantages: this surface was exposed already in most otoplasties, and the smooth anterior surface of cartilage was left intact when the cartilage was thinned or weakened by work on its posterior surface. It was not found difficult after a short while to transpose in one's mind the position of the fold desired in anterior view to where work had to be done on the posterior surface to produce the weakening. Thinning by abrading or rasping was found to be technically easier than shaving or paring with the scalpel or curette. It was all too easy to thin too much in too localized a fashion (Fig. 11-7B). Actually, it was found best in most cases to equally thin the entire area where the curvature was desired, rather than to thin the central line of the desired curvature more than its peripheral edges. Partial scoring, except with multiple beveled cuts, did not weaken evenly and well, and even with them, was less satisfactory than abrading. Morselizing the posterior surface was better than morselizing the anterior surface or both surfaces in our cases, but we found it no better than abrading. It should be kept in mind that these treatments of the posterior surface build into the cartilage a tendency to curve in the direction opposite to that desired. With enough thinning, however, this tendency was easily overbalanced by the actual total weakening accomplished.

3. WEAKENING AND BUILDING DESIRED NEW INTRINSIC CURVATURES BY ABRADING, SCORING, THINNING, AND/OR MORSELIZING THE ANTERIOR SURFACE. Methods used to get to the anterior surface have been described. Examples are shown in Figures 11-21C through F, 11-22A and B, and 11-25A. All were satisfactory. However, it was found easy to leave irregularities from scoring or morselizing through small tunnels (Fig. 11-24D) with limited visualization of the treated surface. To abrade the anterior surface well with motor-driven equipment and over a large enough area, we found it helpful to raise a good-sized flap using an incision at the junction of the scapha with the helix. The helical curl hid the incision line well, except when we made the incision a little too far into the scaphal area or below the curl (Fig. 11-22B). We did not use this flap in any patients without the helical curl.

RESULTS OF TECHNIQUES THAT BEND THE ANTHELIX AND MOVE IT CLOSER TO THE HEAD

This goal is dictated by the combination of underdevelopment or lack of anthelical fold with the presence of prominence of the fold when it is produced by finger pressure on the helix. Prominence is caused by excessive heights of the walls of the fossa triangularis and conchal cup. Both problems had to be treated for satisfactory results. In a given case, we learned that what may be the best solution for part of the problem may make the answer to the other more difficult. Also, the cumulative effect of two or three methods was often found to be more reliable than excessive use of just one modality.

In previous sections, we have listed most of the variables in treatment employed. Here we will discuss certain important observations and conclusions derived from the results of combining techniques to produce improvement of both problems. Almost all patients in the series had some elements of both. Most of the observations mentioned in the section on techniques were derived from the results of treating both problems in the same patient; only a few will be repeated here.

The superior crural part of the anthelical fold is the lateral rim of the fossa triangularis, and the inferior crus and lower part of the anthelical fold with the antitragus make up most of the lateral rim of the conchal cup. All three maneuvers, (1) anterior rotation of the conchal cup and fossa triangularis, (2) flattening of floors and conversion of medial walls into floors, and (3) excisions of interposed tissues, lessened *prominence* of the anthelical *fold* but diminished the effect of attempts to increase anthelical *curvature* when the attempts relied on scaphal pull-in forces coming, in effect, from the mastoid. All three, by permitting the anthelical rim to move closer to the mastoid, allowed relief of the forces tending to bend the anthelix. Therefore, when one or more of these modalities was employed, greater pulls from the mastoid had to be added, the anthelical area had to be weakened, or the scapha to conchal and fossa triangularis wall pulls had to be

added to produce anthelical bending if an appreciable bending effect was required.

Most of the patients shown in this chapter had skin excisions with the medial edge of the defect in the sulcus. A few had some mastoid skin excised as well. Therefore, almost all had some pulls from mastoid exerted on the concha and/or scaphal areas by closure of the skin defect. The only exception shown here is in Figure 11-25A. Almost every author advocating any technique for prominent ear correction in the last 30 years ultimately has concluded that some postauricular skin must be excised or recurrence rates become excessive. We had reached similar conclusions with regard to the techniques tested in our series. It certainly was not found necessary to carry the lateral edge of every skin excision out close to the scapha, nor was it required that every medial edge be at the mastoid. The more the patient's problem involved anthelical bending, and the less it required medial displacement of the anthelical fold, the more confined the skin excision could be to the area near the fold itself. However, since almost all the patients shown here did need some medial displacement of the fold, we placed the medial edge of the skin excision in or near the sulcus. Therefore, the reader should keep in mind as he or she analyzes these cases that, added to the other techniques employed, pulls from mastoid were present in the patients shown here.

The other technique common to most of the patients shown here was undermining of parts of the floor. The exceptions are in Figures 11-7A through C, 11-11, 11-12A and B, 11-23A, and 11-25A. Essentially all other cases had some degree of anterior rotation of the floors beyond the small amount allowed by stretching of floor attachments to mastoid which results from closure of skin excisional defects.

Obviously, some floor flattening occurred in every case from closure of the skin defects, if not additionally from other mastoid to ear pulls introduced with other techniques. Also, because most patients had some pulls on scapha applied by closure of the skin defects, there was some increase in the curvature of the anthelix, unless anthelical displacement toward the head relieved essentially all the bending forces applied.

Disc excisions of cartilage of the floors and, in some cases, of the medial parts of the walls were done in the patients shown in Figures 11-7E and F, 11-8, 11-9, 11-15 through 11-19, 11-23B through F, 11-24, and 11-25B. Mastoid soft-tissue excisions were used in patients appearing in Figures 11-9C,11-13,11-14,11-21C through F, and 11-22A and B.

Pull-in forces exerted by skin-defect closures have been mentioned. Those provided by sutures follow: scapha-concha (Figs. 11-4 and 11-5 [left ear], 11-23, 11-24A through D, and 11-25B), scapha–fossa triangularis (Figs. 11-23A through D,11-24C and D, and 11-25B), scapha-mastoid (Figs. 11-21 and 11-22A and B), fossa triangularis–mastoid (Fig. 11-22C through F), and concha-mastoid (Fig. 11-22C through F). Those provided by perichondrial and soft-tissue flaps follow: flap sutured to concha (Fig. 11-25C through H), and flap sutured to mastoid (Fig. 11-25C through H) (this case was selected because it illustrates both techniques).

The cases showing techniques used to change the anthelical cartilaginous spring to diminish its resistance to bending forces have been listed. To these should be added the one shown in Figure 11-23A.

The other element of prominence found in most of these patients was the unduly protruding lobule. Five techniques for its correction are illustrated in this chapter. Skin excision was involved in correcting almost all. In addition, we used resection of the cauda in patients shown in Figures 11-4 and 11-5 (right ear), 11-7A and B and D through F, 11-8,11-15,11-16,11-18 through 11-20,11-23E and F, and 11-24A and B. Resection of a small segment attaching the cauda to the rest of the auricular cartilage was used in Figure 11-17. Treatment of the enlarged and prominent lobule is shown in Figure 11-8E and F. The rest of the patients either had incisions that separated the cauda from the rest of the cartilage or this was not done because the other techniques used to correct prominence above the lobule corrected the prominence of the lobule as well.

Final Thoughts

Many conclusions can be reached from these results, all long-term enough to illustrate salient points. We have shown that otoplasty does not interfere with adequate growth of the ear. We have demonstrated that more than one technique can be used to correct each of the two main elements contributing to the prominent ear: inadequate anthelical fold curvature and lateral prominence of the anthelical fold itself. It should be apparent that enough variations exist to eliminate the likelihood that any one technique is the best solution to all problems. Based on the long-term results of this study, in which many techniques have been employed, we must conclude that each patient requires meticulous diagnosis and that almost all corrections should involve combinations of technical steps. If modality A, moderately employed, is the best answer for problem 1, and modality B, moderately employed, is the best answer for problem 2, but in its use it lessens the corrective effects of modality A on problem 1, then modality A may have to be employed to a greater degree, or modality B may have to be used to a lesser degree, or other modalities may have to be added to or subtracted from the operative maneuvers. Because so many dynamic concepts are involved, we must admit that individual solutions are complex and we have no final answers. If the sights are set high enough, making "the perfect ear" still remains a challenge for the aesthetic surgeon.

References

1. Courtiss, E.H., Webster, R.C., and White, M.F. Otoplasty: Direct Surgical Approach. In F.W. Masters and J.R. Lewis (Eds.), *Symposium on Aesthetic Surgery of the Nose, Ears and Chin.* St. Louis: Mosby, 1973. P. 127.
2. Ely, E.T. An operation for prominence of the auricles. *Plast. Reconstr. Surg.* 42:582, 1968. (Reprinted from *Arch. Otology* 10:97, 1881.)

3. Furnas, D.W. Correction of prominent ears by concha-mastoid sutures. *Plast. Reconstr. Surg.* 42:189, 1968.

4. Kaye, B.L. A simplified method for correction of the prominent ear. *Plast. Reconstr. Surg.* 40:44, 1967.

5. Luckett, W.H. A new operation for prominent ears based on the anatomy of the deformity. *Plast. Reconstr. Surg.* 43:83, 1969, (Reprinted from *Surg. Gynecol. Obstet.* 10:635, 1910.)

6. Mustardé, J.C. The correction of prominent ears using simple mattress sutures. *Br. J. Plast. Surg.* 16:170, 1963.

7. Mustardé, J.C. The treatment of prominent ears by buried mattress sutures: A ten-year survey. *Plast. Reconstr. Surg.* 39:382, 1967.

8. Rubin, F.F. Permanent change in shape of cartilage by morselization. *Arch. Otolaryngol.* 89:602, 1969.

9. Rubin, L.R., Bromberg, B.E., Walden, R.H., and Adams, A. An anatomic approach to the obtrusive ear. *Plast. Reconstr. Surg.* 29:360, 1962.

10. Sercer, A. Einige Worte über die Ursache und die Korrektur abstehender Ohren. *Pract. Otorhinolaryngol.* 13:9, 1951.

11. Spira, M., McCrea, R., Gerow, F.J., and Hardy, S.B. Correction of the principal deformities causing protruding ears. *Plast. Reconstr. Surg.* 44:150, 1969.

12. Stark, R.B., and Saunders, D.E. Natural appearance restored to the unduly prominent ear. *Br. J. Plast. Surg.* 15:385, 1962.

13. Stenström, S.J. A "natural" technique for correction of congenitally prominent ears. *Plast. Reconstr. Surg.* 32:509, 1963.

14. Stenström, S.J. Cosmetic deformities of the ears. In W.C. Grabb and J.W. Smith (Eds.), *Plastic Surgery* (2nd ed.). Boston: Little, Brown, 1973. Pp. 595–607.

15. Webster, R.C., Davidson, T.M., and Nahum, A.M. Otoplasty (parts I, II, and III). *Classics in Soft Tissue and Cosmetic Surgery* (videocassettes). San Diego, Calif., 1977. (Produced by Educational Foundation of American Academy of Facial Plastic and Reconstructive Surgery.)

16. Webster, R.C., Smith R.C., White, M.F., McCollough, E.G., and Smith, C.W. Otoplasty: Pull-in or pull-back techniques—25 year experience. *Aesth. Reconstr. Facial Plast. Surg.* 1:1, 1974.

17. Wright, W.K. Otoplasty goals and principles. *Arch. Otolaryngol.* 92: 568, 1970.

Melvin Spira

COMMENTS ON CHAPTERS 10 and 11

Comments on Chapter 10

EARLY in his chapter, Mustardé emphasizes that the mattress sutures used in corrective otoplasty must pierce the anterior perichondrium and lie just under, but not in, the anterior auricular skin to be effective. I concur with this advice, but feel that synthetic sutures should be used instead of silk. Braided white nylon does not come undone easily, causes less reaction than silk, and can safely be snipped quite short.

I differ with Mustardé's extension of his technique to patients in whom a well-defined anthelix is present with protrusion secondary to conchal enlargement or angulation. To correct outstanding ears by deliberately obliterating the anthelix in order to achieve a more medially placed lateral conchal rim conflicts with the usual surgical goal—to correct rather than camouflage a defect. Mustardé advises complete removal of all connective tissue and muscle, combined with wide undermining on the posterior surface of the ear. This must be adhered to if one is effectively to employ his technique. I disagree with Webster and Smith and Mustardé about the need for removal of postauricular skin.

Mustardé's remarkably low recurrence rate (1.8 percent) testifies to his skill with this technique, as does his even lower complication rate (1 percent). Worrisome but not serious complications of his method are late bowstringing and extrusion of buried sutures. The author states, and I agree, that the sutures can be removed after 3 to 6 months without fear of relapse of the setback ear. He alludes to, but does not detail, the complication of postoperative wound infection. Treatment of this condition, whether it occurs early or late, should include immediate removal of all buried sutures. Of the 45 patients operated on 10 or more years before who responded to Mustardé's poll, 7 (15 percent) had some degree of reprotrusion. This seems a realistic figure in line with my own results.

Personal Experience with the Late Results of Surgical Correction of Protruding Ears

A retrospective evaluation of my own series of otoplasty patients operated on with the modified Mustardé technique [3,5,6] (Fig. 1A through I) and followed for 3 or more years reveals the following:

1. Overall configuration:
   a. All patients' ears had undergone varying degrees of reprotrusion, ranging in severity from only slight to total reprotrusion (the latter occurred only once) from their immediate postoperative setback position:
   b. The tendency to recurrence seems to be primarily in the upper half of the ear. Greater attention must be paid to this area.
   c. Conchal sutures alone were usually not effective in those ears in which protrusion was due to a very large concha. Without direct conchal excision, a very deep concha will remain deep postoperatively.
   d. Any excess of postauricular skin shrinks and flattens with time.
   e. Regardless of the technique employed, the earlobe generally stays back where it has been placed.
   f. Asymmetry before surgery generally means asymmetry afterward. If asymmetry exists preoperatively, both ears should be corrected. The patient should be forewarned.
2. Untoward results or complications [4]:
   a. Late reprotrusion (6 months or more postoperatively) is always possible, but is unusual. Loss of the surgical setback is usually seen within the first 3 months following operation.
   b. An anthelix that seems excessively sharp

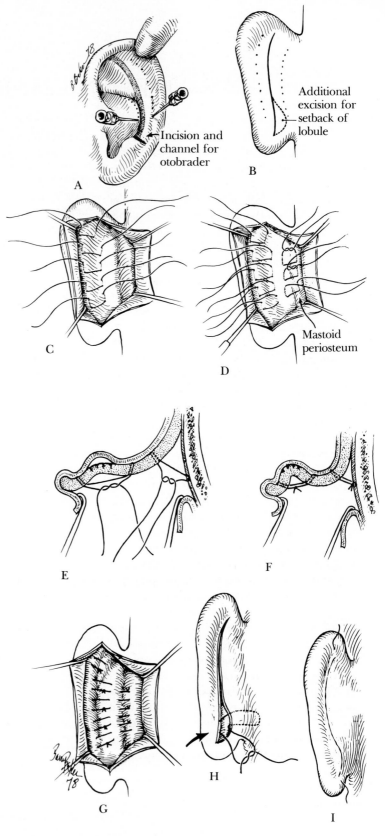

Incision and channel for otobrader

A

Additional excision for setback of lobule

B

C

Mastoid periosteum

D

E

F

G

H

I

early postoperatively will maintain that appearance (Fig. 2A through G).

c. Postauricular bowstringing is still an occasional problem (see 3h).

d. Early postoperatively, the lateral ear skin may be hypoaesthetic, and skin erosion or abrasion secondary to a pressure bandage is occasionally seen.

e. Since all ears reprotrude slightly, the surgeon should overcorrect slightly.

f. Suture extrusions can occur years after surgery. If this happens, the suture should be removed.

3. Suggestions to improve the technique based on long-term follow-up:

a. Stenström's [7] modification of scratching or abrading the anterior ear cartilage is a useful way to weaken the cartilage when recontouring the anthelix, and it creates a soft superior crus. I once considered this technique appropriate only in adults, but now I use it frequently in otoplasties on patients of all ages.

b. I now use fewer sutures and stress the importance of using a noncutting needle on a permanent suture, preferentially 4-0 braided nylon or braided Dacron.

c. To create a superior crus where there is none, place the sutures between the fossa triangularis and the scapha rather than between the concha and the scapha. This differs from Mustardé's original technique.

d. Thoroughly clean the areas over the mastoid in the sulcus before placing conchomastoid sutures.

e. Suturing the tail of the anthelix and lobe to the mastoid area without cutting or excising the cauda helicis effectively corrects the severely protruded earlobe.

FIGURE 1. *(A through I) Author's present technique. (A) Creating outline for insertion of sutures by depressing helix to create normal contour. (B) Dye marks on posterior ear—and skin excisions. (C) Cartilage exposed and lateral sutures placed. (D) Concha set back when needed. (E) Cross section—sutures in position. (F) Concha sutures tied first. (G) Internal closure complete. (H) Dermis to periosteum suture repositioning lobe. (I) Closure completed.*

f. A suture between the root of the helix and the temporalis fascia [1] is a mainstay in setting the root of the helix back against the scalp, especially when preoperative angulation in this area is severe.

g. Anterior skin scars are no problem. If a concha is very large, I do not hesitate to remove a through-and-through crescent of concha just lateral to the external auditory meatus in order to decrease total ear protrusion.

h. The removal of minimal postauricular skin allows some thickening and overlapping and prevents or reduces the incidence of bowstringing. I excise as little tissue as possible from this area.

i. Early reprotrusion can sometimes be aborted if the patient wears a hairband or tennis headband continually for 8 to 12 weeks. This ploy may even reposition the ear as it was immediately after surgery. I routinely prescribe a headband for all patients for a month after surgery.

Comments on Chapter 11

Webster and Smith recognize the protruding ear deformity as being due to a lack of development of the anthelix, to a protruding conchal rim, or to a combination of these two problems. The analysis of this common ear deformity also requires special attention to the protruding lobule and to the auriculocephalic angle of the root of the helix. Webster's and Smith's discussion of auricular anatomy provides the reader with a sound basis for an understanding of the rationale behind the variety of techniques used to treat this problem. The goal common to all methods is the achievement of symmetrical, softly contoured ears with an unoperated appearance. The authors rather uniquely classify the operative procedures to include pull-in, suture, and incision techniques. The surgical combinations they have employed become the foundation for de-

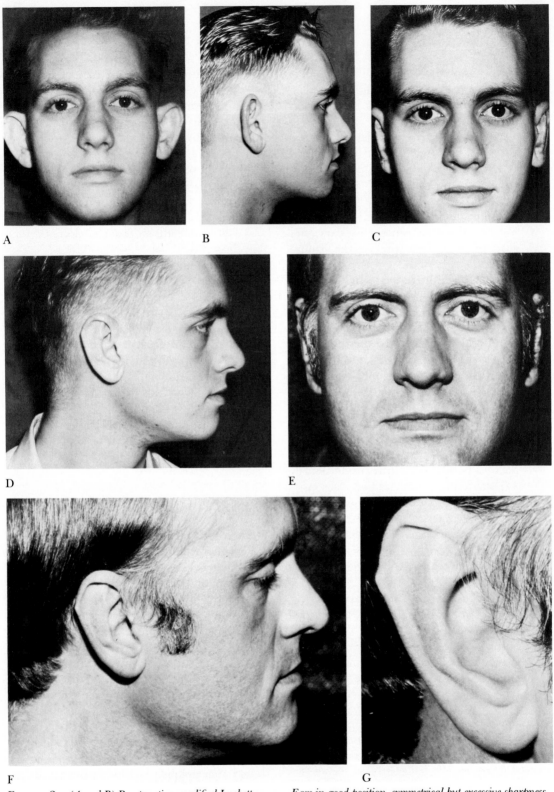

A   B   C

D   E

F   G

FIGURE 2. *(A and B) Preoperative; modified Luckett procedure performed [2]. (C and D) Postoperative; 1 week. (E and F) Postoperative; 18 years. (G) Close-up of part F.*

Ears in good position, symmetrical but excessive sharpness in anthelix and superior crus.

scriptions of years of surgical experience in setting back the protruding ear.

Surgeons agree that simple skin excision alone is ineffectual on a long-term basis for symmetrical repositioning of the protruding ear. These authors present an interesting modification which combines wide undermining with postauricular skin excision and which apparently leads to acceptable and permanent results in patients with well-developed anthelical folds in whom protrusion is secondary to moderate prominence of the conchal rim. My own experience with skin excision is that it is undependable, even as an adjunct. The repositioning of a protruding ear must be accomplished another way; skin excision is only for exposure and removal of redundant tissue.

Unfortunately, Webster's and Smith's highly detailed anatomical critiques of the many techniques they have used over the years make difficult, and sometimes even confusing, reading; a specific procedure may be familiar to an experienced plastic surgeon but incomprehensible to a neophyte. This is particularly true of the technique which combines skin excision and undermining with the excision of mastoid soft tissue and cartilage.

Cartilage weakening or abrading has its drawbacks. I agree with their position that the procedures designed to "break the spring," including abrasion, morselization, and "fish-scaling," when carried deeply enough to be effective, can introduce the problems of ridging and sharp, unsightly irregularities.

Suture techniques in every combination have received attention over the years. Warnings about this technique should be heeded; the surgeon should use enough sutures, and they should be buried deeply and firmly. In addition, the surgeon should overcorrect to allow for later "cutting in" of sutures.

I disagree with Webster's and Smith's treatment of the protruding earlobe. Incising, detaching, and/or excising the cauda has been advocated. In my experience, this has lead to a late, unsightly bend in the helical rim at the site of excision or of manipulation of the cartilaginous tail of the helix. For repositioning of the cauda helicis, I prefer a direct suture between it and the concha.

In accordance with Webster and Smith, I have found that the type of postauricular skin closure makes little difference. Closure of the postauricular sulcus is more easily obtained with a running buried, half-buried, or exposed suture rather than with interrupted sutures, which tend to waste time, both in the operating room and in the office.

Webster's and Smith's observations relative to the beneficial effects of conchomastoid suturing techniques for the correction of conchal prominence secondary to abnormal angulation or enlargement are cogent. Of particular importance is their medial placement of the lateral conchal suture and the posterior angulation into the mastoid area. This avoids buckling of the base of the concha into the external canal with subsequent narrowing near the meatus.

The section in Chapter 11 on the creation or accentuation of an anthelix cites most variables, and the scholarly analysis of nearly every conceivable manipulation of these variables in an attempt to create a soft, normal look is worthwhile reading. Webster and Smith advise that a cartilage-weakening procedure combined with conchoscaphoid sutures requires slight overcorrection in most instances; this is the basis for the technique I have employed for 15 years.

The authors' reiteration that every technique used for correction of prominent ears must be accompanied by some postauricular skin excision or the recurrence rate becomes excessive is in direct variance with my own experience in using the modified Mustardé technique. One wishes that these experienced plastic surgeons would give the reader the benefit of their wide experience with various techniques by describing which particular procedure is best used for which deformity.

Final Impressions

The importance of correct analysis of the deformity prior to surgery cannot be overem-

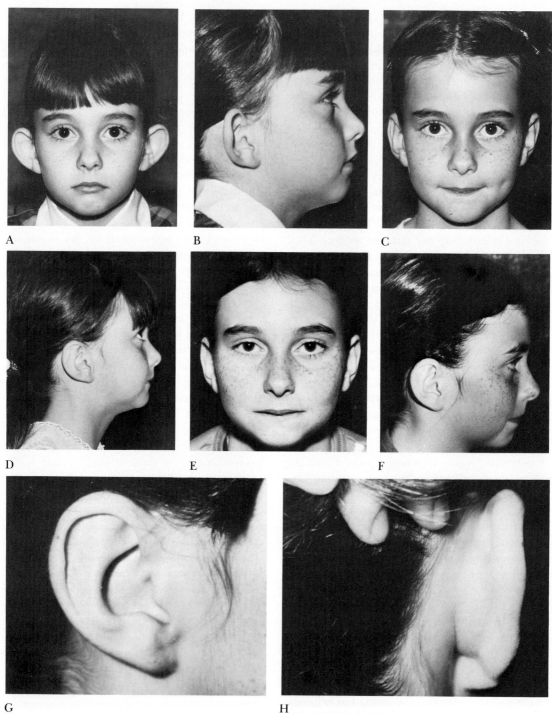

A   B   C

D   E   F

G   H

FIGURE 3. (A and B) Preoperative; technique employed as described in Figure 1. (C and D) Postoperative; 6 months. (E and F) Postoperative; 8 years. (G) Close-up of Part F. Compare with Figure 2G. Softer contour of ant- helix and gentle roll of superior crus evident. (H) Same patient. Posterior surface of ear is smooth; no skin excised at surgery.

phasized. Many protruding ears protrude only because of failure of the anthelix to develop. Other ears have well-developed anthelices but protrude because of a large or angulated concha. Some ears combine both problems; others have these problems together with peculiarities in segmental areas, e.g., a very severely protruding earlobe. Do not do the wrong operation. The surgeon will court failure if he attempts to set back a protruding ear by re-forming the anthelix when the protrusion is secondary to an enlarged and angulated concha; this patient needs a conchal setback. There is no one operation that is useful for all cases. Patient satisfaction is primarily dependent on obtaining a symmetrically setback ear without complications. Thus, while the patient desires a permanent setback with symmetry, the surgeon wants the same, plus a normal appearing ear (Fig. 3A through H). The patient really is not too concerned about the appearance of the ear, particularly about the sharpness or softness of the anthelix. The patient wants his ears to remain closer to his head and not to reprotrude partially or completely. Each technique is limited; to employ an otoplasty technique for repositioning a normal-sized protruding ear for treatment of a classic small-cup ear will result in disappointment for both patient and surgeon. In our search for excellence we will continue to

aim for symmetrical repositioning with normal contour and configuration and no complications. A true evaluation of results, as in many aesthetic procedures, must be made on a long-term basis.*

References

1. Hatch, M.D.   Common problems of otoplasty. *J. Int. Coll. Surg.* 30:171, 1958.
2. Luckett, W.H.   A new operation for prominent ears based on the anatomy of the deformity. *Surg. Gynecol. Obstet.* 10:635, 1910.
3. Mustardé, J.C.   The correction of prominent ears using simple mattress sutures. *Br. J. Plast. Surg.* 16:170, 1963.
4. Spira, M.   Reduction Otoplasty. In R.M. Goldwyn (Ed.), *The Unfavorable Result in Plastic Surgery.* Boston: Little, Brown, 1972. P. 162.
5. Spira, M., McCrea, R., Gerow, F.J., and Hardy, S.B.   Analysis and Treatment of the Protruding Ear. In G. Samvemero-Rosselli and G. Boggio-Rozutti (Eds.), *Transactions of the Fourth International Congress of Plastic and Reconstructive Surgery.* Amsterdam: Excerpta Medica, 1969. P. 1090.
6. Spira, M., McCrea, R., Gerow, F.J., and Hardy, S.B.   Correction of the principal deformities causing protruding ears. *Plast. Reconstr. Surg.* 44:150, 1969.
7. Stenström, S.J.   A "natural" technique for correction of congenitally prominent ears. *Plast. Reconstr. Surg.* 32:509, 1963.

*When photographs of protruding ears before and after surgery are made, there must be sufficient distance between the patient and the camera to prevent foreshortening. This problem is commonly seen when a "normal" focal length 50- to 55-mm lens is used for 35-mm photography. A telephoto lens enables the photographer to obtain a truer and more natural relationship between the ears and head of his subject. Appropriate lighting fully exposes both sides of the subject's head and does not leave one ear partially obscured by shadow.

12

LYMPHANGIOMAS and their subdivision cystic hygroma have been considered rare tumors [9,24,30]. However, the cystic hygroma is the most prominent cervical anomaly or new growth of lymphatic origin [15,33,34,37]. Although 80 percent of these lesions appear in the posterior cervical triangle, they may occur anywhere from the mastoid process to the clavicle [6].

Gross and Goeringer [15] reported that 65 percent of their cases of lymphangiomas were present at birth, another 15 percent appeared within the first year of life, and 10 percent appeared within the second year. In a small number of patients, this tumor may be noticed in the late thirties or when the patients are older [37]. Several studies have been made of the embryology of the cervical lymphatic system in order to understand the nature of lymphangiomas. They may be considered either embryonal malformations or tumors. As tumors, they are usually histologically benign, although they may be clinically aggressive.

Classification

Many attempts have been made to classify the various pathological changes that appear in the lymphatic vessels in the face and cervical regions [1,34] (Table 12-1). The classification of Landing and Farber [20] seems to us to be the most acceptable: capillary lymphangioma, cavernous lymphangioma, cystic lymphangioma (hygroma), and hemangiolymphangioma.

Embryology

Since the purpose of this chapter is not to present all that is known about lymphangiomas,

Bernard Hirshowitz
Isaac Eliachar

TREATMENT OF LYMPHANGIOMA AND CYSTIC HYGROMA

let it suffice for us to mention that the embryology of lymphangiomas is still poorly understood, despite the proliferation of theories [12,14,17,22,27]. It is agreed, however, that the various forms of lymphangiomas result from failure either to maintain or to effect a functional connection between the lymphatic and venous systems. This may be due to obstruction or sequestration of the lymphatic anlage or disconnected sprouting buds of the primitive systems. The hygroma may penetrate adjacent tissues by pushing ahead columns of endothelium which subsequently cannulate, secrete fluid, and form more cysts. This process causes pressure and necrosis of the normal tissues. The cysts may enlarge and extend along and into fascial spaces and planes, into muscles and nerves, or around vital structures, including nerves and blood vessels (Figs. 12-28 and 12-29). If deeper layers are involved, the spread of the cystic hygroma may be into the mouth, pharynx, and larynx above or into the mediastinum below. The chest wall and axilla may also be invaded, and this may occur across the clavicles if the superficial spaces are occupied.

Histopathology

As noted in the previous classification, lymphangiomas may consist of four or more elements, and the ultimate classification may depend on the dominant component within the tumor mass [4,8,16,33,36]. The structural variations that typify these tumors and place them in the several categories depend on the tumor's site of origin, whether central near the main collectors (cystic hygroma) or more peripheral

(capillary lymphangioma). In addition, the histology may vary with the age of the patient, the duration of the lesion, and previous treatments [11]. Older cysts may become thicker and more fibrotic or infected, with resultant cellular proliferation and infiltration of the walls and the stroma [28]. On the other hand, internal pressure may cause atrophy of the walls of the adjacent cysts, resulting in large cavities with a lobular appearance. The lobules may communicate but usually are separated by fibrous septa, a phenomenon that can be demonstrated radiographically [3].

Clinical Appearance

The cystic hygroma, as noted, may be present at birth or appear soon afterward, and it may grow either rapidly or slowly to become a massive tumor. Adjacent structures have to accommodate their enlarging neighbor (Figs. 12-30 and 12-31) [33].

The natural history of hygromas is such that there are periods of regression, but rarely does the cystic hygroma disappear spontaneously. With adolescence, the growth rate of these tumors slows [23]. Sudden appearance and rapid growth may follow upper respiratory tract infections or internal bleeding, producing respiratory and/or deglutitory embarrassment. Although nerves of the face, neck, or brachial plexus are often surrounded, seldom is there pain or motor weakness. The size of the lymphangioma may be so great that it may mask facial movements. The walls of the cyst are usually very close or even adherent to the overlying skin, which is stretched and thinned by pressure from within. In time, when fibrosis secon-

195

TABLE 12-1. *Historical Table Listing the Various Designations Given to Lymphangioma and Cystic Hygroma*

Author/Year*	Etiology and/or Pathology
1. Rendenbacher, 1823 [25]	First reported lymphangiomata
2. Wernher, 1843 [35]	Neoplasm
3. Bruch, 1849 [7]	Not neoplastic, effusion
4. Von Rokitansky, 1855 [32]	Periedematous process
5. Luschka, 1862 [21]	Originating from the ganglion intercaroticum
6. Virchow, 1863 [31]	Neoplasm
7. Arnold, 1865 [2]	Degeneration of connective tissue
8. Koester, 1872 [19]	Cysts with endothelial lining
9. Borst, 1902 [5]	Relation with lymphangioma, disconnection from venous system
10. McClure, 1909 [22]	Sequestration of lymphatic tissue from original relation to venous system
11. Huntington, 1911 [17]	Failure to achieve secondary connection with venous system
12. Sabin, 1912 [27]	Failure to maintain primary connection with venous system
13. Thompson and Keiller, 1923 [29]	Origin in lymph anlages
14. Goetsch, 1938 [13]	Growth sprouts from cyst wall that penetrate and destroy neighboring tissues
15. Havens and Lockhart, 1953 [16]	Coexistence of lymphangiomatous and hemangiomatous tissue elements
16. Willis, 1960 [36]	Variant of hemangioma
17. Bill and Sumner, 1965 [4]	Unified concept of cystic hygroma and lymphangioma
18. Crikelair and Cosman, 1968 [8]	Histologically benign, clinically malignant

*The numbers in brackets refer to the list of references; not all appear in the text.

darily develops, parts of the walls become thick and contain tissues into which the cyst may have penetrated.

Palpation will show the tumors to be fluctuant, diffuse, nontender, and poorly circumscribed. Blue venous coloration and translucency are frequent. Regional lymphadenopathy may occur secondarily. In the mouth, sagolike or papillary excrescences are typical and indicate mucous membrane involvement by the lymphangioma.

Differential Diagnosis

Although it is not difficult to diagnose a lymphangioma, there are other possibilities which should be kept in mind: the plexiform neurofibroma [10,23], cavernous hemangioma, branchial cysts, dermoid and thyroglossal cysts, cystic dysplasia of the thyroid, hematoma, lymphoma, and metastatic lesion.

Treatment

In the series of eight patients discussed here, surgery was the only treatment employed (Table 12-2). It was generally felt that when the tumor was localized, no advantage was to be gained by delay, and the operation was performed shortly after the patient was first seen. In infants, if surgery was considered advisable, it was generally undertaken as soon as pediatric and anesthetic considerations permitted. When the tumor was extensive and generalized, involving a number of important anatomical structures, a more conservative approach was taken.

The morphology, location, and extent of the

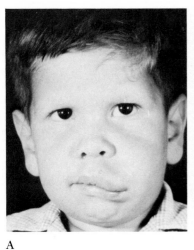 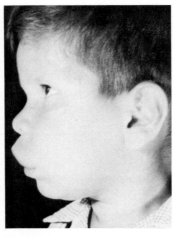 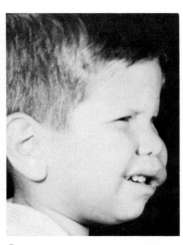

A   B   C

FIGURE 12-1.   (A, B, and C) Photographs of a 4-year-old child with marked swelling of the upper lip and left cheek due to lymphangioma.

tumor dictated the type of surgical procedure. When feasible, total excision was performed. Frequently, however, radical removal of the tumor was precluded by the infiltration of essential structures. Neither beneficial nor detrimental effects were noted when sclerosing agents were used to supplement the surgical

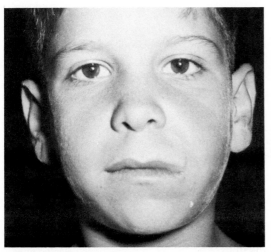

FIGURE 12-2.   Same patient at age 8 after three surgical interventions in which wedge excisions of upper lip and excision of tissues of the cheek were performed.

excision. Application to the operative field of a dilute, half-strength iodine solution aimed at sclerosing residual endothelial lining was routinely performed, but no proof of its effectiveness could be established [18]. In view of the relative radioresistance of lymphangiomas, radiotherapy was not used as a primary or secondary treatment in any of the patients. Interference with growth of both the soft tissues and bone as well as the spectre of late carcinogenesis of the thyroid gland and nasopharynx discouraged this therapeutic modality [18]. In general, successful excision was more likely when the tumor consisted primarily of cystic elements rather than of capillary lymphangiomatous components.

Recurrence or persistence of the tumor was more likely when it extended over several anatomical regions. Because of the difficulty in removing all the involved tissue, only two of the eight patients in this series are free of any evidence of the lymphangioma after 12 years or more. In an additional three patients, the recurrences were relatively small and almost insignificant in comparison to what existed prior to operation. It would appear that recurrences were the result of residual lymphangiomatous tissue left in situ through incomplete removal. Perhaps, because of insufficient lymphatic drainage, the preexisting lymph channels became distended and grew [4]. Kiesewetter [18]

TABLE 12-2. *List of Eight Patients with All Relevant Details Relating to Lymphangiomatous Process*

	Present Age	Sex	First Seen	Type of Lymphangioma and Location	Symptoms
A.L. Figs. 12-1 through 12-4	19	M	1963	Lymphangiomatous infiltration of left cheek and upper lip	Repeated bouts of cellulitis, 1 year
D.M. Figs. 12-5 through 12-7	13	M	1965	Lymphangiomatous infiltration of left cheek and upper lip	Repeated bouts of cellulitis, 9 months
E.S. Figs. 12-8 through 12-14	47	F	1962	Lymphangioma-hemangioma of neck, soft palate, and nasopharynx	Cosmetically deforming appearance of neck, gradually increasing since childhood
B.E. Figs. 12-15 through 12-17	16	M	1960	Cystic hygroma of cheek and lower jaw, chin and floor of mouth	Enlarging in size since age of 6 months
R.W. Figs. 12-18 and 12-19	22	F	1956	Cystic hygroma of neck	Rapid growth following birth
M.A. Figs. 12-20 and 12-21	18	M	1961	Diffuse lymphedema of face, head, and neck. Variant of lymphangioma?	Cosmetically disfiguring since birth
S.G. Figs. 12-22 through 12-24	18	F	1967	Lymphangiomatous infiltration of full thickness of cheek, upper and lower lip, and tongue	Slow growth since age of 2 years
N.A. Figs. 12-25 through 12-27	26	F	1966	Lymphangiomatous infiltration of cheek, side of nose, and upper lip	Slow growth since age of 6 years

Treatment, Number of Operations	Complications at Operations	Length of Follow-up (in Years)	Present Symptoms and Remarks
Wedge excision of upper lip, including excision of involved tissue of lip, cheek, and mucous membrane, 1964, 1965, and 1966	—	15	Active and healthy, no complaints
Excision of wedge of upper lip, including involved tissues of lip, cheek, and mucous membrane, 1965–1967	—	10	Active and healthy, no complaints
Subtotal excision of neck mass, including removal of numerous phleboliths. Emergency tracheotomy performed in 1963	Severe nasopharyngeal bleeding, controlled by two inflated Foley catheters	15	In good health, some growth of nasopharyngeal and palatal components of tumor; minimal recurrence in the neck region
Total excision of cystic mass, 1961. Excision of involved mucous membrane of cheek and lower lip, 1970	Transient right lower facial palsy	14	Has small recurrence on right side of chin; no other disability
Excision of cystic mass at age of 7 months. Recurrence with reexcision, 1971	—	22	Recurrence of cystic hygroma over preauricular and infra-auricular regions during two pregnancies, with some involution after delivery
Biopsy, 1961	—	16	Healthy; no progress of swelling since age of 6 to 7 years; perhaps some involution of lymphedema
Wedge excision of lower lip to reduce bulk, 1969. Reduction of bulk of cheek with complete exposure and preservation of facial nerve. Excision of papillary excrescences of tongue, 1977	Transient weakness of buccal branch of facial nerve	11	Better aesthetic appearance; function of facial musculature and tongue improved
Wedge excision and thinning of upper lip, 1968. Procedure repeated, 1978	—	10	Some discomfort in areas of swelling; appearance of upper lip has been improved by recent surgery

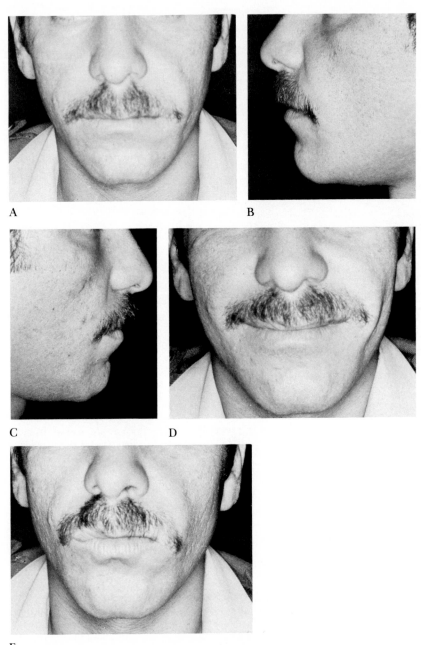

A

B

C

D

E

FIGURE 12-3. *(A through E) Same patient, now at age 18, with no residual disabilities.*

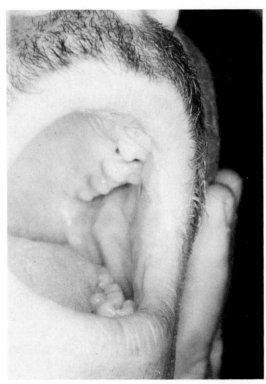

FIGURE 12-4. *Intraoral view showing appearance of mucous membrane following a number of extirpatory procedures for excrescences caused by lymphangioma.*

states that a cystic hygroma, especially under the stimulus of an upper respiratory infection, can grow extensively and can be a dangerous complication causing respiratory obstruction. A rapid increase in size may also follow hemorrhage into a cystic space. In these situations, emergency measures are indicated. In none of the patients in this series, however, even when an extensive hygroma of the neck was present in babies, was it necessary to perform emergency aspiration or drainage of the cyst. Emergency tracheostomy was done for respiratory embarrassment only once in a 2-day-old baby (Fig. 12-32) who did not survive.

Case reports have appeared concerning the rapid growth of extensive lymphangiomas where perhaps the stimulus was a respiratory infection [8, 13, 23, 26]. In these patients, limited partial excisions did not appear to have been justified, since they did not alleviate the symptoms. In addition, these procedures often resulted in unsightly scarring. We would suggest that in such cases combined antibiotic and corticosteroid therapy might be tried prior to surgical intervention. Perhaps a parallel can be drawn to the use of corticosteroids in inducing resolution of extensive, enlarging juvenile hemangiomas that are not amenable to surgical excision [38].

In two of our patients with lymphangiomas of the cheek and upper lip (A.L and D.M.), recurrent cellulitis made the excision of all involved tissue a matter of relative urgency. When this was accomplished, no further inflammatory episodes ensued. In a third patient (S.G., Fig. 12-22), there was no possibility of radical removal of the entire tumor, which involved the tongue, cheek, and upper lip. In this patient, no bouts of cellulitis occurred, perhaps due to prophylactic antibiotic therapy and good oral and dental hygiene.

In patient R.W. (Fig. 12-18), a large cystic

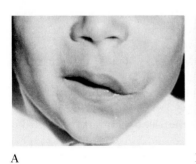
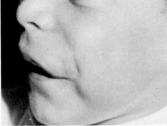
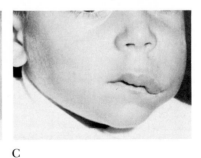

A   B   C

FIGURE 12-5. *(A, B, and C) A 3-year-old boy with lymphangiomatous swelling of the left upper lip and cheek.*

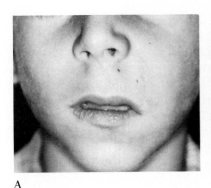
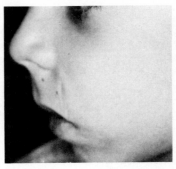
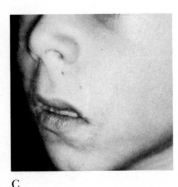

A   B   C

FIGURE 12-6.   (A, B, and C) Same patient at 13 years of age. He has undergone two wedge excisions of the left upper lip and nasolabial fold areas.

hygroma of the neck and angle of the jaw was operated on in infancy. The patient had surgery again at age 18 because of recurrence. At this time, now age 22, she is the mother of two children and has noted that during each pregnancy, there have been recurrent swellings in the preauricular and infra-auricular areas (Fig. 12-19). Swelling decreased after delivery and with the use of antibiotics and steroids.

As mentioned previously, lymphangiomas have little propensity to regress spontaneously. Nevertheless, we have generally employed a cautious attitude when multiple structures have been extensively involved, and we have performed only essential excisions during the growth period of the child, waiting for more definitive surgery when the patient reaches adulthood (patients S.G. and N.A.).

In general, it is our impression from this follow-up that whereas lymphangiomatous tissue may actively infiltrate into and destroy surrounding tissues, the latter suffers mainly from pressure resulting from the distended lymphatic spaces which pervade them (Figs. 12-28 and 12-29) [4]. In a close review of the literature on the histopathology of lymphangioma and cystic hygroma, there is support for both contentions—that these tumors may be either invasive and destructive or expansive and permeating. The fact that there is almost no record of neural involvement, pain, or complete lack of muscular function lends clinical support to the expansive theory.

As a rule, the tumor should be removed as completely as possible, but without compromising function while striving for the best

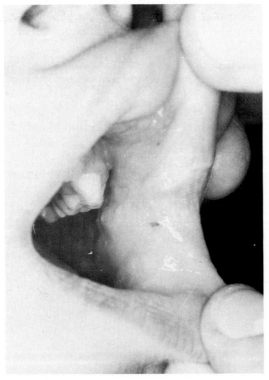

FIGURE 12-7.   Excrescences of the mucous membrane of the left upper lip and cheek due to lymphangioma were also removed.

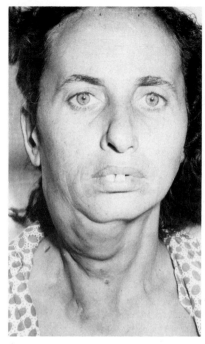
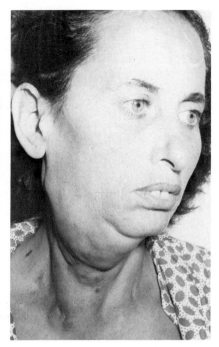

A   B

FIGURE 12-8. *(A and B) Preoperative photographs showing extensive swelling of the right side of the neck due to vascular lymphangioma. (Reprinted, with permission, from B. Hirshowitz, H. J. Birkhahn, and M. Heifetz, A case of vascular lymphangioma of the neck and face. Plast. Reconstr. Surg. 32:620–625, 1963.)*

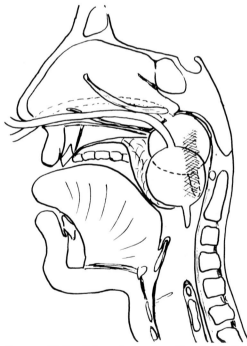

FIGURE 12-9. *Schematic drawing of two inflated Foley catheters located in the nasopharynx and used to control bleeding caused by anesthetic instrumentation. (Reprinted, with permission, from B. Hirshowitz, H. J. Birkhahn, and M. Heifetz, A case of vascular lymphangioma of the neck and face. Plast. Reconstr. Surg. 32:620–625, 1963.)*

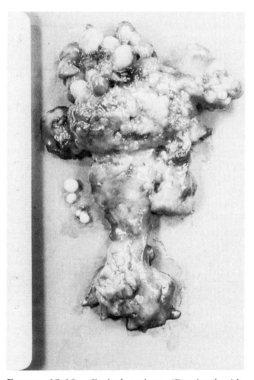

FIGURE 12-10. *Excised specimen. (Reprinted, with permission, from B. Hirshowitz, H. J. Birkhahn, and M. Heifetz, A case of vascular lymphangioma of the neck and face. Plast. Reconstr. Surg. 32:620–625, 1963.)*

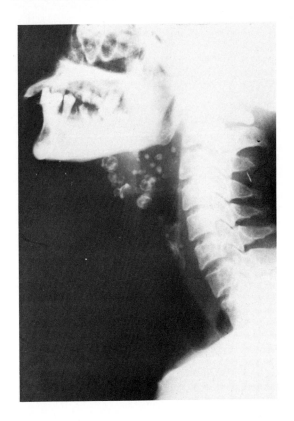

FIGURE 12-11. *Multiple phleboliths seen on x-ray. (Reprinted, with permission, from B. Hirshowitz, H. J. Birkhahn, and M. Heifetz, A case of vascular lymphangioma of the neck and face. Plast. Reconstr. Surg. 32:620–625, 1963.)*

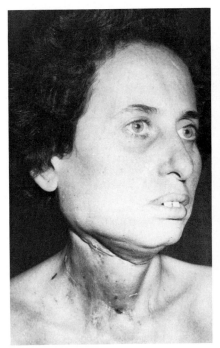

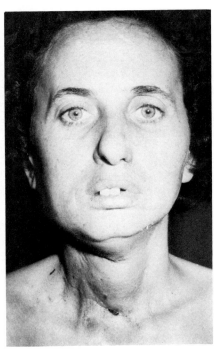

A   B

FIGURE 12-12. *(A and B) Photographs 1 month post-operatively. (Reprinted, with permission, from B. Hirshowitz, H. J. Birkhahn, and M. Heifetz, A case of vas-cular lymphangioma of the neck and face. Plast. Reconstr. Surg. 32:620–625, 1963.)*

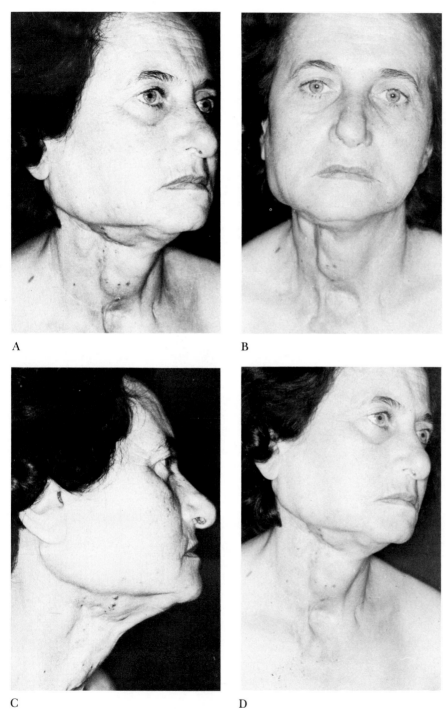

A

B

C

D

FIGURE 12-13. *(A through D) Same patient 15 years later with minimal local recurrences in the neck.*

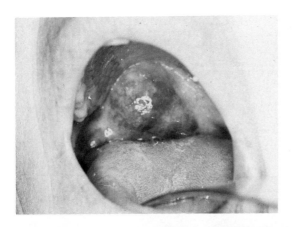

FIGURE 12-14. *The tumor of the soft palate has grown in size.*

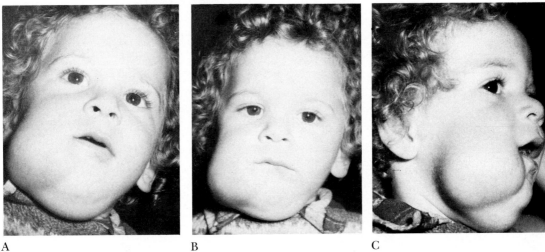

A　　　　　　　　　B　　　　　　　　　C

FIGURE 12-15. *(A, B, and C) Cystic hygroma of the right cheek, lower jaw, chin, and floor of mouth.*

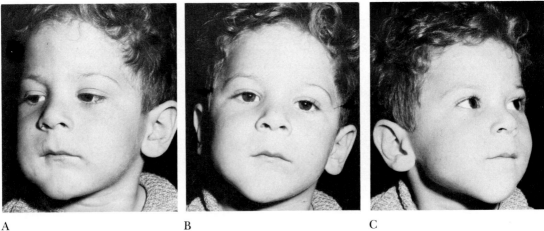

A　　　　　　　　　B　　　　　　　　　C

FIGURE 12-16. *(A, B, and C) Appearance at 6 years of age.*

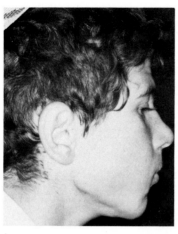 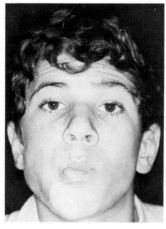 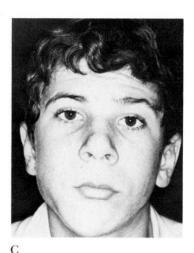

A   B   C

FIGURE 12-17. *(A, B, and C) Same patient at 16 years of age. There is a small recurrence in the right chin.*

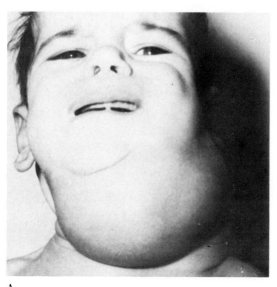 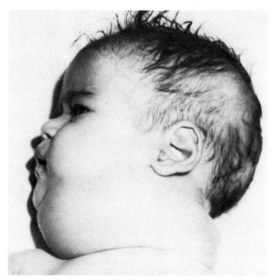

A   B

FIGURE 12-18. *(A and B) Marked swelling due to cystic hygroma of the neck, mainly on the left.*

208

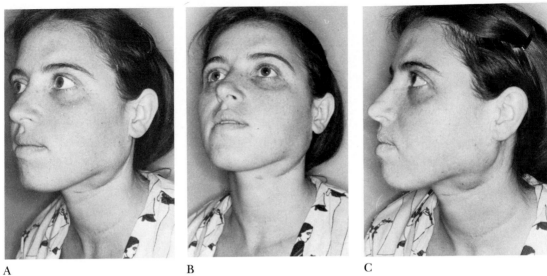

A   B   C

FIGURE 12-19. (A, B, and C) Photographs of the same patient 22 years later. Cystic recurrences are present in the preauricular, infra-auricular, and submandibular regions.

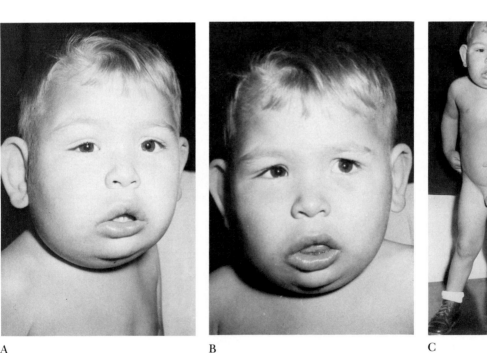

A   B   C

FIGURE 12-20. (A, B, and C) Generalized lymphedema of head and neck since birth. (Courtesy of Professor Simon T. Winter, Head of the Department of Pediatrics, Rothschild University Hospital, Technion, Haifa.)

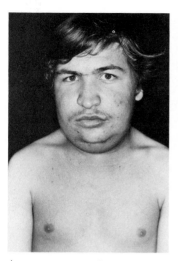
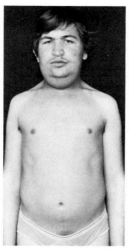
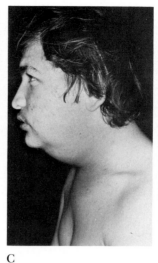
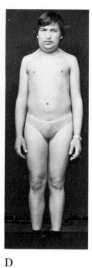

A   B   C   D

FIGURE 12-21.   (A through D) Photographs of the same patient, 17 years of age, with partial involution of the lymphedematous swelling. (Courtesy of Professor Simon T. Winter, Head of the Department of Pediatrics, Rothschild University Hospital, Technion, Haifa.)

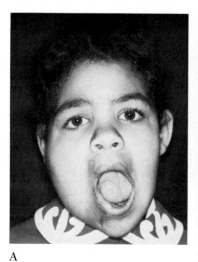
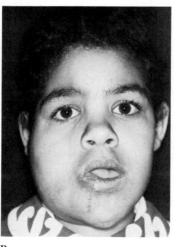
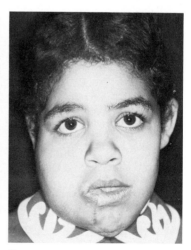

A   B   C

FIGURE 12-22.   (A, B, and C) Photographs of a 7-year-old girl following a large wedge resection of the lower lip, undertaken to reduce bulk caused by lymphangioma.

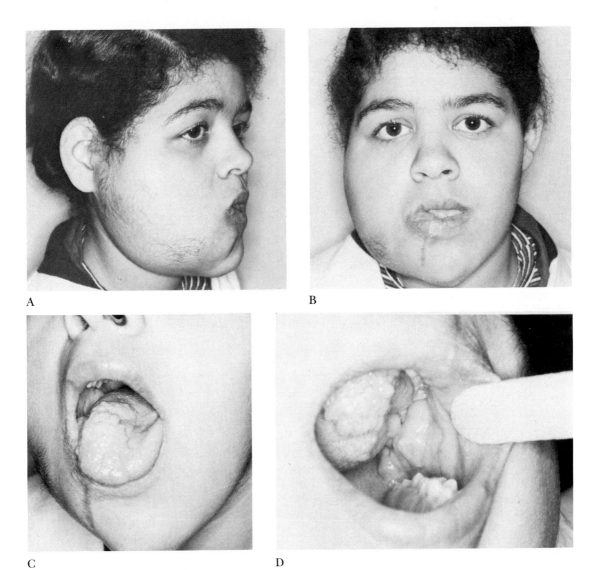

A

B

C

D

FIGURE 12-23. *(A through D) Same patient 11 years later showing some progression of lymphangiomatous involvement of the right side of the face. The tongue shows* *papillary excrescences, characteristic of changes in mucous membrane infiltrated by lymphangioma.*

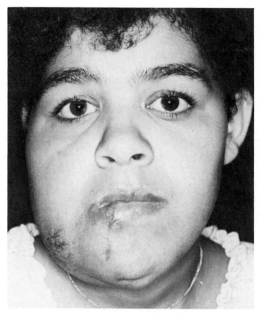 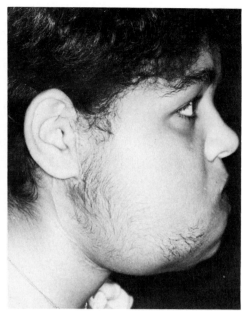

A   B

FIGURE 12-24.   *(A and B) Postoperative photographs following partial excision of lymphangiomatous tissue of the right cheek and lower lip. Further improvement can be expected following correction of lower lip scarring.*

cosmetic result possible. Although extensive surgical procedures were carried out at an early age in some of the patients in this series, our overriding aim was to obtain the most acceptable cosmetic result possible while still retaining full functional integrity.

In patient S. G., because of marked swelling of the lower lip which caused difficulty in eating and talking, only limited excision was done at first to decrease the lip bulk. The diffuse involvement of the tongue by the tumor caused only slight disability, and accordingly, the macroglossia was not operated on at an early age. The patient is now approaching adulthood, and more definitive cosmetic surgery has recently been undertaken.

Patient M.A. was included in this series because congenital lymphedema of the head and neck is considered analogous to lymphangioma [1,34]. This patient had no surgical intervention except for a biopsy from behind the right ear.

Distended thin-walled capillary-sized lymphatic channels were seen widely distributed throughout the subcutaneous tissue. Apart from the grossly swollen facial features, he had no functional disability. He is now 18 years old, and the impression is that there has been a lessening of the swelling with progressing age.

Final Thoughts

Lymphangiomas have minimal tendency to regress spontaneously and are not significantly affected permanently by any treatment other than complete early excision. Following incomplete removal, recurrence is the rule, although malignant transformation has never been demonstrated. Neural and muscular deficiencies related to this tumor are rarely encountered. These tumors, occurring as diffusely permeating growths, cause local deformation, and the earlier and more radical the removal, the more likely the chance of cure. This may be said with full conviction only if the surgical procedures do not seriously compromise function or result in aesthetic deformity which is more severe than that associated

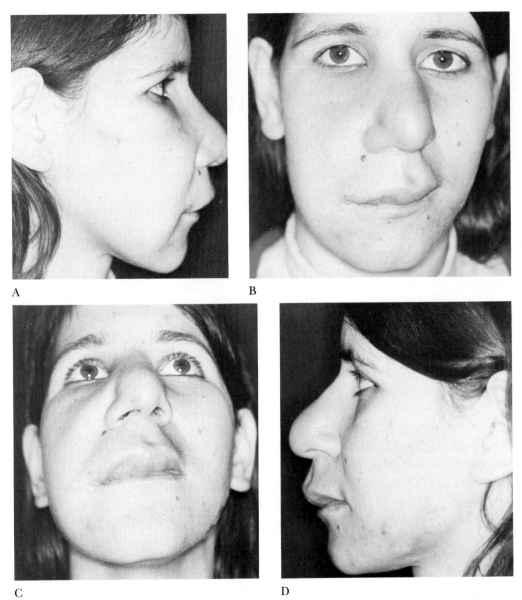

FIGURE 12-25. *(A through D) Photographs of lymphan-giomatous swelling of the right side of the face and upper lip.*

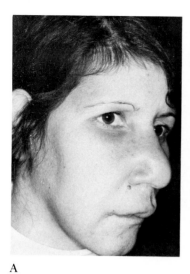

A

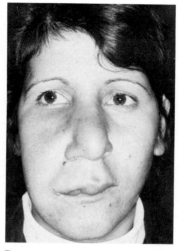

B

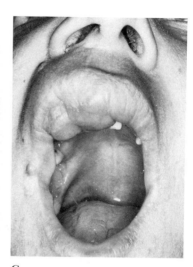

C

FIGURE 12-26. *(A, B, and C) Same patient 10 years later; there is only a slight increase in swelling of the right cheek and side of nose and a moderate increase in bulk of* *the right upper lip since the wedge excision (Kocher incision) performed 10 years previously.*

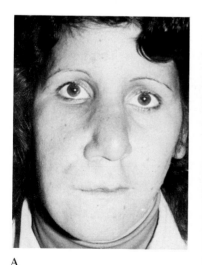

A

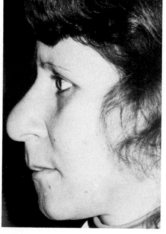

B

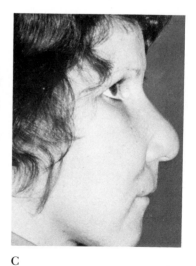

C

FIGURE 12-27. *(A, B, and C) Postoperative photographs following excision of excess tissue of the right upper lip. An improvement in appearance has been obtained.*

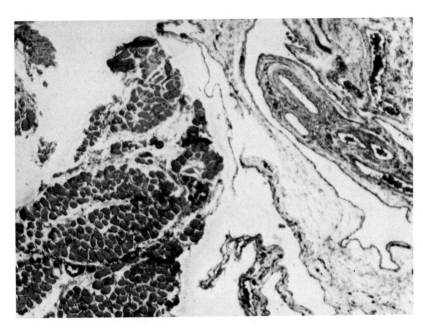

FIGURE 12-28. *Cystic hygroma adherent to and pressing on a striated muscle and vascular bundle without actual penetration or destruction. H&E, 50×. (Courtesy of Dr.* *Yehudith Ben-Arie, Department of Pathology, Rambam Medical Center, Technion, Haifa.)*

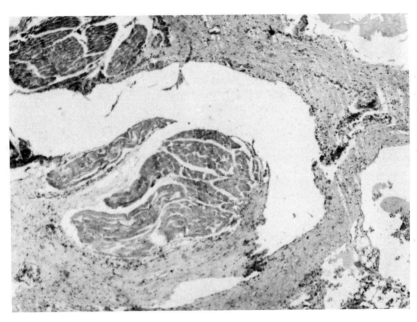

FIGURE 12-29. *Lymphangiomatous spaces infiltrating a striated muscle, separating the muscular bundles with secondary fibrosis. H&E, 50×. (Courtesy of Dr. Yehudith* *Ben-Arie, Department of Pathology, Rambam Medical Center, Technion, Haifa.)*

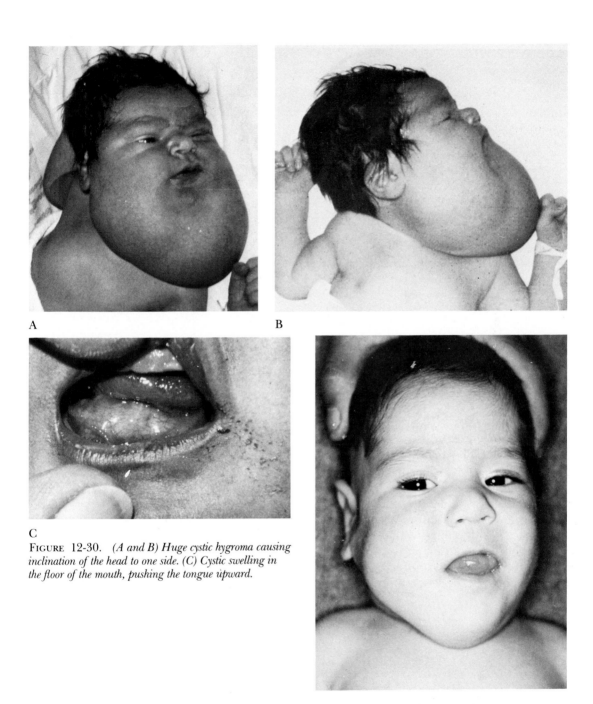

C

FIGURE 12-30. *(A and B) Huge cystic hygroma causing inclination of the head to one side. (C) Cystic swelling in the floor of the mouth, pushing the tongue upward.*

FIGURE 12-31. *Early postoperative appearance.*

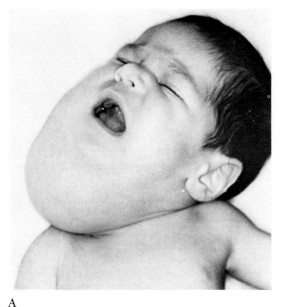

A

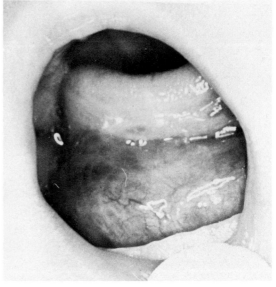

B

FIGURE 12-32. *(A and B) Enormous cystic hygroma of the neck, which caused respiratory embarrassment.*

with the primary lesion. Since growth of the lymphangioma generally ceases after puberty, more definitive surgery for reducing the tumor bulk is best undertaken after that age. Cystic hygromas are far more amenable to surgery than are capillary lymphangiomas, which have a tendency to permeate diffusely into various structures. The preceding characteristics determine the long-term clinical course and may have a direct bearing on the therapeutic and surgical approaches to these tumors.

References

1. Allen, A.C. *The Skin, A Clinicopathologic Treatise.* St. Louis: Mosby, 1954.
2. Arnold, J. Zwei Fälle von Hygroma colli cysticum congenitum und deren fragliche Beziehung zu dem Ganglion intercaroticum. *Arch. Pathol. Anat.* 33:209, 1865.
3. Barrand, K.G., and Freeman, N.V. Massive infiltrating cystic hygroma of the neck in infancy. *Arch. Dis. Child.* 48:523, 1973.
4. Bill, A.H., and Summer, D.S. A united concept of lymphangioma and cystic hygroma. *Surg. Gynecol. Obstet.* 120:79, 1965.
5. Borst, M. *Die Lehre von den Geschwülsten.* Wiesbaden: Bergmann, 1902. Vol. I, p. 191.
6. Broomhead, I.W. Cystic hygroma of the neck. *Br. J. Plast. Surg.* 17:225, 1964.
7. Bruch, C. Zur Entwickelungsgeschichte der pathologischen Cystenbildungen. *Z. Rat. Med.* 8:91, 1849.
8. Crikelair, G.F., and Cosman, B. Histologically benign, clinically malignant lesions of the head and neck. *Plast. Reconstr. Surg.* 42:343, 1968.
9. Dingman, R.O., and Grabb, W.C. Lymphangioma of the tongue. *Plast. Reconstr. Surg.* 27:214, 1961.
10. Dowd, C.N. Hygroma cysticum colli: Its structure and etiology. *Ann. Surg.* 58:112, 1913.
11. Duke-Elder, W.S. Neurofibromatosis. In *Textbook of Ophthalmology.* London: Kimpton, 1952. Vol. 5, p. 5104.
12. Freeman, G.C. Conservative surgical treatment of massive cystic lymphangioma: With the report of eight cases. *Ann. Surg.* 137:12, 1953.
13. Goetsch, E. Hygroma colli cysticum and hygroma axillare: Pathologic and clinical study and report of twelve cases. *Arch. Surg.* 36:394, 1938.
14. Gray, H. *Anatomy of the Human Body* (26th ed.). Philadelphia: Lea & Febiger, 1954. P. 760.
15. Gross, R.E., and Goeringer, C.F. Cystic hygroma of the neck: Report of twenty-seven cases. *Surg. Gynecol. Obstet.* 69:48, 1939.
16. Havens, F.Z., and Lockhart, H.B. Angiomas of

interest to the otolaryngologist. *Ann. Otol. Rhinol. Laryngol.* 62:36, 1953.

17. Huntington, G. *The Anatomy and Development of the Systemic Lymphatic Vessels in the Domestic Cat.* Philadelphia: Wistar Institute, 1911.

18. Kiesewetter, W.B. Cystic Hygroma. In C. Rob and R. Smith (Eds.), *Operative Surgery* (2nd ed.). Philadelphia: Lippincott, 1969. Vol. 6, pp. 12–18.

19. Koester, K. Ueber Hygroma cysticum colli congenitum. *Verh. Phys.-Med. Ges. Würzb.* 3:44, 1872.

20. Landing, B.H., and Farber, S. Tumors of the Cardiovascular System. In *Atlas of Tumor Pathology.* Washington, D.C.: Armed Forces Institute of Pathology, 1956. Sect. 3, fasc. 7.

21. Luschka, H. Ueber die drüsencartige Natur des sogenannten Ganglion intercaroticum. *Arch. Anat. Physiol. Wissensch. Med.* 4:405, 1862.

22. McClure, C.F.W., and Silvester, C.F. A comparative study of the lymphatico-venous communications in adult mammals: I. Primates, carnivora, rodentia, ungulata and marsupialia. *Anat. Rec.* 3:534, 1909.

23. Mustardé, J.C. (Ed.). *Plastic Surgery in Infancy and Childhood.* Philadelphia: Saunders, 1971, Pp. 138, 340, 341.

24. Paletta, F.X. Lymphangioma. *Plast. Reconstr. Surg.* 37:269, 1966.

25. Rendenbacher, E.A.H. *De Ranjla Sub Lingua, Speciali, cum Casu Congenito.* Monachii: M. Lindauer, 1828.

26. Robinson, D.W. Lymphangioma of the lower face and neck involving mandible. *Plast. Reconstr. Surg.* 23:187, 1959.

27. Sabin, F.R. The Development of the Lymphatic System. In F.K.J. Keibel and F.P. Mall (Eds.), *Manual of Human Embryology.* Philadelphia: Lippincott, 1912. Vol. 2, p. 709.

28. Schetlin, C.F., and Stone, P.W. Unilocular cervical cystic hygroma: Report of a case with attachment to the thoracic duct. *Surgery* 32:1006, 1952.

29. Thompson, J.E., and Keiller, V.H. Lymphangioma of the neck. *Ann. Surg.* 77:385, 1923.

30. Vaughn, A.M. Cystic hygroma of the neck: Report of a case and review of the literature. *Am. J. Dis. Child.* 48:149, 1934.

31. Virchow, R. *Die krankhaften Geschwülste.* Berlin: Hirschwald, 1863. P. 170.

32. Von Rokitansky, K. *Lehrbuch der pathologischen Anatomie* (3rd ed.). Vienna: Braumuller, 1855. Vol. I, p. 230.

33. Ward, G.E., and Hendrick, J.W. *Diagnosis and Treatment of Tumors of the Head and Neck.* Baltimore: Williams & Wilkins, 1950.

34. Watson, W.L., and McCarthy, W.D. Blood and lymph vessel tumors: A report of 1,056 cases. *Surg. Gynecol. Obstet.* 71:569, 1940.

35. Wernher, A. Die angeborenen Kysten-Hygrome und die ihnen verwandten Geschwuelste, in anatomischer, diagnostischer und therapeutischer Beziehung. Giessen: Heyer, 1843. P. 76.

36. Willis, R.A. *Pathology of Tumours* (3rd ed.) London: Butterworth, 1960.

37: Woodring, A.J. Cervical cystic hygroma: A review of the literature and report of an unusual case. *Ann. Otol. Rhinol. Laryngol.* 77:978, 1968.

38. Zarem, H.A., and Edgerton, M.T. Induced resolution of cavernous hemangiomas following prednisolone therapy. *Plast. Reconstr. Surg.* 39:76, 1967.

Joseph E. Murray

COMMENTS ON CHAPTER 12

ALTHOUGH the experience reported is relatively limited, the principle of conservatism emerges clearly. Several points are worthy of reemphasis. First, lymphangiomas seldom regress spontaneously as contrasted with the hemangiomas, of which a high percentage do. Second, surgical excision is the only effective treatment, but associated structures should not be sacrificed for fear of damage to nerve and muscular function. The final point is that growth of the lymphangioma in adulthood usually slows, although exacerbations can occur.

The use of steroids is certainly questionable, even for the hemangiomas, and I would feel they are contraindicated in dealing with a lymphangioma because of unpredictable adverse side effects.

The caveat against the use of radiotherapy should be respected because not only is it ineffective, but its use in young children also can often lead to late carcinomas, especially in the head and neck.

13

FOR purposes of this review, we have considered a pigmented nevus to be "giant" when it involves at least 5 percent of the body surface or when it occupies enough area on the head or extremities to create a significant problem in coverage if it were excised.

Clinical Material

The clinical courses of 65 patients with giant nevi were studied, but only 43 whose treatment was completed are included. Three groups could be distinguished:

Group I. Fifteen patients with pigmented lesions of the trunk in one or two locations occupying 5 percent or more of the body surface area.

Group II. Nineteen patients with very large pigmented nevi on the face, scalp, neck, or extremities.

Group III. Nine patients who not only have nevi similar to patients in Group I or II but also have nevi in a spotty distribution (the "Dalmatian child").

Follow-Up

These 43 patients were followed from 2 to 17 years, the majority for 10 years or more.

Treatment

In France, several decades ago, it was almost forbidden to operate on a giant nevus because of the fear of causing malignant transformation. Those who do not believe in such a possibility still were very reluctant to treat these nevi because of the frequent difficulty of resurfacing

Raymond Vilain
Julien Glicenstein
Xavier Latouche

TREATMENT OF GIANT NEVI

the defect, and because of the complexity of multiple operations in young children. Progressively, attitudes have changed, but the problem of managing giant nevi remains. No universally acknowledged optimal procedure has yet evolved.

Dermabrasion

Dermabrasion was proposed as a means of eliminating the nevus and avoiding the problem of skin grafting for coverage. The difficulty with this technique is that the nevus frequently extends into the deep dermis, and complete epithelialization may take a very long time. Hypotrophic scarring is common. One of our patients eventually required excision of the dermabraded areas and grafting (Fig. 13-1). We no longer use dermabrasion.

Serial Excision

Described by Morestin [5] and later by others [2], serial excision, when feasible, offers many advantages: simplicity, a short hospital stay, minimum discomfort in terms of positioning and pain, and usually a good final result (Fig. 13-2). This method, however, does have disadvantages. Numerous procedures over many years may be necessary; the baby or young child requires general anesthesia; frequently the nevus is too large to be removed by this technique because of either size and/or its location near body orifices, on extremities, or on the face. A theoretical liability of this technique is malignant transformation [4] during the time that the nevus is being removed, presumably as a result of surgical trauma. However, in none of our patients having been managed by this method and followed for 15 years has malig-

nancy been noted in an operative site (Figs. 13-3 and 13-4).

Excision and Grafting

The principal advantage of this technique is the speedy elimination of the nevus, rapid coverage of the defect, and one or only a few hospitalizations [1, 6]. The drawbacks of grafting for this condition are well known. Occasionally, the patient may have insufficient donor skin; grafts, no matter how well done, may ultimately give the child a patchwork-quilt appearance; grafts often thicken at their junction with other grafts or normal tissue; grafted skin may remain anesthetic with poor texture and contour; and donor-site scarring can be significant and is usually permanent [3] (Figs. 13-5 through 13-11).

White Zebra Technique

The evolution of this method was based on our observation that scars within nevi, as, for example, from serial excision, were white and not usually hypertrophic [7]. The execution of the technique is simple. By electrocautery, 3- to 4-cm-wide bands of the nevi are excised parallel to the normal skin creases and deep to the nevus. Care must be taken not to place defects where tension on the wound is greatest, or secondary healing will be delayed and scars will widen and thicken, nullifying the advantages of this procedure.

The open areas are covered by tulle gras, soaped off with saline, and changed twice a week. Final epithelialization may take 6 to 8 weeks. After a few days in the hospital, the child may go home where parents can do the dressings, using simply tap water in a bath and tulle

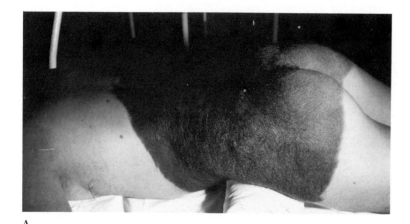

A

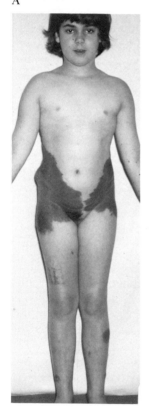

B

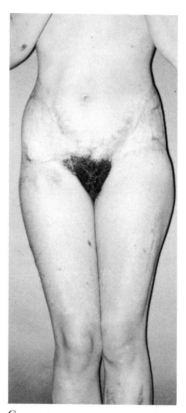

C

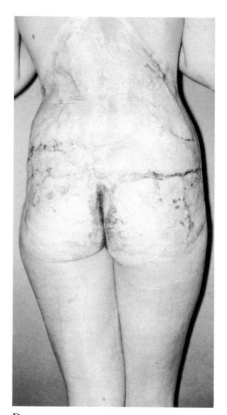

D

FIGURE 13-1. (A and B) Preoperative 9-year-old girl who underwent dermabrasion on the back with a poor result because of severe scarring. (C and D) Ten years after excision and grafting. Donor areas on thighs have healed well. Some pigment has migrated. A portion of the nevus was intentionally left on the pubis and around the anus. The patient is now a mother of one child, born free of abnormal nevi.

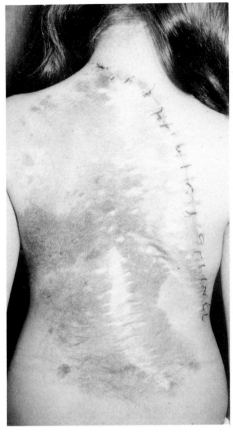
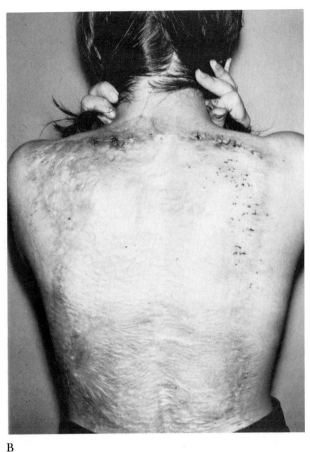

A   B

FIGURE 13-2. *(A) Ten-year-old girl after five serial excisions. (B) Patient 8 years later, after further excision.*

gras. When the excised bands have healed, the result does resemble the coat of a zebra. Sometimes, pigment migrates into the segments of excision. Although this may lessen the cosmetic result, the tumor, as confirmed histologically, no longer remains. After a few months, the patient will undergo another excision—of the remaining bands of nevi. After this procedure, secondary epithelialization is slower because the adjacent scar, not the nevus, provides the new epidermis.

The advantages of this method are its simplicity, the brief hospitalization, and the usually good scarring with more nearly normal skin color and texture than would be the result of excision and grafting. Furthermore, the white zebra technique does allow for the possibility of future serial excisions, if necessary, or dermabrading with overgrafting using extremely thin skin.

The white zebra operation does have its disadvantages. More than one procedure is required; wounds are open for weeks and must be monitored closely; dressings must be done regularly; and a small minority of patients may have moderate pain.

Since 1972, we have used this method on 10

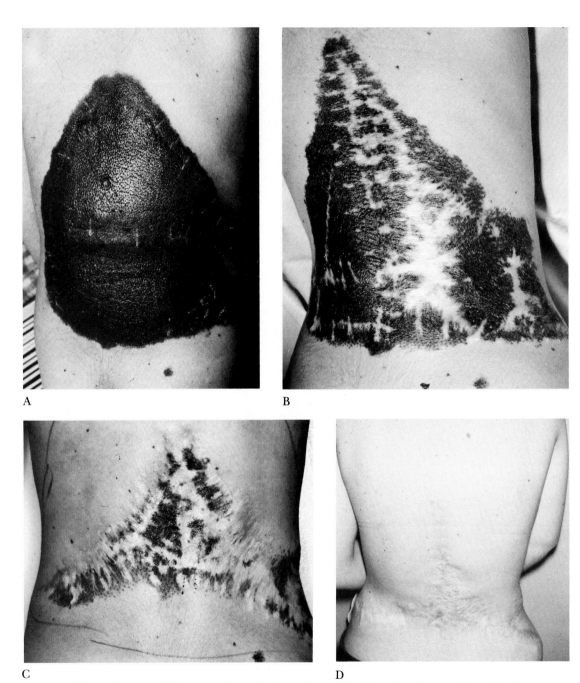

A

B

C

D

FIGURE 13-3. *(A) Six-year-old girl, 1 month after first serial excision. Note scars along the margin of the nevus and in the center. (B) Postoperative: 3 years after a total of five serial excisions. (C) Two years later, after four more excisions. (D) Postoperative: 12 years after the first operation. Patient is emotionally well adjusted and is working.*

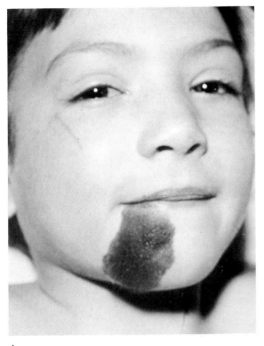

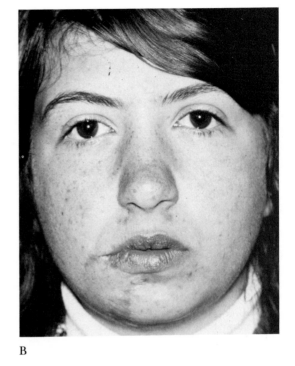

A

B

FIGURE 13-4.   *(A) Preoperative 5-year-old girl. (B) Postoperative: 11 years after five serial excisions. Scar is satisfactory. In a recent letter, the patient said she was married and had two children without abnormal nevi.*

patients, and the results have been most encouraging (Fig. 13-12).

Malignancy

None of the patients who underwent removal of their nevi by any method developed a melanoma. One patient came with a subcutaneous nodule at the elbow that was biopsied and diagnosed as melanoma, but he refused any further treatment, either surgery or chemotherapy (Fig. 13-13). He has been lost to follow-up.

Operative Mortality

In none of the 43 patients were there any operative deaths.

Aesthetic Result

The appearance of the patient after surgery was considered very good in 13 patients, good in 22, and fair in 8.

Final Thoughts

Representative patients have been selected to illustrate the principles of management. Although giant nevi constitute a formidable problem, surgery, if judiciously performed, can improve the quality of life for these unfortunate individuals. Admittedly, we would hope that another backward look in two decades will

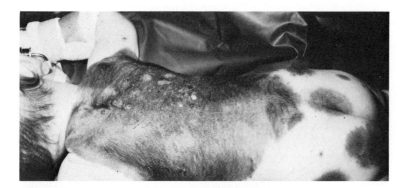

A

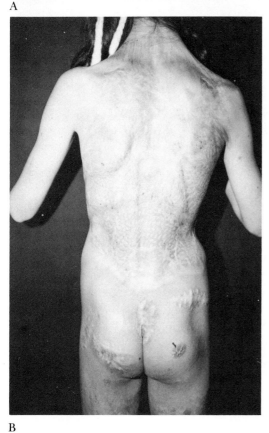

B

FIGURE 13-5. *(A) Preoperative 1-year-old girl with a large hairy nevus as well as nevi in a "Dalmatian" distribution (Group III). (B) Age 10, now 9 years after serial excision of the nevi spots and two episodes of excision and mesh split grafting for the large nevus. Scarring is satisfactory; donor sites are well healed.*

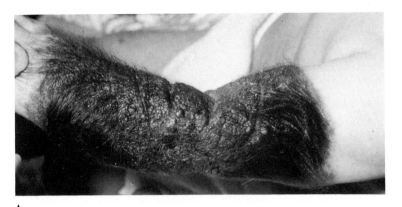

A

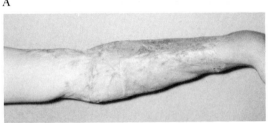

B

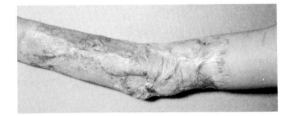

C

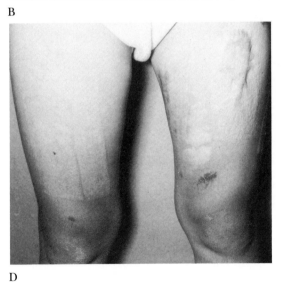

D

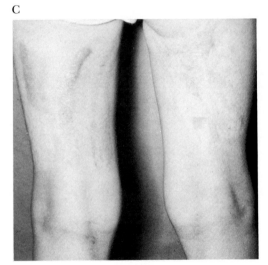

E

FIGURE 13-6.   (A) Preoperative 6-month-old girl with circumferential nevus of the left arm. (B and C) Post-operative: 5 years after excision and grafting in two stages. Recipient sites are hypertrophic, particularly at borders.

Some evidence of pigment migration. Function is normal. (D and E) Donor sites 5 years later. After the second stage, the left thigh donor site became infected.

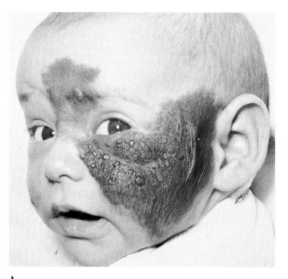

A

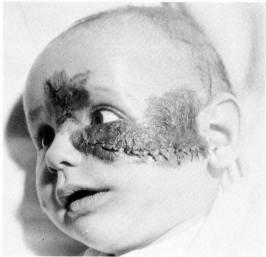

B

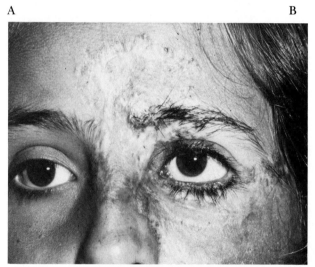

C

FIGURE 13-7. *(A) Preoperative 3-month-old girl. (B) Postoperative: 8 days after partial excision of nevus on left cheek and glabella. (C) Postoperative: 11 years after excision with immediate full-thickness grafts from behind ears and lower neck. To spare the eyebrow, nevus was coagulated. Residual nevus is still present along the ciliary border. The patient has recently married.*

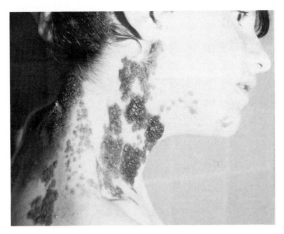

A

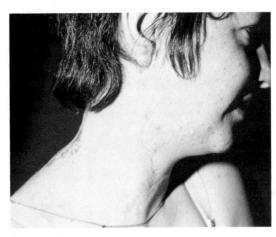

B

FIGURE 13-8. *(A) Preoperative 16-year-old girl with multifocal nevi. (B) Postoperative: 10 years after excision of nevus with thick split-thickness*

graft from abdomen. Patient is the mother of two children without abnormal nevi.

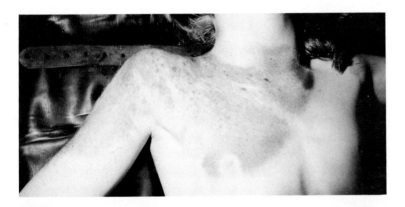

A

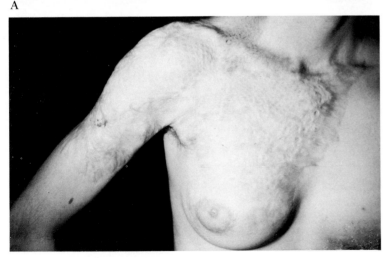

B

FIGURE 13-9. *(A) Preoperative 9-year-old girl. (B) Postoperative: 8 years after excision and split-thickness mesh graft. The breast has developed well.*

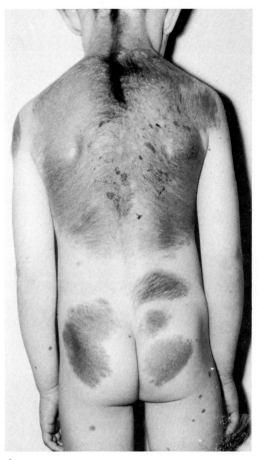

A

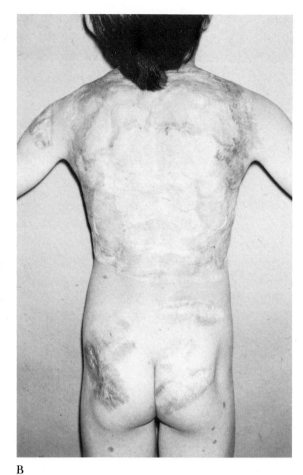

B

FIGURE 13-10. *(A) Preoperative 4-year-old boy with giant nevus as well as large spots of nevi (Group III). (B) Postoperative: 5 years after serial excision for spots and excision with grafts for large nevus. The grafts have been placed in a horizontal rectangular fashion for better healing. Note the absence of hypertrophic scarring at junctions of the grafts. Serial excision could be done for remaining nevus of the left buttock.*

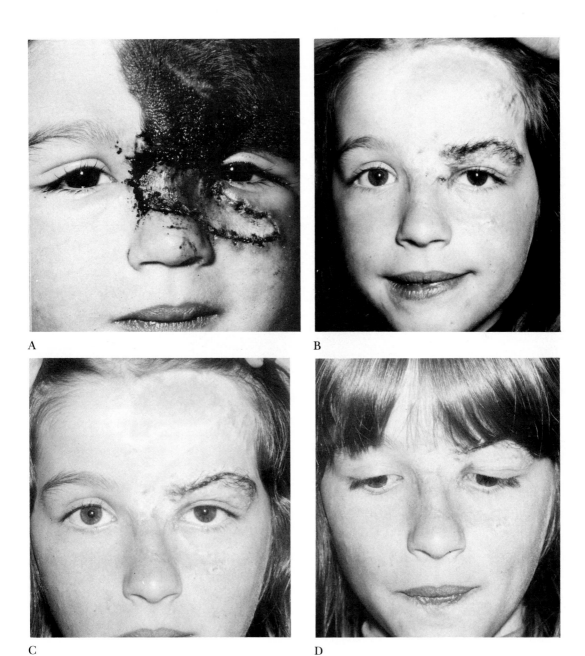

A

B

C

D

FIGURE 13-11. *(A) Two-year-old girl, 8 days after excision and full-thickness retroauricular grafts. (B) Postoperative: 5 years after further excision and more full-thickness grafts from behind ears as well as from the lower* neck. *Nevus was coagulated to spare the eyebrow. (C and D) Postoperative: 8 years. Satisfactory result. Good match in color between grafts from the lower neck and from behind the ears.*

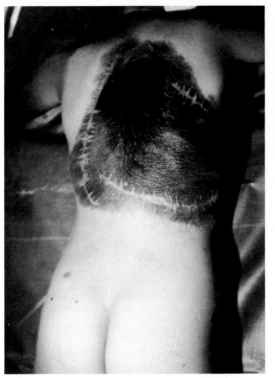

A

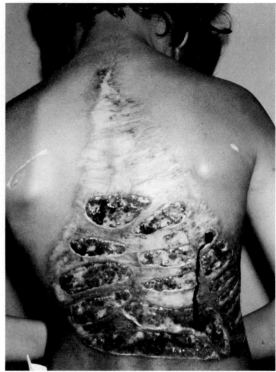

B

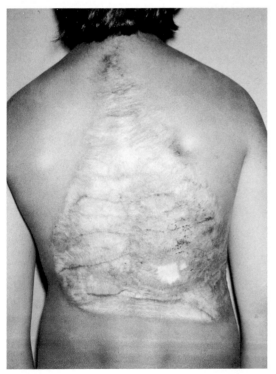

C

FIGURE 13-12. *(A) Three-year-old boy, 3 months after partial excision. Note the white color of scars. (B) Four years later, after the third procedure, using a "white zebra" technique. This view is 1 week after the most recent excision. The patient was sent home on daily dressings and tulle gras. No antiseptic or antibiotic ointments were needed. (C) Five years after the first operation. Scarring is satisfactory. Small dark areas examined histologically show no residual nevus. Further improvement can be obtained by serial excision or dermabrading and overgrafting with very thin skin.*

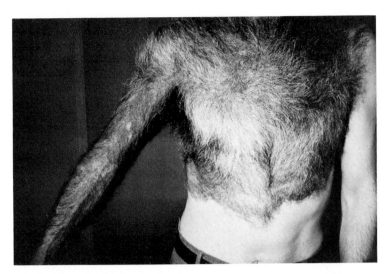

FIGURE 13-13. *A 52-year-old male with giant nevus and a subcutaneous nodule over the right elbow. Biopsy showed metastatic melanoma. Patient refused all treatment and has been lost to follow-up.*

show that progress will have been made in the treatment of giant nevi and, it is hoped, in their prevention.

References

1. Block, L.I., and Conway, H.   Excision and skin grafting of a giant naevus of face and neck. *Plast. Reconstr. Surg.* 31:472, 1963.

2. Davis, J.S.   The removal of wide scars and large disfigurements of the skin by gradual partial excision with closure. *Ann. Surg.* 90:645, 1929.

3. Greeley P.W.   Plastic correction of naevi. *Plast. Reconstr. Surg.* 2:288, 1947.

4. Kaplan, E.N.   Risk of malignancy in large congenital naevi. *Plast. Reconstr. Surg.* 53:421, 1974.

5. Morestin, H.   Cicatrice très étendue du crâne réduite par des excisions successives. *Bull. Mem. Soc. Chir.* (Paris) 42:2052, 1913.

6. Pickrell, K.L., and Clay, R.C.   Giant naevus of the thigh successfully treated by complete excision and primary grafting. *Arch. Surg.* 48:319, 1944.

7. Vilain, R.   Serial excision of skin disfigurements (including giant naevi) by gradual serial excision with closure. *Presse Médicale* 41(2):307, 1965.

Robert M. Goldwyn

COMMENTS ON CHAPTER 13

THE chapter by Dr. Vilain and his associates concerns one of the most formidable problems in plastic and reconstructive surgery. The patient and family, of course, bear the greatest burden, but the surgeon has no light task. The most difficult part of the management is frequently the initial decision—to remove or not to remove. If the nevus is visible and disfiguring cosmetically, the decision is easier than if it is hidden. In the latter situation, the future holds the justification for surgery, since it would be undertaken primarily to prevent malignant transformation rather than removal of an actual existing melanoma. Does the review of patients in Chapter 13 help with regard to who should have an operation? Not really, since the patients with giant nevi have all been treated (except for one patient who had a metastatic melanoma on his forearm). In other words, the data presented by Dr. Vilain and his associates do not give information about the natural history of giant nevi. It can be said from what they have written that after various treatments for giant nevi, none of their patients followed from 1 to 10 years has yet developed a melanoma. Theoretically, this unfortunate event might still occur.

Returning to the question of how frequently giant nevi become malignant, the literature offers no consensus. The incidence of the development of melanomas in giant nevi in various studies ranges from 2 to 31 percent, with an average of about 14 percent [1, 2, 4]. Furthermore, malignancy may arise in large congenital nevi at any age [5]. Although approximately 60 percent of melanomas develop from these nevi during the first decade, another 10 percent appear between the ages of 10 and 20, and 30 percent thereafter. Kaplan [4] has noted that in most reports on malignant giant nevi, patients have been followed for less than 5 years. Complicating the problem is the variation in the definition of a "giant nevus," although most would agree with the criteria given by Dr. Vilain and his co-authors. Another complicating factor is that many authors who have reported on malignancy in giant nevi have assumed wrongly that these were all melanomas; some, in fact, were undifferentiated neural tumors.

Not mentioned by Dr. Vilain and associates but helpful in making the decision regarding operation is the use of biopsies. Kaplan has suggested that if, by biopsy, the nevus is seen microscopically to be intradermal, excision is not advised, but parents are informed of the "unknown potential risk." If the nevus is a junctional, neural, or blue nevus, excision is suggested. In his series, no patient with an intradermal nevus in the reticular dermis (without junctional nevi, blue nevi, or deep dermal "neural" nevi) had a melanoma. Kaplan did note, however, that in 1 out of 14 patients, the histological pattern identified on permanent section was different from that obtained by screening biopsy. Therefore, the preoperative biopsy, while helpful, was not really reliable. In an attempt to define better the malignant potential of the giant pigmented nevus, Dellon and his associates [1] investigated the lesion with light and electron microscopy, tissue culture, and measurements of immunological activity, such as the presence or absence of lymphocytic infiltrates and identification of T and B cells.

If, principally on the basis of the malignant potential of the nevus, the decision is to excise, the next set of judgments concerns how and how much. Since Dr. Vilain and associates have enumerated very well the major therapies along with their advantages and disadvantages, it is of no use to recapitulate that information except to comment on the dissatisfaction with dermabrasion as a method of treatment. While others have also reported disenchantment with dermabrasion, Johnson [3], however, noted success in permanently removing pigmentation from the giant nevus if the dermabrasion was performed *within* the first 2 months of life; if done later, pigmentation returned. Presumably, reduction in pigmentation is accomplished by decreasing the number of melanocytes, and this effect might have prophylactic value. Johnson's observation about dermabrasion early in infancy should be investigated further.

If, in a particular patient, staged excision is chosen to produce the best cosmetic and functional result, is that individual at greater risk by several procedures than by total excision in one stage with grafting and then serial excision of the graft? To answer this possible objection to staged excision, Dr. Vilain and associates observed that none of their patients developed melanoma in any of their nevi during (or even after) their multiple excisions. However, these patients have not been followed for more than 10 years. But even when total excision is done, either in one session or in many, some of the nevus may be intentionally left, as, for example, around orifices, as noted by Dr. Vilain and his colleagues. Is the patient being done a disservice? Is the removal of 98 percent of the nevus enough from the point of view of cancer potential? Is the presence of one tiny nest of tumor sufficient to become a melanoma later? The answer to the last question is probably "yes," but does that justify excising (and reconstructing) the external genitalia in a 5-year-old? Perhaps so, if previous biopsies showed significant malignant potential. However, in dealing with the giant nevus, as with any medical problem, the physician must continually think in terms of probable and possible advantages and disadvantages, as Dr. Vilain and his associates have so ably done. By a review of

their patients in another 25 or 50 years, Dr. Vilain and associates or their successors could obtain important information about the danger of lack of such thinking in electing not to excise totally each giant nevus in each patient.

Dr. Vilain and his co-authors have shown by biopsy that their zebra technique, with its deep planing excision, does remove the nevus, although pigment cells might migrate into the operative sites. Another follow-up in 10 or 20 years with repeat biopsies would be of interest in determining whether there is recurrence of the nevus, and that observation, as well as a much later follow-up, might tell us whether the regrowth of the giant nevus was of significance to the patient's health.

References

1. Dellon, A.L., Edelson, R.L., and Chretien, P.B. Defining the malignant potential of the giant pigmented nevus. *Plast. Reconstr. Surg.* 57:611, 1976.
2. Greeley, P.W., Middleton, A.G., and Curtin, J.W. Incidence of malignancy in giant pigmented nevi. *Plast. Reconstr. Surg.* 36:26, 1965.
3. Johnson, H.A. Permanent removal of pigmentation from giant hairy naevi by dermabrasion in early life. *Br. J. Plast. Surg.* 30:321, 1977.
4. Kaplan, E.N. The risk of malignancy in large congenital nevi. *Plast. Reconstr. Surg.* 53:421, 1974.
5. Lorentzen, M., Pers, M., and Bretteville-Jensen, G. The incidence of malignant transformation in giant pigmented nevi. *Scand. J. Plast. Reconstr. Surg.* 11:163, 1977.

14

IT is unusual to begin a discourse with a summation, but I feel I must in order not to beguile you with expectations of good results. Summing up, the long-term result of any form of hemangioma treatment is not good.* However, the overall result of those treated expectantly is good. It is the exceptions that are discouraging. And who is to know which will be which? Therein lies the dilemma.

During my training, I spent a year as assistant to Frederick A. Figi, M.D., then near the end of his busy career at the Mayo Clinic. He did a fantastic amount of work. His patients all but worshiped him and would return year after year for check-ups and further work, so I had the opportunity of seeing patients treated decades before. I was appalled at the number of patients he had treated by every modality who needed further reconstruction. At that time, he was still inserting radon seeds in some lesions, which admittedly seemed like insurmountable problems; yet other patients were returning with tragic inhibition of bony growth because of radon radiation (Fig. 14-1 A and B).

Some of Dr. Figi's patients had been treated with sclerosing solution, and some, those who had a combined lymphangioma-hemangioma, had received injections of boiling water. Extensive lesions were often managed by several methods. My strong impression was that the long-term results were poor. Those who returned with premalignant actinodermatitis had certainly been done a disservice. I recommend, nevertheless, that you read his papers if you wish a thorough knowledge of this subject.

---

*The term *hemangioma* is of Greek origin, literally meaning "blood tumor." The trend, according to Dr. Frank McDowell, editor of *Plastic and Reconstructive Surgery,* is away from the Greek plurals (in this case, *hemangiomata*) and toward use of the anglicized plural *hemangiomas.* English has always been a living language, so I do not suppose we can buck the trend. Personally, I like *hemangiomata* better.

Hugh A. Johnson

TREATMENT OF HEMANGIOMAS

Seeing some late cases, however, has made me leary of the plea for the *"noli me tangere"* conservative treatment of all hemangiomas.

Twenty years ago I spent an academic year teaching at the Christian Medical College in Vellore, India. Hemangiomas do not seem as common among the dark-skinned, yet I did see untreated and neglected cases. The spontaneous regression seems to apply only to those patients whose hemangiomas have a cavernous element. I saw a few cases of radionecrosis of the mandible, where inexpert and injudicious radiation had been given. These were horrors and healing problems I will not soon forget.

And as I write this introduction while on exchange in Moscow, I have yet another chance to study the results of another senior surgeon near the end of his career, Professor Khitrov. On a head and neck service (Central Institute of Stomatology, Moscow) of more than 60 beds, there are six patients who have or have had extensive hemangioma about the head. Two were adults in the process of repeated excision and grafting, several stages having been done over the years. The results were excellent for this type of treatment, but the problem of skin color and the border of red capillaries that follows excision were there no matter how well done. Two of the six patients treated years previously by radiation were getting final touching up by Filatov tubes to reconstruct mandibles lost from radionecrosis. Another patient had a large defect following excision of the entire lower lip, also in the process of repair by Filatov tube. The last patient was a young female adult with a unilateral exophthalmos and tumor deep in the parotid and masseter regions. She was about to have angiograms prior to exploration.

I state the preceding experience to show that my clinical work is not subject only to my own bias. In a few months I will have been in private practice for 25 years—a quarter of a century of a busy, varied practice of general plastic surgery in a community of 140,000. As a regional medical center, we have a higher than average number of specialists, especially pediatricians. These have been the source of most hemangioma referrals, although some come from family physicians.

In 25 years I have had 378 patients with hemangiomas, most of whom have been infants. I have operated on the majority, since most were referred specifically for surgery, which was usually indicated. The infants' lesions have chiefly been rapidly expanding combined cavernous and capillary hemangioma, often in regions where a feature was endangered by the lesion. Having a few experiences where expanding lesions were "watched," such as one patient whose cranium was penetrated, with extension onto the dura mater (Fig. 14-2A through E), one begins to err on the side of elective excision (Fig. 14-3A through E). I have always given every patient the benefit of the doubt and have "watched" the lesions myself at 2- to 4-week intervals, taking photographs to be certain of progression or regression. A photographic record is most important. If the hemangioma remains static, I always defer surgery.

A paragraph about the classification of hemangiomas is indicated. For those not familiar, I suggest any good text, since most of the literature is full of descriptive terms signifying nothing. Basically, there are capillary hemangiomas, cavernous hemangiomas, and combined lymphangioma-hemangiomas, the last by far the most difficult to treat.

The life history of these lesions is not understood but can be considered as follows. The strictly capillary lesions are present at birth and do not change much, but they often become nodular in adult life, rendering camouflage by makeup difficult. Treatment of capillary hem-

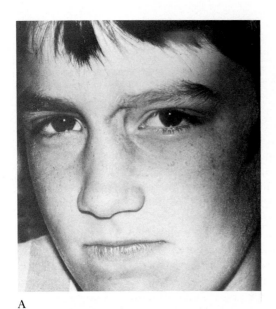

A

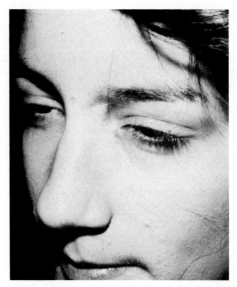

B

FIGURE 14-1. *(A) Failure of bone growth. Radon seeds are visible beneath the atrophic skin. (B) Reconstruction with subcutaneous flap and full-thickness retroauricular graft.*

angiomas is disappointing, as I will demonstrate later. The combined capillary and cavernous lesions often are not present at birth or may be present just as a pinhead that expands rapidly. Payne has described a precursor to hemangioma present at birth, a pale area in which the hemangioma develops. The combined lesions grow rapidly, often to the point of sloughing, then regress, leaving some residual atrophy or redundancy of skin or scarring of varying degrees. This residual may require late repair (Fig. 14-4A and B). By far the majority of lesions regress spontaneously. It is the lesion that does not that gives the heartache.

Another type of very common hemangioma can occur in the sixth decade and onward. These are the senile hemangiomas, often multiple and never over a millimeter or two in size, and they are excised or cauterized easily for strictly aesthetic reasons.

Having observed the failure and iatrogenic deformities that have followed exotic forms of treatment (radiation in all its forms [remember,

x-rays are for taking pictures, and even then one should use care], dry ice, liquid nitrogen, and sclerosing solutions of all types), what treatment have I chosen after reviewing my long-term results?

First, I will discuss some experimental attempts or previously untried methods of treatment. After I had observed the spontaneous regression of some lesions I had partially excised, I wondered whether the lesion released an antigen. Since many sloughed in the process of involution, Arthus's phenomenon came to mind. I convinced a family whose child had an entire right arm involved (Fig. 14-5 A through E) to let me excise part of the tumor, emulsify it, then inject it at weekly intervals. My negative results were reported [7].

To treat the capillary type, it occurred to me that altering the bed of the hemangioma might change the characteristics of the vessels in the hemangioma. I asked two patients to let me try to transplant part of their capillary hemangioma to normal beds and some normal skin to the hemangioma's bed. The results were as shown in Figure 14-6A, B, and C. These negative findings also were published [5].

As you can see, I have given this very difficult

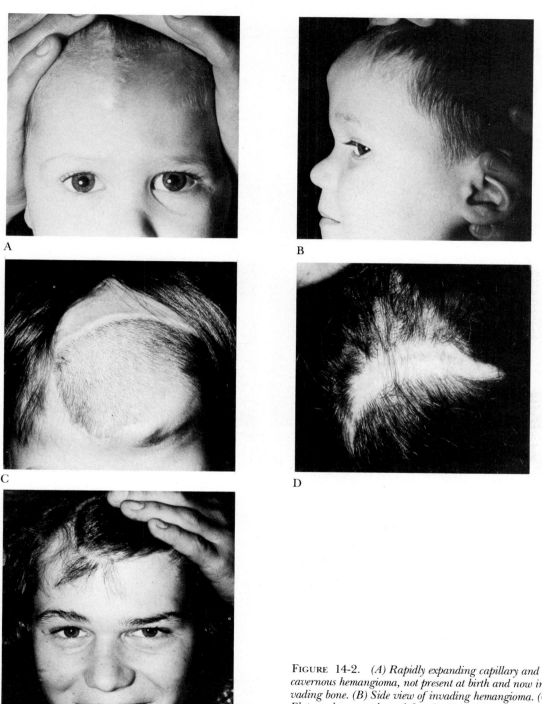

FIGURE 14-2. *(A) Rapidly expanding capillary and cavernous hemangioma, not present at birth and now invading bone. (B) Side view of invading hemangioma. (C) Flap used to cover bony defect. Lesion was just invading dura. (D) Defect after excision of graft. (E) Ultimate result. All could have been avoided if the lesion had been adequately excised at the first attempt.*

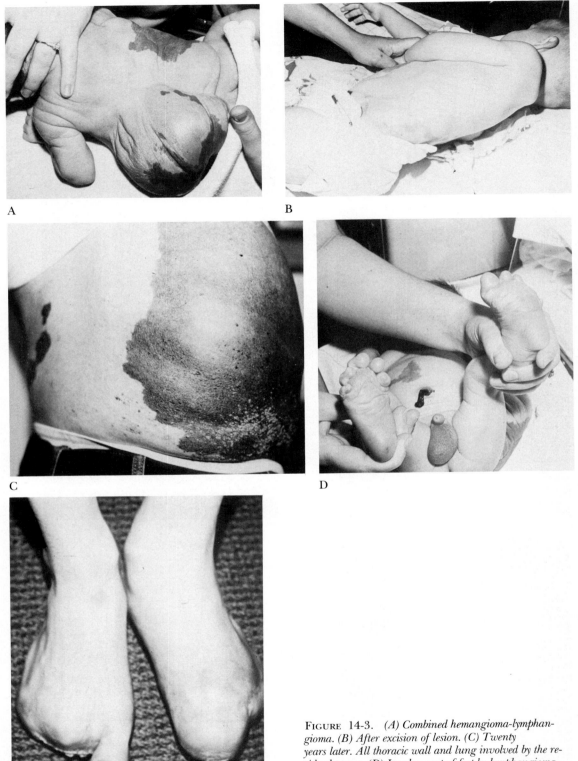

A

B

C

D

E

FIGURE 14-3. *(A) Combined hemangioma-lymphangioma. (B) After excision of lesion. (C) Twenty years later. All thoracic wall and lung involved by the residual tumor. (D) Involvement of feet by lymphangioma. (E) Twenty years later. The patient disguises his feet by wearing large, high tennis shoes.*

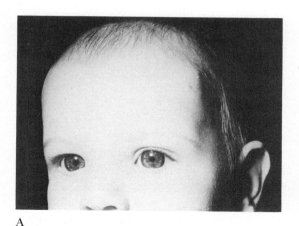

A

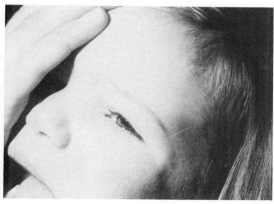

B

FIGURE 14-4. *(A) Area of white atrophy and redundant skin after spontaneous regression of capillary and cavernous hemangioma. (B) After excision of redundant skin.*

problem considerable thought in the belief that there must be an answer. Recent experiments with tetramethylhydrazine hydrochloride in Swiss mice have consistently produced blood vessel tumors. Perhaps a door is opening.

Treatment of Capillary Hemangiomas

When capillary hemangiomas occur on the face, they are tragic. Abrasive surgery should be mentioned, but only after patients are warned that it will probably be unsuccessful. I have had one patient for whom it was successful (Fig. 14-7A and B). I reluctantly suggest doing a patch test to see. If it lightens the lesion considerably, it is worth a try, for although the lesion is still present, lightening makes the task of makeup cover more simple. Small lesions on males, which can be covered with full-thickness grafts, should be excised (Fig. 14-8A and B). Males will not wear makeup and are more willing to accept scars. It is very discouraging to get

a beautiful graft on a female only to find her still wearing makeup. For most females, makeup is the answer. The familiar brand is Covermark.* Mother and child should get professional advice for its use.

With the passage of time, many capillary hemangiomas become nodular. Then extensive resection and skin grafting are indicated. These grafted cases should be followed because even though the excision is done into apparently normal skin, peripheral capillaries dilate, and the graft becomes surrounded by a narrow border of hemangioma. For this phenomenon, I can offer no explanation (Fig. 14-9A and B).

If I see an infant or newborn whose lesion is confined to one extremity, I try long-term pressure with one of the Jobst gloves or stockings.† It is worth a try and certainly less risky than any of the other experimentations I have already described. If parents participate in the decision, there is no problem with the legal aspect. Most people in the world are good; just a few are litigious, and one can usually spot these people ahead of time with some experience.

*Lydia O'Leary, 575 Madison Avenue, New York, New York 10022.
†Jobst Institute Inc., Box 653, Miami St., Toledo, Ohio 43694.

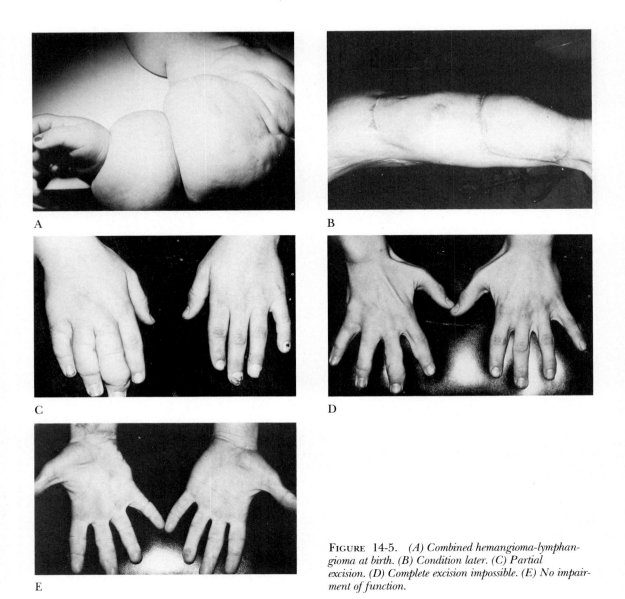

A

B

C

D

E

FIGURE 14-5. *(A) Combined hemangioma-lymphan-gioma at birth. (B) Condition later. (C) Partial excision. (D) Complete excision impossible. (E) No impair-ment of function.*

Treatment of the Combined Capillary and Cavernous Hemangiomas and Expectant Treatment

I would emphasize adding the adjective *watchful* to the waiting or expectant treatment. Two-week intervals are best at first, with pho-tographs recording the change. Subjective im-pressions are unreliable. When one's mood is good, patients look better. Later, if the parents feel reassured and the hemangioma is relatively static, the child can be seen every 2 months. If sloughing occurs and the lesion is resectable, this is an indication for surgical intervention (Fig. 14-10A and B) since these hemangiomas,

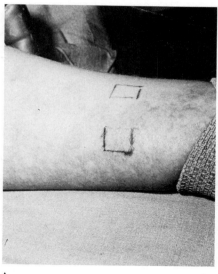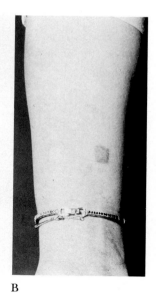

A   B

FIGURE 14-6.   *(A) Areas of normal skin and heman-*
gioma to be exchanged. (B) After exchange. The heman-
gioma remained unchanged on a normal bed, and the
normal skin on the hemangioma bed was not affected.

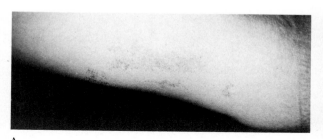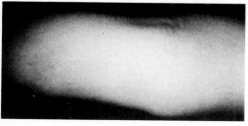

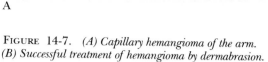

A   B

FIGURE 14-7.   *(A) Capillary hemangioma of the arm.*
(B) Successful treatment of hemangioma by dermabrasion.

if untreated, may heal with disfiguring scars (Fig. 14-11A and B). One cannot predict how far the slough will progress, or whether there will be infection. Infection and bleeding seldom occur. However, oozing is common and is often frightening to parents. There is convincing evi-dence for the efficacy of watchful waiting (Fig. 14-12A and B).

A parent's wishes should theoretically not be an indication for surgery, yet often I have made it one. I recall a case, a beautiful first child with a cherry-like lesion just above the hairline. Each visit was tearfully ended with a plea for surgery. It was so simple and was accomplished on an outpatient basis using local infiltration anes-thesia and minimal inhalation anesthesia. The parents were so grateful. I must admit that I

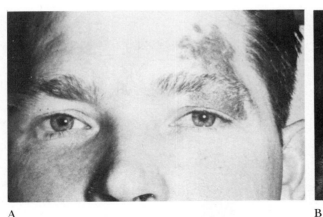

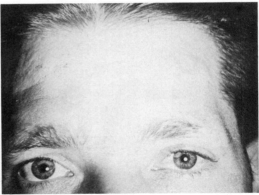

A

B

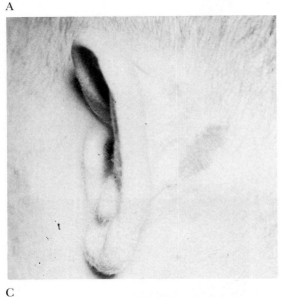

C

FIGURE 14-8. *(A) Capillary hemangioma. (B) Hemangioma excised and replaced with full-thickness retroauricular graft. (C) Hemangioma, transplanted to a normal bed, remained unchanged.*

made my decision to operate after my experience with a child (Fig. 14-13A and B) whose family physician had "watched" the frontal lesion grow, invade bone, and ultimately penetrate down to the frontal lobe. Clairvoyance is needed in the selection of cases for surgery in this disease (Fig. 14-14A and B). I have little (Figs. 14-12 through 14-14).

Actually, excision of cavernous lesions is straightforward. The blood supply is the normal blood supply to the area, so one need not worry if dissection is done just outside the le-

sion. The hemangioma comes out as if it were encapsulated. The closure problem varies with the region involved, but is managed according to plastic surgical principles (Figs. 14-15A through D, 14-16A through C, 14-17A through C, 14-18A and B and 14-19A and B).

Because of my bad experiences, certain areas, I feel, should not be treated expectantly; the breast is one. Operate early and shell the lesion out in order to not remove any breast tissue. I have seen tragedies also around the ear, eyelid, and nose that could have been avoided

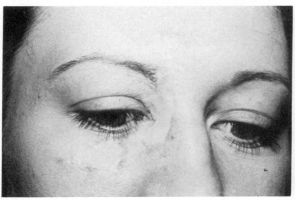
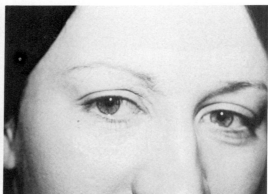

A

B

FIGURE 14-9. *(A) Capillary hemangioma at the border of a graft, which appeared even though 2 to 3 mm of normal-colored skin was excised with the hemangioma. (B) Result after a secondary excision.*

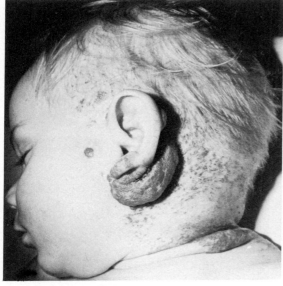
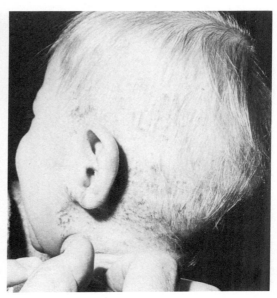

A

B

FIGURE 14-10. *(A) Sloughing lesion, rapidly growing, treated by partial excision. (B) After partial excision. This was involuting when lost to follow-up.*

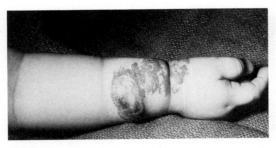

A

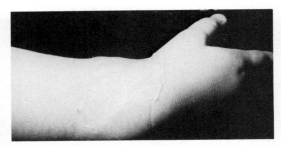

B

FIGURE 14-11. *(A) Sloughing combined lesion. (B) Scarring that followed slough corrected with thick split-thickness skin graft.*

by very early excision. I admit that my reasons are not well documented, but it is a philosophy evolved from experience.

Cavernous Hemangioma and Thrombocytopenia

This is extremely rare, and were I presented with a case, I would certainly try continuous pressure to see its effect on the thrombocyte count. The case I reported in 1959 [5] was treated before the reports on effectiveness of pressure (Fig. 14-20A through C). The lad is now 25 years old, works as a laboratory technician in a hospital, is married, and walks with a slight limp. He recently had a seminoma removed and has been well for 2 years. In view of this case and another patient who developed a brain tumor (malignant, but apparently cured), one wonders if there is some inhibitory mechanism missing—something that should be investigated.

Continuous pressure has been suggested for these cavernous hemangiomas with throm-

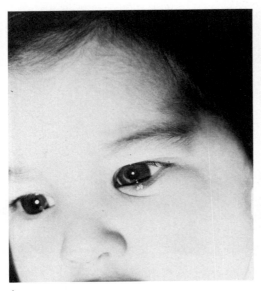

A

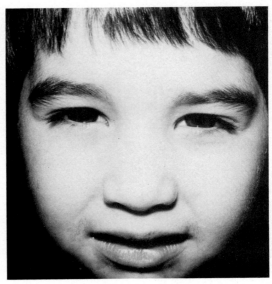

B

FIGURE 14-12. *(A) Lid involvement. (B) Spontaneous involution of lesion of left lower lid.*

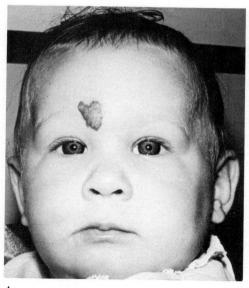

A

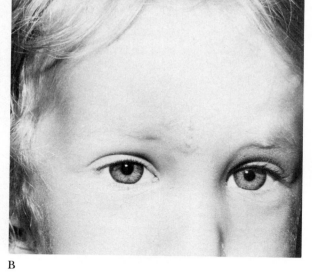

B

FIGURE 14-13.   (A) Combined capillary and cavernous hemangioma. (B) Spontaneous regression, but some residual deformity.

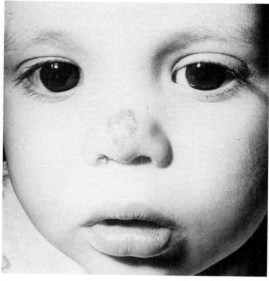

A

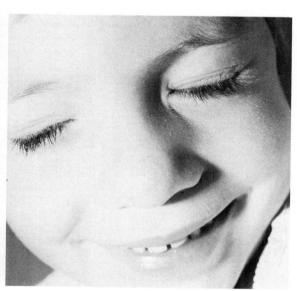

B

FIGURE 14-14.   (A) The gray look that often accompanies regression. (B) Some residual, but minor.

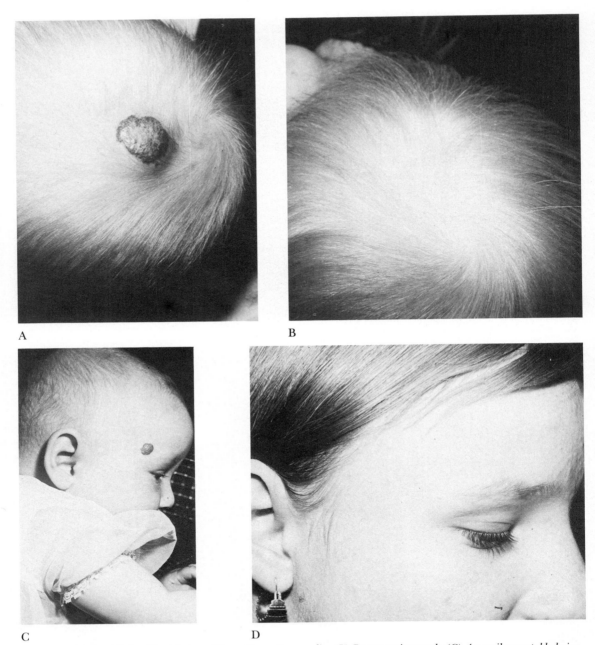

A

B

C

D

FIGURE 14-15. (A) Combined lesion of the scalp, easily resectable under minimal general anesthesia and local infiltration with 0.5% Xylocaine with 1:200,000 adrenalin. (B) Postoperative result. (C) An easily resectable lesion that causes much concern to young parents. (D) Widened scar; the result 18 years later.

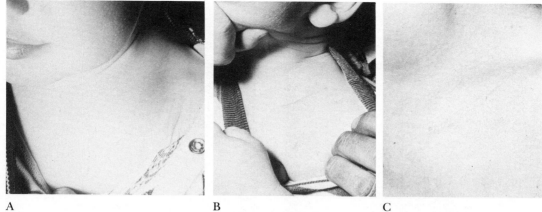

A   B   C

FIGURE 14-16. *(A) Cavernous lesion thought to communicate with an internal portion. (B) Early postoperative result. Although deep and extensive, the lesion shelled out easily and did not enter the chest. (C) Result 20 years later.*

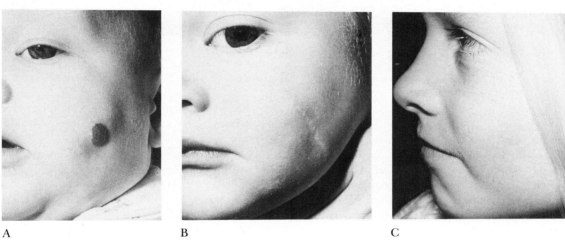

A   B   C

FIGURE 14-17. *(A) Rapidly expanding lesion. (B) Early postoperative result. (C) Result 4 years later.*

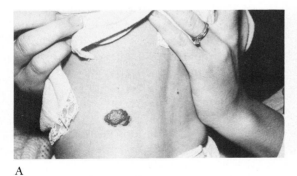

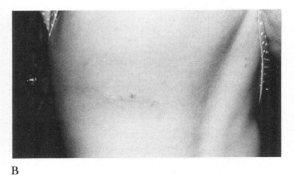

A   B

FIGURE 14-18. *(A) Multiple lesions not present at birth. (B) Capillary elements were not visible at the time of excision but are now present, a common occurrence despite careful removal with a rim of apparently normal tissue.*

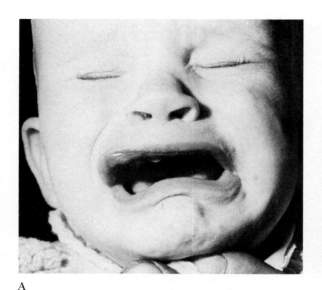

A

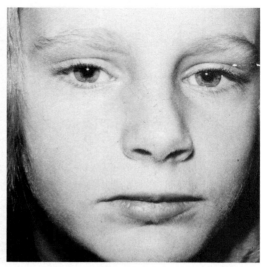

B

FIGURE 14-19. *(A) Present at birth and expanding rapidly. (B) Result 17 years later.*

bocytopenia and is certainly worth a try. If the pressure does not work, then one must give blood with thrombocytes at the time of excision. Some have reported the use of cortisone. I have no experience and hope that I am never faced with such a case, which fortunately is extremely rare.

Treatment of Combined Lymphangioma and Hemangioma

The combination of lymphangioma and hemangioma presents an extremely difficult situation. Basically, I believe that there is little connection in etiology, that the hemangiomatous part is merely incidental to the lymphangioma. Nothing short of excision is effective in these lesions. Fortunately, lymphangioma is rare, 27 cases compared with 378 hemangiomas in my 25 years of practice. I believe that surgery should be undertaken as soon as feasible because of the overgrowth of the involved parts (Figs. 14-15 through 14-19).

In conclusion, I offer the following thoughts:

1. The long-term results of treatment for hemangioma are poor no matter what the modality.
2. Certain forms of treatment used in the past produce iatrogenic deformities and/or premalignant lesions, e.g., radiation in any form (Figs. 14-21 A through D and 14-22 A and B), dry ice, or sclerosing solutions.
3. Combined capillary and cavernous hemangiomas are usually absent or small (or preceded by a depigmented area) at birth, grow rapidly, often to the point of slough, then regress, leaving no or some residual deformity such as a scar or redundant tissue. These lesions are best treated by careful follow-up at frequent intervals, with *photographs*. If there is no growth, or if involution occurs, no treatment is given. After involution, reconstructive procedures may be indicated.
4. A few expanding lesions encroaching on a feature perhaps can be approached best by excision, if resectable, before that feature is destroyed. There is no way to predict the rate and extent of growth (Figs. 14-23A and B and 14-24A and B).
5. Capillary hemangiomas are best not treated.

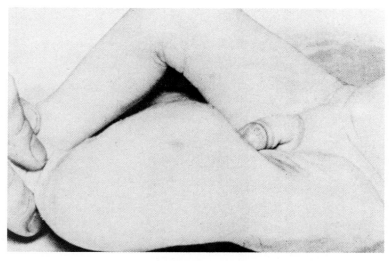

A

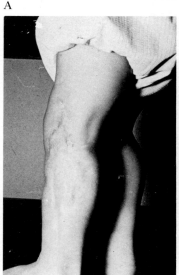

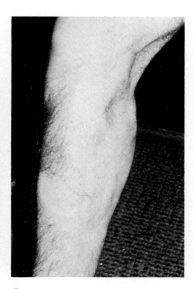

B   C

FIGURE 14-20.   *(A) Expanding hemangioma with thrombocytopenia. (B) After excision (fraught with complications). (C) Twenty-two years later. There is some vascular insufficiency and some loss of function. Two years ago* *the patient developed a seminoma but is presently well. (Reprinted, with permission, from H.A. Johnson, Expanding hemangioma with associated thrombocytopenia. Br. J. Plast. Surg. 12:69, 1959.)*

An extremely small percentage is helped by abrasive surgery, thus I suggest a test patch under local anesthesia. Do not give the parents false hopes. Small lesions may be treated by excision and reconstruction done with local tissues and/or full-thickness grafts. Females may end up wearing makeup to hide the scars and graft. Makeup generally conceals this lesion effectively.

6. Later in life, capillary hemangiomas may become nodular, and excision with grafting can be done with advantage.

7. Combined lymphangioma-hemangioma is best treated surgically.

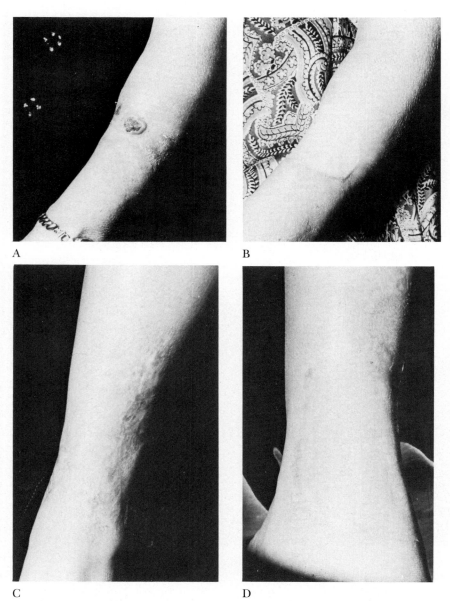

FIGURE 14-21. *(A) Epithelioma arising in a postir-radiated hemangioma. The average time for development of malignancy is 20 years. The lesions contain squamous cell and basal cell components. The basal cell lesions often show spindling and can be misdiagnosed as sarcoma. (B) Wide excision and split-thickness skin graft. (C) Beginning breakdown of an area of actinodermatitis 17 years after x-ray treatment. (D) Area excised and grafted.*

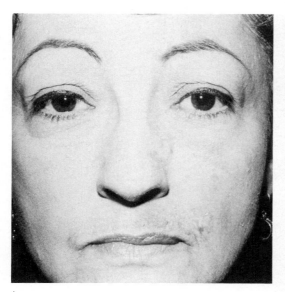
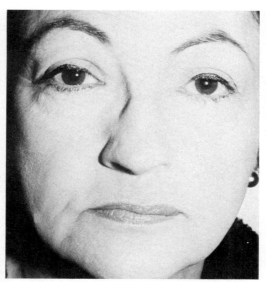

A

B

FIGURE 14-22.   *(A) Radiation changes in an area of capillary hemangioma irradiated 25 years previously. (B) Area excised and grafted with full-thickness skin grafts.*

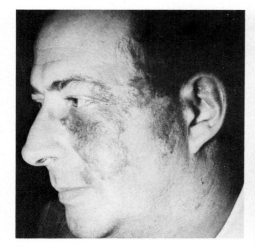
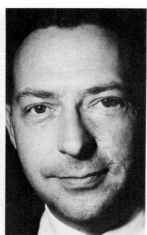

A

B

FIGURE 14-23.   *(A) Beginning thickness in an area of previously flat capillary hemangioma. (B) All the hemangioma was excised and grafted with a thick split-thickness* *dermatome graft. The color match is not good, but more acceptable than the hemangioma.*

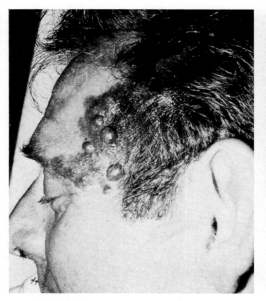

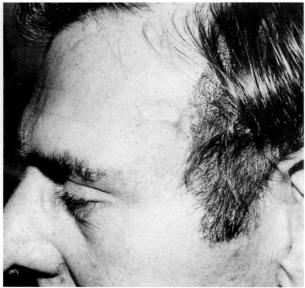

A   B

FIGURE 14-24. *(A) Thickening capillary hemangioma in an untreated lesion. (B) Lesion excised and grafted with a full-thickness graft.*

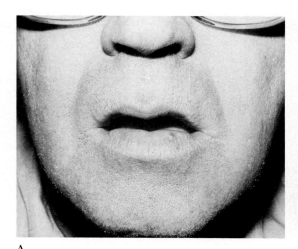

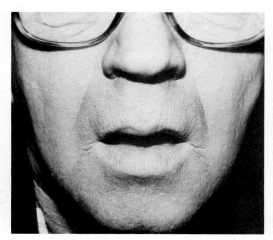

A   B

FIGURE 14-25. *(A) Senile hemangioma of the lip. These are often multiple. Most can be destroyed easily with diathermy, but they should be marked first with Bonney's blue* *before injecting anesthetic; otherwise, they will be obscured. (B) This lesion was excised. Cautery was not used because it leaves a white scar.*

8. Hemangioma with thrombocytopenia is rare, but can be life-threatening. Continuous pressure should be given a fair trial before undertaking excision, which is usually a dangerous procedure unless fresh blood with platelets is administered.

9. Senile hemangiomas appear from the sixth decade onward. They are of no significance except aesthetic, are usually never more than a millimeter or two in diameter, are often multiple, and are easily excised (Fig. 14-25A and B) or destroyed by cautery.

References

1. Blackfield, H.M., Morris, W.J., and Torrey, F.A. Visible hemangiomas: A preliminary statistical report of a 10-year study. *Plast. Reconstr. Surg.* 26:326, 1960.
2. Blackfield, H.M., Torrey, F.A., Morris, W.J., and Low Beer, B.V.A. The management of hemangiomata: A plea for conservatism in infancy. *Plast. Reconstr. Surg.* 20:38, 1957.
3. Figi, F.A. The treatment of hemangiomas of the head and neck. *Plast. Reconstr. Surg.* 3:1, 1948.
4. Figi, F.A., and O'Brien, R.W. Treatment of angiomas. *Plast. Reconstr. Surg.* 18:448, 1956.
5. Johnson, H.A. Expanding hemangioma with associated thrombocytopenia. *Br. J. Plast. Surg.* 12:69, 1959.
6. Johnson, H.A. Transplantation's effect on capillary hemangiomas. *Plast. Reconstr. Surg.* 26:330, 1960.
7. Johnson, H.A. Lymphangioma and Arthus' phenomenon. *J.A.M.A.* 191:602, 1965.
8. Payne, M.M., Moyer, F., Marcks, K.M., and Trevaskis, A.E. The precursor to the hemangioma. *Plast. Reconstr. Surg.* 38:64, 1966.
9. Stout, A.P. Tumors of the Soft Tissues. In *Atlas of Tumor Pathology.* Washington, D.C.: Armed Forces Institute of Pathology, 1967, Sect. 2, fasc. 5.
10. Toth, B., Nägel, D., Erickson, J., and Kupper, R. Tumorigenicity of tetramethylhydrazine hydrochloride in Swiss mice, *J. Natl. Cancer Inst.* 57:1179, 1976.

Robert M. Goldwyn

COMMENTS ON CHAPTER 14

IN his usual piquant and unambiguous style, Dr. Johnson has given us the distillate of 25 years of experience with one of the unsolved major problems in medicine. The etiology of these vascular abnormalities is obscure, their classification confusing, and their treatment haphazard.

Wherever there is a blood vessel, a hemangioma has the potential of forming. From a pragmatic and simplistic viewpoint, hemangiomas are either minor or major with respect to function and/or cosmesis. They may regress, stay the same, or progress. Because of the unpredictability of their behavior, careful observation of most hemangiomas is mandatory, as Dr. Johnson suggests. Since we lack a valid method of classifying hemangiomas according to their biological activity, we can advise parents only in terms of a hemangioma's *probable* behavior. Numerous studies have documented the fact that about 60 percent of hemangiomas are present at birth, 30 percent appear in the first few weeks of life, about 8 percent come within the next 5 months, and another 2 percent appear afterward [12].

The most common type is the capillary hemangioma (strawberry or raspberry marks) [12]. Those appearing on the face, particularly the eyelids, nose, ears, lips, and mucous membranes, are of most concern cosmetically. It is not unusual for the capillary type to have a cavernous component. Usually, the strawberry and/or cavernous hemangioma grows rapidly for the first 6 months of life, reaches a plateau, then spontaneously regresses. As Dr. Johnson has emphasized, it is the exceptions to this sequence that cause the nightmares. A hemangioma, for example, encroaching upon an infant's vision forces a decision about treatment: what or when? Biopsies during a period of growth may cause undue concern and unwarranted surgery in some cases. Reviewing about 6,500 patients with hemangiomas, MacCollum and Martin [12] stated that biopsies in 68 instances were diagnosed as hemangioen-

dothelioma; yet all lesions from which these biopsies were taken subsequently proved to be benign. In addition to them, however, six patients with highly malignant hemangioendotheliosarcoma were encountered, and these patients died soon afterward.

Usually a biopsy is not done on a patient whose hemangioma is expanding, as on the eyelid in the instance just cited. Surgical excision is the obvious method of treatment, and the plastic surgeon is asked for an opinion. Frequently, excision, if done, might produce gross disfigurement because of the area requiring removal and might still fail to extirpate the hemangioma. For this situation, radiation therapy (200 to 300 rads in air) has been used at many centers to good advantage. However, the ultimate effects and complications of radiation may become evident only after many years, for example, an increase in the likelihood of cancer of the thyroid or any organ in the radiation field, leukemia, underdevelopment of facial bones, and even birth defects in progeny. Furthermore, there is always the possibility that the hemangioma would have regressed if untreated. Even radiotherapy enthusiasts, however, generally withhold treatment when a hemangioma infarcts, causing slough accompanied by infection. Although this phenomenon may represent the ultimate in involution, gross disfigurement may be the outcome if a facial feature has rotted away and if secondary healing has been accompanied by significant wound contracture. Caution in the use of radiation is the message, not necessarily abandonment of this form of treatment which, for the majority of patients, may have helped their problem or at least not have harmed them. Administration of x-rays at very low dosage and proper shielding of the patient are crucial.

Another means of therapy for the rapidly growing hemangioma causing concern is the use of steroids. Despite reports [4] of the successes of steroid therapy, many pediatricians fear its consequences if administration is continued for more than 2 weeks, particularly in a very young child, because of possible late effects on growth and endocrine development, not to mention immediate dangers of gastric ulcers.

Another alternative method of managing the proliferating hemangioma is the use of cryotherapy by the application of liquid nitrogen through probes [8, 9]. This technique involves little present or future risk to the patient and can cause remarkable regression of the hemangioma without danger of bleeding.

In addition to surface hemangiomas, there are others whose type, size, and location cause the most severe problems for the patient, the family, and the doctor: cavernous hemangiomas of the orbit [10], cranium, pharynx [9], esophagus [5], larynx, and sinuses. Invasive hemangiomas of the head and neck may persist despite herculean surgery [11]. The decision has to be made whether to attempt to extirpate the tumor or to settle for reducing its size in order to control its growth and prevent infection and hemorrhage. Naturally, meticulous follow-up is necessary, since the biological behavior of these tumors is unpredictable.

Confusing the species *hemangioma* is the genus *vascular malformation,* which can be predominantly venous, predominantly arterial, predominantly arterial-venous, or predominantly lymphatic [13]. Although these vascular problems most often affect the extremities [1], they can involve solely the head and neck, the trunk, and other sites. Trauma can initiate savage growth in what was once a small, dormant lesion. Not only can these vascular malformations and large hemangiomas encroach upon vital structures, but they also can be accompanied by giantism, local ulceration and hemorrhage, cardiac failure and pulmonary edema, as well as coagulopathy [3, 15]. Disseminated intravascular coagulation may arise. Microthrombi form in the small vessels and remove fibrinogen and platelets from the circulation [3, 15]. Factors II, V, VIII, X, and XII may be reduced systemically, bleeding may occur, and fibrinolysis may exceed new fibrinogen production. Abnormalities of a minor nature also have been detected in surface hemangiomas,

where local intravascular coagulation is well compensated for by a proportionate increase in fibrinogen [3]. The long-term course of any hemangioma, but particularly those of large size, is unpredictable because a hemangioma may increase alarmingly as a result of trauma, as mentioned, or simply of the phases of puberty and adolescence and, later, pregnancy.

Concerning another difficult problem— congenital arterial venous fistulae—a book, not simply a chapter or commentary, could be written. These fistulae are usually composed of hundreds of small communications and have been considered of two types: arterial hemangiomas and hemangiomatous giantism, the latter associated with marked regional overgrowth usually in the extremity but occasionally in a portion of the face. Despite repeated surgical attack, a massively involved extremity may eventually have to be amputated. Dr. Johnson discussed also the condition of combined lymphangioma and hemangioma. Others would agree completely with his statement that "there is little connection and etiology, and the hemangiomatous part is merely incidental to the lymphangioma." When feasible, surgical excision may be the only effective treatment for this variety, as it is for the solitary lymphangioma. Although the treatment of hemangiomas during the past 75 years has been disappointing, as noted by Dr. Johnson, the next 25 years seem more hopeful. Dr. Johnson noted his own imaginative efforts to regulate the hemangioma with immunotherapy. Doubtless more sophisticated attempts will be made, and hopefully some might succeed. We should have a better understanding of the tumor angiogenic factor [16]. which is mitogenic for capillary endothelium. Perhaps it may someday be used to arrest and reverse the growth of a hemangioma. The status of angiography becomes more elegant each year, and it would not be a surprising development to have available predictable methods of selectively closing the vascular channels that feed arteriovenous fistulae. Someday perhaps we shall have the means of manipulating the clotting mechanism to thrombose designated vessels locally and regionally without causing systemic problems. Already for the port wine stain there is an encouraging alternative to simply using makeup, and this is the laser [6, 7]. Its effect might be maximized by appropriate pharmacological agents. The development also of the carbon dioxide laser may make the surgery for hemangiomas less bloody for the surgeon and safer for the patient. Laboratory investigation of hemangiomas during growth and involution may provide clues to a useful classification based on biological activity. Hopefully, perhaps through tissue cultures, it will be possible to predict accurately the behavior of every hemangioma and, more important for the patient, to treat it effectively. Maybe the treatment should begin in the earliest stage of the hemangioma with the entity mentioned by Johnson and described by Payne et al. [14] as a "precursor" to the hemangioma: a pale, well-demarcated, nonelevated area, visible on careful examination but more apparent when the newborn cries, causing the adjacent skin to become suffused. Possibly cryosurgery, the argon laser, or microsurgical excision will effectively eliminate the hemangioma.

Also not to be dismissed from this utopian vision is the possibility of understanding the etiology of the hemangioma and preventing prepartum its occurrence.

References

1. Allen, P.W., and Enzinger, F.M. Hemangioma of skeletal muscle: An analysis of 89 cases. *Cancer* 29:8, 1972.
2. Apfelberg, D.B., Maser, M.R., and Lash, H. Argon laser treatment of cutaneous vascular abnormalities: Progress report. *Ann. Plast. Surg.* 1:14, 1978.
3. Dube, B., Pillai, P.H., Singhal, G.D., and Khanna, N.N. Blood coagulation studies in children with surface hemangiomas. *Int. Surg.* 60:524, 1975.
4. Edgerton, M.T. The treatment of hemangiomas with special reference to the role of steroid therapy. *Ann. Surg.* 183:517, 1976.
5. Feist, J.H., Siconolfi, E.P., and Gilman, E. Giant cavernous hemangioma of the esophagus. *J.A.M.A.* 235:1146, 1976.
6. Goldman, L. Effects of new laser systems on the skin. *Arch. Dermatol.* 108:385, 1973.
7. Goldman, L., and Dreffer, R. Laser treatment of extensive mixed cavernous and port-wine stains. *Arch. Dermatol.* 113:504, 1977.
8. Goldwyn, R.M. Evaluation of Cryosurgery for Hemangiomas. In S.A. Zacarian (Ed.), *Cryosurgical Advances in Dermatology and Tumors of the Head and Neck.* Springfield, Ill.: Thomas, 1977. Pp. 235–248.
9. Goldwyn, R.M., and Rosoff, C.B. Cryosurgery for large hemangiomas in adults. *Plast. Reconstr. Surg.* 43:605, 1969.
10. Habal, H.B., and Murray, J.E. The natural history of a benign locally invasive hemangioma of the orbital region: Case report. *Plast. Reconstr. Surg.* 49:209, 1972.
11. Hoehn, J.G., Farrow, G.M., Devine, K.D., and Masson, J.K. Invasive hemangioma of the head and neck. *Am. J. Surg.* 120:495, 1970.
12. MacCollum, D.W., and Martin, L.W. Hemangiomas in infancy and childhood: A report based on 6479 cases. *Surg. Clin. North Am.* 36:1647, 1956.
13. Malan, E. (Ed.). *Vascular Malformations (Angiodysplasias).* Milan: Carlo Erba Foundation, 1974. Pp. 1–58.
14. Payne, M.M., Moyer, F., Marcks, K.M., and Trevaskis, A.E. The precursor to the hemangioma. *Plast. Reconstr. Surg.* 38:64, 1966.
15. Shim, W.K.T. Hemangiomas of infancy complicated by thrombocytopenia. *Am. J. Surg.* 116:896, 1968.
16. Wolf, J.E., Jr., and Hubler, W.R., Jr. Tumor angiogenic factors and human skin tumors. *Arch. Dermatol.* 111:321, 1975.

15

PRIOR to 1960 our management of epistaxis as a manifestation of hereditary hemorrhagic telangiectasia had been more than disappointing. There were no long-term good or even fair results. Emergency measures such as intranasal packing, posterior pharyngeal packs, and inflatable cuffs generally controlled acute hemorrhage, but, of course, they were only temporary measures. Roentgen therapy, radium, venom, rutin, vitamins, hormones, escharotics, sclerosing agents, and ethmoidal or carotid artery ligations had all been advocated. Some of these modalities we had tried; the unpredictable and usually unsatisfactory results of others we had observed or seen recorded.

In 1942 Figi and Watkins [4] reported on treatment of the 20 patients with hereditary hemorrhagic telangiectasia seen at the Mayo Clinic during the previous 20 years. Epistaxis was the chief complaint in all these cases. Figi and Watkins considered electrocoagulation the most effective local means of controlling the nasal hemorrhage associated with hereditary hemorrhagic telangiectasia. They described their experience with this modality as follows:

In our practice, electrocoagulation has given better results than any other form of therapy. This has usually been carried out following cocainization of the nasal fossae but in a few instances general anesthesia has been necessary because of the patient's inability to tolerate the discomfort associated with it. For this purpose, pentothal sodium has been administered

Gordon Letterman
Maxine Schurter

THE SURGICAL MANAGEMENT OF HEREDITARY HEMORRHAGIC TELANGIECTASIA IN PERSPECTIVE

intravenously. The coagulation requires extreme patience, persistence and gentleness. Before using it, the bleeding should be controlled with liberal applications of epinephrine and a 10 percent solution of cocaine, and the site of the points of hemorrhage must be carefully noted. In the face of active bleeding, the current is likely to be dissipated so rapidly that coagulation progresses very slowly and when it does take place excessive adherent crusting forms. As the electrode is then moved, the bleeding point is reopened. Often this will occur repeatedly and only persistent, thorough electrocoagulation will control it. Frequently, too, after one has checked the bleeding at one point it will become active at another point well removed until one is tempted to insert a pack rather than spend more time. However, this usually is not a wise policy for even Vaseline gauze is likely to adhere sufficiently so that further hemorrhage will develop upon its withdrawal.

Figi and Watkins [4] described Houser's experience as follows:

Houser noted that in one of his cases, regardless of how thoroughly the nevi were destroyed, new ones promptly formed in the adjacent mucosa and these showed just as much tendency to bleed as did the original lesions. This was observed in several of our cases and was a most discouraging feature, for at times the patients' economic situations did not permit their remaining under prolonged observation or returning later for treatment. At times, too, because of this the patients became convinced that the situation was hopeless and stopped the treatment.

Our early experience with coagulation as a means of treating heredity hemorrhagic telangiectasia had been similar to that of Houser.

At the October 1959 meeting of the American Academy of Ophthalmology and Otolaryngology, Saunders [15] presented a paper and motion picture describing "septal dermoplasty" for the control of nasal hemorrhage associated with hereditary hemorrhagic telangiectasia. The technique [14] was subsequently summarized as follows:

Briefly, . . . a split-thickness skin graft is removed from the thigh or buttock under local anesthesia. After excision of septal mucosa, the graft is fixed to the anterior third of both sides of the nasal septum. The graft extends from dorsum to floor of the nose, and comes far enough anteriorly to be sutured to vestibular skin. Posteriorly it extends about one-third of the length of the septum.

The removal of nasal mucosa dotted with telangiectases and its replacement with a split-thickness skin graft seemed to us a logical way to control and prevent the severe nasal bleeding associated with hereditary hemorrhagic telangiectasia [8, 9]. We [10] tried the procedure, but with experience it seemed equally logical that complete elimination of the episodes of severe nasal hemorrhage required removal of all nasal mucosal surfaces bearing telangiectatic lesions. Obviously, to accomplish this it was necessary to extend the "septal dermoplasty" (Figs. 15-1 through 15-4).

In our experience, the telangiectatic lesions which were the source of nasal hemorrhage in this disease had not been confined to a limited

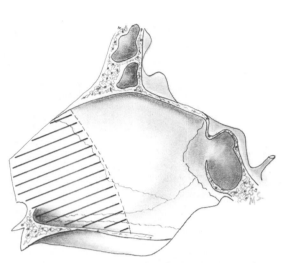

FIGURE 15-1. *Sagittal view of the nasal septum. The diagonally lined area shows mucosa to be removed according to our early concepts. (Reprinted, with permission, from G. Letterman and M. Schurter, The split-thickness skin graft in the management of hereditary hemorrhagic telangiectasia involving the nasal mucosa.* Plast. Reconstr. Surg. *34:126–135, 1964.)*

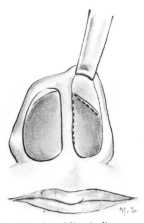

FIGURE 15-2. *The dotted line indicates excision not only of septal mucosa, but also of the mucosa on the under surface of the lateral cartilage. (Reprinted, with permission, from G. Letterman and M. Schurter, The split-thickness skin graft in the management of hereditary hemorrhagic telangiectasia involving the nasal mucosa.* Plast. Reconstr. Surg. *34:126–135, 1964.)*

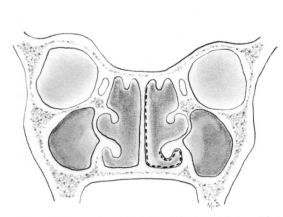

FIGURE 15-3. *Coronal section of the internal nose. The dotted line represents mucosa to be excised from the septum, floor of the nose, and inferior turbinate. (Reprinted, with permission, from G. Letterman and M. Schurter, The split-thickness skin graft in the management of hereditary hemorrhagic telangiectasia involving the nasal mucosa.* Plast. Reconstr. Surg. *34:126–135, 1964.)*

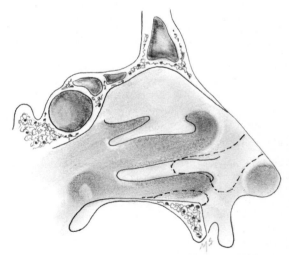

FIGURE 15-4. *Internal view of the lateral wall of the nasal cavity. The dotted lines indicate the mucosa to be excised from the inferior turbinate and the floor of the nose. (Reprinted, with permission, from G. Letterman and M. Schurter, The split-thickness skin graft in the management of hereditary hemorrhagic telangiectasia involving the nasal mucosa.* Plast. Reconstr. Surg. *34:126–135, 1964.)*

area of the septum. Telangiectases were widely and indiscriminately distributed within the mucosa not only of the septum, but also within the mucosal coverings of the nasal cartilages, floor of the nose, lateral nasal walls, and over the turbinates.

Furthermore, we learned early that skin grafts on the septum as used by Saunders [16, 17] had a definite tendency to contract, pulling mucosa over from the lateral cartilages and up from the floor of the nose onto the septum. Thus, once again, involved mucosa was brought into a position that subjected it to drying and crusting.

In our experience, bleeding from telangiectatic lesions of the inferior turbinates and floor of the nose was common. Indeed, the mucosa in these areas, as well as the septum, is subjected to great eddies of air currents. This results inevitably in drying and crusting of the membrane. Such trauma is the forerunner of nasal bleeding in the patient afflicted with hereditary hemorrhagic telangiectasia.

Our experience over the next several years led to ever more extensive removal of the involved nasal mucosa. This was accomplished by a series of modifications of the original operative procedure. Ideally all diseased and irreversibly damaged tissue should be resected and replaced by vital cells. We attributed our past poor results in treating hereditary epistaxis to our failure to apply this surgical principle.

A small but significant group of patients with hereditary telangiectasia were operated on to control nasal hemorrhages between 1961 and 1966. In each case, diseased nasal tissue was resected and the denuded surface replaced by split skin grafts. The operative procedures varied; they became more radical. Each patient's operative procedures are presented in some detail to provide a better basis for evaluating the operations and for predicting the course of the disease following operation. It is our hope that the mistakes, failures, and successes of the past will point the way to more successful therapeutic management of hereditary epistaxis in the future.

In May 1961 the authors [10] of this chapter presented a paper on hereditary hemorrhagic telangiectasia at a New York meeting of the American Association of Plastic Surgeons. In 1962 Hueston and Willis [7] reported on their experience in treating hereditary epistaxis. In 1964 Crawford, Adamson, and Horton [3] described a patient seen postoperatively who lost his nose following resection of the nasal septal mucosa for the control of hereditary epistaxis. This unfortunate result they attributed not necessarily to the surgical procedure, but in large part to the repeated cauterizations and x-ray and radium therapy of the part.

Case Reports

CASE 1

H.M. was born April 20, 1894 and died at the Veterans Administration Hospital in Martinsburg, West Virginia on May 4, 1969 at the age of 75 years. The cause of death was arteriosclerotic heart disease. His complete record was not available. In 1960 the patient was admitted to this veterans' hospital because of recurrent severe nasal hemorrhages. The nasal mucosa was spotted with telangiectases typical of Osler's disease. At that time, a large area of the involved septal mucosa was resected on the left side of the nose. It was replaced with a split skin graft which took well. It was our first experience with this operative approach in the management of hereditary hemorrhagic telangiectasia.

In 1965, on a follow-up visit, it was noted that the patient had had only slight oozing from his nose since the operation. However, on July 13, 1967, H.M. entered the hospital with profuse bleeding, again from the left nostril. The skin graft was intact, but telangiectases were prominent in the mucosa covering the lower alar cartilage. Adhesions joined the right inferior turbinate with the septum. Bleeding was controlled with packing. Not quite 2 years later the patient died of arteriosclerotic heart disease. The severe bleeding so characteristic of hereditary telangiectasia had been controlled for almost 10 years, with the exception of the recurrent episode in 1967.

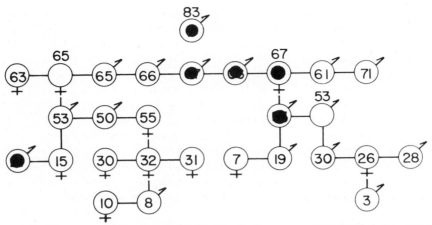

FIGURE 15-5. *Family history of case 2. Numbers indicate age at the time the patient was first seen, and the black spots indicate members with hereditary hemorrhagic telangiectasia. (Reprinted, with permission, from G. Letterman and M. Schurter, The split-thickness skin graft in the management of hereditary hemorrhagic telangiectasia involving the nasal mucosa. Plast. Reconstr. Surg. 34:126–135, 1964.)*

CASE 2

F.H. had a characteristic family history of hereditary hemorrhagic telangiectasia with its epistaxis and telangiectases (Fig. 15-5). He had himself first noted telangiectases of his facial skin at the age of 23 years. When he was 40 years old, episodes of epistaxis began, but they occurred only occasionally. By the age of 42 his nasal bleeding had become frequent and profuse. Nitric acid applications, electrocoagulation, transfusions, vitamin K, and a submucous septal section were all used in efforts to control the hemorrhages. During this period, telangiectases of the hands and feet appeared.

F.H.'s nosebleeds became ever more frequent and severe [11]. At the age of 54 years he was admitted to the George Washington University Hospital. On January 9, 1961, the septal mucosa on the left side of this patient's nose was resected, and the denuded surface was covered with a split-thickness skin graft. Exposure was obtained by a through-and-through incision which followed the left alar crease. Intraoperative bleeding was profuse (Fig. 15-6A through F). The graft took and healed promptly (Fig. 15-7). The patient was discharged. Two months later he had two episodes of hemorrhage in the left knee joint.

For nearly 2 years' time F.H. had no further episodes of epistaxis. Then, to our great disappointment, he bled profusely from the same left side of his nose. There was a conglomerate patch of telangiectases on the left side of the septum above the skin graft. The graft had contracted and pulled mucosa from the under surface of the left nasal bone and lateral cartilage onto the septum. At the age of 56 he was readmitted to the hospital. On December 5, 1962, the original left alar crease incision was reopened, and the mucosa overlying the dorsal and posterior septum was removed. A split-thickness skin graft was applied, and healing was uneventful.

The patient was free of nasal bleeding for only about 2 months. For the next 5 months F.H. had frequent hemorrhages from the left

FIGURE 15-6. *(A) Epistaxis noted while the patient was on the operating room table, before starting the surgery. (B) Alar crease incision marked with methylene blue. (C) Ala elevated for intranasal exposure. (D) Septum and floor of the nose after removal of the mucosa. (E) Split-thickness skin graft over the septum. Sutures have been placed through the mobile septum, and packing has been inserted. (F) Surgery completed and skin incision reapproximated. (Reprinted, with permission, from G. Letterman and M. Schurter, The split-thickness skin graft in the management of hereditary hemorrhagic telangiectasia involving the nasal mucosa. Plast. Reconstr. Surg. 34:126–135, 1964.)*

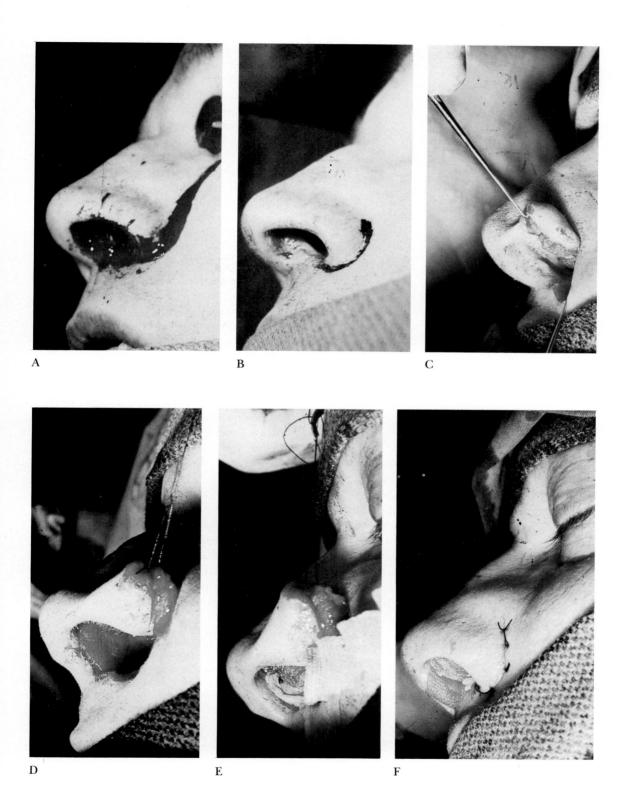

A

B

C

D

E

F

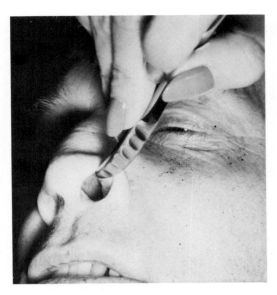

FIGURE 15-7. *Same patient (case 2) 2 months after surgery with a grafted septum in view. (Reprinted, with permission, from G. Letterman and M. Schurter, The split-thickness skin graft in the management of hereditary hemorrhagic telangiectasia involving the nasal mucosa. Plast. Reconstr. Surg. 34:126–135, 1964.)*

nasal cavity, and these required two hospitalizations for observation, nasal packing, and transfusion.

At the age of 57 he was again admitted to the hospital. On January 20, 1965, a left lateral rhinotomy was performed, and all accessible mucosa was stripped from the septum and turbinates (Fig. 15-8A through G). The raw areas were covered with split-thickness skin grafts. The anterior two-thirds of the left nasal cavity had now been completely replaced with skin grafts.

The patient continued to have frequent and severe episodes of epistaxis from the left side and was readmitted within 2 months of the previous surgical procedure. The left external carotid artery was ligated.

For the next 5 years he had only occasional bleeding from the left side of the nose, but progressively more severe and frequent hemorrhage from the right side. At the age of 62 he

was admitted to the hospital for replacement of the mucosa of the right nasal cavity.

On January 24, 1969, a right lateral rhinotomy incision gave access to the septum, turbinates, and undersurfaces of the right nasal bone and lateral cartilage. All mucosa was excised and replaced with a split-thickness skin graft (Fig. 15-9A through F).

Although there was complete healing of the skin graft, the patient continued to bleed from the right nasal cavity. This became progressively more severe. Within 2 months of the previous surgical procedure the patient was readmitted to the hospital with a hemoglobin of 7.8. Multiple blood transfusions were administered, but he continued to hemorrhage. After 12 days of unsuccessful conservative treatment, the right external carotid artery was ligated under local anesthesia. Three days later he was found on the floor with slurred speech, left hemiplegia, and an abrasion of the left forehead. Treatment was supportive. Two days later he had a cardiac arrest but was resuscitated successfully. Another 2 days later a tracheostomy and feeding pharyngotomy were performed under local anesthesia. He continued to bleed profusely from the right side of the nose, became comatose and died at the age of 62.

The autopsy examination revealed atherosclerosis of the coronary arteries and a recent infarct of the right frontoparietal region of the brain in the area of distribution of the right middle cerebral artery. The pathologist postulated that there had been an episode of hypotension from hemorrhage. The hypotensive state, together with atherosclerotic nar-

FIGURE 15-8. *(A) Incision marked with methylene blue for a left lateral rhinotomy. (B) The frontal process of the left maxilla has been exposed. (C) Frontal process of the left maxilla being cut with a Joseph nasal saw. (D) The nasal bones have been separated, and the left side of the nose has been reflected medially. The septum and lateral nasal wall are well visualized. (E) The mucosa has been removed, and a split-thickness skin graft is sutured in place. (F) Nasal packing helps to apply pressure to the grafted areas. (G) Left lateral rhinotomy incision reapproximated with fine silk sutures.*

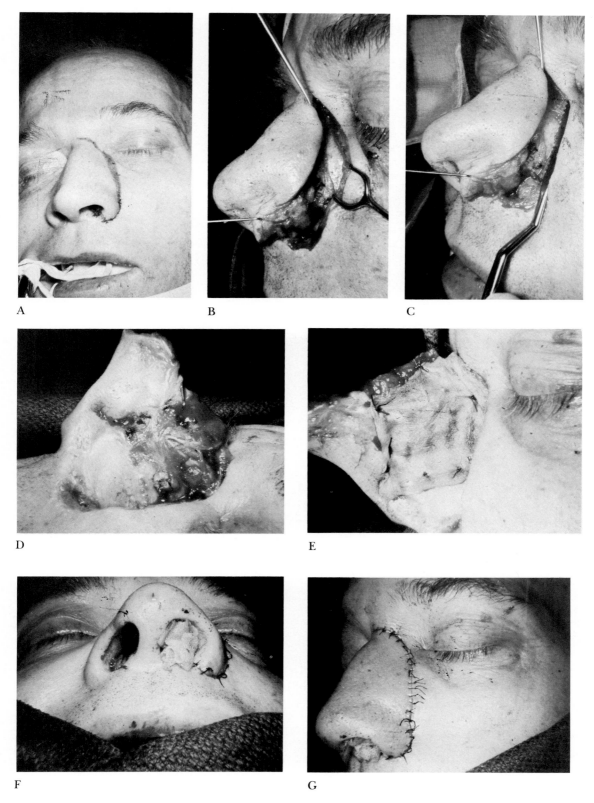

A

B

C

D

E

F

G

269

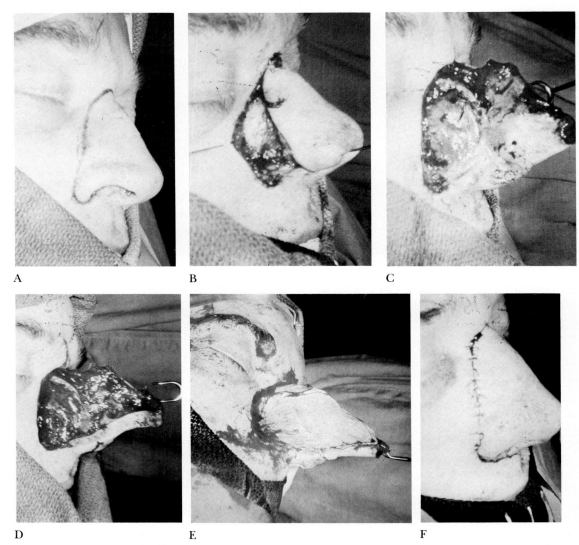

A   B   C

D   E   F

FIGURE 15-9. *(A) Right lateral rhinotomy incision marked with methylene blue. (B) Right nasal bone exposed and ala elevated. (C) The frontal process of the right maxilla has been cut with a Joseph saw and the nasal bones separated. The nose has been reflected medially. (D) The mucosa has been excised from the septum, floor of the nose, inferior turbinate, and under surface of the lateral cartilage and nasal bone. (E) Split-thickness skin graft in place over the denuded area. (F) Original rhinotomy incision reapproximated.*

rowing of the right middle cerebral artery and internal carotid, could well have led to cerebral necrosis. Additionally, three duodenal ulcers were found. There were many telangiectatic areas of the skin and mucosa of the mouth, colon, and subcapsular area of the liver. Many calcific plaques existed in the abdominal aorta.

CASE 3

J.S. was unaware of any bleeding problems in other members of her family. When she was 33 years old, this patient was found to be anemic, but the etiology was not determined. Her blood loss was marked at the time of delivery of twins at the age of 37.

After the age of 46, J.S. had many hospitalizations for epistaxis, and when 48 years old, she suffered with cholecystitis, and diagnosis of cholelithiasis was made on the basis of roentgenography. The episodes of nasal bleeding continued. At the age of 54 a diagnosis of psychoneurosis was made. This presumably was based on her frequent, recurrent hospital admissions.

At the age of 56 it was necessary to extract her teeth. At that time she was found to have hypochromic anemia. J.S. also continued to have epistaxis; the bleeding was most severe and most frequent from the left nostril.

Because of weakness, she was hospitalized at the age of 59 and found to have anemia (type and source not determined). Bone marrow examination showed erythrocytic hyperplasia. A GI series was negative. The ECG showed coronary artery insufficiency.

J.S. continued to have epistaxis; the nose bleeds were devastating. On one hospital admission at the age of 60 her hemoglobin was 8.5 gram-percent. The patient was again hospitalized at the age of 62 for shortness of breath. At that time the ECG showed ventricular extrasystoles, myocardial damage, coronary insufficiency, and posterior myocardial ischemia.

When 63 years old J.S. was admitted to the George Washington University Hospital with the chief complaint of dysphagia. She was unaware of any rectal bleeding, but occult blood was found on stool examination. Her hemoglobin was 5.0 gram-percent. She continued to have moderately severe epistaxis and received multiple transfusions of whole blood. Her liver could be palpated two finger breadths below the right costal margin. Telangiectases were noted on the tongue, lower lip, ears, finger, and beneath the nail beds. Hematological consultation revealed a chronic iron deficiency anemia; it was attributed to epistaxis. Finally, after 30 years of nasal hemorrhage, the diagnosis of hereditary hemorrhagic telangiectasia was made. The patient was referred to the plastic surgery service for surgical removal of the telangiectases of the internal nose.

At last, at the age of 63 the patient was treated definitively. On May 31, 1962 the mucosa on both sides of the septum was resected, and the septum was resurfaced with split-thickness skin grafts. Exposure was obtained by bilateral alar incisions. The visible septal mucosa was removed (Fig. 15-10A through C).

Healing of the grafts was complete (Fig. 15-10D). The patient had no further nasal bleeding for 12 years, when she died suddenly at the age of 74. An autopsy examination was performed, and the findings were as follows: massive small bowel bleeding (estimated more than 3 liters in the lumen), irreversible shock (clinical), and bilateral pulmonary edema. Heart disease was not found, and the central nervous system was not examined.

CASE 4

J.H.S.'s father and two sisters had telangiectasia. He began having occasional nosebleeds at the age of 26. They became more and more frequent over the next 15 years and required periodic hospitalizations. Rectal bleeding was also present. He had chronic hypochromic microcytic anemia. At the age of 46, telangiectases of the septum and inferior turbinates were noted. He also had telangiectases of the upper thorax, face, and neck.

The patient was admitted to the hospital and operated upon on April 23, 1963. Under local anesthesia the mucosa was removed from both sides of the nasal septum through alar incisions (Fig. 15-11A through C). The septum was resurfaced with split-thickness skin grafts.

There was no further epistaxis for 2 years, when he had one episode which was considered minimal. However, he had been jaundiced during that interim. His liver was palpable two finger breadths below the right costal margin, and the spleen was palpable two finger breadths below the left costal margin.

For the next 8 years he was hospitalized many times for gastrointestinal bleeding of an undetermined origin. A GI series was normal, and esophagoscopy revealed no varices. At the age of 52 he was found to have diabetes mellitus.

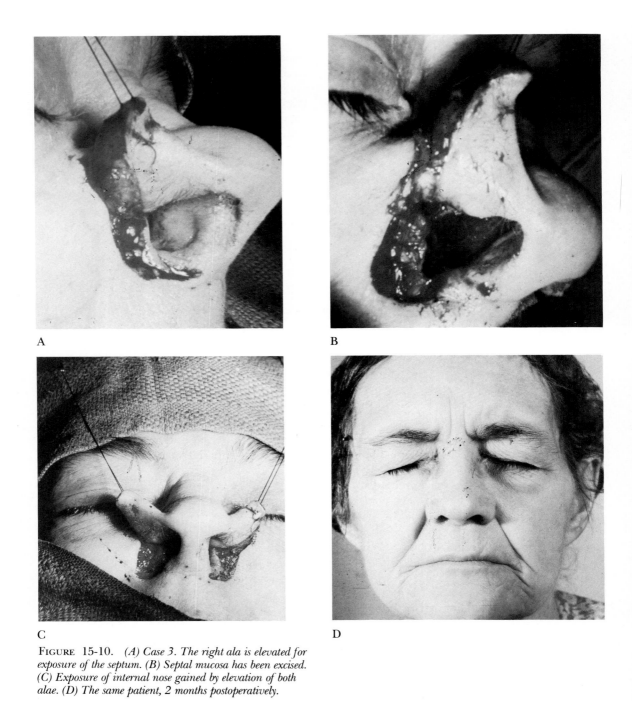

A

B

C

D

FIGURE 15-10. (A) Case 3. The right ala is elevated for exposure of the septum. (B) Septal mucosa has been excised. (C) Exposure of internal nose gained by elevation of both alae. (D) The same patient, 2 months postoperatively.

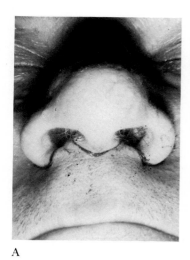
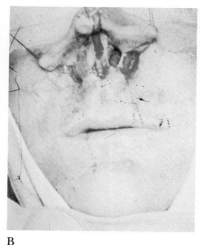
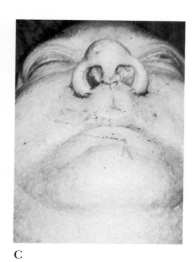

A   B   C

FIGURE 15-11.   *(A) Case 4. Bilateral alar crease and columellar base incision outlined with methylene blue. (B) Alae and columella elevated. (C) Original incisions reapproximated after grafting.*

On his final hospital admission (February 20, 1973) he had some minimal nasal bleeding and the usual gastrointestinal bleeding. During a transfusion he became short of breath and expired. An autopsy examination was not conducted. For almost 10 years after the intranasal skin grafting he had remained free of serious nasal hemorrhage.

CASE 5

J.C.T.'s mother and brother's son had epistaxis and visible telangiectases. The patient himself had epistaxis at the age of 15 and was found to have a perforated nasal septum shortly thereafter. He had several episodes of nasal bleeding from the age of 15 to 25, at which time bleeding became progressively more severe and frequent. At the age of 44 he was hospitalized for transfusions following severe episodes of epistaxis. He exhibited telangiectases of the conjunctiva, nasal cavity, tongue, and beneath the fingernails. Bleeding had always been from the left side of the nose. He was admitted to the Veterans Administration Hospital in Mar-

tinsburg, West Virginia for definitive surgery of the internal nose at the age of 46.

On February 9, 1965, under local anesthesia, an incision was made on the left side of the nose from the level of the glabella laterally down to and through the alar crease after separating the nasal bones. The frontal process of the maxilla was cut, and the entire left side of the nose was reflected medially. The mucosa was resected from the left side of the septum, the left inferior turbinate, the under surface of the left nasal bone, and the lateral cartilage. The raw surfaces were resurfaced with a split-thickness skin graft taken from the thigh (Fig. 15-12A through E). The microscopic findings of the mucous membrane showed papillomas and telangiectasia.

Healing was uneventful, and the patient had no further epistaxis until the age of 49, when he was again admitted to the hospital with moderate epistaxis, severe microcytic anemia, sore throat, and cough. He was found to have an anaplastic bronchogenic carcinoma. He underwent a left pneumonectomy on March 29, 1968, at which time it was found that the carcinoma involved the left lung and hilum. A tracheostomy was also performed. After surgery the patient pulled out the fresh tracheotomy tube, suffered a cardiopulmonary arrest, and died.

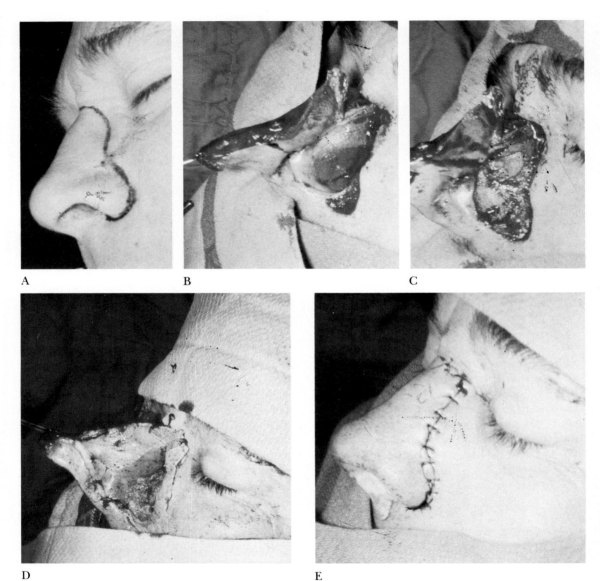

FIGURE 15-12. (A) Case 5. Left lateral rhinotomy incision marked with methylene blue. (B) Elevation of the left side of the nose after cutting the frontal process of the maxilla and separating the nasal bones. (C) The mucosa has been removed from the septum and lateral wall of the nasal cavity. (D) A split-thickness skin graft is sutured in place. (E) Lateral rhinotomy incision closed with interrupted sutures.

An autopsy examination was performed; the cause of death was congestive heart failure due to pericarditis from metastases of anaplastic carcinoma of the left lung. There was also bronchopneumonia of the upper lobe of the right lung. Besides the previously described telangiectases, there was also a small hemangioma of the liver.

CASE 6

C.F.R., Sr. was unaware of any bleeding problems in other members of his family. He had occasional epistaxis and gastrointestinal bleeding until the age of 50, when these episodes became increasingly more frequent and severe. He was hospitalized on multiple occasions for transfusions. There were many visible telangiectases of the nasal cavity, tongue, palate, and oropharynx.

At the age of 70 he was admitted to the Veterans Administration Hospital in Martinsburg, West Virginia with severe epistaxis. His hematocrit was 28 percent. He continued to bleed, and it was necessary to give 9 units of packed cells to maintain a hematocrit of 31 percent. It was decided to proceed with skin grafting of the nose. Under local anesthesia the right nasal cavity was opened with a lateral rhinotomy from the glabella down through the alar crease (Fig. 15-13). The frontal process of the maxilla was cut and the nasal bones separated. The mucosa was excised as far back as possible from the right side of the septum, turbinates, inferior surfaces of the right nasal bone, and lateral cartilage. Bleeding was profuse during this procedure, and it was necessary to interrupt the operation and pack the nose while pumping packed cells intravenously. When his condition stabilized, the raw surfaces were covered with a split-thickness skin graft taken from the thigh.

Healing was uneventful, but postoperatively the patient had several episodes of bleeding from the other side of the nose and also from the gastrointestinal tract. When bleeding stopped, he was discharged from the hospital.

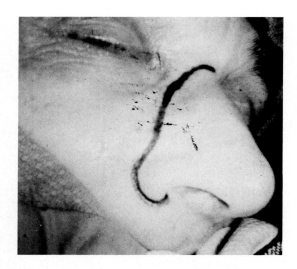

FIGURE 15-13. *Case 6. Right lateral rhinotomy incision marked with methylene blue.*

Four months later, still at the age of 70, the patient was readmitted for resurfacing of the left side of the nasal cavity, which was performed in the same manner as that of the right. Healing was again uneventful, and he was discharged from the hospital.

One month later he returned with severe gastrointestinal bleeding, although there had been no further epistaxis. It was decided that the bleeding was from the gastric mucosa. A hemigastrectomy and vagotomy were performed, carrying out a Billroth I procedure with end-to-end anastomosis.

During the next 8 years there was no further epistaxis, but there were at least 10 hospital admissions for gastrointestinal bleeding. At the age of 78 he was admitted to the hospital with a hemoglobin of 4 gram-percent. He was transfused frequently, but continued to bleed and died 2 months later of exsanguination.

An autopsy examination was performed, and the cause of death was determined to be hemorrhage from hemorrhagic ulceration and atrophy of the gastric mucosa. There was also extensive lobular pneumonia of the upper lobe of the right lung and both lower lobes. *Diplococcus pneumoniae* was cultured. There was also evidence of severe hemorrhagic cystitis. The heart was hypertrophied and showed moderate sclerosis of the coronary arteries. Telangiectases were found on the hard palate, tongue, oropharynx, cardia, small intestines, and left adrenal gland.

Discussion

HEREDITY

Hereditary hemorrhagic telangiectasia is commonly referred to as Osler's or Rendu-Osler-Weber disease. In 1865, Babington [1] reported on a hereditary form of nasal bleeding occurring in five generations of a family. In 1896, Rendu [13] differentiated hereditary epistaxis from hemophilia. In 1901, Osler [11] published his classical account of the disease in a paper entitled "On a Family Form of Recurring Epistaxis Associated with Multiple Telangiectases of the Skin and Mucous Membranes." In 1907, Weber [18] described a family affected with hereditary nasal bleeding.

In 1907, after a thorough study of Osler's disease, Hanes [6] concluded his treatise on the subject with the following paragraph:

The disease is a definite clinical entity, and as such deserves a specific name. I suggest that the affection be called "hereditary hemorrhagic telangiectasia," the name which I believe not only adequately describes the condition, but conforms to the strictest rules of medical nomenclature.

The diagnosis of hereditary hemorrhagic telangiectasia should rarely be made without a family history of nasal bleeding. It was not possible to obtain such a history in all the cases included in this series. Several of the patients were older and unfamiliar with the illnesses of their deceased relatives. Others had lost track of their siblings, uncles, aunts, or cousins. However, when a reliable family history could be obtained and verified, it was always quite typical of hereditary hemorrhagic telangiectasia (Fig. 15-5). Hereditary hemorrhagic telangiectasia is a dominant trait. Atavism is believed to account

for a lack of a characteristic family history of the disease in some patients.

HEMORRHAGE

Hemorrhage is considered the sine qua non of hereditary hemorrhagic telangiectasia. Physiological hemostasis is initiated by an organism's vascular response. Vascular constriction, retraction, and collapse, together with the agglutination of a vessel's lining, contribute to the clotting mechanism. The nasal bleeding which is so diagnostic of hereditary hemorrhagic telangiectasia can be attributed to an inherent vascular defect. Functionally, vascular contraction and retraction of the vessels are minimal in patients afflicted with this disease. The rigidity of the intranasal structures further limits retraction and constriction and prevents collapse of blood vessels. Minimal trauma produced by drying and crusting makes the involved nasal mucosa a prime area for hemorrhage in patients with this disease.

Epistaxis is the prominent initial complaint in hereditary hemorrhagic telangiectasia. All the patients in this follow-up study had severe and frequent epistaxis prior to operation. With the exception of case 2, all the patients were relatively free of nasal bleeding for the remaining years of their lives. Interestingly, the patient discussed in case 6 died of exsanguination from gastrointestinal bleeding attributed to telangiectases, but for the 8 years prior to death, he had no significant nasal bleeding. In our experience no form of therapy has proven so successful in managing hereditary nasal bleeding as resection of diseased tissue and resurfacing with split-thickness skin grafts.

TELANGIECTASES

The essential and characteristic lesion in telangiectases [12] is an arteriovenous fistula. Sharp-

FIGURE 15-14. *Typical skin and mucosal lesions seen in hereditary hemorrhagic telangiectasia. (A) Lower lip, case 2. (B) Tongue, case 3. (C) Chin, case 4. (D) Palate, case 6. (E) Ear, case 6. (F) Finger, case 6.*

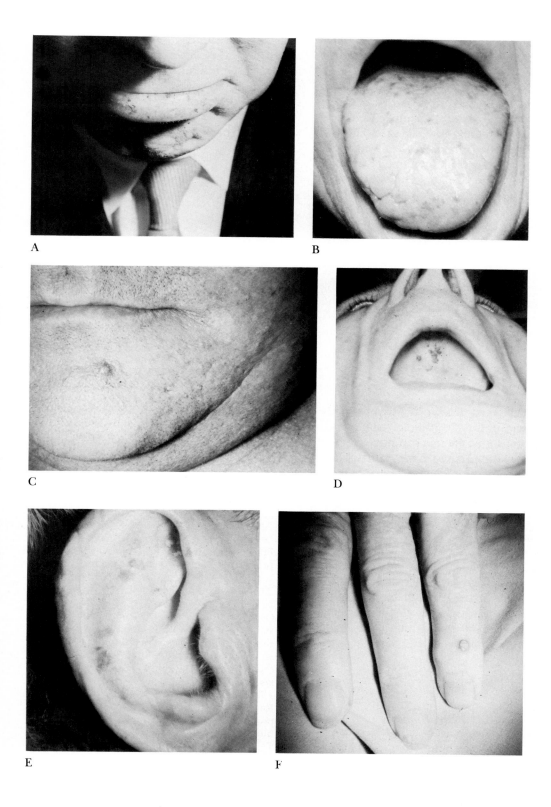

ly demarcated vascular spots are generally smooth or slightly depressed. The central area of the lesion is larger than that usually seen in cutaneous spiders, and the efferent vessels are more numerous. There is either a total lack or a pronounced deficiency of the connective tissue and muscular elements. Indeed, the wall of a lesser vessel may be composed of only a single layer of endothelial cells and a minimal amount of connective tissue. Telangiectases are seen most frequently in the mucous membranes and skin. Kesselbach's area and the hands are often the site of vascular spots, but the lesions have been seen in almost every organ of the body. Even pulmonary arteriovenous aneurysms have been considered but another variant of Osler's disease. All the patients operated on by us had telangiectatic lesions scattered over the skin and mucous membranes (Fig. 15-14A through F). At autopsy such lesions were found in many organs.

CLINICAL COURSE

In all these patients, diagnosis was not made until quite late in life. So often a diagnosis of chronic hypochromic anemia of undetermined etiology was made. Many of the patients had guaiac-positive stools long before actual hemorrhage. This was probably due either to blood swallowed from small nose bleeds or slight bleeding from the gastrointestinal mucosa. These patients were very long in finding someone who could make the correct diagnosis.

Many of these patients also had associated arteriosclerosis, which led either directly or indirectly to their death. It might be postulated that sclerosis of the vessels was the final insult to the already deficient vessel walls and made clotting an impossibility.

Final Thoughts

If nasal hemorrhage is to be controlled in patients with hereditary hemorrhagic telangiec-

tasia, exposure to the inside of the nose must be adequate, and resection of mucosa must be extensive. The operative resection of diseased nasal mucosa and resurfacing with split-thickness skin grafts have proven to be successful in the management of bleeding in hereditary hemorrhagic telangiectasia.

References

1. Babington, B.G. Hereditary epistaxis. *Lancet* 2:362, 1865.
2. Brown, J.B., and McDowell, F. *Plastic Surgery of the Nose.* St. Louis: Mosby, 1951. Pp. 299–300.
3. Crawford, H.H., Adamson, J.E., and Horton, C.E. Hereditary hemorrhagic telangiectasia. *Plast. Reconstr. Surg.* 34(2):136, 1964.
4. Figi, F.A., and Watkins, C.H. Hereditary hemorrhagic telangiectasia. *Ann. Otol. Rhinol. Laryngol.* 52(2):330, 1943.
5. Fitz-Hugh, T., Jr. The importance of atavism in the diagnosis of hereditary telangiectasia. *Am. J. Med. Sci.* 166:884, 1923.
6. Hanes, F.H. Multiple hereditary telangiectases causing hemorrhage (hereditary hemorrhagic telangiectasia). *Bull. Johns Hopkins Hosp.* 20:63, 1909.
7. Hueston, J.T., and Willis, R. Excision of nasal lining and split-skin graft replacement in Osler's disease. *Br. J. Plast. Surg.* 15:314, 1962.
8. Letterman, G.S., and Schurter, M. The split-thickness skin graft in the management of hereditary hemorrhagic telangiectasia involving the nasal mucosa. *Plast. Reconstr. Surg.* 34(2):126, 1964.
9. Letterman, G.S. Schurter, M., and Prandoni, A. Prophylactic anticoagulation in the cross-leg flap procedure. *Plast. Reconstr. Surg.* 27:520, 1961.
10. Letterman, G.S., Schurter, M., and Prandoni, A. The use of split-thickness skin grafts in patients receiving anticoagulants. *Am. Surg.* 27:762, 1961.
11. Osler, W. On a family form of recurring epistaxis, associated with multiple telangiectases of the skin and mucous membranes. *Bull. Johns Hopkins Hosp.* 12(128):333, 1901.
12. Osler, W. On multiple hereditary telangiectases with recurring haemorrhages. *Q. J. Med.* 1:53, 1907–1908.
13. Rendu, M. Epistaxis répétées chez un sujet porteur des petits angiomes cutanês et muqueux. *Bull. Mém. Soc. Méd. Hôp.* (Paris) 13:731, 1896.

14. Saunders, W.H.   Permanent control of nose-bleeds in patients with hereditary telangiectasia. *Ann. Intern. Med.* 53(1):147, 1960.

15. Saunders, W.H.   Septal dermoplasty for control of nosebleeds caused by hereditary hemorrhagic telangiectasia or septal perforations. *Trans. Am. Acad. Ophthalmol. Otolaryngol.* 64:500, 1960.

16. Saunders, W.H.   Hereditary hemorrhagic telangiectasia: Control of nosebleeds by septal dermoplasty. *J.A.M.A.* 174(15):1972, 1960.

17. Saunders, W.H.   Hereditary hemorrhagic telangiectasia. *Arch. Otolaryngol.* 76:245, 1962.

18. Weber, F.P.   Multiple hereditary development angiomata (telangiectases) of the skin and mucous membranes associated with recurring haemorrhages. *Lancet* 2:160, 1907.

Robert M. Goldwyn

COMMENTS ON CHAPTER 15

HEREDITARY hemorrhagic telangiectasia may be "fascinating" to the medical student or resident, but for the patient, it may be lethal. Of the six cases chronicled by Drs. Letterman and Schurter, at least two, and possibly three, died of their disease, with preterminal bleeding from the nasal cavity and/or the gastrointestinal tract. The nature of this affliction is such that while it may be controlled in the nose, it usually cannot be controlled in the gut.

Patients with hereditary hemorrhagic telangiectasia must live in fear of exsanguination, at worst, or annoying, recurrent bleeding, at least. Their additional concern is the transmission of this malady to their offspring. In their excellent discussion, Drs. Letterman and Schurter note that the basic lesion is an arteriovenous fistula. Because these anomalies are minute, multiple, and widespread, they are difficult, if not impossible, to identify. These vascular spots lack connective tissue and muscle and will neither contract nor clot normally. They may be susceptible to arteriosclerotic plaque formation, as also noted by the authors.

Another disquieting aspect of hereditary hemorrhagic telangiectasia is that diagnosis is often delayed or never made. Its possibility should be considered in every patient with epistaxis or gastrointestinal bleeding. A carefully taken family history may easily establish its presence.

Recent reports on the use of cryotherapy— liquid nitrogen [1] or estrogens [2]—for this disease have been encouraging, although long-term follow-up, such as we have here, is not yet available.

Incidentally, the reader would enjoy the original paper describing the disease, as cited by Drs. Letterman and Schurter. In addition to the writings of Babington, Rendu, Osler, and Weber is the article by Sutton [3], who in 1864, a year before Babington, noted a familial syndrome of epistaxis and gastrointestinal bleeding (no mention of telangiectasia). Moreover, with Sir William Gull in 1872, he first clearly described arteriosclerotic atrophy of the kidney ("arteriocapillary fibrosis").

References

1. Cahan, W.G. Five Years of Cryosurgical Experience: Benign and Malignant Tumors with Hemorrhagic Conditions. In R.W. Rand, A.P. Rinfret, and H. von Leden (Eds.), *Cryosurgery.* Springfield, Ill.: Thomas, 1968. Pp. 404–505.
2. McCaffrey, T.V., Kern, E.B., and Lake, C.F. Management of epistaxis in hereditary hemorrhagic telangiectasia: Review of 80 cases. *Arch. Otolaryngol.* 103:627, 1977.
3. Sutton, H.G. Epistaxis as an indication of impaired nutrition and of degeneration of the vascular system. *Med. Mirror* 1:769, 1864.

16 General Considerations

The evaluation time necessary for any survey to be regarded as final depends on the pathology. In congenital malformations, as, for example, in cleft lips and cleft palates, a long-term evaluation can be made when growth is completed.

However, in genitourinary malformations, the final assessment should be postponed until much later. The end result must not only be considered in terms of the morphology of the reconstructed urethra, the location of the meatus, and the aesthetic appearance of the genitals, but also in terms of the sexual function, which depends on the curvature of the penis and the capability for erection. Moreover, the psychosexual condition of the patient with relation to his partner must be considered as well. In addition, the reconstructed urethra must have the same growth potential as the penile tissues in order to adapt to the increasing urinary-flow requirements, or it may have late repercussions on the proximal urinary tract that may not be detectable until much later.

Nevertheless, we do not know of any technique in which all these requirements for final evaluation are included. This is due mainly to the time limitations imposed on both the surgeon and the patient by life circumstances. It applies also to the present evaluation, primarily because the techniques evaluated were first utilized in 1965, with a limited follow-up of a maximum of 11 years for the main technique of penis tunnelization. Nevertheless, we believe that the objectivity of our survey may contribute some valuable data, although it is not a final report.

After a minimum of 2 years following the final surgery, it is possible to appreciate with a relatively small margin of error how the future evolution will be. In 1960, Backus and De Felice

Ulrich T. Hinderer
Francisco Rodríguez Durán
Matías Pradas Caravaca

HYPOSPADIAS REPAIR

[3] had already recorded over 150 techniques. The reason for such a variety is that many surgeons have changed the original techniques, thus creating "modified" methods to correct factory results. To this moment, the clear superiority of any technique has not been statistically demonstrated. Usually the results obtained with one method differ according to the surgeon's experience, being best in the hands of the originator.

Of our series with completed repair, 27.9 percent were patients in whom up to 22 previous attempts at repair made in other clinics had failed. This illustrates primarily the difficulty of hypospadias repair. In the literature reviewed we found most papers give the mistaken impression that the techniques described are easy to perform, thus inducing surgeons with less experience in this field to approach the problem with unrealistic optimism. It does not matter who performs hypospadias repair, whether urologists, plastic surgeons, or pediatric surgeons. However, it is indispensable that the surgeon possess a wide experience in plastic surgery technique and a basic knowledge of urology in order to be able to cope with possible complications.

Moreover, we believe that hypospadias should be treated in specialized genitourinary units that have a sufficient number of cases, a plastic surgeon in charge of the surgery itself, and a well-trained medical and nursing staff.

The overall goal in hypospadias surgery must be to use techniques that are safe and provide the best results with fewer operations and hospitalizations. This requires a comparison of the long-term results obtained by different genitourinary units based on the same classifications and objective criteria.

With this purpose in mind, we also report the preoperative condition and classification of hypospadias. The techniques used in our unit are briefly described and the results are analyzed. Judgment is made according to our criteria for evaluation of results, which we propose for general acceptance as a basis for future comparisons of different techniques.

Goals of Repair in Hypospadias Surgery

As goals of repair in hypospadias surgery we include with the attainment of normal sexual function and orthostatic micturition, the prevention of an abnormal personality, which requires that a normal appearance of the genitals be obtained and that the repair be performed prior to school age, since adverse comparison with other boys may interfere with the normal emotional development. The basic steps of repair are as follows:

1. Correction of defects of the urethral wall and the meatus (meatoplasty).
2. Correction of the penile curvature (orthoplasty).
3. Reconstruction of a wide, uniform, elastic, and hairless urethra with a normal growth potential up to the tip of the glans (urethroplasty).
4. Shifting of the dorsally redundant penile and preputial skin to the deficient ventral surface of the penis (skinplasty).
5. Correction of associated malformations (scrotum, testes, etc.).

Evaluation of Results

Comparison of results obtained with different techniques requires that the same objective cri-

TABLE 16-1. *Classification of the Results of Hypospadias Repair*

		Excellent	Good	Satisfactory	Unsatisfactory
Urinary function	Micturition	Normal	Moderately deviated stream	Deviated, fanlike, or slightly narrowed stream	Completely abnormal micturition, in sitting postion, narrowed
	Width and uniformity of urethra (urethrography)	Normal	Wide, only minor irregularities	Irregular	Strictures with retrograde dilatation
	Urinary flow	According to age	Within the normal spectrum	Reduced with regard to the age, but without proximal urinary tract complications	Reduced, with proximal urinary tract complications
	Intraurethral hair growth	No hair	No hair	Occasional hair tufts	Diffuse hair and calculi
Sexual function	Erection	Penis straight and erection of normal hardness	Slight curvature or torsion, not causing intercourse difficulties	Diminished strength of erection, intercourse difficult but possible; curvature less than 20 degrees	Impotent during intercourse
Aesthetic appearance	Meatus	At tip of glans	At glans	Close to the coronary sulcus	Below coronary sulcus
	Penoscrotal skin	Normal	Inconspicuous	Irregular, asymmetric, or with mobile scars	Immobile scars, abnormal
Psychosexual evaluation	Partner relationship	Normal	Satisfactory	Occasional difficulties	No relationship because of lack of self-confidence
	Self-confidence	Normal	Occasional emotional disturbances	Decreased	

teria be used. With this purpose in mind, a classification of the results in four groups, judged by morphological and functional assessment, including objective criteria such as urethrography and urinary-flow measurement, as well as some indication of the psychological effect, was published by Farkas, Hinderer, and Wilkie [17], in 1971. Since then, it has been further developed by Hinderer (Table 16-1). Only completed cases, a minimum of 2 years after repair, should be evaluated, and the evaluation should be repeated until adulthood. However, the number of operations and the total hospitalization time required also must be considered. Although of secondary importance compared with the results obtained by a specific technique, a minimal number of operations and hospitalizations are important from the physical, psychic, and economic points of view (Table 16-2).

TABLE 16-2. *Schema for Evaluation of Results*

Technique				Evaluation Period: _____ to _____ Years after Repair		
	Results					
Number of cases	Excellent	Good	Satisfactory	Unsatisfactory	Average operations per case	Average hospitalizations for all surgeries per case (in days)

Classification

In hypospadias, the morphological findings vary from the mildest to the most severe types with different involvement of the genital structures. In balanic hypospadias, the malformation seems to be due to an abnormal canalization of the invading ectoderm. In the prebalanic types also, the formation of the corpus spongiosum is arrested, thus resulting in a premeatal subepidermal cleft, in most cases present in varying extensions.

The missing mesenchymal ingrowth, distally from the end of the corpus spongiosum, and the abnormal disintegration of the urethral plate (missing or abnormal formation of the primary and secondary urethral grooves and fusion of the ectodermal integument) give rise to fibrous tissue, which causes the downward curvature. In some cases this resembles true chordee. Paraurethral ducts (and also the urethra duplex) are the result of anomalies of the resorption of the urethral plate. The formation of the penile and preputial skin is completed by the ingrowth of the mesenchyme from proximal to distal and from the dorsal aspect to the ventral surface, finally resulting in the medial fusion or raphe.

The base of the genital tubercle seems to suffer a cranial displacement when the corpora cavernosa develop and the genital swellings, which form the scrotum, fuse caudally. The caudally displaced penis (in perineal position) in two patients in our series seems to confirm this theory [58].

In hypospadias, the penile and preputial skin distribution is also affected. Distally to the end of the corpus spongiosum, the normal developing skin remains dorsally redundant, and the penile raphe divides in Y form or to either side. The prepuce does not join and may be adhered to the glans and contain cysts.

The frenulum is represented by two raphe-like sutures which run from the glans in a proximal and lateral direction. The abnormal skin distribution may cause by itself, even in the balanic type of hypospadias, chordee of the penis or glans when the skin is pulled proximally, thus later impairing intercourse. In more severe forms of hypospadias, the scrotum may be bifid, and the scrotal raphe may also deviate in Y form at the base of the penis. In other cases, the scrotum has lateropubic insertions at the root of the penis and adopts a vulviform aspect; even a peno-scrotal transposition may be present.

In some cases, despite a location of the meatus close to the tip of the glans, the deviation of the raphe shows evidence of a defect of the corpus spongiosum. At the level of the subepidermal cleft, fibrous tissue is present between urethra and corpora cavernosa, and the thinner urethral wall itself is retracted and short. The penis may show a torsion resulting from an asymmetrical skin distribution and mesenchyme ingrowth.

Hypoplasia of the penis was recorded in 108 patients (15.4 percent), and a clitoris-like penis was found in 6 patients (0.9 percent).

The migration of the testes may also be affected in hypospadias.

Extragenital malformations may also be associated with hypospadias. In our 703 patients, malformations of the extremities were found in 16 (2.3 percent), facial malformations in 15 (2.1 percent), hernia in 9 (1.3 percent), cutaneous malformations in 8 (1.1 percent), psychic retardation in 7 (1 percent), malformations of internal organs in 6 (0.9 percent), malformations of the upper urinary tract in 2 (0.3 percent), malformations of the spinal cord in 2 (0.3 percent), and anal malformations in 1 (0.1 percent). The combination of these multiple genital morphological findings with their functional repercussions make any detailed classification difficult.

Therefore, we have grouped our cases in this chapter according to the most commonly adopted classification in order to facilitate a possible comparison of results. With regard to diagnosis, we use the level of the meatus after orthoplasty (balanic, proximal balanic, and prebalanic coronal, penile, penoscrotal, scrotal, and perineal hypospadias). Subdivisions have been made according to the techniques used, also separating primary from secondary cases (Table 16-3).

TABLE 16-3. *Classification of Hypospadias*

Type	Technique	Primary Repair	Secondary Repair	
With more than 2 years of follow-up:				
Balanic hypospadias	Meatoplasty, skinplasty	34	3	
Proximal balanic hypospadias	Eventual meatoplasty, urethroplasty at glans, and skinplasty	10	3	
Prebalanic hypospadias	Initial technique	3	6	
	Hinderer's penis-tunnelization technique	214	79	
Short urethra	Distal displacement of urethra	6	2	
	Two-stage urethroplasty	—	1	
	Hinderer's "island flap urethroplasty"	1	—	
Congenital urethral fistulae	Fistulae closure	1	1	
Secondary repairs with remedial operations		—	9	
		269	104	
With less than 2 years of follow-up and uncompleted hypospadias of all types:		294	36	Total
		563	140	703

Balanic Hypospadias

THE PREOPERATIVE CONDITION

This type of hypospadias corresponding to the "intranavicular" type described by Ombrédanne [48] was seen in 37 patients. Chordee of the glans when pulling the penile skin in a proximal direction was recorded in 24 patients; 2 patients urinated in the sitting position. The prepuce was circular in 14 patients, phimotic in 4, dorsally redundant in 16, and missing, as a result of a previous circumcision, in 3. The meatus, in 13 patients located close to the tip of the glans and in 24 more proximal, was normal in 19, stenotic in 6, and showed a web or transverse bar distally to the meatus, causing deviation of the urinary stream, in 12. In 5 patients, the urethra was more superficially located at the glans, and a subepidermal cleft, proximal to the coronary sulcus, was recorded. The penis was normal in 35 and hypoplastic in 1 patient. In one patient, a torsion of the penis was present. The scrotum and testes were normal in all of them.

One patient had ectopic testes, and in one patient, one testicle was located at the inguinal canal. Three patients had paraurethral canals at the glans; and one patient, at the penis. Two patients exhibited retarded physical development, while all others had a normal body configuration.

TREATMENT

Treatment was performed according to the morphological findings: in 4 patients only a meatoplasty was performed, in 9 patients a meatoplasty and circumcision were needed, and in 24 patients, besides a meatoplasty, the dorsally redundant skin was shifted to the inferior surface in order to correct the cutaneous chordee produced when pulling the skin backward (see Fig. 16-1 and Table 16-4).

Proximal Balanic Hypospadias

THE PREOPERATIVE CONDITION

In this type of hypospadias, which was seen in 13 patients, the meatus was localized at the base of the glans close to the coronary sulcus. The meatus was normal in eight patients and

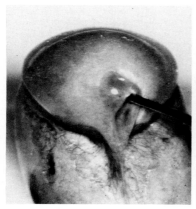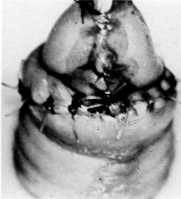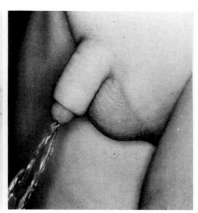

FIGURE 16-1. *Distal balanic hypospadias with distal transverse bar causing a deviated urine stream, circular prepuce, and short frenulum. A meatoplasty and circumcision with elongation of the frenulum were performed.*

presented a distal web or transverse bar in five. Three patients had been operated on before. Only two patients presented short paraurethral canals. The frenulum was missing, because of the location of the meatus, and the prepuce was dorsally redundant. The penis was normal in 12 patients and hypoplastic in 1. One patient exhibited a torsion of the penis. The scrotum was normal in all of them. However, in one patient the testes were hypoplastic. One patient presented testes migrans. All had a normal body configuration.

TREATMENT
In this type of hypospadias, it was felt that the balanic urethra had to be reconstructed in order to place the meatus at the tip of the glans. In addition, the dorsally redundant skin was shifted to the ventral side in order to correct the ventral deflection when pulling the penile skin in proximal direction. The transverse bar, when present, was excised at the same time. In eight patients, the technique shown in Figure 16-2 was used, and in five patients Del Pino's modification of the Barcat technique was used (see Table 16-5).

Prebalanic Hypospadias

THE PREOPERATIVE CONDITION IN PRIMARY CASES
Included in this group are 362 hypospadias in which, after orthoplasty, the meatus was localized at the coronary sulcus, the penis, the scrotum, or the perineum. In 217 patients, treatment is concluded with a follow-up of a minimum of 2 years; 145 patients have been

TABLE 16-4. *Results in Balanic Hypospadias*

| Technique | Number of Primary Repairs | Number of Secondary Repairs | Total | Number of Complications | End Results | | | Average Operations per Case | Average Hospitalizations per Case (in Days) |
					Excellent	Good	Satisfactory		
Meatoplasty or excision of transverse bar and circumcision	11	2	13	—	13	—	—	1	1.9
Meatoplasty and skin orthoplasty	23	1	24	—	23	1	—	1	3.2

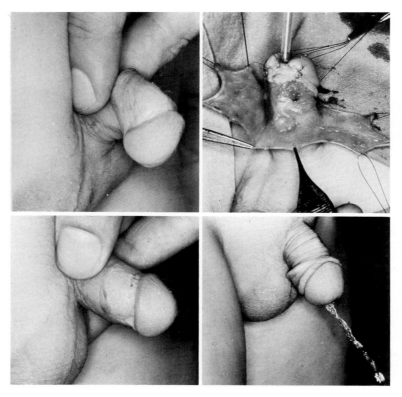

FIGURE 16-2. *Proximal balanic hypospadias with meatus close to the coronary sulcus and incurvation caused by the abnormal skin distribution, which becomes apparent when skin is retracted proximally (upper left). Urethroplasty at the glans is performed by means of a rectangular, distally based penile skin flap, which is partially displaced to the tip of the glans and sutured to lateral incisions made in the glans (the proximal free border of the urethral flap must always remain below the meatus in order to prevent* *stenosis). The dorsal prepuce is incised, opened, shifted to the inferior surface, and sutured with Z-plasties. After surgery, the penis remains straight when skin is retracted (below left). Postoperative result (below right). (Reprinted, with permission, from E. Schmid, W. Widmaier, and H. Reichert,* Wiederherstellung von Form und Funktion organischer Einheiten der verschiedenen Koerperregionen—Behandlung der Hypospadie. *Stuttgart: Thieme, 1977.)*

repaired during the last 2 years. The following data were recorded: The meatus was of normal width in 38 patients (10.5 percent), presented a distal transverse bar in 8 (2.2 percent), and was divided (meatus duplex) in 1 (0.3 percent). A stenosis with or without a premeatal subepidermal cleft was seen in 78 patients (21.5 percent). In 237 patients (65.5 percent), the meatus was of normal width, but a premeatal subepidermal cleft was present. In 86 patients (23.8 percent), the severe degree of the chordee and malformation permitted only micturition in the sitting position.

Accessory paraurethral ducts were present in 176 patients (48.6 percent): one duct at the glans in 98 (27.0 percent), various ducts at the glans in 16 (4.4 percent), one duct at the penis in 41 (11.3 percent), various ducts at the penis in 15 (4.1 percent), and ducts at the glans and the penis in 6 (1.7 percent). The prepuce was circularly surrounding the glans in 19 patients (5.2 percent) and redundant and hooded dorsally in 343 (94.8 percent). The penis was normally developed in 282 patients (77.9 percent), hypoplastic in 63 (17.4 percent), and clitoris-like in 3 (0.8 percent). In 14 patients (3.9 per-

TABLE 16-5. *Results in Proximal Balanic Hypospadias*

Technique	Number of Primary Repairs	Number of Secondary Repairs	Total	Number of Complications	End Results			Average Operations per Case	Average Hospital-izations per Case (in Days)
					Excellent	Good	Satisfactory		
Balanic ure-throplasty and skinplasty with Del Pino's modification of the Barcat technique	5	—	5	—	4	1	—	1	9.4
Balanic ure-throplasty and skinplasty with Hinderer's technique	5	3	8	—	8	—	—	1	5.1

cent), a torsion with deviation of the raphe to the opposite side was present.

The raphe was normal and midline in 64 patients (17.6 percent); deviated to the right in 124 (34.3 percent), to the left in 38 (10.5 percent), and divided in Y form in 133 (36.7 percent); and a penoscrotal plica was present in 3 (0.8 percent). So far we have not found an explanation for the greater amount of deviations of the raphe to the right, also observed by Farkas [13] with regard to penile hypospadias. The scrotum was normal in 326 patients (90 percent), hypoplastic in 10 (2.8 percent), bifid in 12 (3.3 percent), labial-like and joined over the root of the penis in 9 (2.5 percent), and labial-like in 5 (1.5 percent). The testes were normal in 344 patients (95 percent), considerably hypoplastic in 9 (2.5 percent), and both not palpable in 5 (1.4 percent). In four patients (1.2 percent), one testicle (in two the right and in two the left) was not palpable, while the other was at the scrotum. With regard to the localization of the testes, both were at the scrotum in 321 patients (88.7 percent), both were at the inguinal canal in 14 (3.9 percent), and 12 (3.3 percent) had testes migrans. In six patients (1.6 percent), one testicle was at the inguinal canal and the other was at the scrotum. In all, 347 patients (95.8 percent) had a normal body configuration, 4 (1.1 percent) were obese,

4 (1.1 percent) presented a configuration resembling the adiposogenital syndrome, and 7 (1.9 percent) were dystrophic. The level of the meatus before, and its proximal displacement after, meatoplasty and straightening of the penis, representing the diagnosis of the level of the hypospadias, is shown in Table 16-6.

The psychic effects of the malformation were judged by our team simply by observation of the behavior of the child and by interrogation of the family. The results were grouped in four categories: children reacting with indifference to the malformation, those who showed a clear adaptation, those who reacted with aggression, and those with a tendency to introversion and isolation. We do not pretend this to be more than a general impression as opposed to a scientific evaluation. Nevertheless, the results obtained in 362 primary cases as compared with 126 secondary cases in which previous attempts at repair had failed show that the percentage of children reacting with indifference is clearly less than that of the other groups. Several factors seem to be involved: the older age of the patients, now more conscious of the malformation; the increased psychic involvement resulting from the stress of multiple surgeries; and concern with regard to the final result. In some cases, psychotherapy was indicated (see Table 16-7).

TABLE 16-6. *The Level of Meatus before and after Orthoplasty in 276 Prebalanic Hypospadias*

Before Meatoplasty and Orthoplasty			Diagnosis of the Level of Hypospadias	After Meatoplasty and Orthoplasty	
	14	5.0%	H.G.	—	—
	95	34.4%	H.J.G.	14	5.0%
	99	35.9%	H.P.D.	35	19.9% ⎫
138 50%	32	11.6%	H.P.M.	106	38.4% ⎬ 198 71.6%
	7	2.5%	H.P.P.	37	13.4% ⎭
	12	4.3%	H.P.S.	28	10.1%
	10	3.6%	H.S	27	9.8%
	7	2.5%	H.P.R.	9	3.3%

TREATMENT

Treatment of prebalanic hypospadias was performed in 1965 with the initial two-stage technique of urethroplasty, which was replaced in 1966 by the penis-tunnelization technique, used with preference as a one-stage, and in some instances, a two-stage, procedure in both primary and secondary cases. The more severe and secondary cases were operated on by the senior author, while some other primary cases were operated on by the first coauthor and other assistant plastic surgeons at St. Raphael's Hospital.

CRITERIA OF OPERABILITY AND PLAN OF TREATMENT

1. Satisfactory general condition for a surgical treatment under general anesthesia.

2. Sex determination, including chromosomal investigation, hormonal status, and laparotomy with biopsy of the gonads, if necessary, in all doubtful cases and specifically if one or both testes are not palpable. In 27 patients in our series, some of these investigations were necessary, and the following cases of intersex were diagnosed: four patients with pseudohermaphroditism, one with dysgenic male pseudohermaphroditism, one with Reifenstein syndrome, one with mosaicism (48 XYYY/47 XYY/45 X), and one with hermaphroditism. In a total of six patients, the female legal sex adopted at birth had to be changed to male. In cases of genital malformations at birth, we consider an exact diagnosis by teamwork indispensable, and it should not be post-

TABLE 16-7. *The Psychic Effect of the Malformation*

Number	Indifference		Adaptation		Aggression		Introversion	
	Number	Percent	Number	Percent	Number	Percent	Number	Percent
362 primary cases	205	56.6	82	22.6	32	8.8	43	11.9
126 secondary cases	20	55.8	62	42.2	22	13.5	22	13.5

poned beyond the age of 2 years, when the child becomes conscious of his sexual identity. Once the legal sex has been decided, the child should be remitted to a genitourinary unit in order to set up the treatment schedule, which will depend on the morphological findings and functional disorders. The family should be informed accordingly.

3. Urography for detection of eventual associated upper urinary tract malformations and cystourethrography in order to detect obstacles to urination (such as valves, which should be treated by transurethral resection).

4. Exploration of the meatal region. The family is interrogated with regard to the quality of the urinary stream; the diameter of the meatus is checked with a catheter, and the premeatal urethral wall is examined with a metal probe in order to diagnose subepidermal clefts and stenosis. When the tip of the metal probe glides in a distal direction, the end of the corpus spongiosum is detectable by a decreased resistance, while the metal probe becomes more visible since it is covered only by the urethral lining and thin epithelium. Externally the limit coincides with the division or the deviation of the raphe. In cases of stenosis of the meatus, anomalies at the region of the meatus, subepidermal clefts, or the presence of hair follicles or scars of previous operations close to the meatus, a Y-V meatoplasty, mostly at between 1 and 3 years of age, is performed [28, 32].

5. Adequate size of the penis. The preferred age for urethroplasty in our unit is between 3 and 5 years, because we wish to prevent the emotional problems caused by the child's comparing himself to other boys at school. However, the majority of patients operated on are older because of delayed referral. This is even more the case when previous operations in other clinics have failed (see Fig. 16-3). In cases of hypoplasia of the penis, the operation is postponed if this does not cause psychological difficulties to the child. In this last instance, we prefer a treatment with chorionic gonadotrophic

hormone (CGH) (two cycles of 8.0 to 500 U twice per week, with a 2-month interval). Of course, pertinent additional examinations for prevention of complications resulting from the administration of CGH should be made. The augmentation of penis length obtained with this treatment (Fig. 16-4) is shown in 40 children. We felt that this treatment was necessary, despite the fact that the average length of the penis, measured with the same technique, was superior to the figures published by Farkas et al. [17] with regard to healthy Central European boys of the same age. The average in these seems rather small compared to Spanish boys. Between the end of the treatment and urethroplasty, we waited an interval at least 6 months, since we had the impression that the penile tissues became "softer" with increased bleeding.

6. Before surgery, micturition should be evaluated by means of uroflometry. In all cases, the width of the meatus (which should correspond to the width of the normal urethra) is rechecked.

EVALUATION OF RESULTS

Results are evaluated according to the criteria presented in Table 16-1. A clinical examination with uroflometry and voiding photography is made at regular intervals, depending on the progress and problems of each case (preferably after 6 months, 1 year, 2 years, at the ages of 12 and 18, and after marriage). In case of a decrease in urinary flow, the test is repeated, and if it is confirmed, a cystourethrograph is performed. Any stenosis with prestenotic dilation or a diverticulum should be corrected, especially if the cystography reveals proximal urinary tract difficulties.

UROFLOMETRY

Micturition is influenced by the detrusor muscle, the bladder neck, the proximal urethra, the pelvic floor, the abdominal wall and diaphragm, and any other accessory muscles of

Number of cases

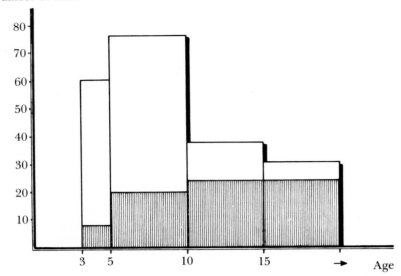

FIGURE 16-3. *Age of repair of prebalanic hypospadias operated with Hinderer's technique of penis tunnelization.*

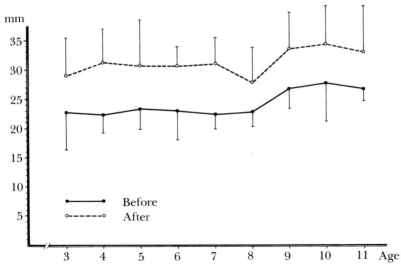

FIGURE 16-4. *Length of penis in 40 children before and after treatment with CGH.*

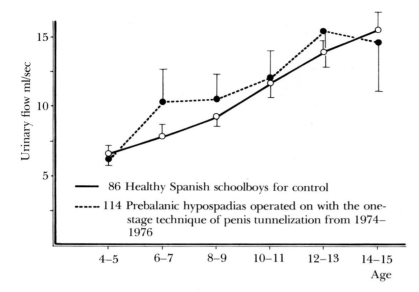

FIGURE 16-5. *Urinary flow in preglandular hypo-spadias operated on with Hinderer's technique of penis tunnelization.*

micturition. For purposes of preoperative evaluation and assessment of the operative result and the follow-up in hypospadias, we believe that the flow-rate profile, which captures in image the micturition action and shows the peak and mean flows, is the easiest and best test for determining such lower urinary tract obstructions as meatal and urethral stenosis or urethral valves. Since the profile image varies with regard to quantity, a minimum of 100 ml of urine is necessary for proper evaluation. The boy should urinate in a separate room in order to avoid inhibition [2, 8, 54].

Since we did not possess until recently a cystourethroflometer, we decided to use timed micturition, knowing, nevertheless, that this was not the most accurate test. The urine is collected in a graduated cylinder, and the time is measured with a stopwatch.

In order to have normal figures for comparison with boys of the same age, one of our nursing staff, José Ramón Mora, checked the urinary flow in 86 healthy Spanish schoolboys for control (see Fig. 16-5). Although the test is not accurate, comparison with the values in these

normal boys has shown it to be valuable in practice, since the conditions of measurement were similar. Checking with the flowmeter confirmed the results of timed micturition. In patients with decreased flow rates, a cystourethrograph was made and another operation performed, if indicated (Fig. 16-6).

TREATMENT WITH THE INITIAL TWO-STAGE URETHROPLASTY

In the two-stage urethroplasty technique, in the first stage (modified from Planas [49]) and after the chordee has been corrected, the urethra is reconstructed with a longitudinal flap of the penile-preputial skin and placed in the ventrally incised glans. In the second stage, after perineal urethrostomy, the intermediate urethra, between the meatus and the neourethra at the glans, is constructed by tubing of a longitudinal cutaneous strip. The remaining prepuce is unfolded according to Byars [8] and used for cover. For results, see Table 16-8.

TREATMENT WITH HINDERER'S TECHNIQUE OF PENIS TUNNELIZATION

The different steps of the penis-tunnelization technique are shown in Figure 16-7. (Figure 16-12 is a patient with prebalanic hypospadias of the middle third of the penis.) The operation

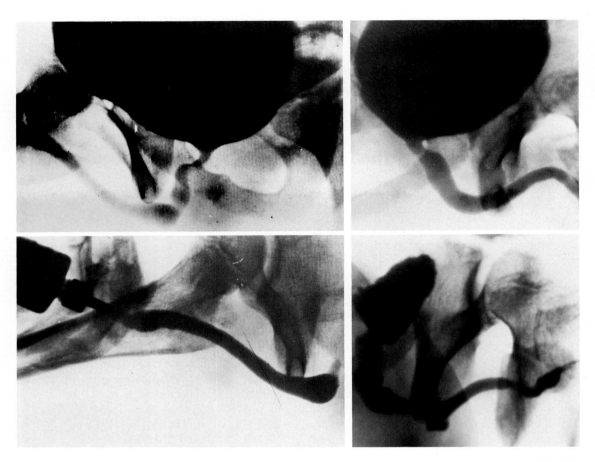

FIGURE 16-6. *Seven-year-old boy with hypospadias of the proximal third of the penis, operated on when 5 years old (above left). The mictural cystourethrography shows a bladder of normal capacity, without urethral reflux and postmictural residue. The retrograde urethrography shows a normal caliber and uniformity of the urethra (below left). Urinary flow (timed micturition) 1 year after surgery was 6 ml/s, and 2 years after surgery, 11 ml/s. Secondary case of penile hypospadias operated on four times elsewhere; boy is 9 years old (above right). The mictural cystourethrography shows a uniform filling of the urethra, which is of normal caliber and uniformity. Bladder contour is normal. Uri-*nary flow (timed micturition) 1 year after surgery is 6 ml/s; 4 years after surgery, 12 ml/s. Penoscrotal hypospadias operated on five times before at another clinic, with obliteration of the urethra (below right). Repair was performed with the technique of penis tunnelization. The mictural cystourethrography, taken a few months after closure of the perineal urethrostomy because of a low urinary flow (4 ml/s), shows moderate modifications of the bladder's contour as a repercussion of the stenosis of the distal part of the neourethra and a diverticulum. The patient has to be reoperated on in order to repair the stenosis of the distal part of the neourethra.*

TABLE 16-8. *Results with the Initial Two-Stage Urethroplasty Technique*

| Primary Repairs | Number of Secondary Repairs | Total | Number of Complications | Results | | | Number of Operations per Case | Total Hospitalizations per Case (in Days) |
				Excellent	Good	Satisfactory		
3	6	9	6	8	1	—	2.9	26

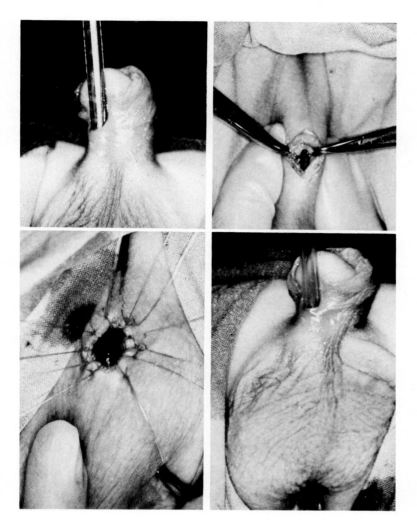

FIGURE 16-7. *Hinderer's technique of penis tunnelization (see text).*

begins with a perineal urethrostomy; then a bladder catheter is inserted. A metal probe, introduced in the catheter, helps tilt the urethra at the desired level of the perineal urethrostomy, while the assistant holds the urethra at the midline raphe. Skin, subcutaneous tissue, and urethra are incised by electrocautery. The urethra is grasped with forceps and sutured with 3-0 Dexon to the skin. The bladder catheter is removed through the perineal urethrostomy, leaving the metal probe in place to serve as a guide for insertion of a catheter of the

same size in the opposite direction (from the perineal urethrostomy to the meatus) (see Fig. 16-8).

Three traction sutures are applied, one on each side and one dorsally to the tip of the glans. The flap for the neourethra is marked and superficially incised on the hairless penile skin along the border of the prepuce of one side, its width being slightly greater than the circumference of the circular catheter. When measuring the length of the flap, the proximal displacement of the meatus resulting from orthoplasty has to be considered. The surrounding skin proximal to the flap is dissected at a very superficial level in order to preserve the

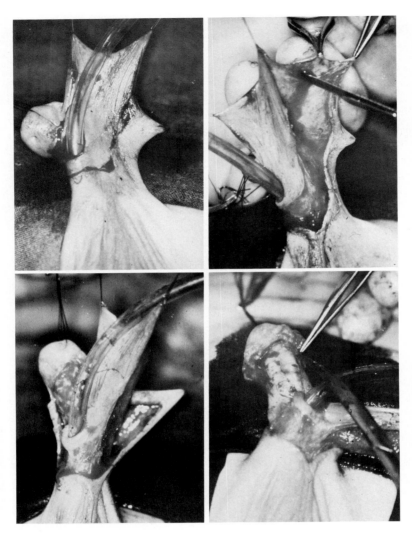

FIGURE 16-8. *The technique of penis tunnelization (continued).*

subcutaneous tissue and vessels supplying the neourethral flap.

Deep dissection separates the neourethral flap with its subcutaneous tissue from the corpora cavernosa down to a level between 1 and 2 cm below the meatus. The chordee is completely excised, not only at the midline, but also on both sides, until the corpora cavernosa appear bluish and soft and a complete

straightening of the penis and glans is achieved (Fig. 16-9).

The flap is sutured around the catheter placed in the hypospadiac meatus using 4-0 Ethilon as a nonperforating, continuous, and removable suture; this starts at the proximal end, where the suture is passed through the scrotal skin and 2 or 3 times through the subcutaneous tissue close to the meatus. Any excess skin of the neourethral flap is trimmed in order to obtain a perfect adaptation of the borders. This first suture line is covered by a second layer of the subcutaneous tissue, which is rotated around the urethra, as shown in the

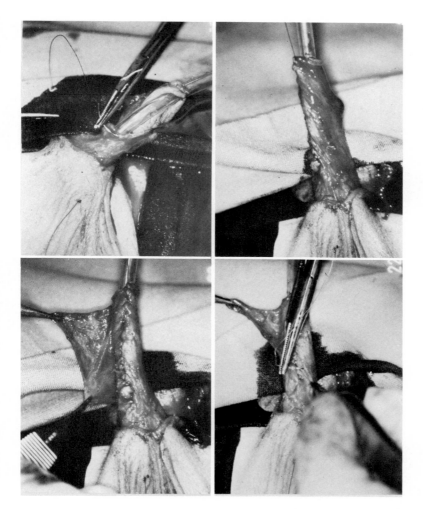

FIGURE 16-9. *The technique of penis tunnelization (continued).*

lower left of Figure 16-10. The suture is performed with interrupted stitches of 5-0 Dexon.

A central lumen is now created from the tip downward, obliquely through the glans and upper part of the penis in the midline, by means of a special cutting trocar*, which is rotated until it surfaces at the albuginea. The trocar is passed through a trapdoor, made with scissors, and the coned balanic and corpora cavernosa tissues are removed from the interior

*Available at Ad. Krauth, 2 Hamburg 70 Wandsbeker Königsstr, 27–29, West Germany.

of the trocar. In the case shown, the level of emergence of the trocar is at the coronary sulcus. Usually (see Fig. 16-12), we prefer a somewhat lower location, approximately 1 cm below the coronary sulcus.

A second instrument* for pulling the urethra through is inserted into the trocar and passed through the penile tunnel as the trocar is removed. A double-ended traction suture is passed through the end of the neourethra and catheter, the catheter being somewhat longer than the tubed flap. Both ends of the traction are passed through holes at the end of the instrument, and the distal end of the removable suture is also passed through one of the holes. The end of the neourethra, with the catheter, is

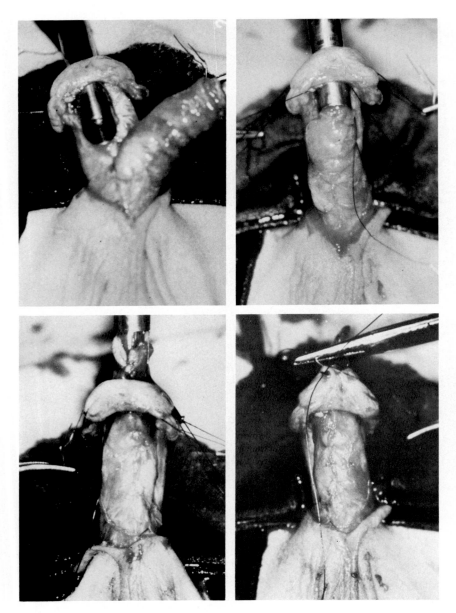

FIGURE 16-10. *The technique of penis tunnelization (continued).*

now inserted into the end of the instrument, facilitated by pulling the threads of the traction sutures downward.

Keeping the 3–0 Ethilon traction sutures under tension, the instrument and the inserted neourethra with catheter are then passed through the lumen created at the penis until they emerge at the tip of the glans. The traction thread is then removed, the neourethra and penis are stretched, and the excess neourethra is trimmed off.

The end of the removable suture is passed through the glans, and the end of the urethra is stitched to the top of the glans with 5–0 Dexon

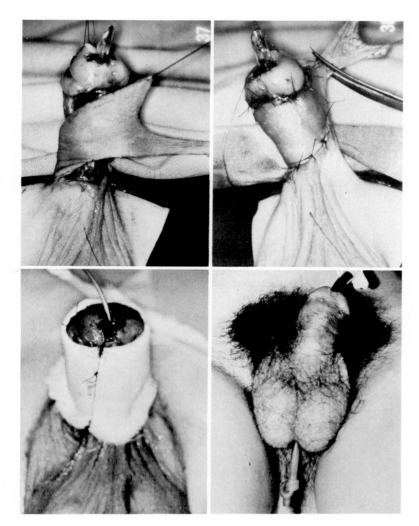

FIGURE 16-11. *The technique of penis tunnelization (continued).*

interrupted sutures. Finally, the trapdoor is sutured with a few interrupted Dexon sutures to the neourethra (Fig. 16-11).

The remaining penile and preputial skin is incised at approximately 2 to 3 mm from the coronary sulcus, the inner blade of the prepuce is unfolded, and the penile-preputial flap is wrapped around the penis and neourethra in the same direction that the neourethral flap was marked.

Suturing with 4–0 Ethilon interrupted stitches starts at the proximal corner and is finished at the coronary sulcus, taking care that no torsion of the penis occurs. Any excess skin is trimmed off. A narrow intravenous silicone catheter is inserted in the urethral catheter while the latter is being removed. This thin intravenous catheter does not interfere with the blood supply when edema starts to develop, nor does it cause necrosis or irritation of the urethra; rather, it acts as an interior lining. Tincture of Merthiolate is applied to the penis, an adhesive is sprayed on the penile surface, and a circular dressing is applied without tension. This is fixed at the dorsum with paper tape and at the inferior side by knotting over

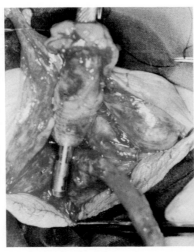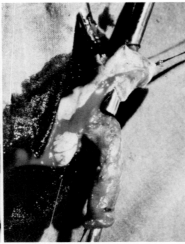

FIGURE 16-12. *Tunnelization of the glans and shaft of the penis down to 1 cm below the level of the meatus, as used in most patients between 1966 and 1973 (left). Site of tunnelization (from the tip of the glans down to approxi-* *mately 1 cm below the coronary sulcus), as used in most patients since 1974 (right). Note the "trapdoor" entrance to the corpora cavernosa.*

the ends of the neourethra's removable suture, which in this way is maintained under tension (Fig. 16-12).

PENIS-TUNNELIZATION TECHNIQUE AS A TWO-STAGE PROCEDURE

In cases where hair follicles are close to the meatus or where there are skin irregularities such as a hypertrophic raphe division or scar tissue from previous operations in secondary repairs, the penis-tunnelization technique is used as a two-stage procedure. After perineal urethrostomy and orthoplasty, tunnelization of the neourethral flap is performed as in the one-stage procedure. However, the tubing of the neourethral flap does not include the meatal region and starts about 1 cm above in order that hairless or scarless penile tissue can be placed between the meatus and the proximal opening of the neourethra. In the second stage, the meatal region is also tubed, and in some cases, the perineal urethrostomy is closed at the same time.

POSTOPERATIVE TREATMENT

Usually Furadantin and anti-inflammatory medication are given. Micturition occurs through the perineal urethrostomy, but some urine may, after a few days, pass through the neourethra and leak through the new meatus. The Melolin dressing is removed as late as possible, around the twelfth day, and the stitches are also removed then. However, the presence of major secretions is an indication for earlier removal of the dressing. In this case, wet chamomile or antiseptic dressings (Rivanol) may be used. The patient is usually discharged the fourth or fifth postoperative day. Three to four weeks after surgery, the fine intravenous catheter is replaced by a urethral catheter (No. 8 Charrière), which is knotted at the proximal end and perforated with a safety pin at the distal end to avoid its slipping into the urethra. Every 2 to 4 weeks, the catheter is replaced by successively larger ones, until the size used during surgery is reached. The purpose of placing the catheter between the perineal urethrostomy and the tip of the glans is to maintain the width of the neourethral flap during the healing period and to promote a uniform lumen. However, it is not for dilation purposes. The patients do not complain about any discomforts caused by the catheter; they go to school and engage in sports such as swimming, and so on. Only twice in 458 urethroplasties did urethritis occur. The catheter is removed after 9 months, when the perineal urethrostomy is closed (circumcision of the urethrostomy and closure in three layers with Dexon under local anesthesia as an outpatient procedure or with general anesthesia and a 1-day hospitalization). It is important that the patient urinate with little pressure in the first postoperative days.

COMMENTS WITH REGARD TO THE TECHNIQUE

When we first presented the technique of penis tunnelization, we reviewed the literature to find out if other similar techniques had been published before. Here we wish to acknowledge previous techniques based on a similar principle of repair: the use of a proximally based penile flap for reconstruction of the urethra.

The first publication we found was by Russell [52] (1900), followed by Thompson [56] (1917) and McWorther [41] (1940), who reported on two cases. Especially we wish to mention the method of Broadbent, Woolf, and Toksu [5, 6] (1961, 1965), which combined the proximally based flap urethroplasty with the orthoplasty in the same stage and incised the glans in order to bring the meatus to the tip.

Theoretically there are advantages to proximally based flap urethroplasties. This is especially true of the penis-tunnelization technique as compared with other methods. However, only comparisons of series of patients operated on with different methods can prove the validity of this hypothesis.

ADVANTAGES OF PENIS TUNNELIZATION

1. The penile skin used for urethroplasty, having the same growth potential as the other penile tissue, will enlarge with the flow requirement according to age.

2. The quality of the urethral wall resulting from primary healing of a flap is regarded as better than in the case of a secondary epithelialization of skin strips (method of Browne [7] and others). In addition, the possibility of retraction of flaps is supposed to be less than that of free grafts.

3. Proximally based penile flaps provide a better blood supply than those based distally (Ombrédanne method [47, 48] and following procedures). If the meatus is at the proximal third of the penis or below, the use of scrotal skin is required, with the danger of inclusion of hair follicles, despite a careful previous electrocoagulation.

4. The transition from the normal urethra to the neourethra does not require a circular or oblique suture, which would increase the possibility of stenosis resulting from scar retraction, as free-graft urethroplasty methods do (Nové-Josserand method [46], McIndoe [40], Horton and Devine [33, 34, 35, 36], and so on).

5. The creation of a central space at the glans and the region of the coronary sulcus rather than merely a perforation (as in other methods mistakenly called "tunnelization") by removal of tissue with a specially designed cutting trocar contributes to an avoidance of stenosis of the neomeatus and neourethra.

6. The method reproduces as far as possible the anatomical and physiological conditions of a normal urethra: from the meatus up to the tunnel, the neourethra is surrounded by a layer of subcutaneous tissue with numerous blood vessels. The quality and resistance of the neourethral wall are therefore comparable to those of a normal urethra with its corpus spongiosum. In addition, more distally the neourethra is surrounded by the glans.

7. The trapdoor-like entrance through the albuginea stabilizes the neourethra without bending. If fistulae occur, they are therefore more proximally located and easier to repair.

8. The use of a catheter from the urethrostomy to the tip of the glans, kept in place during the healing period, results in an even and uniform lumen of the neourethra.

Some of the details of the technique are improvements introduced in 1973 after evaluation of the previous cases, such as the second layer of subcutaneous tissue around the neourethra, the limitation of the tunnelization to the glans and coronary sulcus region in order not to diminish the erectile tissue of the corpora cavernosa, and the trapdoor entrance. The actual evaluation of results has proven the validity of these changes.

SECONDARY REPAIRS

In 1972 we reported on 43 patients with secondary repairs of hypospadias failures [28]. Our statistics now include 140 patients, of whom 104 have been followed for 2 or more years and whose treatment has concluded (Table 16-3). In 54 patients, one operation had been performed previously elsewhere; in 25 patients, two; in 22 patients, three; in 13 patients, four; in 10 patients, five; in 3 patients, six; in 4 patients, seven; in 3 patients, eight; and in 6 patients, ten or more operations, up to twenty-two.

The influence of the number of previous operations on the percentage of urethral complications in 79 secondary cases, reoperated on by us with the one- or two-stage technique of penis tunnelization, has been examined. The incidence of complications in the group with four or more operations is significantly higher than in the group with only one operation (65 percent to 25.7 percent; $X^2 = 1.18$; $p = 0.05$) or the groups with two or three operations (65 percent to 25 percent; $X^2 = 7.11$; $p = 0.008$).

In 66 patients a urethroplasty had been previously attempted. The complications encountered in the urethroplasty are presented in Table 16-9. In these 66 patients, the meatus was placed at the tip of the glans in 4 patients (6 percent), at the glans in 3 patients (4.5 percent),

TABLE 16-9. *Complications of the Neourethra in 66 Secondary Cases of Failed Urethroplasties Performed in Other Clinics*

Types of Complications	Number	Percent
Obliteration	14	21.2
Stenosis	3	4.5
One fistula	13	19.7
Various fistulae	10	15.1
Diverticulum	2	3.0
Combination of various complications	16	24.2
Combination of various complications with urethritis	4	6.0
Overly wide urethra	4	6.0

at the coronary sulcus in 11 patients (16.6 percent), and at different levels of the penis in 48 patients (72.7 percent), thus showing that many surgeons still do not consider the placement of the meatus at the tip of the glans to be a necessary goal in hypospadias surgery.

In 103 patients, orthoplasty had been attempted but was not properly performed in 93 (90.3 percent). This demonstrates that the first and most important step in hypospadias repair, the straightening of the penis, in many cases is not being performed properly.

In 96 cases requiring a secondary procedure in which orthoplasty was performed by our unit, the level of the hypospadiac meatus (after straightening) was at the coronary sulcus in 3 patients (3.1 percent), the distal third of the penis in 9 (9.4 percent), the middle third of the penis in 22 (22.9 percent), the proximal third of the penis in 16 (16.6 percent), the penoscrotal angle in 21 (21.9 percent), the scrotal region in 21 (21.9 percent), and the perineal area in 4 (4.2 percent).

TECHNIQUES USED IN SECONDARY REPAIRS

In the treatment of secondary repairs, the same techniques were used as for primary repairs, giving preference to the penis-tunnelization technique (see Fig. 16-13). Up to now it has not been necessary to use a free-graft technique

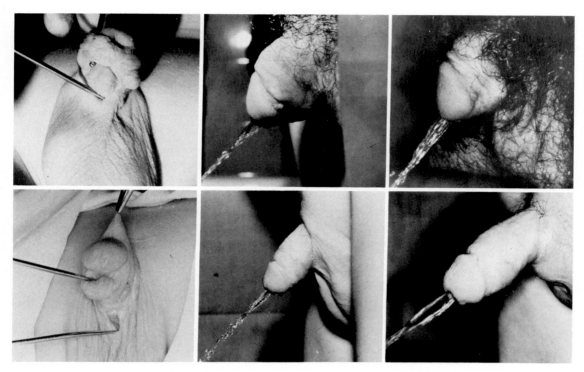

FIGURE 16-13. *Average result with Hinderer's technique of penis tunnelization in secondary cases. This patient, 12 years old, was operated on four times at other clinics, with meatus at proximal third of the penis, chordee, (above left) partial obliteration and diverticulum of the urethra, and immobile scars (above). Two operations were necessary to complete the repair. Postoperative result (above center), 1 and 4 years (above right) after surgery. Note the* *improved urinary stream: urinary-flow measurements (timed micturition) of 10 ml/s and 17 ml/s, respectively. This patient, 9 years old, was operated on five times before at another clinic, with chordee, meatus at the coronary sulcus, stenosis, diverticulum, and fistula (below). Repair was completed in two operations. Urinary flow (timed micturition) 1 year after surgery (lower center) was 7 ml/s, and 3 years after surgery (lower right), 12 ml/s.*

such as the Horton-Devine [33, 34, 35, 36] technique which we suggested in our 1972 publication, since we have always found sufficient hairless skin available for urethroplasty. However, in some patients it was first necessary to shift the remaining hairless dorsal skin to the inferior surface for reconstruction of the urethra, using then the two-stage repair. For skin closure in cases where there is a shortage of skin, the scrotum (or in one patient, pubic flaps) is used.

In nine patients, only remedial operations, such as fistula closure, treatment of stenosis, treatment of diverticula, or the removal of hair follicles and calculi as well as skin plasties, were necessary to complete the repair. The results

obtained in these cases are shown in Table 16-10.

COMPLICATIONS WITH HINDERER'S PENIS-TUNNELIZATION TECHNIQUE

In a previous report, published in 1977 [32], the results were presented with regard to 237 primary repairs. In addition, recent cases, 2 months after urethroplasty, in which the urethrostomies were not yet closed were included. The evaluation of results and the percentages of complications were therefore more favorable than in the present report, in which only 204 consecutive cases with a minimum of 2 years follow-up are regarded.

TABLE 16-10. *Results of Remedial Operations in Secondary Cases*

		Results			Number of Operations per Case	Total Hospitalizations per Case (in Days)
Number	Complications	Excellent	Good	Satisfactory		
9	6	5	3	1	1.8	10.3

Other reasons were that one assistant plastic surgeon in charge of primary cases at St. Raphael's Hospital (October 1975 to June 1977) did not accurately follow the indications for surgery (performing urethroplasties in cases of hypoplasia or meatal stenosis) and delegated the postoperative treatment to an insufficiently experienced nursing staff. This emphasizes once more the importance of the cooperation of a well-trained nursing staff, since the postoperative treatment is as essential as surgery itself.

Complications may concern the skin cover, the penis, and the new urethra. The last two are more important because they interfere with urinary and sexual functions and require more important surgeries for repair. However, we do not feel that the percentage of complications is an important factor. The basis for comparison of different methods is the final result.

However, complications may increase the number of operations and hospitalization, which, on the other hand, is compensated when a technique requires fewer stages. We always inform the family of the possibility of complications and the additional stages required if a complication arises.

Cutaneous complications occurred with the penis-tunnelization technique, cutaneous complications such as hematoma, infection, breakdown of the suture line, or partial skin necrosis, which healed in all cases within 1 month after surgery. However, the importance of cutaneous complications is that in most cases they give rise to urethral complications such as fistula formation.

The number of urethral complications is shown in Table 16-11. In none of our patients did we observe hair growth in the urethra or calculi formation. In addition, no meatal

TABLE 16-11. *Urethral Complications with Hinderer's Technique of Penis Tunnelization in 214 Primary and 79 Secondary Repairs of Prebalanic Hypospadias*

	Number of Cases	Partial Obliteration or Stenosis		Fistula		Diverticula		Total Urethral Complications	
		Number	Percent	Number	Percent	Number	Percent	Number	Percent
Primary repairs:									
One-stage repair, 1966–1973	49	1	2.0	18	36.7	2	4.1	21	42.9
One-stage repair, 1974–1976	153	8	5.3	33	21.6	1	0.6	42	27.5
Two-stage repair, 1966–1976	12	1	8.3	6	50	2	16.7	9	75.0
Secondary repairs:									
One-stage repair, 1966–1973	18	1	5.6	11	61.1	1	5.6	13	72.2
One-stage repair, 1974–1976	40	—	—	13	32.5	—	—	13	32.5
Two-stage repair, 1966–1976	21	1	4.8	4	19.0	2	9.5	7	33.3

TABLE 16-12. *Urethral Complications and Final Evaluations with Relation to the Level of the Meatus in 196 Primary Repairs Concluded with Hinderer's Technique of Penis Tunnelization*

Level of the Meatus after Orthoplasty	Number of Cases	Urethral Complications		Results					
				Excellent		Good		Satisfactory	
		Number	Percent	Number	Percent	Number	Percent	Number	Percent
Coronary sulcus	14	3	21.4	13	92.9	1	7.1	—	—
Penile	142	48	33.8	140	98.6	1	0.7	1	0.7
Penoscrotal	18	10	55.5	16	88.9	1	5.6	1	5.6
Scrotal and perineal	22	11	50.0	19	86.3	3	16.6	—	—

stenosis occurred. The recorded fistulae were all situated below the coronary sulcus, thus being easier to repair. Fistulae in primary repairs decreased significantly after 1974 (36.7 percent to 21.6 percent; $X^2 = 4.5$; $p = 0.025$), as did the total number of urethral complications (42.9 percent to 27.5 percent; $X^2 = 4.10$; $p = 0.046$). The comparison of one-stage repair in primary cases with that of secondary cases in the same periods of time proves that fistulae formation and urethral complications are significantly higher in secondary repairs (36.7 and 61.1 percent, respectively; $X^2 = 3.19$; $p = 0.083$).

If we compare the one-stage technique (1966–1973) with the two-stage repair (1966–1976), the total number of urethral complications is significantly higher with the two-stage repair (42.9 percent versus 75 percent; $X^2 = 3.98$; $p = 0.046$). This proves our previous statements, at least with regard to our technique, that the total number of urethral complications increases with the number of stages required for repair, since in each stage compli-

cations may occur [27, 32]. However, the number of cutaneous complications is lower in secondary repairs.

Urethral complications were examined with regard to the level of the meatus in prebalanic hypospadias (Table 16-12). The number of urethral complications proved to be statistically more significant in penoscrotal hypospadias than in penile hypospadias (55.5 percent versus 33.8 percent; $X^2 = 3.27$; $p = 0.083$). Also, the comparison between coronal hypospadias and penoscrotal hypospadias (21.4 percent to 55.5 percent; $X^2 = 3.80$; $p = 0.046$) and between coronal hypospadias and scrotal-perineal hypospadias (21.4 percent to 50.0 percent; $X^2 = 2.94$; $p = 0.083$) showed a significantly higher percentage of complications when the meatus was more proximally located.

The urethral complications in 214 primary repairs with the penis-tunnelization technique have also been examined with regard to the size of the penis (see Table 16-13). It has been found that the number of complications increases significantly when the penis is hypo-

TABLE 16-13. *Urethral Complications and the Final Evaluations with Relation to the Size of the Penis in 214 Primary Repairs of Prebalanic Hypospadias with Hinderer's Technique of Penis Tunnelization*

	Number of Cases	Total Number of Urethral Complications		Results					
				Excellent		Good		Satisfactory	
		Number	Percent	Number	Percent	Number	Percent	Number	Percent
Penis of normal size	173	49	28.3	167	96.5	4	2.3	2	1.2
Hypoplastic or clitoris-like penis	41	23	56.1	36	87.8	4	9.8	1	2.4

plastic (28.3 percent to 56.1 percent; $X^2 = 11.45$; $p = 0.001$). This suggests that it is indicated to delay the urethroplasty until the size of the penis is large enough for an easy performance of the technique.

TREATMENT OF COMPLICATIONS

In cases of fistulae, repair is postponed until 6 months later, when the tissues have recovered their elasticity and softness. A three-layer closure is performed with a continuous and removable 4–0 nylon suture, taking care not to perforate the urothelium. This layer is covered with subcutaneous and skin sutures.

DIVERTICULA

Diverticula usually result from irregularity or a different thickness and resistance of the neourethral wall, stenosis distal to the diverticulum, a superficially and spontaneously closed fistula, use of hair-bearing skin for the neourethra, causing a secondary deposit of urine crystals (calculi), or use of scar tissue for the neourethra with a lower growth potential. Our technique usually precludes these causal factors.

Mictural and retrograde urethrographies help to establish the diagnosis. During surgery, the urethra is carefully examined with a catheter and metal probes, especially in order to detect postdiverticular stenosis. The urethra is incised, and the cause treated (excision of the urothelium with hair follicles, of the stenosis, etc.). The diverticulum is reduced by means of partial excision of its wall, and the opening is closed with a three-layer suture.

TABLE 16-14. *Two- to Ten-Year Postrepair Evaluation of 352 Hypospadias (1965–1976)*

| Type of Hypospadias | Technique | Surgical Period | Number | | |
			Primary Repairs	Secondary Repairs	Primary and Secondary Repairs
Balanic hypospadias	Meatoplasty and circumcision	1965–1976	11	2	13
	Meatoplasty and skin orthoplasty	1965–1976	23	1	24
Proximal balanic hypospadias	Del Pino–Barcat	1965–1970	5	—	—
	Hinderer	1971–1976	5	3	8
Prebalanic hypospadias	Initial two-stage urethroplasty (Hinderer)	1965–1966	3	6	9
	Hinderer's penis tunnelization: in one stage	1974–1976	153	—	—
	In one and two stages	1966–1976	214	—	—
	In one and two stages	1966–1976	—	79	—
	In one and two stages	1966–1976	—	—	293
Total Balanic and prebalanic hypospadias	All previous techniques	1965–1976	261	—	—
		1965–1976	—	91	—
		1965–1976	—	—	352

Evaluation of Results in Hypospadias

The efficiency of a method is judged by its results, but the more operations and hospitalizations needed, the more significant are the physical, psychic, and economic stresses. The results obtained in 352 hypospadias operations from 1965 to 1976, with a follow-up of a minimum of 2 and up to 10 years, are shown in Table 16-14.

With the penis-tunnelization technique, used in 293 primary and secondary repairs, the level of the new meatus in 287 patients (98 percent) was situated at the tip of the glans, in 1 (0.3 percent) at the distal half of the glans, and in 2 (0.7 percent) at the coronary sulcus. With regard to 153 primary cases operated on with the penis-tunnelization technique (1974 to 1976), in 146 patients (95.4 percent), an excellent result, according to the criteria of evaluation, was obtained (Fig. 16-14).

The average of operations per patient for meatoplasty, orthoplasty, urethroplasty, and the repair of complications necessary to obtain these results was 2.3, and the average of hospitalizations per patient in days was 9.5, thus demonstrating that the technique can be regarded as safe and beneficial because the physical, psychic, and economic stresses are low.

In these statistics, the closure of the perineal urethrostomy, used only for cases of prebalanic hypospadias, has not been included, since it was performed either with local anesthesia or at the same time as the repair of a complication, if present.

Results						Average Operations per Case for Meatoplasty, Orthoplasty, Urethroplasty, and Repair of Complications	Average Hospitalizations per Case (in Days)
Excellent		Good		Satisfactory			
Number	Percent	Number	Percent	Number	Percent		
13	100.0	—	—	—	—	1.0	1.9
23	95.8	1	4.2	—	—	1.0	3.2
4	80.0	1	20	—	—	1.0	9.4
8	100.0	—	—	—	—	1.0	5.1
8	88.8	1	11.1	—	—	2.9	26.0
146	95.4	5	3.3	2	1.3	2.3	9.5
203	94.8	8	3.7	3	1.4	2.2	12.4
69	87.3	10	12.6	—	—	2.2	15.4
272	92.8	18	6.1	3	1.0	2.2	13.2
248	95.0	10	3.9	3	1.1	2.0	10.0
80	87.9	11	12.1	—	—	2.1	16.1
328	93.2	21	6	3	0.8	2.0	12.3

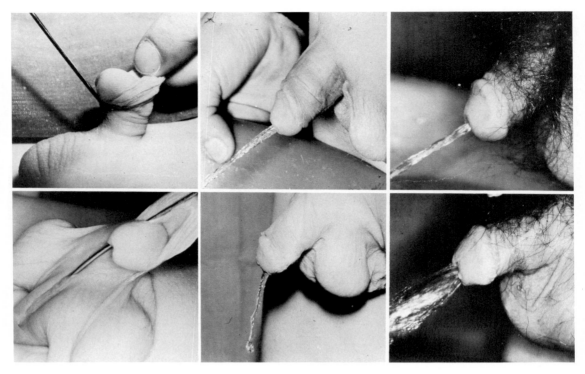

FIGURE 16-14. *Average results with Hinderer's technique of penis tunnelization in primary repairs. This patient was 10 years of age, with meatus at the distal third of the penis, chordee, and a dorsally redundant prepuce (above left). Two years after surgery (above center) timed micturition was 12 ml/s; and 7 years later (above right), 23 ml/s. Scrotal hypospadias with chordee, subepidermal cleft, multiple ducti, and bifid scrotum with scrotal fold over* *the root of the penis (below left). After meatoplasty, the new location of the meatus was perineal. Urethroplasty and orthoplasty were performed in one stage, together with the correction of the repair of the scrotal anomalies. Nine months later, the urethrostomy was closed. Urinary flow after surgery was 8 ml/s; 2 years later (below center), 14 ml/s; and 4 years later (below right), 22 ml/s.*

Short Urethra

This condition was found in 10 patients. The meatus, of normal width, was located at the tip of the glans in seven patients and close to it in three. In all patients, a pronounced incurvation of the penis was present. This was so severe in four patients that they urinated in the sitting position. The prepuce was circularly distributed in two patients and dorsally redundant in six. The penis was normal in seven patients and hypoplastic in three. The scrotum and testes were normal. In one patient, a paraurethral duct at the penis was recorded. One patient had an adiposogenital body configuration; the rest were normal. In all patients, a subepidermal cleft was noted, coinciding with a deviation or division of the raphe. A more or less retracted fibrotic tissue was present between the urethra and albuginea.

TREATMENT

Three different techniques were used for treatment (Table 16-15): in eight patients the urethra was dissected down to the scrotal region and displaced in distal direction after re-

TABLE 16-15. *Short Urethra*

| Technique Performed | Number of | | | Number of Complications | End Results | | | Number of Operations per Case | Total Hospitalizations per Case (in Days) |
	Primary Repairs	Secondary Repairs	Total		Excellent	Good	Satisfactory		
Distal displacement of the urethra	6	2	8	1	7	1	—	1.3	5.6
Two-stage urethroplasty	—	1	1	—	1	—	—	5.0	34.0
Island-flap urethroplasty (Hinderer)	1	—	1	1	—	1	—	2.0	10.0

moval of the fibrotic tissue. In addition, the shortage of skin at the inferior surface was treated by displacement of the redundant dorsal skin. In seven patients, a straight penis was obtained. However, in one patient, a slight curvature persisted, but it did not interfere with intercourse (Fig. 16-15). This patient is now married and the father of two children.

In one secondary case, a two-stage urethroplasty was used: in the first stage, the urethra was sectioned at the coronary sulcus and the orthoplasty performed. Hairless penile skin of the dorsum was then placed between the retracted ends of the urethra. In a second stage, the intermediate urethra was constructed by means of tubing, according to Duplay.

In one patient, Hinderer's "island-flap urethroplasty" in one stage, shown in Figs. 16-16, 16-17, and 16-18, was used with good result.

Congenital Urethral Fistulae

Only two patients were seen with urethral fistulae (Table 16-16). One was situated close to the coronary sulcus, and the other located at the middle third of the penis. In this case, the divided raphe surrounded the fistulae. In both patients closure of the fistulae was performed. In one, the fistula recurred, and closure had to be repeated.

Final Thoughts

The overall goal in the investigation of hypospadias must be to determine which techniques are safe and provide best results with fewer operations and hospitalizations. This requires the comparison of long-term results, from 2 years after repair, with revisions, until adulthood, made by different genitourinary units and based on a comparable classification and the same criteria for evaluation. The authors propose for general acceptance classification according to the level of the meatus after orthoplasty (balanic, proximal balanic, coronal, penile [in thirds], penoscrotal, scrotal, and perineal hypospadias), besides short urethra, urethra duplex, and congenital fistulae. This classification scheme is the one most commonly used.

For evaluation of results, we suggest Hinderer's classification into four groups judged first by the urinary function (micturition, width and uniformity of the urethra, and urinary flow), second by the sexual function (erection), third by the aesthetic appearance of the genitals (final location of the meatus and quality of the peno-scrotal skin), and fourth, whenever possible, by psychosexual evaluation (partner relationship and self-confidence). The final evaluation of a method should also include the average number of operations and hospitalizations required for repair, because this is im-

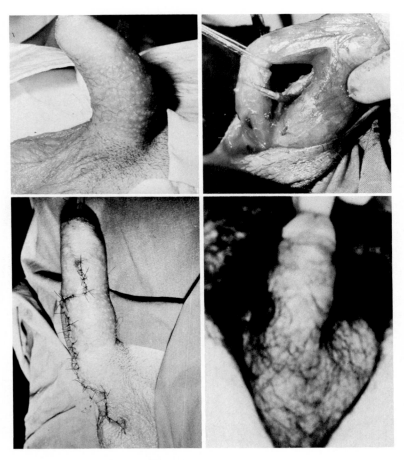

FIGURE 16-15. *Short urethra with meatus at the tip of the glans and circular prepuce. The incurvation of approximately 60 degrees during erection impeded sexual intercourse. The urethra and corpora cavernosa were exposed through a longitudinal incision, the urethra was dissected from the coronary sulcus down to the scrotal perineal level, and the fibrous tissue between the urethra and the corpora cavernosa was completely excised to achieve, together with the distal displacement of the penoscrotal urethra, a complete straightening of the penis. Finally, the skin of the lower surface was elongated with Z-plasties. Final result: a satisfactory straightening of the penis was obtained. An incurvation of approximately 15 degrees was still appreciable, although not interfering with intercourse. The patient subsequently fathered two children.*

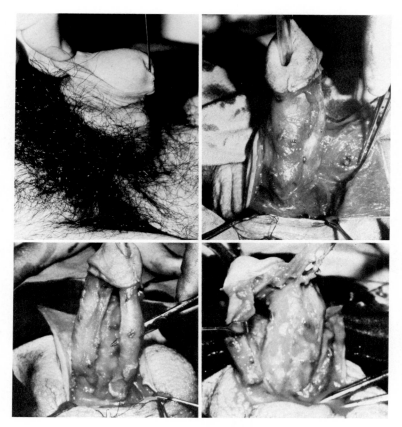

FIGURE 16-16.   *Hinderer's "island-flap urethroplasty" for short urethra, also used for urethral stenosis. Short urethra with considerable chordee and superficial location of the balanic urethra (above left). After dissection of penile and preputial skin (above right). The urethra, with inserted catheter, is dissected from the corpora cavernosa and its covering of fibrotic tissue (lower left). The fibrotic tissue between the urethra and the albuginea is excised from below to above (below right). (Reprinted with permission from E. Schmid, W. Widmaier, and H. Reichert,* Wiederherstellung von Form und Funktion organischer Einheiten der verschiedenen Koerperregionen—Behandlung der Hypospadie. *Stuttgart: Thieme, 1977.)*

portant from the physical and psychological as well as economic points of view.

The preoperative findings in 703 patients with hypospadias are presented and the techniques used are described. A 2- to 10-year evaluation is made with regard to the procedures used in 352 patients, including Hinderer's technique of penis tunnelization for prebalanic hypospadias, which is considered a safe and satisfactory procedure.

In 214 primary and 79 secondary repairs, 94.8 and 87.3 percent excellent results, respectively, were obtained with the one- and two-stage procedures, requiring for meatoplasty, orthoplasty, urethroplasty, and the repair of complications (not including the closure of the perineal urethrostomy) an average of 2.2 operations per patient and an average of 12.4 and 15.4 days hospitalization for primary and secondary cases, respectively.

Concerning 153 patients operated on with the one-stage technique of penis tunnelization

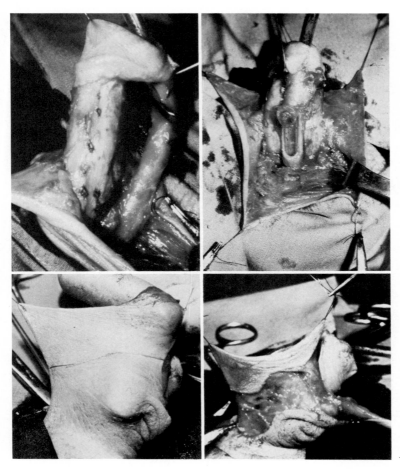

FIGURE 16-17. *Continuation of the "island-flap ure-throplasty." Dissection completed (above left). The urethra is being transected in an oblique direction to obtain a complete straightening of the penis (above right). A rectangular flap, its length corresponding to the length of the missing urethra and its width corresponding to the circumference of the urethra, is marked on the hairless penile skin of one side (below left). The flap is incised and the proximal skin dis-* sected at a very superficial level in order to preserve the subcutaneous tissue with the blood vessels nourishing the island flap (below right). (Reprinted with permission from E. Schmid, W. Widmaier, and H. Reichert, Wiederherstellung von Form und Funktion organischer Einheiten der verschiedenen Koerperregionen–Behandlung der Hypospadie. Stuttgart: Thieme, 1977.)

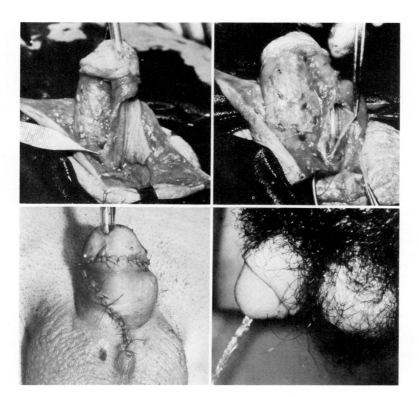

FIGURE 16-18. *Continuation of the "island-flap ure-throplasty." The island flap's surface is placed around the catheter and its ends are sutured to the ends of the transected urethra with Dexon. The longitudinal suture of the urethra, almost closed in the figure, is also performed with Dexon, and the suture line covered by a second layer of the island flap's subcutaneous tissue (above right). The penis is covered with the remaining penile and preputial skin flaps (below left). Postoperative result (below right). (Reprinted with permission from E. Schmid, W. Widmaier, and H. Reichert, Wiederherstellung von Form und Funktion organischer Einheiten der verschiedenen Koerperregionen—Behandlung der Hypospadie. Stuttgart: Thieme, 1977.)*

TABLE 16-16. *Congenital Urethral Fistulae*

| Technique Performed | Number of | | | Number of Complications | End Results | | | Average Operations per Case | Average Hospitalizations per Case (in days) |
	Primary Repairs	Secondary Repairs	Total		Excellent	Good	Satisfactory		
Closure of the fistula and skinplasty	1	1	2	1	2	—	—	1.5	16

from 1974 to 1976, an excellent result was obtained in 95.4 percent, with an average of 2.3 operations and 9.5 days of hospitalization per case.

References

1. Anger, T. Hypospadias péno-scrotal, compliqué de condure de la verge: Redressement du pénis et uréthro-plastic par inclusion cutanée. *Bull. Mem. Soc. Chir. Paris* 1:179, 1875.
2. Avellán, L., and Johanson, B. Preoperative and Postoperative Evaluation. In C.E. Horton (Ed.), *Plastic and Reconstructive Surgery of the Genital Area*. Boston: Little, Brown, 1973. P. 370.
3. Backus, L.H., and De Felice, C.A. Hypospadias—then and now. *Plast. Reconstr. Surg.* 25:146, 1960.
4. Boyarsky, S., and Weinberg, S. Urodynamic Concepts. In W. Lutzeyer and H. Melchior (Eds.), *First International Symposium on Urodynamics*. Berlin: Springer, 1973. P. 1.
5. Broadbent, T.R., and Woolf, R.M. Hypospadias: One-stage repair. *Br. J. Plast. Surg.* 18:406, 1965.
6. Broadbent, T.R., Woolf, R.M., and Toksu, E. Hypospadias: One-stage repair. *Plast. Reconstr. Surg.* 27:154, 1961.
7. Browne, D. Observations on the Treatment of Hypospadias. In A.B. Wallace (Ed.), *Transactions of the Second International Congress of Plastic Surgery* Edinburgh, Engl.: Livingstone, 1960. P. 370.
8. Byars, L.T. Hypospadias and Epispadias. In J.M. Converse (Ed.), *Reconstructive Plastic Surgery*. Philadelphia: Saunders, 1964. Vol. 5, p. 2021.
9. Dickie, W.R., and Sharpe, C. Crypto-hypospadias: A review of 38 cases. *Br. J. Plast. Surg.* 26:227, 1973.
10. Dieffenbach, J.F. *Die Operative Chirurgie*. Leipzig: Brockhaus, 1845. P. 518.
11. Duplay, S. De l'hypospadias périnéo-scrotal et de son traitement chirurgical. *Arch. Gen. Med.* 6 (23): 513, 1874.
12. Edmunds, A. Pseudo-hermaphroditism and hypospadias. *Lancet* 1: 323, 1926.
13. Farkas, G.L. *Hypospadias*. Prague: Academia, 1967.
14. Farkas, G.L. Urethra constructed in hypospadias from the skin of the shaft of the penis and/or scrotum complemented by dermoepidermal graft. *Panminerva Med.* 9:458, 1967.
15. Farkas, G.L. Problems of Surgical Treatment of Hypospadias. In J.T. Hueston (Ed.), *Transactions of the Fifth International Congress of Plastic and Reconstructive Surgery*. Sydney: Butterworth, 1971. P. 306.
16. Farkas, G.L. Konstruktive, Rekonstruktive und Ästhetische Chirurgie des Männlichen Urogenitaltraktes. In J. Gabka (Ed.), *Handbuch der Plastischen Chirurgie*. Berlin: De Gruyter, 1973. Vol. 2, number 51.
17. Farkas, G.L., Hinderer, U., and Wilkie, T. Coded Surgical Chart for Hypospadias. In J.T. Hueston (Ed.), *Transactions of the Fifth International Congress of Plastic and Reconstructive Surgery*. Sydney: Butterworth, 1971. P. 313.
18. Glenister, T.W. The origin and fate of the urethral plate in man. *J. Anat.* 88:413, 1954.
19. Hamilton, W.I., Boydt, J.D., and Mossmann H.W. *Embriología Humana*. Buenos Aires: Intermédica, 1968.
20. Hinderer, U. Coded chart for hypospadias. Unpublished manuscript. Madrid, 1968.
21. Hinderer, U. Hipospadias. *Rev. Esp. Cir. Plást.* 1:53, 1968.
22. Hinderer, U. Hipospadias: II. Técnica de tunelización del pene. *Rev. Esp. Cir. Plást.* 2:115, 1968.
23. Hinderer, U. Hipospadias Técnica Mediante Tunelización del Pene en un Tiempo. In P. Martinez (Ed.), *II Curso Monográfico de Urología, Cirugía Próstato Uretral*. Madrid: Liade, 1969.
24. Hinderer, U. New One-Stage Repair of Hypospadias (Technique of Penis Tunnelization). In J.T. Hueston (Ed.), *Transactions of the Fifth International Congress of Plastic and Reconstructive Surgery*. Sydney: Butterworth, 1971. P. 283.
25. Hinderer, U. Discussion on the Subject "Chirurgia Riparatrice dell' Uretra." In V. Consiglio (Ed.), *Atti del Simposio di Chirurgia Riparatrice dell' Uretra*. Bari, Rome: Arti Grafiche Favia, 1970. P. 33.
26. Hinderer, U. Discussion on the Subject "Il Problema dell' Intersesso." In V. Consiglio (Ed.), *Atti del Simposio di Chirurgia Riparatrice dell' Uretra*. Bari, Rome: Arti Grafiche Favia, 1970. P. 55.
27. Hinderer, U. One-Stage Repair of Hypospadias: Technique of Penis Tunnelization. In J.T. Hueston (Ed.), *Transactions of the Fifth International Congress of Plastic and Reconstructive Surgery*. Sydney: Butterworth, 1971. P. 283.
28. Hinderer, U.T. Secondary repair of hypospadias failures: Another use of the penis tunnelization technique. *Plast. Reconstr. Surg.* 50:13, 1972.
29. Hinderer, U. La Cirugía Plástica en el Tratamiento del Intersexo. In J.P. Marañes Pallardo (Ed.), *Jornadas de Endocrinología Infantil*. Madrid: Liade, 1973.

30. Hinderer, U. La cirugía plástica en el tratamiento del intersexo. *Acta Soc. Endocrinol.* (Madrid) 6 (3):39, 1974.

31. Hinderer, U. Die Plastische Chirurgie der Intersexualität und der Missbildungen des Urogenitaltraktes: Allgemeine Richtlinien und Eigene Behandlungsmethoden. In E. Schmid, W. Widmaier, and H. Reichert (Eds.), *Wiederherstellung von Form und Funktion Organischer Einheiten der Verschiedenen Körperregionen.* Stuttgart: Thieme, 1977. P. 295.

32. Hinderer, U. Behandlung der Hypospadie und der Inkompletten Hypospadieformen nach Eigenen Methoden von 1966 bis 1975. In E. Schmid, W. Widmaier, and H. Reichert (Eds.), *Wiederherstellung von Form und Funktion Organischer Einheiten der Verschiedenen Körperregionen.* Stuttgart: Thieme, 1977. P. 264.

33. Horton, C.E., Adamson, J.E., Mladick, R.A., and Devine, C.J., Jr. Hypospadias Repair. In J.T. Hueston (Ed.), *Transactions of the Fifth International Congress of Plastic and Reconstructive Surgery.* Sydney: Butterworth, 1971. P. 333.

34. Horton, C.E., Devine, C.J., Jr., Crawford, H.H., Adamson, J.E., Devine, P.C., and Devine, C.J., Sr. A One-Stage Hypospadias Repair. In T.R. Broadbent (Ed.), *Transactions of the Third International Congress of Plastic and Reconstructive Surgery.* Amsterdam: Excerpta Medica, 1964. P. 900.

35. Horton, C.E., Devine, C.J., Jr., Crawford, H.H., and Adamson, J.E. Hypospadias. In T. Gibson (Ed.), *Modern Trends in Plastic Surgery* (Series 2). London: Butterworth, 1966. P. 268.

36. Horton, C.E., Devine, C.J., Jr., Crawford, H.H., and Adamson, J.E. One Hundred One Stage Hypospadias Repairs. In G. Sanvenero and G. Boggio-Robutti (Eds.), *Transactions of the Fourth International Congress of Plastic and Reconstructive Surgery.* Amsterdam: Excerpta Medica, 1967. P. 962.

37. Johanson, B. Reconstruction of the male urethra in strictures. *Acta Chir. Scand.* [Suppl.] 176:1, 1953.

38. Johanson, B. Treatment of the Ruptured Male Urethra. In V. Consiglio (Ed.), *Atti del Simposio di Chirurgia Riparatrice dell' Uretra.* Bari, Rome: Arti Grafiche Favia, 1970.

39. McCormack, R.M. Simultaneous chordee repair and urethral reconstruction for hypospadias. *Plast. Reconstr. Surg.* 13:257, 1954.

40. McIndoe, A.H. An operation for the cure of adult hypospadias. *Br. Med. J.* 1:385, 1937.

41. McWhorter, G.L. Operative treatment for extensive hypospadias. *Surg. Clin. North Am.* 10:275, 1930.

42. Mirabet-Ippolito, V. Modificación de la técnica de McIndoe para el tratamiento de los hipospadias. Ph.D. thesis, University of Valencia, 1964.

43. Moore, F.T. A review of 165 cases of hypospadias. *Plast. Reconstr. Surg.* 22:525, 1958.

44. Mustardé, J.C. Personal communication, November 21, 1969.

45. Mustardé, J.C. Discussion. In V. Consiglio (Ed.), *Atti del Simposio di Chirurgia Riparatrice dell' Uretra.* Bari, Rome: Arti Grafiche Favia, 1970.

46. Nové-Josserand, G. Traitement de l'hypospadias: Nouvelle méthode. *Lyon Med.* 85:198, 1897.

47. Ombrédanne, L. Hypospadias pénien chez l'enfant. *Bull. Mem. Soc. Chir.* 37:1076, 1911.

48. Ombrédanne, L. *Précis Clinique et Opératoire de Chirurgie Infantile.* Paris: Masson, 1923.

49. Planas, J. L'hypospadias. *Acta Urol. Belg.* 30: 357, 1962.

50. Planas, J. Hypospadias. In J.T. Hueston (Ed.), *Transactions of the Fifth International Congress of Plastic and Reconstructive Surgery.* Sydney: Butterworth, 1971. P. 7.

51. Rochet, R. Nouveau procédé pour refaire le canal pénien dans l'hypospadias. *Gaz. Hebd. Méd. Chir.* 4:673, 1899.

52. Russell, R.H. Operation for severe hypospadias. *Br. Med. J.* 2:1432, 1900.

53. Scatafassi, S. *L'Ipospadia.* Bari, Rome: Arti Grafiche E. Cossidente, 1965.

54. Scott, F.B. Correlation of Flow Rate Profile with Diseases of the Urethra in Man. In W. Lutzeyer and H. Melchior (Eds.), *First International Symposium on Urodynamics.* Berlin: Springer, 1973.

55. Stark, D. *Embryologie* (3rd ed.). Stuttgart: Thieme, 1975.

56. Thompson, J.E. A study of modern operations in hypospadias from an anatomical and functional standpoint. *Surg. Gynecol. Obstet.* 25:411, 1917.

57. Van der Meulen, J.C. *Hypospadias.* Springfield, Ill.: Thomas, 1964.

58. Van der Meulen, J.C. Hypospadias and cryptospadias. *Br. J. Plast. Surg.* 24:101, 1971.

59. Wood-Smith, D. Hypospadias: Some Historical Aspects and the Evolution of Methods of Treatment. In J.M. Converse (Ed.), *Reconstructive Plastic Surgery.* Philadelphia: Saunders, 1964. Vol. 5, p. 2010.

60. Young, F., and Benjamin, J.A. Repair of hypospadias with free inlay skin graft. *Surg. Gynecol. Obstet.* 86:439, 1948.

17

HYPOSPADIAS is generally defined as a congenital anomaly in which the meatus is situated on the ventral surface of the penis or in the perineum, owing to anomalous development of the urethra. This simple definition, however, is hardly an adequate description of the complex nature of hypospadias, with its widely varying morphology in which different components are present to varying degrees. To elucidate the problems associated with hypospadias, studies of the etiology and morphology were carried out in a nonselected clinical material comprising 220 primary cases of hypospadias of all types: 4 cryptohypospadias (congenital short urethra), 105 glandular, 87 penile, 7 penoperineal, 10 perineal, and 7 perineal without bulb (Fig. 17-1). Micturition, puberal development, sexual début, and sexual function were investigated in consecutive series in this material, in which the patients were treated during the period 1965 to 1969 and followed up for 8 to 12 years.

Incidence in Sweden

Since the incidence of hypospadias has varied greatly in different investigations, and since these variations were assumed to be due to failure to register the mildest cases of hypospadias, a study of the incidence of hypospadias in Sweden, totally and by type, was carried out [1].

The study was based on cases of hypospadias continuously reported to central malformations registers during the period 1965 to 1968 and extended by follow-up of hypospadiacs treated at specialist departments up until 1973. Altogether 666 live male infants with hypospadias were identified among 480,607 live births of both sexes. The mean incidence of hypospadias was 13.9 per 10,000 births of both sexes, or 2.7 percent, or 1 hypospadias per 371 male infants.

Bengt Johanson
Lars Avellán

OPERATED HYPOSPADIAS

Of the 666 hypospadias, 62 percent were glandular, 30 percent were penile, 2 percent were penoperineal, 3 percent were perineal, and 2 percent were cryptohypospadias; 93.5 percent of the hypospadias were single, and 6.5 percent of the patients had simultaneous malformations.

Etiology

Since Sørensen's study [20] of the etiology of hypospadias showing a familial occurrence of hypospadias in 28 percent of the cases, cytogenetic investigation has been introduced, and the influence of hormonal factors on the etiology has been discussed. It was therefore thought to be of interest to analyze genetic and nongenetic factors in the clinical material [3].

The study showed that heredity was the most important factor, two or more hypospadiacs being identified in 28 families of the 213 index patients. In one family, 10 patients with hypospadias associated with bilateral clinodactyly were identified. This family suggests an autosomal dominant gene as the cause of the hypospadias, and it seems probable that the two malformations were genetically coupled (Fig. 17-2). In the remaining 185 of 213 index patients, the probable etiology was known in 11; in 3 patients, there were chromosomal aberrations (46 XY/45 X0); in 2 there were well-defined syndromes with a known genetic background (G syndrome and Laurence-Moon-Biedl syndrome); in 1 there was maternal diabetes; in 2 maternal rubella; and 2 of the hypospadiacs were born after use of anticonvulsant drugs by the mothers and 1 after use of thalidomide by the mother. In the great majority of cases (174 of 213), neither genetic nor nongenetic factors could be identified.

Morphology

Morphological investigation has been performed by, e.g., Farkas [10], but in view of the complex nature of hypospadias and the consequent variability in treatment and treatment results, an analysis of the morphology in the clinical material was considered necessary [4].

EXTERNAL GENITALIA

The most common shape of the meatus was transverse or longitudinal fissural, followed by the pinpoint type and the type in which the terminal ventral side of the urethra was covered with a thin membrane, the pellucid roof of the urethra (Fig. 17-3). In some hypospadiacs with meatus of the pinpoint type, the meatus was surrounded by soft, yielding tissue which dilated during micturition, while in others it was surrounded by taut, fibrous tissue which was not dilated by the urinary flow. The meatus was judged to be clinically adequate in 50 of 220 patients and inadequate in 170 of 220.

The *depth of the glandular groove* was normal in 66 of 220 patients, shallower than normal in 67, shallow in 77, and marked only in 10.

Vestiges of a *frenulum* were found in 12 patients: in four cryptohypospadias and in eight glandular, in which an undivided prepuce surrounded the glans. In the remaining 208 patients, the frenulum was absent and the prepuce was hooded dorsally.

The *penis* was normally developed in 213 of 220 patients. In one penoperineal hypospadiac with the Laurence-Moon-Biedl syndrome, hypogenitalism was present. In two perineal hypospadiacs with 46 XY/45 X0, the penis was hypoplastic, and in one perineal hypospadiac without bulb with 46 XY/45 X0, and in three with normal male chromosomal composition, the penis was clitoridean.

317

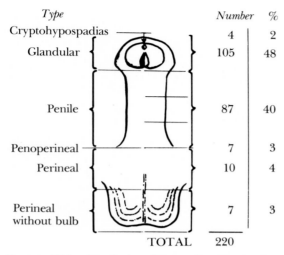

Type	Number	%
Cryptohypospadias	4	2
Glandular	105	48
Penile	87	40
Penoperineal	7	3
Perineal	10	4
Perineal without bulb	7	3
TOTAL	220	

FIGURE 17-1. *Distribution of hypospadias. (Reprinted, with permission, from L. Avellán, On aetiological factors in hypospadias.* Scand. J. Plast. Reconstr. Surg. *11:115–123, 1977.)*

Curvature was observed in 151 of 220 patients (69 percent), 56 of whom were glandular, 67 penile, 7 penoperineal, 10 perineal, 7 perineal without bulb, and 4 cryptohypospadiacs. No curvature was present in 69 of 220 patients.

Torsion was registered in 35 of 220 patients (16 percent), the degree of torsion varying be-

tween 20 and 90 degrees (Fig. 17-4). The rotation of the shaft to the left side was found in 28 and to the right side in 7. The penile raphe deviated in a contralateral direction to the torsion in all 35 hypospadiacs.

The scrotum was of normal appearance in 205 of 220 patients. A partially bifid scrotum was observed in three hypospadiacs: one penoperineal and two perineal. Total bipartition of the scrotum was present in four perineal and seven perineal hypospadiacs without bulb.

In 43 of 220 patients, the scrotal skin completely surrounded the root of the penis, while in 67 patients, it surrounded two-thirds of the root; in 11 patients, it surrounded half the root. In 99 patients, the root of the penis was normal and completely free from scrotal skin.

Normal *testes* were present in the scrotum in 192 of 220 patients; 32 of these were *retractile*, 22 were bilateral, and 10 were unilateral.

Cryptorchism was found in 23 of 220 hypospadiacs, undescended testes being present in the inguinal canal bilaterally in 9 and unilaterally in 14.

One penile hypospadiac (1 of 220 patients) with normal male chromosomal composition had a eunuchoid physical constitution and he showed total anorchism. The diagnosis

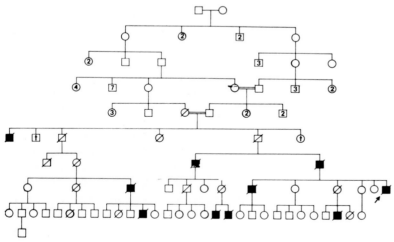

FIGURE 17-2. *Family with 10 penile hypospadiacs, all associated with clinodactyly of the little fingers. Consanguinous marriage is indicated by double lines. ■ indicates the hypospadias and / indicates the clinodactyly. The index patient is indicated by the arrow. (Reprinted, with permission, from L. Avellán, On aetiological factors in hypospadias.* Scand. J. Plast. Reconstr. Surg. *11:115–123, 1977.)*

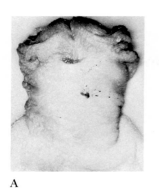
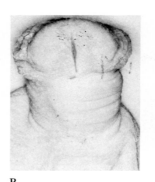
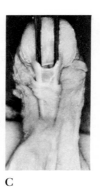
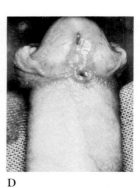

A   B   C   D

FIGURE 17-3.   *Types of meatus. (A) Transverse fissural meatus. (B) Meatus of pinpoint type. (C) Meatus with pellucid roof of the urethra. (D) Meatus of pinpoint type with a fibrotic ring. (Reprinted, with permission, from L. Avellán, Morphology of hypospadias.* Scand. J. Plast. Reconstr. Surg. *In press.)*

was established after bilateral exploratory laparotomy, and the entire area from the scrotum to the inferior pole of the kidney was examined without finding the testes. Aortography revealed bilateral absence of spermatic arteries, and hormonal analysis showed high

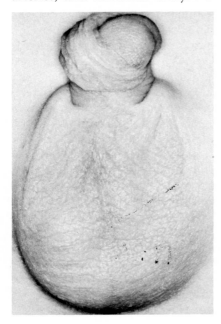

FIGURE 17-4.   *Glandular hypospadias with torsion: 90-degree rotation of the shaft to the left side. (Reprinted, with permission, from L. Avellán, Morphology of hypospadias.* Scand. J. Plast. Reconstr. Surg. *In press.)*

gonadotropin values as further verification of the diagnosis. After substitution hormone therapy, the patient underwent puberty.

Disturbances in gonad differentiation were observed in 4 of 220 hypospadiacs. In one perineal hypospadiac with normal male chromosomal composition, a streak gonad was found on one side and a testis of normal size in the inguinal canal on the other; in one perineal hypospadiac with 46 XY/45 X0, a streak gonad was found on one side and a testis of normal size in the scrotum on the other. In a perineal hypospadiac without bulb with normal male chromosomal composition, a streak gonad was found on one side and a hypoplastic testis in the inguinal canal on the other; and in a perineal hypospadiac without bulb with 46 XY/45 X0, a streak gonad was found on one side and an intra-abdominal fetal testis on the other. All four of these cases were diagnosed as mixed gonadal dysgenesis.

INTERNAL GENITALIA

The internal genitalia were investigated by means of micturition urethrocystography, urethroscopy, or exploratory laparotomy.

Congenital urethral valves (Fig. 17-5) were found in 4 of 220 hypospadiacs, only cases with definite obstruction being counted as valves [16]. Enlargement of the *prostatic utricle* (Fig. 17-6) was found in 3 of 220 patients: in two glandular and one perineal hypospadiac. In 9 of 220 hypospadiacs, a *vagina* opened into the segment of the urethra normally forming the bulb. In two perineal hypospadiacs (Fig. 17-7) and one perineal hypospadiac with 46 XY/45

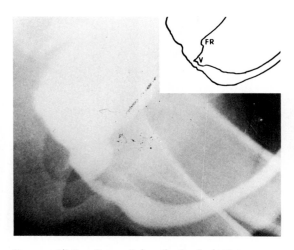

FIGURE 17-5. *Congenital urethral valve with prestenotic dilatation (FR, fundus ring; V, valve). (Reprinted, with permission, from L. Avellán, Morphology of hypospadias. Scand. J. Plast. Reconstr. Surg. In press.)*

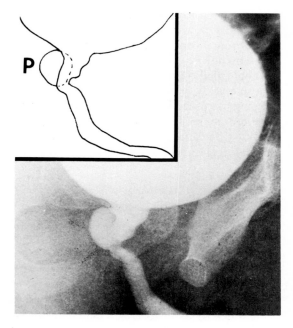

FIGURE 17-6. *Glandular hypospadias with enlarged prostatic utricle (P). (Reprinted, with permission, from L. Avellán, Morphology of hypospadias. Scand. J. Plast. Reconstr. Surg. In press.)*

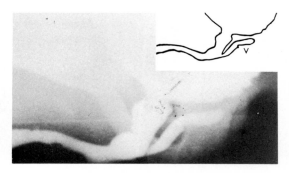

FIGURE 17-7. *Perineal hypospadias without bulb, with vagina (V) from the dorsal part of the bulbous urethra. (Reprinted, with permission, from L. Avellán, Morphology of hypospadias. Scand. J. Plast. Reconstr. Surg. In press.)*

X0 and diagnosed as mixed gonadal dysgenesis, the vagina terminated in a *fetal uterus with a unilateral fallopian tube* with a streak gonad. A vagina was found in six perineal hypospadiacs without bulb and, in two of these patients, diagnosed as mixed gonadal dysgenesis, the vagina terminated in a fetal uterus, a unilateral fallopian tube being present in one case and bilateral fallopian tubes in the other (46 XY/45 X0) (Fig. 17-8). Both patients with unilateral fallopian tubes had on the contralateral side a vas deferens leading from a testis in the scrotum or in the inguinal canal.

Congenital aplasia of the prostate was diagnosed in one perineal hypospadiac with normal male chromosomal composition, 1 of 142 patients who had reached fertile age. Vasovesiculography showed that the vesicles and ejaculatory ducts were longer than normal and that the latter discharged directly into the urethra, which lacked a colliculus but contained an enlarged prostatic utricle. The patient had normal spermiogenesis, verified by aspiration biopsy of the testis, but a functional anomaly in the form of retrograde ejaculation, verified by analysis of a two-glass urine sample after ejaculation.

Absence of the internal sphincter mechanism was found in 2 of 220 hypospadiacs: one glandular and one perineal. Urethroscopy revealed a broad communication between the bladder and the funnel-shaped segment of the urethra, extending to the colliculus, in both cases. Normal spermiogenesis was found in both these hypo-

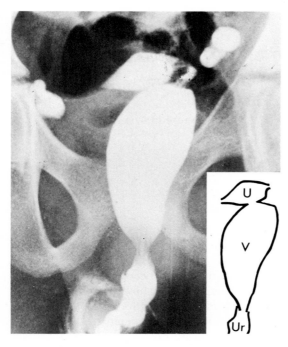

FIGURE 17-8. *Perineal hypospadias without bulb, with vagina (V) from the dorsal part of the urethra (Ur), uterus (U), bilateral fallopian tubes, and a streak gonad on one side and a fetal testis on the other. (Reprinted, with permission, from L. Avellán, Morphology of hypospadias.* Scand. J. Plast. Reconstr. Surg. *In press.)*

spadiacs. The absence of the internal sphincter mechanism led to retrograde ejaculation in both cases, since there was nothing to prevent the semen from being forced backward into the bladder during ejaculation [11, 19]. None of the three patients with retrograde ejaculation had diabetes or neurogenic disorders [9].

Preoperative urography revealed simultaneous malformations in the upper urinary tract in 7 of 220 hypospadiacs, as follows: a double renal pelvis and double ureters in one glandular and one perineal hypospadiac, a unilateral double renal pelvis and single ureter in two penile hypospadiacs, a high ureter insertion of the Östling type in one penile and one penoperineal hypospadiac, and a unilateral ectopic kidney in one penile hypospadiac.

Congenital malformations outside the urogenital system were found in 15 of 220 hypospadiacs. In 5 patients, *multiple* simultaneous

malformations were found: hydrocephalus, cleft lip and cleft palate (with congenital diabetes), unilateral cleft lip and cleft palate and hypertelorism (G syndrome), congenital loss of hearing and coarctation of the aortic isthmus or persistent ductus arteriosus (rubeolaembryopathy) in two hypospadiacs, and polydactyly of both hands and feet, obesity, and mental retardation (Laurence-Moon-Biedl syndrome). In 10, *singular* simultaneous malformations were found: hydrocephalus, unilateral cleft lip and cleft palate, unilateral cleft lip, cleft palate, congenital megacolon (Hirschsprung's disease), ventricular septal defect, unilateral pes valgus, bilateral hypoplasia pollicis and hallucis, bilateral syndactyly of the feet, and unilateral postaxial polydactyly.

Treatment Principles

The aim when correcting hypospadias was to enable the boy to urinate in a normal manner from early childhood and to create conditions for normal development of the penis as a functional sexual organ in adulthood. In order to meet these objectives, a special treatment schedule was drawn up [6] (Table 17-1). This schedule requires hypospadias to be *diagnosed* during the first year of life, preferably at the maternity hospital.

Opinions differ as to the *optimal time* for initiation of surgical treatment, but we have been unable to find objective evidence in support of any of these views. Our study of micturition in hypospadiacs [5] showed that in 18 of 61 hypospadiacs, changes occurred preoperatively as a result of infravesical obstruction in the form of trabeculation, diverticula, vesicoureteral reflux, and dilation of the ureters as early as at the age of 2 to 4 years, and that the highest incidence of changes (22 of 51) occurred between the ages of 4 and 10 years. The most marked regression of these changes was observed when surgical treatment was started at the age of 2 to 4 years.

An *obstruction in the urethra* is the only absolute indication for surgical treatment of hypospadiacs during early childhood. It is therefore

TABLE 17-1. *Treatment Schedule*

Test	Age		Operation
Uroflometry			Meatotomy
Urography	3	Stage 1	Resection of valve
Micturition urethrocystography			Straightening or urethral construction
	4	Stage 2	Urethral construction
Uroflometry	5		
Uroflometry	12		
Micturition urethrocystography	17		

important above all to determine whether or not an obstacle to urination is present. In the study of micturition using a Brotherus uroflometer [7] in a consecutive series of 148 of 220 hypospadiacs, the maximal flow preoperatively was within the normal range for age in a control material in 72 of 148 patients (49 percent), above the upper limit in 57 of 148 (38 percent), and below the lower limit in 19 of 148 (13 percent). The value of preoperative uroflometric investigation, therefore, seemed questionable. The most important information on obstruction, its location and any effect on the urinary tract, is obtained by micturition urethrocystography.

When the obstruction was caused by *meatal stenosis*, meatotomy was performed. But meatotomy was also carried out when the meatus was nearly adequate, in view of the fact that urethral construction was to be performed at the second stage. The chief objective of this procedure was to construct a urethra with the same lumen as the normal, proximal urethra, and a prerequisite for this was that the meatus of the proximal urethra had a sufficiently large lumen and was surrounded by corpus spongiosum.

When the obstacle to flow consisted of a *congenital urethral valve*, transurethral resection of the valve was performed.

In order to achieve the objective of normal development of the penis as a functional sexual organ in adulthood, *curvature with or without torsion* had to be corrected at the same time that

obstacles to urination were eliminated. Curvature and torsion were determined by examining the boy in the morning when he awoke and a normal physiological erection occurred. This reliable method also showed whether or not only a glandular curvature was present. Correction of curvature was performed in all cases, even in those with only a glandular curvature, because untreated glandular curvature can cause sexual difficulties in adulthood. Torsion was always corrected simultaneously with the curvature.

Method of Operation

During the years 1946–1949 Browne [8] used his method with a buried strip of intact epithelium for urethral construction in 51 hypospadiacs operated on at The Hospital for Sick Children, London. In 1950, Johanson [13] was given an opportunity to follow-up 48 of these patients and concluded that the method had given a functional urethra in all types of hypospadias, that the caliber was adequate with respect to the patient's age, that the tube had grown without causing strictures or curvature, and that the tube was sufficiently elastic for normal erection.

In view of these experiences, Johanson continued to develop the method and has used it since 1950 [14].

The surgical treatment has been performed in *two stages*: meatotomy or meatotomy in combination with straightening in stage 1 and urethral construction according to Browne in stage 2. In occasional patients with meatal stenosis in which the urethra after meatotomy drained on the ventral side of the glans or into the coronal sulcus, urethral construction was not indicated, and in a few cases with adequate meatus and absence of curvature, the only surgical procedure at stage 1 was urethral construction according to the Browne method.

FIRST STAGE

Meatotomy (Fig. 17-9).   The distal extension of a circular corpus spongiosum is determined, via the meatus, using fine-tissue forceps. A suture is then applied, via the meatus, in the midline through the anterior wall of the urethra, where the corpus spongiosum is circular, and marks the proximal limit of the incision. The incision is complete when an adequate lumen with circular corpus spongiosum has been achieved. The suture is tied, and the mucosa is attached to the skin by means of two or three more sutures.

Straightening (Fig. 17-10).   The incision in the coronal sulcus on the ventral side, including

half the circumference, is made with a knife. The first short cuts are made on the ventral side with small, straight, sharp-pointed scissors via the incision while maintaining traction with a towel clip in the opposite direction to the curvature. The curvature is caused by a connective tissue-spongioid plate on the ventral surface of the penis, continued laterally on either side. The plate is separated from its fixation to the shaft of the penis by multiple short cuts, taking care to leave the tunica albuginea intact. Careful separation is also carried out for a considerable distance on both sides, where the plate consists of connective tissue only. As the plate is separated, the curvature is successively corrected and the plate retracts toward the base of the penis, the tissue accumulating just distal to the meatus. The so-called chordee is thus not excised. When the area between the coronal sulcus and meatus has been completely freed from the fixation and the tunica albuginea is denuded, the curvature has been eliminated. With this technique, the shaft of the penis is lengthened longitudinally, but at the same time the transverse fixation within the ventral half of the circumference is released, so that the diameter of the shaft also increases. Skin flaps, consisting mainly of the inner layer of the pre-

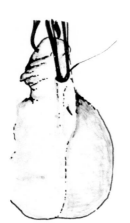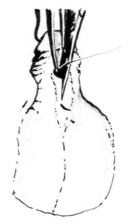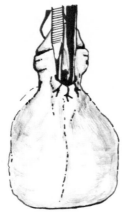

FIGURE 17-9.   *Meatotomy. The body of the penis is held during operation by a towel clip fixed in the glans. Suture is inserted via meatus in the midline to indicate the location of circular corpus spongiosum and to fix the mucosa. Using ordinary straight operating scissors, the ventral wall of the*   *urethra is cloven in the midline in a proximal direction into a lumen of normal caliber and circular corpus spongiosum. The mucosa is sutured to the skin with chromic catgut (4-0) around the meatus.*

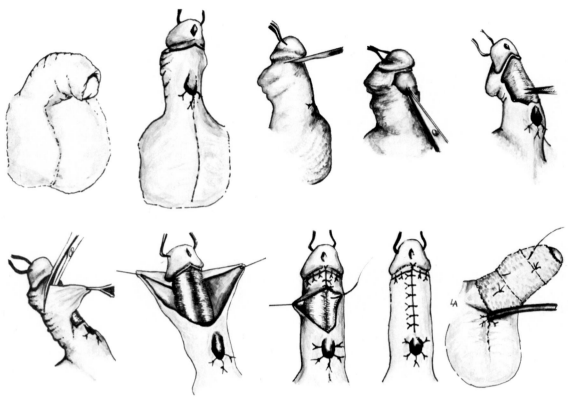

FIGURE 17-10. *Straightening. Incision in the coronal sulcus is indicated. The incision is made with a knife. The connective-tissue spongioid plate is separated by multiple, short cuts with small, straight, sharp-pointed scissors from the fixation to the shaft of the penis, keeping the shaft stretched by means of a towel clip with traction in the opposite direction to the curvature. The connective-tissue spongioid plate is completely separated within the area between the coronal sulcus and meatus and for a considerable distance on either side, and the curvature is corrected. The connective-tissue spongioid tissue is retracted and accumu-* *lates just distal to the meatus. Rotation flaps mainly consisting of the inner layer of the prepuce are mobilized bilaterally. The apices of the flaps are sutured with chromic catgut (4-0) to one another and to the coronal sulcus in the midline. Within the midline the flaps are sutured to one another and to the shaft of the penis. Suturing is completed. The bladder is drained by means of an indwelling catheter in the urethra. The penis is wrapped in ribbon gauze soaked with paraffin and flavine and fixed with nylon sutures (4-0) to the fascia of the penis.*

puce, are mobilized bilaterally and rotated inward over the defect on the ventral side of the penis. Using chromic catgut, the apices of the flaps are sutured to one another and to the coronal sulcus in the midline, and then along the coronal sulcus. In the midline the flaps are sutured to one another and to the shaft of the penis.

When the defect on the ventral side of the penis is longer than the skin flaps, the flaps are extended by bilateral incisions before being sutured to one another and to the shaft of the penis. In order to achieve temporary hemostasis during the operation and to provide a clear view of the operation field, the surgeon compresses the dorsal part of the shaft of the penis between the thumb and index finger of his left hand.

Diversion of Urine. The bladder is drained by means of an indwelling catheter in the urethra. Free urination is permitted after 1 week.

Dressing. The penis from the glans is wrapped in ribbon gauze soaked with paraffin and flavine and fixed with sutures to the fascia of the penis for 1 week.

Correction of Torsion. Torsion is caused by connective tissue extending from the base of the penis on one side diagonally across the ventral side of the penis to the contralateral, distal part of the shaft. It is corrected at the same time as the curvature by separating the diagonal, connective tissue so that the shaft rotates into the normal position.

SECOND STAGE

The following factors must be borne in mind when carrying out urethral construction. In order to achieve a perfect urethra according to Browne's method, the buried strip of epithelium has to be of good quality. Since the strip of epithelium will include the scar in the midline after straightening, the scar must be soft. The urethral construction is therefore performed after an interval of 1 year.

The buried strip must be left intact with its bed. Its breadth along the shaft of the penis, where the strip is firmly attached to the underlying tissue, should be equivalent to about two-thirds of the inner circumference of the constructed tube; the remaining one-third is obtained by secondary epithelialization [13].

Urethral construction is carried out, provided that the meatus has been adequately preserved. If the clinical assessment and uroflometric investigation have given the least evidence of a nonadequate meatus, remeatotomy is performed before urethral construction terminates the treatment 1 to 2 months later.

Urethral Construction (Fig. 17-11). When marking the incision lines for the buried strip of epithelium from the meatus to the tip, the breadth of the strip should be taken into consideration. The lumen of the proximal, normal urethra provides a good guide for assessment.

The skin on the ventral side of the penis must not be stretched during marking, because a strip which appears to be adequate during tension will prove too narrow after relaxation of the skin. The incision is started with scissors proximally in the skin over the normal urethra, taking care to avoid damaging the corpus spongiosum urethrae. When the scissors have incised the skin over the urethra, they are situated in the right tissue layer and the continued incision in a distal direction can be made without difficulty. Care must be taken to leave the tunica albuginea intact. The right tissue layer having been reached, the bilateral penile or penoscrotal flaps can be mobilized without difficulty, and good viability is ensured. The angle at the apex of the flaps should be 90 degrees.

To secure a broad adaptation of the flaps along the ventral side and so relieve the tension on the skin edges during healing, special double-stop sutures, designed by Browne, are employed. This entails the use of glass beads next to the skin, outside of which aluminum cylinders are threaded on and crushed upon the sutures. The suture material for the skin edges consists of chromic catgut in the coronal sulcus and nylon along the ventral side. The knots should not be tied too tightly. A relaxation incision should always be made on the dorsal side of the penis.

Diversion of Urine. In cases with penile localization of the meatus, diversion of urine is accomplished by means of perineal urethrostomy with a Malecot catheter, according to the method reported by Browne, and in cases with penoperineal and perineal localization of the meatus, by means of a suprapubic trocar cystostomy. The catheters are removed after 10 days, and free micturition is permitted.

Dressing. The penis is wrapped in ribbon gauze soaked with paraffin and flavine and fixed with nylon sutures to the fascia of the penis. The circular dressing is removed after 1 day. Careful checks that no blood or seroma

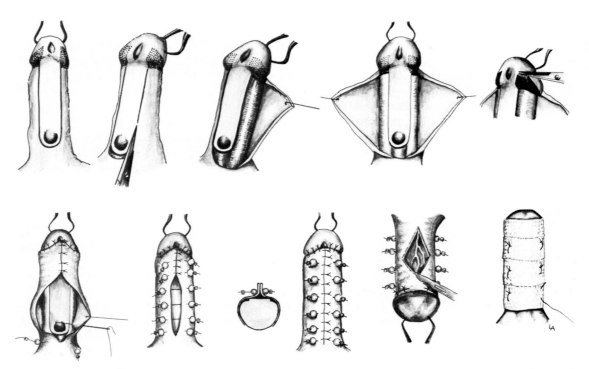

FIGURE 17-11. *Urethral construction. The line of the incision and the area that will be deepithelialized on either side of glandular groove are marked. For the incision, small, straight, sharp-pointed scissors are used. The incision is started in the skin over the normal, proximal urethra and continued distally. The flaps are prepared by stripping them off the very adherent glandular skin on either side of the groove. The first suture with chromic catgut (4-0) fixes the apices of the flaps, which are right-angled, to the two deepithelialized areas. Double-stop suture with nylon (4-0) is inserted, showing the distance to the skin margin.*

Suturing is completed: in the coronal sulcus, chromic catgut (4-0), and in the skin edges in the midline exactly, by fine sutures with nylon (5-0). The cross section shows the localization of the buried strip and the distance between the crushed aluminum cylinder and glass bead. The dorsal relaxation incision is spread wide open. The incision just goes through the skin, leaving the subcutaneous venous plexus intact. The penis is wrapped in ribbon gauze soaked with paraffin and flavine and fixed with nylon sutures (4-0) to the fascia of the penis.

remains under the flaps, and that the skin under the glass beads is not exposed to too much pressure, are made each day. The double-stop sutures are removed after 1 week. No medication is given during this postoperative phase.

At *closure of a postoperative fistula*, the fistulous track should be excised in toto, and the surrounding skin should be freely undermined and broadly adapted, using double-stop sutures, to bury the hole in the urethral wall. A suprapubic trocar cystostomy is performed for urinary diversion. The catheter is removed after 10 days, and free micturition is permitted.

The Treated Series

THE FIRST SERIES, 1950–1955

The first series of hypospadiacs was operated on with this method by Johanson during the years 1950–1955 at Karolinska Hospital, Serafimer Hospital, and Kronprinsessan Lovisa's Children's Hospital, Stockholm, and the University Hospital in Lund and Malmö, Sweden. The series comprised altogether 276 hypospadiacs: 220 primary cases (3 cryptohypospadias, 76 glandular, 94 penile, 14 penoperineal, 20 perineal, and 13 perineal without bulb) and 56 secondary cases. Among the primary hypospadiacs, meatal stenosis was noted in 61 of 220 (28 percent) and curvature in 152 of 220 (69 percent). In stage 1, meatotomy was performed in 24 patients, straightening in 113, meatotomy in combination with straightening in 39, urethral construction in 35, and only reduction of the dorsal prepuce in 9. Stage 2—urethral construction—was performed in 162 patients. After urethral construction, complications occurred in 8 of 220 patients, in the form of separation of the skin flaps, and in 12 of 220 as fistulae. Reoperation with urethral construction was performed in 8 and fistula closure in 12, all with fully satisfactory results. The short-term results (5 months to 1½ years after operation) were very satisfactory with respect to clinical findings and function. No systematic follow-up of these patients has been performed because of their geographical distribution over the whole country.

THE SECOND SERIES, 1957–1969

During the years 1957–1969, 299 primary cases of hypospadias (6 cryptohypospadias, 155 glandular, 110 penile, 10 penoperineal, 11 perineal, and 7 perineal without bulb) were treated by the same method at the Department of Plastic Surgery, Sahlgrenska sjukhuset, Göteborg, Sweden. Meatal stenosis was noted in 121 of 299 patients (40 percent), curvature in 201 of 299 (67 percent), and torsion in 36 of 299 (12 percent) (Table 17-2). Congenital urethral valves were found in 10 of 299 patients (3 percent). In stage 1, meatotomy was performed in 95 patients, meatotomy in combina-

TABLE 17-2. *Distribution of Meatal Stenosis, Curvature, and Torsion*

Number		Meatal Stenosis	Curvature	Torsion
271		121	173	36
28			28	

TABLE 17-3. *Operations*

Number		Stage I			Stage II
		Meatotomy	Meatotomy and Straightening	Urethral Construction	Urethral Construction
271		95	173	3	258
28			28		28

tion with straightening in 201, and urethral construction in 3. Stage 2—urethral construction—was performed in 286 patients (Table 17-3). Transurethral diathermic cutting of the valves was performed in 10 patients.

Complications. After meatotomy in combination with straightening, remeatotomy was considered indicated in 8 of 299 patients: in 5 on clinical grounds, although the maximal flow was within the normal limits, and in 3 because the maximal flow was below the lower normal limit. After urethral construction, complications occurred in *5 of 299 patients (2 percent) in the form of separation of the skin flaps and in 6 of 299 (2 percent) as fistulae.* Reoperation with urethral construction was performed in five patients and fistula closure in six, all with fully satisfactory results.

Follow-up of the Results of Operation

The conventional follow-up of the results of surgical treatment in hypospadiacs has mainly consisted of clinical observations without detailed analysis of the *functional results.* Our treatment schedule entailed follow-up with uroflometric control at the ages of 5 and 12 years and micturition urethrocystography at the age of 17. For assessment of the functional results of urethral construction, continuous uroflometric follow-up of the maximal flow was necessary, while for assessment of the functional results of straightening, determination of the age of sexual début and information on sexual function were required. For these assessments, *consecutive series* were subjected to annual control examinations.

Micturition studies were performed preoperatively, interoperatively, and postoperatively in a consecutive series comprising 148 of 220 hypospadiacs, both short-term results (on average 1.25 years after the last operation) and long-term results (on average 6.25 years after the last operation) being recorded. In our investigation [5] a Brotherus uroflometer [7] (Fig. 17-12) was used which, by means of a special chair, enables uroflometric investigations to be performed even in small children.

The clinical material was subdivided into six age groups, and the results were compared with a control material comprising 176 males. High maximal flow values were consistently recorded preoperatively in the hypospadiacs: in

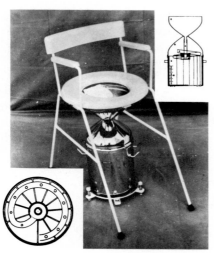

FIGURE 17-12. *Components of the Brotherus uroflometer with chair-pot. Sagittal section of the segmented collector with a scale in each compartment (upper right). Transverse section of the spiral distributing tube with outlets into compartments (lower left). (Reprinted, with permission, from L. Avellán, Morphology of hypospadias. Scand. J. Plast. Reconstr. Surg. In press.)*

38 percent the values were above, in 49 percent within, and in 13 percent below the normal limits for the corresponding age group in the control material. Interoperatively, after meatotomy had been performed in all cases, a further increase of the maximal flow was recorded. Both the short- and long-term postoperative results showed a successive decline in maximal flow toward the control levels (in the long-term results 26 percent of the values were above the upper normal limit and 76 percent within the normal range). The scatter around the regression lines was greatest preoperatively, as a result of the great variations in meatus caliber, with a gradual decrease after urethral construction, as a result of more uniform caliber.

Preoperative *micturition urethrocystography* revealed pathological changes in 48 of 148 patients: trabeculation only in 29, trabeculation and diverticula in 5, vesicoureteral reflux in 14, 3 of them having dilated ureters in addition to changes of the bladder. The highest incidence of changes (22 of 51) was found in the age group 4 to 10 years and the second highest (18 of 61) in the age group 2 to 4 years. Among these patients with pathological lesions, maximal flow was within the normal range in 27 of 48 and above the upper limit for age group in the control material in 18 of 48. Postoperative micturition urethrocystography revealed a successive regression of the pathological changes. After, on average, 10.6 years, vesicoureteral reflux was present in two hypospadiacs only, one of whom had a slightly dilated ureter unilaterally. The most marked regression of the changes was recorded when surgical treatment was started at the age of 2 to 4 years.

Because of the consistently high maximal flow values, the value of preoperative uroflometry seemed questionable, but follow-up of the results of surgical treatment showed it to be an objective method of investigation. For follow-up in older children and adults, *timed micturition*, introduced by Johanson [13], is a simple and useful method of objective flow measurement.

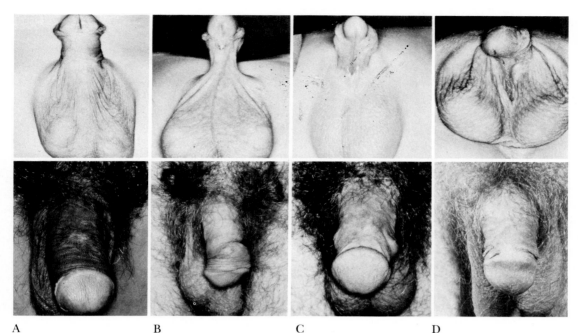

A   B   C   D

FIGURE 17-13.   *The development of the genitals in hypospadiacs is evaluated according to Tanner. Preoperatively, they are all in stage 1, aged 8 to 9 years. At follow-up, they are all in stage 5, aged 18 years. Types of hypospadias: (A) glandular, (B) penile, (C) penoperineal, (D) perineal. The flaccid penises in parts A through D are* *of normal size. At follow-up the erection was examined in all cases at age 18 years or more, and the size in the erect state was normal. (Reprinted, with permission, from L. Avellán, The development of puberty, the sexual début and sexual function in hypospadiacs. Scand. J. Plast. Reconstr. Surg. 10:29–44, 1976.)*

SEXUAL DÉBUT AND SEXUAL FUNCTION

Israel, Gustavsson, Eliasson, and Lindberg [12] have shown that an early sexual début is dependent on early puberty. Our investigation, therefore, included puberal development for assessment of the sexual début and sexual function in hypospadiacs [2].

In a consecutive series, *puberal development* was followed for a decade, and a longitudinal study of height and weight, development of pubic hair, and development of the genitals and testes was performed. With regard to *height and weight,* development was normal in 175 of 220 hypospadiacs followed, except for six patients, three of whom had chromosomal aberrations (46 XY/45 X0).

For assessment of *pubic hair,* Tanner's [21] classification was used. The results of the investigation of 127 of 220 hypospadiacs were compared with the findings in a normal material reported by Marshall and Tanner [17] and showed normal development of pubic hair in the hypospadiacs, except in five patients, three of whom had chromosomal aberrations.

The development of the *genitals* was investigated in a consecutive series consisting of 124 of 220 hypospadiacs (3 cryptohypospadias, 64 glandular, 53 penile, 1 penoperineal, 2 perineal, and 1 perineal without bulb) aged 10 to 18 years (Fig. 17-13). Tanner's classification, consisting of five stages, was used. In *stage 1,* preadolescent, testes, scrotum, and penis are of about the same size and proportion as in early childhood. In *stage 2,* enlargement of scrotum and testes, the skin of the scrotum reddens and changes in texture. Little or no enlargement of penis occurs at this stage. In *stage 3,* enlargement of penis occurs, at first mainly in length. Further growth of testes and scrotum occurs. In *stage 4*, increased size of the penis occurs, with growth in breadth and development of glans. Further enlargement of testes and scrotum occurs, and there is an increased darkening of scrotal skin. In *stage 5*, the genitals obtain adult size and shape. No further enlargement takes place after stage 5 is reached. On the contrary, it seems that the penis decreases slightly in size from the immediate postadolescent peak.

The mean values for the different stages in hypospadiacs were in agreement with those in normal subjects, except for retardation in 5 of 124 patients. Of the latter, three patients with chromosomal aberrations remained underdeveloped, while the other two patients showed retarded development and reached stage 5 at 21 and 23 years of age, respectively.

Testicular growth was followed in a consecutive series consisting of 177 of 220 hypospadiacs in the age group 8 to 18 years. The longitudinal axis of the testes was measured with a sliding caliper, as described by Quaade [18], and the results were compared with findings in normal subjects. Testicular development in the hypospadiacs was found to be normal, except for 16 of 177 patients (12 with cryptorchism, 1 with total anorchism, and 3 with chromosomal aberrations).

The age at first ejaculation, *ejacularche*, is an important criterion of biological maturity. The first ejaculation is observed at masturbation. Of 192 of 220 hypospadiacs aged 10 years or above, 117 stated when they had first observed ejaculation. The median age at ejacularche was 12.9 years. The cumulative distribution by age at ejacularche in hypospadiacs showed good agreement with a corresponding distribution in a normal population reported by Kinsey, Pomeroy, and Martin [15]. Lack of ejacularche was recorded for three hypospadiacs with retrograde ejaculation and one with total anorchism.

On the basis of these investigations, hypospadiacs were judged to undergo normal puberty, except for the three hypospadiacs with chromosomal aberrations.

Of the 117 hypospadiacs who had had the ejacularche, and the 3 with retrograde ejaculation and 1 with total anorchism, altogether 121 of 220 patients aged between 13 and 30 years, 66 (55 percent) had had sexual intercourse, while 55 (45 percent) had had no experience of sexual intercourse. The median age for the *sexual début* was 16.9 years. The cumulative distribution by age at the sexual debut in hypospadiacs showed good agreement with the findings in Zetterberg's study [22]. The median age in Zetterberg's material was slightly lower, 16.6 years. The 55 hypospadiacs who had had no experience of sexual intercourse showed no significant deviation from the pattern in the normal population, except in the age group 16 to 20 years, where the percentage was lower in hypospadiacs than in the normal population.

The influence of surgical treatment on the sexual début was investigated in 121 of 220 hypospadiacs, divided into two groups: one group in which treatment was terminated at the age of 12 or earlier and another group in which treatment was completed at the age of 13 or above. The age for the sexual début was lower in the first group (median age 15.5 years) than in the second group (median age 17.6 years).

Of the 55 of 220 hypospadiacs who had had no experience of sexual intercourse, five patients (two penoperineal, one perineal, and two perineal without bulb) stated that this was a direct result of the hypospadias and felt that their penises were underdeveloped. Of these five patients, the penis was of clitoridean type in two perineal hypospadiacs without bulb; in one penoperineal hypospadiac with the Laurence-Moon-Biedl syndrome, there was a hypogenitalism; and in the other two hypospadiacs, the penis was of normal size, both in the flaccid and erect states. The remaining 50 hypospadiacs who had had no experience of sexual intercourse stated that their sexual abstinence was not due to the hypospadias.

Sexual Function. All 66 of 220 hypospadiacs who had had sexual intercourse stated that they had continued their sexual activity more or less regularly after the sexual début. In seven hypospadiacs who had had their début at age 13 to 14, there was a delay of 1 to 2 years before taking up regular sexual activity, while in the age group 15 to 20 years, the level of sexual activity was high in 46. Among patients aged 21 years or above, 13 reported regular sexual activity.

Forty-one hypospadiacs were married (62 percent). Twenty-four of them had children. In 17 cases, the marriage was childless. This was involuntary in five cases only: two cases with retrograde ejaculation, one with total anorchism, one with a streak gonad and an intra-abdominal testis, and one with cryptorchism and bilateral hypoplastic testes. The remaining 12 hypospadiacs exhibited normal spermiograms and normal ejaculate volumes.

The study showed that correction of hypospadias enables the penis to develop normally into a functional sexual organ.

Long-Term Results

At first operation, the mean age of the 220 hypospadiacs was 8.5 years, the median age 4.4, and at the latest control the mean age was 18.4 years, the median age 15.1 (Table 17-4). The mean interval between operation and follow-up was 7.1 years.

CLINICAL FINDINGS
The meatus was vertically positioned in the glans in 76 of 220 patients, transversally positioned in the coronal sulcus in 133, and was lying directly proximal to the sulcus in 11. The position and extent of the meatus accorded with the depth of the glandular groove: in 66 patients the depth was normal, in 144 it was shallow, and in 10 it was marked.

DORSAL RELAXATION INCISION
In 210 of 220 hypospadiacs in whom urethral construction was carried out, the scar after the relaxation incision on the dorsal side of the penis was mostly broad, always soft, and yield-

TABLE 17-4. *The Age at First Operation and the Latest Control*

Age Group	The First Operation (Number)	The Latest Control (Number)
1–3	78	—
4–7	70	—
8–11	29	18
12–15	10	91
16–19	12	56
20–29	13	38
≥30	8	17
Total	220.0	220.0
Median age	4.4	15.1
Mean age	8.5	18.4

ing without signs of keloid. In 9 patients, the area showed slightly increased pigmentation.

DEVELOPMENT OF THE PENIS
In 213 of 220 hypospadiacs, the penis was normally developed for age. In 138 the penis had reached Tanner's stage 5: genitals of adult size and shape. In 7 patients, the penis was underdeveloped: hypogenitalism in a penoperineal hypospadiac with the Laurence-Moon-Biedl syndrome, hypoplastic penis in two perineal hypospadiacs with chromosomal aberrations, and clitoridean penis in four perineal hypospadiacs without bulb, one of these with chromosomal aberrations.

MICTURITION
In all 220 hypospadiacs, the maximal flow values were within the normal range for the relevant age group in the control material. *Significant bacteriuria* (at least 100,000 bacteria per milliliter of urine) was found postoperatively in 6 of 220 patients, and prostatitis was diagnosed in two of these patients. We have not seen a single case of prostatitis since we started advising the patients at routine controls to urinate after intercourse. All 220 hypospadiacs were free from bacteria at the latest control.

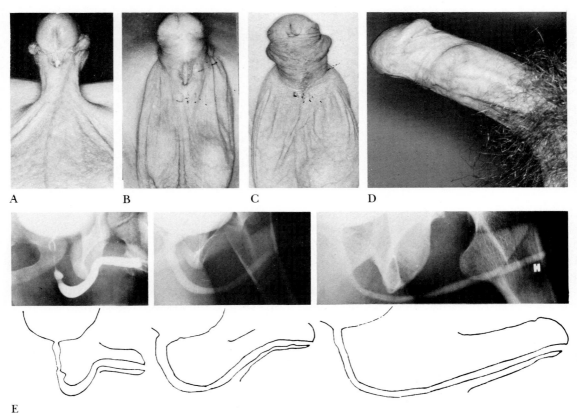

E

FIGURE 17-14. *Penile hypospadias. (A) Preoperatively, age 8 years; (B) after meatotomy and straightening, age 9 years; (C) after the urethral construction, age 10 years; (D) normal size of penis in the erect state, age 18 years; (E) micturition urethrocystography in the same hypospadiac after the urethral construction, age 10, 14, and 18 years.*

The *erection* was examined in all 220 hypospadiacs and no signs of curvature or torsion could be detected (Fig. 17-14). Of 220 hypospadiacs, 142 have reached fertile age with the ejacularche within the normal age period.

The latest *micturition urethrocystography* showed an adequate urethra without signs of stricture within the area between the proximal, normal, and constructed urethra. Bilateral vesicoureteral reflux was still present in two hypospadiacs; both of them had had bilaterally dilated ureters preoperatively, but regression had occurred, and at the latest control a slightly dilated ureter was found unilaterally in one patient only.

Conclusions

When assessing the long-term results, we found that the conclusions drawn by Johanson 28 years ago after following up Browne's hypospadias patients were also valid for the present study.

Complications necessitating additional surgical measures occurred during the treatment: after stage 1, remeatotomy was performed in eight hypospadiacs, and after stage 2, urethral reconstruction was carried out in five and closure of fistulae in six of 299 patients.

The complications after stage 2 were a direct consequence of inadequate observation during the 10 days of diversion of the urine. Johanson emphasized the importance of this point in connection with reconstruction of the male urethra in strictures, with regard both to the diversion of the urine and to the local area of operation.

References

1. Avellán, L. The incidence of hypospadias in Sweden. *Scand. J. Plast. Reconstr. Surg.* 9:129, 1975.
2. Avellán, L. The development of puberty, the sexual début and sexual function in hypospadiacs. *Scand. J. Plast. Reconstr. Surg.* 10:29, 1976.
3. Avellán, L. On aetiological factors in hypospadias. *Scand. J. Plast. Reconstr. Surg.* 11:115, 1977.
4. Avellán, L. Morphology of hypospadias. *Scand. J. Plast. Reconstr. Surg.* To be published.
5. Avellán L. Micturition studies in hypospadiacs. *Scand. J. Plast. Reconstr. Surg.* To be published.
6. Avellán, L., and Johanson, B. Preoperative and Postoperative Evaluation. In C.E. Horton (Ed.), *Plastic and Reconstructive Surgery of the Genital Area.* Boston: Little, Brown, 1973.
7. Brotherus, J.V. Über die Uroflowmetrie. *Urol. Int.* 15:205, 1963.
8. Browne, D. An operation for hypospadias. *Proc. R. Soc. Med.* 42:466, 1949.
9. Ellenberg, M., and Weber, H. Retrograde ejaculation in diabetic neuropathy. *Ann. Intern. Med.* 65:1237, 1966.
10. Farkas, L.G. *Hypospadias.* Prague: Academia, 1967.
11. Hotchkiss, R.S., Pinto, A.B., and Kleegman, S. Artificial insemination with semen recovered from the bladder. *Fertil. Steril.* 6:37, 1955.
12. Israel, J., Gustavsson, N., Eliasson, R.-M., and Lindberg, G. Sexuelle Verhaltungsformen der Schwedischen Gross-Stadtjugend. In H. Giese (Ed.), *Modellfall Skandinavien? Sexualität und Sexualpolitik in Dänemark und Schweden.* Hamburg: Rowohlt, 1970.
13. Johanson, B. Reconstruction of the male urethra in strictures. *Acta Chir. Scand.* [Suppl.] 176:5, 1953.
14. Johanson, B., and Avellán, L. Hypospadias: A review of 299 cases operated 1957–69. *Scand. J. Plast. Reconstr. Surg.* To be published.
15. Kinsey, A. C., Pomeroy, W. B., and Martin, C.E. *Sexual Behavior in the Human Male.* Philadelphia: Saunders, 1948. P. 182.
16. Kjellberg, S.R., Ericsson, N.O., and Rudhe, U. *The Lower Urinary Tract in Childhood.* Stockholm: Almqvist & Wiksell, 1957. P. 204.
17. Marshall, W.A., and Tanner, J.M. Variations in the pattern of pubertal changes in boys. *Arch. Dis. Child.* 45:13, 1970.
18. Quaade, F. Estimate of testis volume by measurement of testis length in an autopsy material. *Acta Endocrinol.* (Kbh.) 20:268, 1955.
19. Rose, S.S. An investigation into sterility after lumbar ganglionectomy. *Br. Med. J.* 1:247, 1953.
20. Sørensen, H.R. *Hypospadias, with Special Reference to Aetiology.* Copenhagen: Munksgaard, 1953.
21. Tanner, J.M. *Growth at Adolescence* (2nd ed.). Oxford: Blackwell, 1962. P. 1.
22. Zetterberg, H.L. *Om Sexuallivet i Sverige.* Stockholm:Nordiska Bokhandeln, 1969.

Alan D. Perlmutter

COMMENTS ON CHAPTERS 16 AND 17

TRULY long-term data on the results of hypospadias repair, including psychosexual adjustment and reproductive capability, have been sparse. Both these comprehensive reviews, demonstrating very different operative approaches and management, make a substantial contribution to the literature on hypospadias. Both reinforce the conviction of many of us that hypospadias surgery is indeed complex and challenging and best done under the supervision of experts. These reports raise a number of practical and philosophical questions that are not yet resolved.

How necessary is a glandular meatus? It is certainly not essential for directed voiding or insemination when the orifice is sufficiently distal. Hinderer and associates feel that an intraglandular urethra is aesthetically important, and his results are impressive. The price, however, to achieve this is an elaborate operative procedure with a significant complication rate and a prolonged course of management, including an indwelling catheter through the defunctioned neourethra for 9 months and the need for a final, albeit minor, procedure to close the mature perineal urethrostomy.

Alternatively, Johanson and Avellán, using the classic Browne repair, bring the meatus onto the glans by triangular denudation of glans epithelium on either side of the glans groove at the time of urethroplasty. There are remarkably few complications, and the results seem very satisfactory, although the cosmetic appearance of the ventral glans is slightly compromised at times. Ultimately, the meatus in their series assumed a coronal sulcus position in somewhat over half their patients, presumably from dehiscence or retraction, and was positioned in the glans in the remainder. Sommerlad [7], in a long-term follow-up of 60 hypospadias repairs, 24 by the Browne technique, observed the new meatus to be retracted more than 1 cm proximal to the glans pit in almost half the patients. Although he felt that the patients generally did not seem concerned about

the retracted meatus, it is my clinical impression that many older children, when given a choice, will elect to have a retracted meatus advanced.

Regardless of the type of hypospadias repair, if skin has been attached to either side of the glans groove at the initial procedure, such as described by Smith [6] or as utilized in a variety of one-stage repairs, then it is very simple to revise the retracted meatus using the ventrolateral skin attachments still flanking the glans groove to advance the meatus and snug it across the groove. I have even done this as an ambulatory surgical procedure at times. One advantage of having skin flaps attached to denuded glans triangles is to allow for construction of a meatus on the glans even when the glans groove is shallow.

I have only infrequently used glans-penetrating or glans-splitting procedures to position a neomeatus. I have generally preferred to place the meatus on the glans, but not within it, by using the glans pit as the roof and sides of the meatus. The floor may be a tiny flap of skin turned up from the ventral shaft or the lateral edges can be closed directly as in a Thiersch-Duplay procedure, but in either instance the ventral-shaft skin defect is replaced with a rotation flap of skin, generally from one side of the preputial hood, which is advanced onto the ventral glans to cover the meatoplasty. This approach is applicable to distal shaft hypospadias, including release of minor chordee, as a one-stage procedure. Appropriate trimming of the flap allows for a snug and cosmetically satisfactory meatus and glans.

The issue of what effort is justified in creating an intraglandular meatus must remain unresolved, although from an aesthetic standpoint a normally positioned meatus is the ultimate achievement.

Is preoperative urethral obstruction a significant problem? Johanson and Avellán, on the basis of urinary flow measurements, observed a diminished flow rate in 13 percent of boys preoperatively. While such data is sobering, and while we can offer no data to refute their findings, the significance must be questioned. In a series of over 300 cases of hypospadias, our group has not been impressed that urethral obstruction in the untreated patient often poses a clinical problem with either obstructive symptoms or disturbances of micturition. Some boys will have a narrow-appearing but rubbery and elastic hypospadic meatus which causes no apparent alteration of urinary flow. A few, of course, do have true meatal stenosis. Aside from these, we have not, in our series, routinely done preliminary meatoplasty. When severe chordee is present, we have elected in a one-stage procedure to extend the urethra by a tubed pedicle graft from the prepuce, such as described by Hodgson [3] or Toksu [8]. If necessary, the proximal meatus can be incised or resected as far as needed to create an adequate lumen before anastomosing the skin-tube extension.

More measurements of urinary flow rates are needed to determine the significance, if any, of the observed reduction below the mean of some unoperated boys with hypospadias. Postoperatively, this study should be an excellent and objective means of assessing the adequacy of urethroplasty.

The literature on psychosexual adjustment after hypospadias repair is somewhat contradictory. Farkas and Hynie [1] published a follow-up report on 130 previously operated adults which was pessimistic in tone, indicating that, although normal sexual function could be expected after adequate repair, many men abstained from sexual relations because of feelings of abnormality and inferiority. However, this article did not detail the ages at surgical repair, the kinds and numbers of operations required, and the functional and cosmetic results. Sommerlad [7], in long-term follow-up of 60 patients repaired by the Browne or Ombrédanne technique, reported generally satisfactory sexual function, but observed that about one-third of the group had been sufficiently self-conscious about their deformity to avoid changing clothes publicly at school. Half had

suffered adolescent anxiety regarding future sexual function and fertility, and a majority still regarded their penises as abnormal. A recent, optimistic report by Kenawi [4] was based on a retrospective mail survey. However, a response rate of only 23 percent may bias his data. Because of its detailed observations, the current report by Johanson and Avellán is particularly reassuring with regard to the normalcy of sexual function and practice after repair and thus is a most valuable reference. Those patients whose repair was completed by the age of 12 years had an earlier onset of sexual activity, comparing favorably with normal peers.

Nevertheless, there are patients who have problems adjusting. We need more studies on body-image perceptions in people with hypospadias, relating them to such objective findings as the aesthetic and functional results of repair, age at surgery, the type and number of procedures, and complications. This might resolve the discrepancy among reports in the literature.

For those few patients with severe hypogenitalism, what is an adequate phallus? Objectively, a penile size which allows for satisfactory sexual performance and partner satisfaction is adequate, but subjectively, the patient may feel inadequate. To develop criteria for penile adequacy, we have been recording measurements of penile size at various ages using the nomograms of Schonfeld [5] for stretched penis length and width for children and adults and the nomograms of Feldman and Smith [2] for newborns. We feel this is a valid approach, since the stretched penis closely approximates the erected penis in length.

On the basis of data thus far available, it appears that skillful and appropriate hypospadias repair in early childhood is least likely to result in later sexual dysfunction; most patients will function normally as adults. These two fine chapters make significant contributions to the art of hypospadias surgery and address themselves to a number of issues which should stimulate further investigations from other centers.

References

1. Farkas, L.G., and Hynie, J.   Aftereffects of hypospadias repair in childhood. *Postgrad. Med.* 47:103, April 1970.
2. Feldman, K.W., and Smith, D.W.   Fetal phallic growth and penile standards for newborn male infants. *J. Pediatr.* 86:395, 1975.
3. Hodgson, N.B.   A one-stage hypospadias repair. *J. Urol.* 104:281, 1970.
4. Kenawi, M.M.   Sexual function in hypospadias. *Br. J. Urol.* 47:883, 1976.
5. Schonfeld, W.A.   Primary and secondary sexual characteristics: Study of their development in males from birth through maturity, with biometric study of penis and testes. *Am. J. Dis. Child.* 65:535, 1943.
6. Smith, D.   A de-epithelialised overlap flap technique in the repair of hypospadias. *Br. J. Plast. Surg.* 26:106, 1973.
7. Sommerlad, B.C.   A long-term follow-up of hypospadias patients. *Br. J. Plast. Surg.* 28:324, 1975.
8. Toksu, E.   Hypospadias: One-stage repair. *Plast. Reconstr. Surg.* 45:365, 1970.

18

TWENTY years ago the repair of hypospadias was considered one of the most difficult of all reconstructive operations. Multiple-staged procedures followed by a high incidence of complications were the rule. The good end result was usually typified by a straight penis, with the meatus in an abnormal position under the glans. Frequently, the skin was redundant and uneven. The aesthetic appearance was not considered to be of much importance. Surgery was not usually contemplated in infancy and was deferred until the patient was of school age or older. Chordee was felt to be difficult to correct, and recurrence of chordee, resulting from new growth of abnormal fibrous tissue in the penile area, was a concept accepted by many. All authorities agreed that urethroplasty should not be done if any chance of recurrence of chordee existed. Therefore, the urethroplasty was customarily completed in older-aged individuals where erections and urinary diversion with bladder spasms and pain were the expected, not the unusual. Meatal stenosis frequently complicated every attempt to bring the urethra to the tip of the glans, causing most surgeons to accept a standard of normalcy if the meatus was reconstructed to any site near the coronal sulcus. Older patients retained bad memories of painful, complicated healing. An occasional innovative surgeon had previously reported single-stage repairs of hypospadias; however, this concept was considered dangerous and improper by most plastic and urological surgeons who performed the majority of hypospadias repairs.

It was about this time that the authors elected to collaborate on all hypospadias repairs, to combine the specialty talents of both plastic surgery and urology. McCormack [6] had re-

Charles E. Horton
Charles J. Devine
John B. McCraw

THE EVOLUTION OF A HYPOSPADIAS REPAIR

ported simultaneous urethroplasty and chordee release, but no series of one-stage hypospadias repairs were available for consideration and evaluation (Table 18-1). Our first efforts were directed toward procedures allowing adequate exposure of the ventral penile surface to remove (effectively) all restricting bands causing chordee. A graft was utilized for urethral reconstruction since it was felt that local flaps would have impaired vascularity because of the wide surgical dissection.

All repairs done since by the authors have been characterized by wide surgical exposure with adequate chordee release (Fig. 18-1). We conclude that if adequate resection of all abnormal tissue is performed, no tissue regrowth of congenital chordee will appear, and the penis will be straight unless hematomas or external skin scarring produces curvature. This conclusion has been verified in over 750 cases of hypospadias repair performed subsequently.

The grafts we first used for urethroplasty were thick split-thickness grafts which had a tendency to contract to a size smaller than was acceptable. In 1956 we changed our technique to employ a full-thickness graft from a hairless area of the body, usually the upper inner arm or groin. At that time we felt it was essential to preserve all tissue of the prepuce, which might be required later for penile coverage. Full-thickness grafts taken in areas other than from the penis mature and soften more slowly than preputial skin grafts. We noted that the inner leaf of the folded prepuce was thin, hairless, and would make an ideal graft for urethroplasty. In addition, the vascularity of this tissue, when used as a flap, is not good. In the usual hypospadias case, this graft tissue available from the prepuce will form a tube extending

from the perineum to the tip of the glans, leaving adequate additional preputial tissue for ventral coverage of the penis. Preputial skin became our choice of full-thickness graft tissue for urethroplasty, and only in extremely unusual cases of previous loss of prepuce and penile tissue will we construct a urethra from other skin. If necessary, we will take a full-thickness graft from the dorsum of the penis for urethroplasty and cover the defect of the penile surface with a split-thickness graft.

For ventral skin coverage we first utilized the well-popularized "buttonhole" perforated preputial flap. This technique left prominent dog ears laterally and usually required secondary scar revisions. Later the technique of midline splitting of the prepuce, as popularized by Byars, was adopted as routine. This gave well-vascularized surface coverage and less tissue distortion. Most flap tissue transferred was still left in excess in early cases, always with the consideration that fistula repair and other surgical procedures "might" be necessary and extra tissue needed.

Another problem noted infrequently concerned the anastomosis between the graft and the existing urethra. Although an oblique union was normally constructed, a stricture occasionally occurred at this site as a result of the semicircular anastomosis. A much larger "tongue in groove" anastomosis was utilized as we developed confidence in the basic technique. This radical oblique anastomosis now is rarely a source of difficulty.

As confidence was gained with this early technique, it was found that each operation was proving to be easier with wider and more unlimited exposure. The entire shaft of the penis was routinely uncovered and the entire pre-

TABLE 18-1. *Evolution in Our Surgical Treatment of Hypospadias*

1. Simultaneous release of chordee and urethroplasty
2. Split-thickness grafts (STG) urethroplasty
3. Full-thickness grafts (FTG) urethroplasty
4. Preputial full-thickness grafts
5. Ombrédanne buttonhole flaps
6. Division of prepuce in midline with lateral flap coverage
7. Large, oblique "tongue in groove" anastomosis of skin grafts
8. Wide surgical exposure of entire shaft
9. Use of adrenalin to aid hemostasis
10. Early operations (ages 2 to 3)
11. Use of 6-0 chromic catgut throughout repair and in skin
12. Elastoplast four-tailed dressing
13. Frequent tubbing after 3 days
14. Ophthalmic-tipped tube with ointment in meatus postoperatively
15. Lateral glandular flaps
16. Midline glandular flaps
17. Release of chordee beneath the glans
18. Flip flap
19. Careful tailoring of skin, leaving no excess "tabs"
20. Lateral reinforcing subcutaneous flaps
21. Artificial distention of penis with saline
22. Flaps taken from a distance for "cripples"
23. Early removal of urethral diversion of distal cases
24. Fluorescein dye to evaluate flap viability
25. Dermal grafts to tunica albuginea
26. Voiding urethrogram
27. Circumcision approach to fistulae
28. Cold compresses and elevation of penile area postoperatively

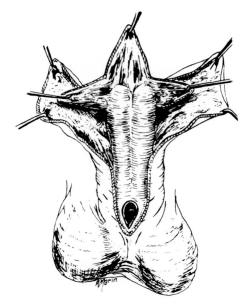

FIGURE 18-1. *Wide exposure of corporal bodies and existing urethra allows complete resection of all tissue causing chordee.*

puce unfolded, thereby allowing a better evaluation of the problem by the surgeons.

With wider exposure it became increasingly necessary to consider the problem of hemostasis. Initially a tourniquet was used around the base of the penis. However, this restricted exposure and did not seem to aid in the total control of bleeding. This was abandoned. The judicious use of 0.5 ml of 0.5% Xylocaine with adrenalin 1:200,000 injected in the area of sur-gery, supplemented with pressure by flexing the penis over a finger, has given superior hemostasis over the years. The patient must be deeply anesthetized, for light anesthesia causes straining and bucking of the patient, with filling of the penis with blood and excess blood loss.

The routine use of the cautery for hemostasis is recommended. However, in over half of our cases, we do not encounter a bleeding vessel large enough to require coagulation. If a drain is deemed desirable, we do not hesitate to drain. However, most cases do not need this.

As experience was gained, it was noted that older patients were harder to manage. We felt the tissue causing chordee became more fibrotic with age, that patients bled more with the more difficult dissection required, and that post-operative erections were more common. Suture removal was more difficult, pain and memory recall were more intense, and the fear of surgery was more real in children of older ages. We concluded that since clinical and laboratory data demonstrated that full-thickness grafts grow without restricting growth, earlier hypo-spadias repair would be desirable. So at the present time, when the phallus is large enough to operate on, we do the surgery. This is usually at 1 to 2 years of age, although we have operated as early as 8 months on a well-developed penis. If the penis is not large, we recommend deferral of surgery. The use of systematic or local testosterone is not usually necessary.

Another refinement of technique includes the use of chromic catgut for all skin sutures in order to avoid holding a struggling child to remove permanent skin sutures. We first used 4-0 and 5-0 chromic catgut in the skin. However, this persisted in the skin for 2 to 3 weeks and caused local irritation. We tried 6-0 chromic catgut, but the usual 6-0 chromic catgut was difficult to see. It was noted that dyed ophthalmological blue suture was available on a small cutting needle, which allowed easy visualization of the suture. Spontaneous early dissolution of 6-0 chromic catgut suture in the skin occurs and makes this our suture of choice. Newer types of absorbable sutures which are hydrolized are retained in the skin too long if used for skin sutures. However, we frequently use them for subcutaneous repair.

Securing a bandage to the penile area can be difficult. By cutting a 4-in. elastoplast into a four-tailed strip, the top area can be used to place accurate but limited pressure around the penis postoperatively, while the "tails" secure the bandage to the area at the base of the penis. When a catheter is used postoperatively, it is desirable to carry the catheter superiorly onto the abdomen to prevent constant pressure on the glans flaps, which may cause dehiscence of the glans suture line. By incorporating the catheter into the elastoplast bandage on the abdomen, stabilization of the catheter in the proper direction is obtained. Bleeding into the bandage can cause a firm clot with pressure necrosis of underlying tissue. The bandage is now being removed on the first day postoperatively after pressure and a cold sterile compress have been applied for a few hours.

The skin of the penis is thin and does not gain wound strength rapidly. It can be easily pulled apart after 3 to 4 days of healing. Because the anus is nearby and can contaminate, because urine must be evacuated through or near the repair, and because erections which pull on the incision areas postoperatively occur even in infants, the suture lines must be given particular attention. We found that massive penile skin edema occurred when no bandage was applied. When a bandage is removed, care must be taken to avoid pulling the incisions apart. After the initial dressing is removed, the patient is tubbed three times a day to soak away the remaining bandages and to keep the area clean. No further bandages are used.

When a catheter is left in place postoperatively for several days, we have routinely been using a voiding cystourethrogram to determine whether or not the urethra is intact after the catheter is withdrawn from the bladder and urethra. By allowing the patient to void, we can see if fistulous tracts are imminent because the dye will appear in the subcutaneous tissues of the penis. If the dye does extravasate beyond the urethra, a new catheter is put into the hypospadias repair and retained for another 5 to 7 days to allow the weakened area of the urethra to heal more properly. We feel this technique has reduced the number of complications by preventing fistulae which were not well developed but which were likely to occur in the future had not the catheter been replaced.

An infrequent cause of fistulae formation appeared to us to be the formation of bloody crust in the penile meatus, effectively "corking" the urethra so that when urination is attempted, back pressure occurs and a proximal leak (fistula) results. Tubbing three times daily helps to prevent crusting. Further prevention is obtained by instructing the nurse and mother to take an ophthalmic-tipped tube of antibiotic ointment and apply the ointment to the meatus several times a day while gently inserting the tip of the tube into the meatus. This cleans, softens, and clears the discharge which would otherwise accumulate, dry, and plug the meatus.

Until 1966, no totally new concept of hypospadias repair had been incorporated into our technique. Only modifications and extended uses of previously described techniques were

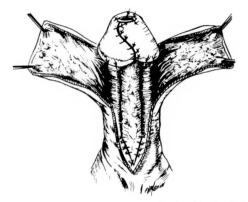

FIGURE 18-2. *Urethroplasty completed, with glandular flaps for distal coverage of the tubed full-thickness graft. The preputial flaps will be brought ventrally for closure of the skin.*

employed at one time to produce a one-stage repair. Several attempts had been made to penetrate the glans using a "punch" to "core out" tissue to construct the meatus to the tip, but most cases had postoperative meatal stenosis in the glans. We then decided to mobilize the glans, to produce a flap which could be inserted into the distal circular anastomosis (Fig. 18-2). We first used two lateral flaps, but then later combined them into a large central flap. This allowed adequate mobilization of the lateral glandular wings, which provided an unexpected bonus in that, for the first time, it could be seen that the bands causing chordee inserted into the glans and actually produced a flexion of the glans onto the shaft of the penis. Other operations had been described which suggested excision of the dorsal tunica albuginea to prevent glans flexion. However, we feel that if the chordee is released adequately by exposing the undersurface of the glans, then flexion is automatically corrected. The plastic surgical principle that insertion of a flap into a circular incision prevents contracture in the glans has been noted, and no major loss of glans from the elevation of the glandular flap has occurred. This permitted changing the shape of the abnormal flat glans to a normal conical appearance and the construction of the urethral meatus at the tip of the glans. We con-

tinue to use this technique and feel it is one of our most important contributions to hypospadias repair [1–4].

At this time, enough confidence has been gained to change from a conservative attitude to a more confident approach regarding the external appearance of the penile shaft. Previously we had left all excess skin tissue, rationalizing that if the repair "broke down," we would need all possible skin for subsequent surgery. Realizing that we had never had a complete "breakdown" and that the 20 percent complication rate (10 years ago) which had occurred in approximately 250 primary cases usually consisted of a small fistula 1 to 2 mm in size, we decided to discard all excess skin and make the penis appear as normal as possible at the initial operation. Actually, the tissue we then began to discard was the least substantial, less well vascularized tissue, and the remaining tissue healed even better and more uneventfully.

As we discarded skin, it became apparent that one flap of the denuded prepuce could be identified as having better blood supply by simply observing the vessels that supply the prepuce. This one flap was usually sufficient to resurface the penis in distal cases. Instead of totally discarding the other preputial flap, the subcutaneous tissue was carefully dissected from the skin and used as a subcutaneous tissue flap to give double coverage to the urethroplasty area (Fig. 18-3). The excess skin over the subcutaneous flap was then excised. This has helped reduce the fistulae rate in our last 100 cases to 6 percent. This technique is not always possible in more proximal cases.

Recently, several authors have reported that chordee is usually caused by a skin shortage ventrally and that deeper fibrous tissue does not cause chordee in some cases. To determine this, we have effectively used artificial erection of the penis with saline to produce an erection in the operating room [5]. We conclude that in some cases which appear to have no deep chordee and are distended, true deep chordee can be demonstrated by this technique. We also use the artificial distention technique routinely to

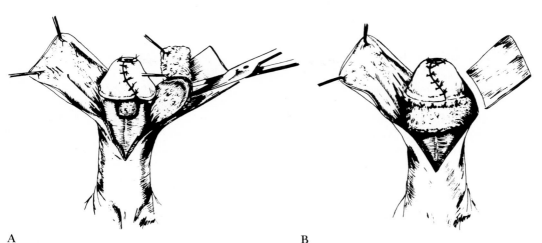

A

B

FIGURE 18-3.   *In distal hypospadias cases, when one flap from half the prepuce will be adequate for ventral coverage, we use a subcutaneous flap from the opposite preputial area, which would otherwise be discarded. This* *gives double coverage for the urethroplasty. (A) Dissecting the subcutaneous tissue from the preputial flap. (B) Subcutaneous closure over urethroplasty.*

check all patients before beginning the urethroplasty to make certain the penis is straight. This technique is essential in hypospadias cripples and in cases of penile curvature with diverse etiologies.

When previous surgery has caused extensive scarring of the tunica albuginea resulting in a permanent chordee which cannot be corrected by the removal of congenital dysplastic tissue, then a decision must be made whether or not the central tunica albuginea should be elongated with a dermal graft or the dorsal tunica albuginea shortened by excision of an ellipse of normal tissue. Each case must be individualized and a decision made according to the circumstances existing. However, we frequently employ dermal grafts to elongate a scarred ventral surface to correct chordee.

In complicated cases where chordee is not present and multiple fistulae exist, we feel that external inspection of the old constructed urethra is important. We routinely look through the lumen of the urethra with a cystoscope to check its internal configuration, and we commonly get dye contrast studies to see where the urethra is deficient. However, it has only been recently that we have made a circumcising-like incision and retracted all the

skin of the penis down from over the urethra so we can accurately look at the length of the abnormal and insufficiently repaired urethra. This allows us to identify diverticula, strictures, flow disturbances from valves, scar torsion, and other problems which contribute to fistulae formation. By retracting the penile shaft skin proximally and looking at the urethra in its entire length, an accurate diagnosis of the problem can be made, and the problem can be corrected by simple closure of the urothelium, by adding a patch graft of free full-thickness preputial or penile skin onto the urethra, or by excising the diverticulum and releasing the scar tissue. When the penile shaft skin has been retracted over the repaired urethra, it can be rotated slightly to the side so the original fistulae openings can be closed a distance from the underlying fistulae stricture repairs.

Although this chapter is primarily concerned with technique development over a long term for hypospadias patients, it should be mentioned that as experience is gained in genital reconstructive techniques, much benefit is derived in approaching complicated failure cases after many previous unsuccessful operations. We have not hesitated to employ large scrotal flaps, island groin flaps based on the superficial circumflex iliac artery, or the gracilis-muscle-skin island flap recently described by McCraw [7]. We do not hesitate simultaneously to (1) correct chordee, (2) construct the urethra from penile skin, and (3) resurface from local or distant areas when necessary.

A most valuable technique which has offered assistance in this complicated problem is that of using fluorescein for determination of the vascularity and viability of skin flaps and glandular tissue. If we have doubt regarding the blood supply of the flap for penile resurfacing, 5 ml of fluorescein dye is injected IV (in the usual 1- to 2-year-old patient). Directing an ultraviolet light on the surgical area in a darkened operating room will identify viable tissue, which fluoresces, and allows discarding of nonviable skin flaps. Local adrenalin must not be used in these cases.

We have recently changed our dressing technique. The penile skin is thin and acts similarly to eyelid skin, which swells with edema as a response to local trauma. To combat the postoperative edema, we used occlusive dressings for many years. We allowed the patients to ambulate early and rest in bed with the head elevated and the penile area dependent. It was no wonder that the postoperative edema was not successfully handled with this treatment. We would not expect blepharoplasty patients to sleep with the head down, and most surgeons now use cold compresses to combat edema. Employing these same principles, we elevate the foot of the bed, place a pillow under the buttocks, and use cold sterile saline continuous compresses postoperatively for 3 days. We have been amazed at the lack of edema, the patient acceptance, and the good healing which has occurred in these patients.

We have followed our hypospadias repairs for many years and have noted normal growth of the penis and urethra in all cases. Many patients have become fathers in the interim. No patient has complained of sexual inadequacy in any way after a successful repair of hypospadias in infancy. All patients feel normal and look normal. While none of our patients have had children with hypospadias, we have had several twins with hypospadias and several brothers and father-son combinations with hypospadias.

Most operative techniques do not develop spontaneously and instantaneously. We owe a great debt to the many surgeons who contributed building blocks that have allowed us to construct our present hypospadias technique. This technique has now progressed so that it is reproducible by the experienced hypospadias operator. It has been successful in 92 of the last 100 cases done by us.

Conscientious surgeons must now determine whether they can in good faith continue to offer to their patients a philosophy requiring many operations for hypospadias repair, which in the best hands still has a high complication rate postoperatively, or whether they will adapt to a new time and technique which produces less trauma, less risk, and a better cosmetic and functional result with one-stage surgery for hypospadias.

Not all surgeons should do hypospadias repairs. The occasional operator will unintentionally harm or produce complications which are difficult to correct. Scarring and loss of local tissue which can be used for urethroplasty and penile resurfacing cannot be overcome; the tissue lost is not returnable or reproducible elsewhere in the body.

Interested teams made up of members of the specialties of plastic surgery, urology, and pediatric surgery should be formed to provide centers for care for this complicated problem. We have an obligation as physicians to prevent hypospadias cripples who have had multiple surgeries for hypospadias and whose prognosis for total effective rehabilitation is forever diminished.

References

1. Devine, C.J., and Horton, C.E. Hypospadias repair. *J. Urol.* 118:188, 1977.
2. Horton, C.E., and Devine, C.J. Hypospadias and

Epispadias (a Ciba Foundation Clinical Symposium). Vol. 24, No. 3. Summit, N.J.: CIBA Pharmaceutical Co., 1972.

3. Horton, C.E., and Devine, C.J., Jr.   One-stage Repair. In C.E. Horton (Ed.), *Plastic and Reconstructive Surgery of the Genital Area.* Boston: Little, Brown, 1973. Pp. 273–289.

4. Horton, C.E., and Devine, C.J.   Simulated erection of the penis with saline injection: A diagnostic maneuver. *Plast. Reconstr. Surg.* 59:138, 1977.

5. Horton, C.E., Devine, C.J., and Gursu, K.G.   Review of recent advances in hypospadias surgery. *Hacettepe Bull. Med. Surg.* 7:37, 1974.

6. McCormack, R.M.   Simultaneous chordee repair and urethral reconstruction for hypospadias. *Plast. Reconstr. Surg.* 13:257, 1954.

7. McCraw, J.B., Massey, F.M., Shanklin, K.D., and Horton, C.E.   Vaginal reconstruction with gracilis myocutaneous flaps. *Plast. Reconstr. Surg.* 58:176, 1976.

Robert M. Goldwyn

COMMENTS ON CHAPTER 18

THE authors have given us the distillate of more than two decades of treating the difficult problem of hypospadias. In addition to the valuable content of their chapter, the authorship itself is instructive. It represents the union of two specialties, the summation of whose talents has been responsible for the numerous innovations in this field by the senior authors.

As noted by Drs. Horton, Devine, and McCraw, the principal development in the evolution of hypospadias repair has been the realization that a one-stage procedure at an early age is feasible [1, 6]. No longer is it necessary in the majority of cases to perform multiple operations before completing the job in adolescence [5]. This does not mean that even today, there might not be some patients who would require more than one procedure, but at least, many more will not.

Furthermore, over the past 20 years, standards regarding the end result are much higher than they were. The patient is no longer expected to endure, for example, persistent chordee, once a fairly common finding.

The previous chapters by Drs. Johanson and Avellán and by Dr. Hinderer as well as the comments by Dr. Perlmutter refer to other investigations of late results after hypospadias repair. One of these few studies [8] already mentioned was by Farkas and Hynie [2] of 130 Czech patients age 18 years or older who had had either an Ombrédanne or a Nove-Jossèrand repair. They found that the penis was straight in all patients and that micturition was unobstructed. Although they did not assess fertility, they found diminished sexual activity in many patients and attributed it to psychological factors. Helmig [3], however, in an 8- to 29-year follow-up of 103 of 349 patients who had surgery for hypospadias found that their "sexual lives were those of the average population" in terms of masturbation, intercourse, orgasm, and fertility. Most of these patients did complain about the absence of medical guidance in these matters and attributed their lack of inferiority complex to "understanding partners."

In another excellent review of 113 patients, cited by Dr. Perlmutter, Sommerlad [7] was able to recall for examination 60 patients, of whom 24 had the Browne repair and 30 the Ombrédanne procedure. Only 20 percent of the 60 patients who returned had "unpleasant memories" of their hospitalization. A large majority, 43 of the 60, still regarded their penes as abnormal. In general, those who had had Browne repairs were most concerned about the size, and those who had had the Ombrédanne procedure were distressed about the shape, particularly the redundant skin. By measurement, 9 of the 60 patients had an abnormally small penis in the flaccid state. The Browne procedure was associated with more chordee. Also, the new meatus was rarely at the level of the pit in the glans and was more than 1 cm proximal to it in almost half the cases, no matter what type of surgery had been performed. Urethral fistulae were present in five patients, four of whom declined treatment for it. In more than half the patients, the meatal size was larger than normal. With regard to micturition, the urinary stream was deflected downward from the line of the penis in most patients. Of more annoyance to the patients was spraying, which occurred in over two-thirds of each group. In those who had the Ombrédanne repair, there was a correlation between meatal size and spraying: the larger the meatus, the worse the spraying. No such correlation was found in the Browne group. Because of spraying, over a quarter of the patients, particularly those who had the Ombrédanne repair, found it difficult to use a urinal, and several habitually sat down to urinate. Over two-thirds of the individuals in each group had had sexual intercourse, and only four complained of pain during it, presumably related to abnormal skin tightness. Of interest was the finding that in Sommerlad's patients there was little difference in penile size and chordee and psychological trauma (not assessed in depth) between those who had had numerous procedures and those who had only one or two.

Long-term observations of patients may

347

yield unsuspected information. Hörmann and Brandt [4], for example, using retrograde urethrography, found that several patients who had a perineal urethrostomy in conjunction with the hypospadias surgery developed a stricture, a fistula, or a diverticulum attributable to the urethrostomy and not to their condition of hypospadias or to the repair.

This chapter by Drs. Horton, Devine, and McCraw is, in their words, an account of the evolution of their thinking about hypospadias and their methods of correction. Evolution, of course, is not finite, and with time their already excellent results will be even further improved.

References

1. Broadbent, T.R., Woolf, R.M., and Toksu, E. Hypospadias: One-stage repair. *Plast. Reconstr. Surg.* 27:154, 1961.

2. Farkas, L.G., and Hynie, J. Aftereffects of hypospadias repair in childhood. *Postgrad. Med.* 47:103, 1970.

3. Helmig, F.-J. Langzeitergebnisse nach Hypospadie-Operationen. *Klin. Paediatr.* 186:421, 1974.

4. Hörmann, D., and Brandt, R. Spatveranderungen von Harnrohren nach Perinaler Ableitung in Kindesalter. *Z. Urol.* 66:585, 1974.

5. MacCollum, D.W., Longino, L.A., and Meeker, I.A., Jr. The treatment of hypospadias. *Surg. Clin. North Am.* 36:1, 1956.

6. Mustardé, J.C. One-stage Repair. In C.E. Horton (Ed.), *Plastic and Reconstructive Surgery of the Genital Area.* Boston: Little, Brown, 1973. Pp. 290–297.

7. Sommerlad, B.C. A long-term follow-up of hypospadias patients. *Br. J. Plast. Surg.* 28:324, 1975.

8. Tamir, D., Hirshowitz, B., and Mahler, D. Treatment of hypospadias. A 10 year follow-up study. *Harefuah* 81:370, 399, 1971.

19

THE age of hair transplantation actually began in the early 1960s following the publication in 1959 of Orentreich's classic paper entitled "Autografts in alopecias and other selected dermatological conditions" [6]. Orentreich described the results of transposing multiple, free, skin-punch grafts to areas of alopecia and other sites having certain dermatological disorders. Similar punch grafts for treatment of alopecia had been done many years before Orentreich by other investigators, notably Okuda [5]. He constructed metal punch-graft instruments with diameters of 2 to 4 mm, and with these he transplanted hair-bearing grafts to areas of alopecia in exactly the same manner as described by Orentreich. Because of the war, his work was not noticed, and his original procedures have not been acknowledged. Other surgeons [1, 3] described several types of local flaps for transposing hair to bald areas of the scalp. These techniques did not receive popular acceptance, however.

Orentreich's experiments were done to study the site factors in the pathogenesis of certain skin conditions. As a result of these experiments, he coined the terms *donor dominant* and *recipient dominant*. Donor dominance was used to denote skin autografts which maintained their integrity and characteristics independent of the recipient site. Donor dominance was demonstrated with hair-bearing grafts transposed to areas of alopecia. When a graft containing hair was transplanted in a bald area of the scalp, it retained the hair and continued to grow hair indefinitely. The hair also kept the same color, density, and texture as its donor origin. Moreover, the hair continued to grow at the same rate and with the same period of anagen that regulated the inherent character of the hair in the donor site. This suggested that the pathogenesis of common male baldness is inherent in each individual hair follicle. Oren-

Charles P. Vallis

HAIR TRANSPLANTS

treich felt that each hair follicle is genetically predisposed to respond or not to respond to androgenic and/or other influences that inhibit its growth.

The fact that the transplanted hairs grow indefinitely and will continue to live as long as they would have lived in their original donor site refutes the theory that human baldness is due to "chronic activity of the scalp muscles leading to shearing stresses in the dermis of the scalp and consequent ischemia" [8]. The circulation in the areas of baldness is not diminished. It really has nothing to do with the onset of baldness in the male. After hundreds of transplant procedures, I have been convinced that the circulation in the areas of baldness is just as good as, if not better than, the areas where hair growth has persisted. Transplants also have been done to replace hairs in traumatically scarred areas of the scalp. In areas of scarring, the circulation is obviously markedly diminished, and yet when hair-bearing autografts are transplanted in these areas, the hair follicles will survive and will continue to grow hair indefinitely.

Until recently, baldness was always treated as a disease. Every concoction conceivable has been recommended since the dawn of history for the treatment of baldness. Baldness has always been looked upon by many as a condition caused by a sickness, infection of the scalp, poor circulation, lack of vitamins, poor nutrition, lack or oversupply of hormones, emotional tension, etc. Consequently, someone is always looking for a cure. There is nothing to cure. Male pattern baldness is a natural phenomenon [4], like being tall or short, left-handed or right-handed, blond or brunette. The enigma of baldness lies in the fact that it affects men at different ages and rates and assumes different patterns of hair loss. Many men become severely bald before the age of 21, while others

still have dense hair growth in their late sixties and seventies. In some men baldness proceeds gradually, while in others it occurs as a rapid and even precipitous loss of hair.

Male pattern baldness is controlled by normal male hormone (androgen) levels. However, a man will develop male pattern baldness only if he has a genetic predisposition, i.e., he inherits a gene for baldness from either his father or his mother or both. Hair follicles on the scalp have different periods of longevity depending on their genetic makeup, and consequently, they will respond to the male hormone stimulus under different timetables during the man's life. Women also commonly lose hair in a pattern fashion. Their loss is usually a diffuse thinning throughout the entire scalp. A pattern similar to the male may show up in some women. Women usually produce less male hormone (androgen) than the male, thereby lessening the hormonal effect on the hair follicle. It has been shown that when women are treated with the male hormone testosterone, as in certain forms of cancer, approximately 30 percent will demonstrate some diffuse loss of scalp hair. Some investigators also think that the gene for baldness is dominant in the male and recessive in the female.

Until we understand the complexities of the inherited predisposition to baldness and the action of the male (androgenic) hormones, as well as the effect of the normal aging process, we will continue to flounder in our attempts to arrest or at least retard baldness. It is probable that further progress in the prevention of male pattern baldness will not take place until we have a better understanding of the effect of the male hormone on hair follicles. If the aging effect of the male hormone on the hair follicle could somehow be blocked without disturbing its other more important functions, then a medical cure for baldness would be in the making. At the present time we have to be satisfied with hair transplantation as the only method available that will replace healthy, normal-growing hair to the bald areas of the scalp. In the past two decades we have come closer to a better understanding of hair growth, hair genetics, and the effects of the intrinsic hormones on the hair cycle. The realization has finally dawned that baldness is a natural phenomenon and not a scourge or disease to be simply treated by the topical application of some worthless remedy.

The surgical methods of treating baldness are satisfactory but obviously limited. However, they are the only methods available for the natural treatment of baldness at the present time. As our knowledge of hair loss and hair growth increases, and as new facts are discovered, the surgical methods for treating baldness will eventually be replaced by a better scientific understanding and medical control of all manifestations of hair growth. It has been shown that male pattern baldness is controlled by a single dominant sex-limited gene, the expression of which is dependent on the level of circulating androgen. Recent studies [7] have shown that the androgen inhibition of the growing phase of the hair follicle on the scalp is amenable to treatment. Experiments have shown that dihydrotestosterone (DHT) seems to be the specific hormone responsible for male pattern alopecia. In the normal male there is a circulating enzyme, called 5-alpha-reductase, which converts testosterone to dihydrotestosterone. Steroids such as progesterone safely reduce the production of dihydrotestosterone from testosterone. These experiments have shown that both testosterone and progesterone compete with each other for the 5-alpha-reductase enzyme that converts testosterone to dihydrotestosterone. It is possible that in the near future progesterone and other steroids may offer some hope for safely preventing or retarding male pattern baldness.

After 17 years of performing hair transplants for male pattern baldness, careful observation has shown that the transplants in the recipient sites are still growing hair with the same char-

acteristics of the hair in the original donor sites. In thousands of transplant procedures performed by me and by hundreds of other physicians, there has been no instance of hair-bearing grafts failing to continue the hair growth initially accomplished, if the donor site came from an area of the scalp that was still growing hair. Great care must be taken to select the donor area with an eye toward the future pattern of alopecia formation.

Before discussing the long-term results of hair transplants performed during the past 17 years, a general description of the types of patients seen in consultation would be relevant. From November 4, 1969, to December 29, 1976, a total of 690 patients were seen in consultation for hair transplantation. Of these patients, 668 were men and 22 were women. Of the total number seen, 333 were eventually operated on and 357 did not have any surgery.

Of the 357 patients not operated on, 342 were men. The reasons for not having surgery were varied but significant.

1. One hundred and twelve patients had minimal or no recession. The great majority complained of losing considerable amounts of hair daily, and some of them did have moderate thinning. Their complaints were more subjective than objective, and they were all considered premature candidates and advised to return at a later date when the recession was more obvious.

2. Sixty-five had severe baldness with minimal donor hair left. These patients were told that at best only a moderate amount of hair could be transplanted, and they were dissuaded from having any surgery.

3. Forty-eight were thought to be good candidates, but they did not schedule. It is very important to inform every patient during the consultation of the realities of hair transplantation. When they learn that they have to undergo a long series of tedious and sometimes painful operations, many patients, unless they are highly motivated, will not initiate the series.

4. Ninety-four patients were actually scheduled for surgery, but they apparently had sec-

ond thoughts and canceled the operation. The reason was probably the same as for those who did not schedule.

5. Sixteen patients had generally sparse hair throughout, especially in the donor sites, and they were considered poor candidates and were dissuaded from surgery.

6. Five patients were considered poor candidates for reasons of general health problems, such as previous coronary attack, diabetes, and so forth.

7. Two patients were over 70 years of age and were considered too old for this type of surgery.

As stated, a total of 15 women of the 22 seen were not operated on. The reasons for their not having surgery are also significant.

1. Six patients were not done because their hair was either normal, or there was only minimal thinning of the scalp.

2. Six others were not acceptable because their hair was generally thin and sparse throughout. This is the usual pattern for hair loss in women, making most women unlikely candidates for hair-transplant procedures.

3. Two other patients were scheduled, and for reasons unknown, they canceled their operations.

4. One patient had alopecia areata with patchy baldness, and I felt that she was not a good candidate for hair transplants since in many of these patients the hair may grow again in the areas where it has fallen out.

The ages of the 333 patients that were operated on ranged between 18 and 63 (see Table 19-1).

Of the 333 patients, 48 had strip grafts in addition to the punch grafts. A total of 1,189 punch-graft procedures and 98 strip grafts were done. In a previous publication [10], a survey of patients operated on between October of 1966 and November of 1968 was reported. A total of 75 patients underwent hair-transplant procedures during that period of time. A total of 243 operative procedures were

TABLE 19-1. *Ages of Patients Treated for Baldness*

Age in Years	Number of Patients
Under 20	11
20 to 25	71
26 to 30	76
31 to 35	45
36 to 40	50
41 to 45	29
46 to 50	31
51 to 55	12
56 to 60	5
Over 60	4

done, and of these, there were 64 strip grafts and 179 punch-graft procedures. Of the 75 patients, 30 had a combination of strip grafts and punch grafts, 3 had only strip grafts, and 42 had only punch grafts.

The strip-graft procedure is usually done on patients who have obvious complete frontal recession requiring a totally new frontal hairline. When I first began doing hair transplants, the frontal hairline was first reconstructed with the strip grafts, and the punches were done subsequently as fill-ins behind the strip. This often resulted in a prominent graft at a distant level below the existing hairline. During the past 10 years, practically all the new patients have been started with a series of punch-graft procedures beginning at the existing hairline and gradually working faceward until a new frontal hairline is established. In the great majority of cases, the patient will be content with the result accomplished with the punch grafts alone. However, for those patients who are concerned about the tufted effect produced by the punch grafts, and for those patients who are anxious for a more dense frontal hairline, the strip graft will be suggested and usually done.

The strip graft is occasionally inserted in other areas of the scalp besides the frontal region, e.g., a strip may be placed along the part line of the parietal scalp with the hair angulated medially, thereby providing more coverage for the crown. It also may be placed in a transverse semicircular position on the occipital scalp for the coverage of occipital baldness.

A general description of the seven women who underwent hair transplants follows.

1. Five women had a form of male pattern baldness in the midfrontal scalp. One patient had four procedures totaling 160 plugs, one had two procedures totaling 80 plugs, and three each had one procedure averaging 40 plugs. No strip grafts were done in any of my women patients.

2. Two patients were children, one 8 years of age and one 10 years of age, both with severe scarring of the scalp resulting from healed third-degree burns. One had four procedures totaling 120 plugs, and the other had five procedures totaling 150 plugs.

Objective Survey

To judge properly the long-term results of an operation, an objective as well as subjective evaluation of patients should be done. A complete objective survey of every patient would obviously be impossible because of time limits. From the objective viewpoint, I was especially interested in determining whether the transplanted hair had remained, and whether the patient was still able to style his hair properly. Four patients whose hair-transplant procedures began over 10 years ago were selected. These patients were contacted and asked to come to the office for examination and photographs.

I considered it apropos to include the first patient that had undergone hair transplants in my office. He was a 38-year-old white male who first presented in July of 1961 with the complaint of gradual increasing recession of the frontal temporal areas of the scalp. His first procedure, which was a strip graft, was done in August of 1961. He subsequently underwent several more procedures and was reported in 1964 [9]. This patient eventually had a total of 4 strips and 400 punch grafts over a period of 5 years. His last visit to the office was 10 years ago. He was recently contacted and examined,

and additional photographs were taken (Figs. 19-1 and 19-2). The patient is now 55 years of age. Examination of the scalp reveals that the major portion of the transplanted hair had remained and continued to flourish. He was questioned about the degree of hair loss from the transplanted hair. He stated that the loss was minimal. The scarring at the site of the transplants was insignificant and was easily camouflaged by the growing hair. He was able to style his hair quite well, and he said that he was completely satisfied with the results and was happy that he had undergone the large number of procedures. As already mentioned, this patient was originally treated for frontal temporal recession of the hairline. During the past 10 years he has continued to lose hair behind his transplanted hair, and at the present time he shows considerable baldness over the crown of his scalp. He has allowed the transplanted hair to grow quite long and through expert styling is able to cover the bald areas of the scalp, thereby giving a semblance of a full head of hair.

The second patient was a 26-year-old white male who first came to my office in August of 1967 with marked frontal temporal recession of his scalp (Figs. 19-3 and 19-4). He was advised at that time that he would need about six hair-transplant procedures to give him a significant growth of hair. He had a total of two strip grafts and four sets of punch grafts, each averaging 30 punch grafts per procedure. All six operations were done during November and December of 1967 and January of 1968. He had excellent hair growth from all six procedures. He had 30 more punch grafts in September of 1969. This patient is interesting in the sense that he has had additional punch-graft procedures as his hairline has continued to recede behind the original transplants. He had 30 more punch grafts in September of 1970 and also in September of 1971. He had 40 more punch grafts in October of 1973 and also in July of 1974. The patient continued to lose his original hair slowly, and he was anxious to replace it with additional punch grafts. He had an additional 50 punch grafts in January of 1976 and again in December of 1976. His last

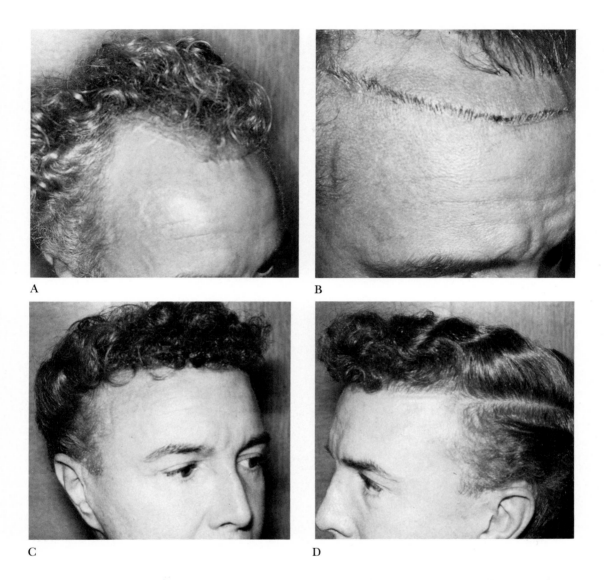

FIGURE 19-1. *(A) Frontal temporal recession in 38-year-old man, July 1961. (B) Position of strip graft. (C) and D) Completed result.*

procedure was in October of 1977, at which time he had an additional 50 punch grafts. This patient has had a total of 2 strip grafts and 435 punch grafts during the past 11 years. He is one of many who have continued the hair-transplant surgery in an attempt to replace hair that is lost as the scalp continues to recede. He has been seen at least once or twice a year dur-ing the past 10 years, and it was interesting to note that although he continued to show nor-mal recession of the scalp, the transplanted hair has remained and has continued to grow. The original strip grafts, which were placed in the frontal area of the scalp in November of 1967, continue to show a full, dense growth of hair. This patient is typical of several other patients who have continued to have hair-transplant procedures over a number of years in a success-ful attempt to remain one step ahead of the in-evitable increasing baldness.

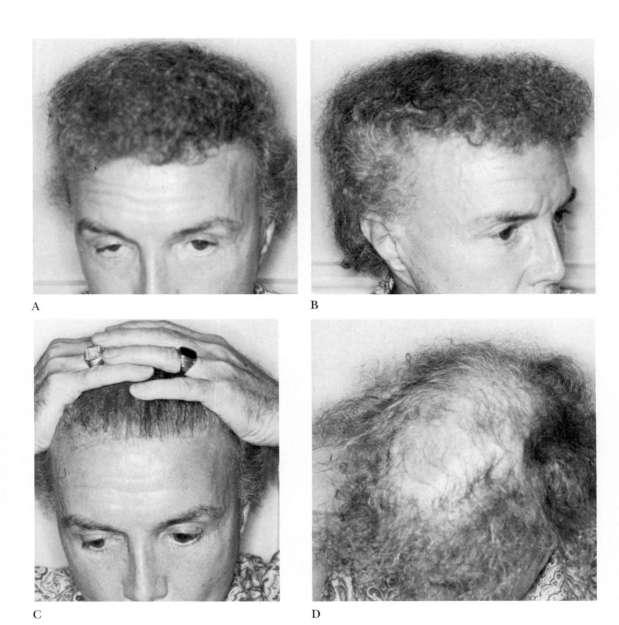

FIGURE 19-2. *(A, B, and C) Same patient, present appearance of scalp, March 1978. (D) Note increased loss of hair on crown.*

The third patient was a 38-year-old white male who first came to my office in December of 1967 with moderate frontal temporal recession of the scalp. Examination revealed that he had dense hair growth on the crown and also on the parietal and occipital areas of the scalp. The patient underwent two strip grafts in January and February of 1968 for reconstruction of the frontal hairline, and during the next 3 years, he had a series of punch-graft procedures. He received a total of 300 punch grafts. His last operation was in May of 1971. He was last seen in my office in June of 1971. The patient was recently contacted. He came to my

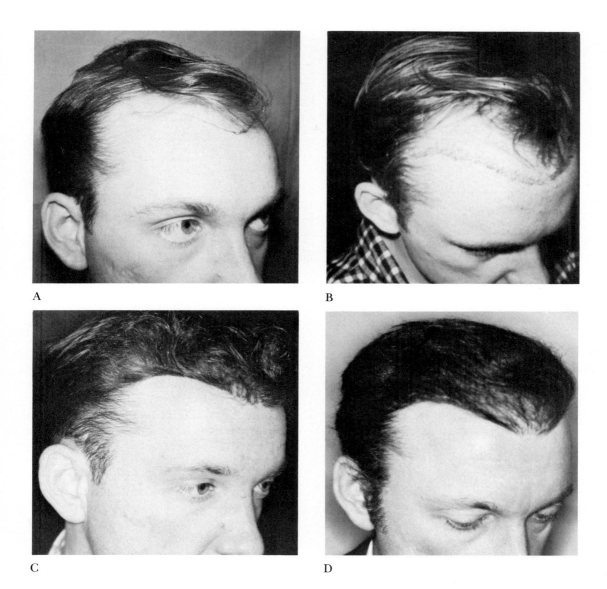

A

B

C

D

FIGURE 19-3. *(A) Frontal temporal recession in 26-year-old man, August 1967. Note marking of proposed frontal hairline. (B) Strip grafts in place. (C) Frontal scalp, September 1969. (D) Appearance, July 1974.*

office for examination in March of 1978 (Figs. 19-5 and 19-6). It was gratifying to note that the hair in the transplants had continued to survive and grow. He had shown only minimal recession of the hair behind the transplants, and he was able to style his hair in a natural manner.

The last patient was a 44-year-old white male who first presented with severe frontal recession of the scalp in December of 1967. This patient had two strip grafts in January of 1968 for reconstruction of the frontal hairline and then underwent a series of punch-graft procedures beginning in February of 1968 until March of 1971 (Fig. 19-7). He had 13 punch-graft procedures, making a total of 540 punch grafts. This patient was seen again in March of 1977, at which time he showed additional recession of

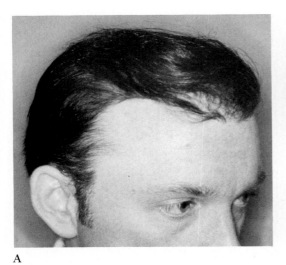
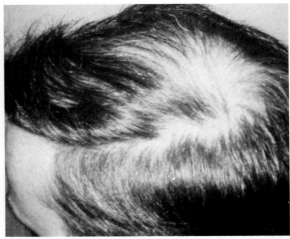

A   B

FIGURE 19-4. *(A and B) Present appearance of scalp, April 1978.*

the scalp behind and lateral to the original hair transplants. He underwent a total of three punch-graft procedures in 1977, making an additional 150 punch grafts (Fig. 19-8). Again it was gratifying to note that he had no loss of hair from the transplants (Fig. 19-9). Like many other patients in my practice, this man developed a certain mania and greed for additional hair. The aversion to baldness in some of these patients is so great that they are willing to undergo the chronic discomfort of multiple hair-transplant procedures in a never-ending attempt to hold back probably the most obvious sign of advancing age. This case also shows how it is possible to take a very large number of punch grafts from the parietal-occipital areas of the scalp without leaving any obvious disfiguring scars (Fig. 19-10). It has been my impression that at least 50 percent of the hair can be removed from these donor areas of the scalp and the patient will still have enough hair in these areas to maintain an apparent normal growth of hair without obvious scarring.

Subjective Survey

The hair-transplant operation has proved to be an effective method for replacing a significant amount of hair on balding areas of the scalp. A large number of these operations are being done by dermatologists and plastic surgeons. All surgeons believe and hope that they are bestowing beneficial effects on their patients when performing any cosmetic procedure. It is true, however, that occasionally a surgeon may think that he has performed a successful operation only to learn to his great chagrin that the patient has not been satisfied with the results.

The only way that a surgeon can evaluate the success and benefits of a particular operation is to determine the opinion and attitudes of the individuals who have undergone the operation. A questionnaire similar to one devised by Farber [2] (Table 19-2) was mailed to all my patients who had had hair-transplant surgery up to 1 year ago. Their answers would supply me with subjective information as to the success or failure of the operations. Their opinions would also give me a better understanding of and insight into the operation from the patient's point of view. All this would result in better patient-surgeon relationships and could possibly aid me in improving my techniques.

A total of 563 questionnaires were mailed, of which 198 were returned completed. One hundred and twenty were returned unopened because of changes of address or the inability of the post office to deliver them. Two hundred and forty-six were never returned. It was con-

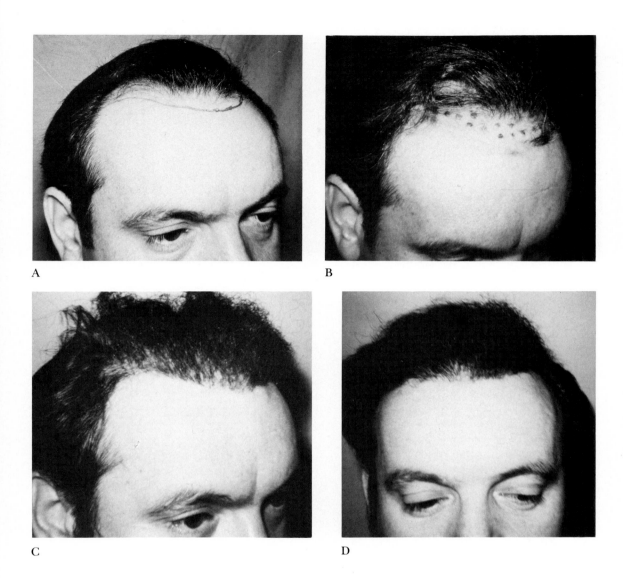

A

B

C

D

FIGURE 19-5. *(A) Frontal temporal recession in 38-year-old man, December 1967. (B) Strips and a few punch grafts in place. (C and D) Completed result, June 1971.*

jectured that those patients who did not return the questionnaire probably did not wish to report unfavorable results. Twenty of these patients were chosen at random and were contacted and asked why they did not respond to the questionnaire. Their reasons were rather mundane. They either misplaced the questionnaire or simply forgot about it. A few claimed that they did not have time to fill it out. Most of these patients stated that they were satisfied with the procedure and apologized for not returning the questionnaire.

The questionnaires were all carefully surveyed, and an attempt was made to determine the cause for each patient's dissatisfaction. This would be of great benefit to me in the handling and treatment of future hair-transplant patients.

The survey showed the following results. A total of 198 patients responded to the survey. They returned the questionnaire completed.

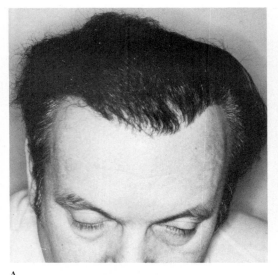

A

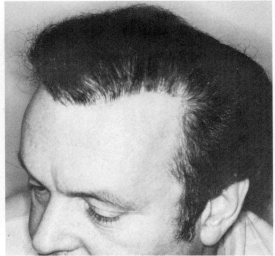

B

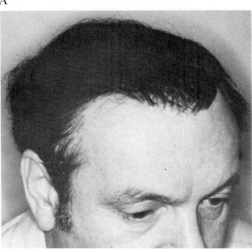

C

FIGURE 19-6. *(A, B, and C) Present appearance of scalp, March 1978.*

Of the 198 patients, 181, or 91.4 percent, reported that the results of the hair transplants were satisfactory. Of the group reporting satisfactory results, a total of 105, or 53 percent, indicated that they were completely satisfied with the results of the operations, and a total of 76, or 38.4 percent, stated that they were partially satisfied. A total of 17, or 8.6 percent, reported complete dissatisfaction with the procedure.

Each of the questionnaires that were returned with the not satisfied response was analyzed very carefully in order to determine the source of dissatisfaction. Two patients who had a series of punch grafts along with two strip grafts expressed a 100 percent failure of the operation. One alleged that he now has a scalp of scars and no hair, while the other claimed that he had very little if any hair at all. These two patients had been reported previously as unsuccessful results [11]. Both these patients wore large hairpieces before the hair transplants were started, and they continued to wear

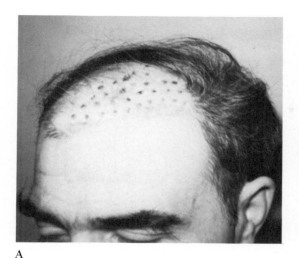

A

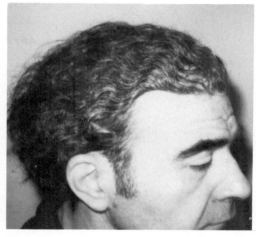

B

FIGURE 19-7. (A) Severe recession of scalp in 44-year-old man, February 1968. Strip grafts and punch grafts recently placed. (B) Appearance in March 1971.

the hairpiece after the hair transplants. It was thought at one time that patients with hairpieces were good candidates, since the hairpiece would camouflage the transplants during the course of treatments. However, it was realized that the hairpiece stifles the growth of hair in the transplants. The hairpiece actually dries the hair and makes the hair brittle, causing it to fracture. When patients with hairpieces come in, they are first told that no matter how

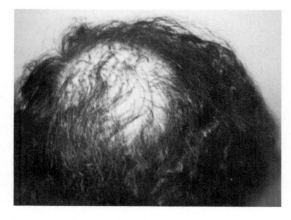

FIGURE 19-8. Punch grafts for coverage of increasing baldness on crown.

many operative procedures they undergo, they will never achieve the density of hair that is provided by a hairpiece. If these patients decide to undergo hair transplants, they are also informed that the continual wearing of the hairpiece will stifle the growth of hair in the transplants, and that unless they are willing to discard the hairpiece within a few months after the first operation, additional hair-transplant procedures will not be carried out.

Three other patients also had a combination of strip and punch grafts. All three complained that the frontal hairline was unnatural, and that there was obvious scarring in the front of the scalp. All three also stated that the hair was too thin, and that there was considerable loss of transplanted hair—as much as 30 percent. This apparent loss of hair may not be real; rather it probably represents additional loss of existing hair. All three claimed that they were unable to satisfactorily style their hair, and all three indicated that they would not recommend this procedure to their friends, nor would they undergo any more transplants if needed. Two of them stated that the procedure was too painful and too costly. These three patients were studied carefully, and it became obvious that they were poor candidates from the start. The hair in their donor sites was rather sparse, resulting in a sparse growth of hair in the transplants. Additional transplants, including strips,

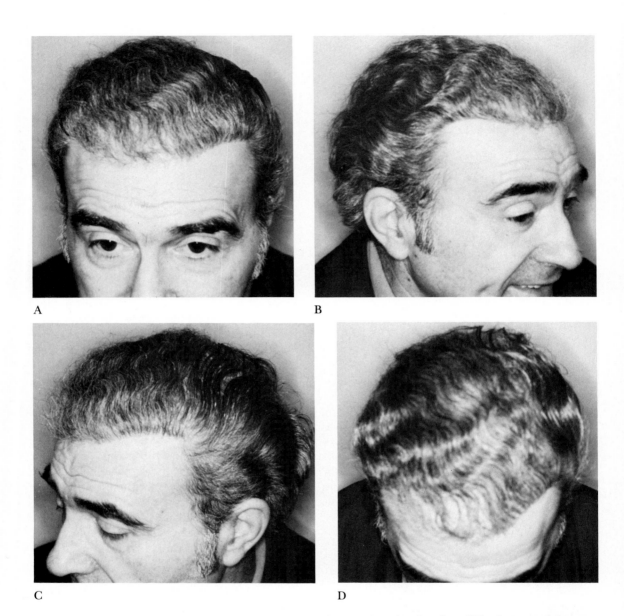

A

B

C

D

FIGURE 19-9. *(A through D) Present appearance of scalp, March 1978.*

simply did not give enough hair growth, thereby contributing to the patients' dissatisfaction. The mistake is too frequently made by the hair-transplant surgeon that if the initial transplants show sparse growth, additional ones will necessarily increase the density of the growth. It is true that the density will be increased, but not significantly. It is a fallacy to assume that a large number of hair-transplant procedures will eventually bring about the dense growth of hair desired by the patient if the first set of transplants resulted in a sparse growth. It is very likely that additional ones will be no more successful.

When a patient first presents himself to me now and examination of his donor site shows a

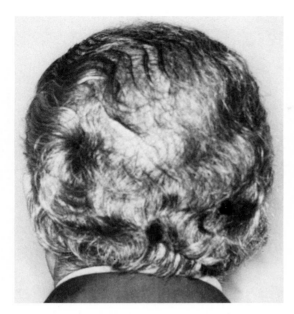

FIGURE 19-10. *Appearance of donor site after two strips and 690 punch grafts.*

low density of hair, and despite this he still insists that he wants hair transplants, I will initially recommend a test procedure of no more than 10 punch grafts. If these test grafts show a growth of at least 10 hairs per 4-mm graft, and if the hair is of good quality, I will then recommend additional hair transplants.

Of the 17 dissatisfied patients, 12 had only punch grafts. It was interesting to note that three of these patients had only one set of punch grafts. One had a test procedure of 10 plugs, and he claimed that he had completed the series of procedures proposed by the doctor. He also stated that he got no results from the transplants, and yet he would recommend this procedure to his friends and would undergo more transplants if needed. The other two had one set of punch grafts totaling 50 plugs. One stated that he completed the series of procedures proposed by the doctor, and the other thought that he had completed the series. Both complained of thin hair with an unnatural frontal hairline. Both felt that they somehow needed more dense coverage. These patients obviously represent a communication block

between the patient and the physician. They somehow did not grasp the information which was presented to them in the initial consultation. It is quite obvious that more than one set of punch grafts is needed before a significant growth of hair can be achieved.

Three other patients had only two sets of punch grafts with a total of 60 plugs. All three complained that the frontal hairline was unnatural, and that the hair was too thin. One stated that the plugs were not close enough, and that they gave the appearance of doll's hair, while the other claimed that the transplanted hair was totally impossible to style. All three patients admitted that they did not complete the series of procedures proposed by the doctor. They also declared that they would not recommend this procedure to their friends, nor would they undergo more transplants if needed. All three felt that the procedure was totally unsatisfactory. It is rather difficult to clearly define what constitutes a completed series of procedures. At my initial consultation with patients, I frequently estimate a certain number of procedures, e.g., four, six, or eight, totally, that will reasonably give a significant growth of hair depending on the amount of recession that exists. However, I always qualify this by asserting that every patient has a different image of what a significant growth of hair actually is, and that frequently a larger or smaller number of procedures will be required to satisfy a particular patient.

Of the remaining six dissatisfied patients, four had three grafts totaling 150 plugs, and two had four grafts totaling 200 plugs. Three said that they did not complete the series of procedures proposed by the doctor, while the other three indicated that they did complete the series. All six felt that the frontal hairline was unnatural and that there was obvious scarring in the front of the scalp. Three claimed that the hair was too thin, and all six stated that they did not lose any transplanted hair. Two mentioned that the hair was too curly, and two actually said that they would recommend this procedure to their friends, and that they would also undergo more transplants if needed. In reviewing these

TABLE 19-2. *Survey Questionnaire*

CHARLES P. VALLIS, M.D., INC.
480 LYNNFIELD STREET
LYNN, MASS. 01904

Dear _____,

The only way that a surgeon can evaluate the success and benefits of a particular operation is to determine the opinion and attitude of the individual who has undergone the operation.

Would you kindly answer the following questions regarding your hair transplant surgery.

Your answers will be confidential and your name will not be used in any survey.

Most questions can be answered with a check mark. A few will require a small explanation.

Your answers are important to me so please take a few moments and complete the following:

1. Are you satisfied with the results?
   a. Completely _____
   b. Partially _____
   c. Not satisfied _____

2. If answer to question 1 is not satisfied, answer following:
   a. Appearance of frontal hairline
      1. Unnatural _____
      2. Natural _____
   b. Obvious scars of scalp
      1. Front of scalp _____
      2. Back of scalp _____
      3. Both _____
   c. Condition of transplanted hair
      1. Too straight _____
      2. Too curly _____
      3. New color _____
      4. Same color _____
      5. Too coarse _____
      6. Too thin _____
      7. Other _____
         (Explain) _____

3. Did you complete the series of procedures proposed by the doctor?
   a. Yes _____
   b. No _____

4. If answer to question 3 is no, complete following:
   a. Too costly _____
   b. Too painful _____
   c. Didn't need anymore _____
   d. Too long _____
   e. Other reason _____
      (Explain) _____

5. Has there been any hair loss in the transplanted hair?
   a. No _____
   b. Yes _____
      1. Minimal _____
      2. Considerable _____
         a. percentage _____

6. Are you able to style your hair satisfactorily?
   a. Yes _____
   b. No _____
      (If answer is no, explain why.) _____

7. Have you had any problems with your scalp since having the transplant?
    a. Numbness _____
       1. How long? _____
       2. Still present? _____
    b. Redness _____
    c. Dandruff _____
    d. Itching _____
    e. Scaling _____
    f. Other _____
      (Explain) _____
8. Overall effect of hair transplant procedure on:
    (Answer: Good, bad, or no effect)
    a. Your job or career _____
    b. Your attitude _____
    c. Your friends _____
    d. Your family _____
9. Would you recommend this procedure to your friends?
    a. Yes _____
    b. No _____
      (Explain) _____
10. Would you undergo more transplants, if needed?
    a. Yes _____
    b. No _____
      (Explain) _____
11. Do you have any suggestions as to how the procedure could be improved?
    _____

six cases, it was obvious that these patients had very severe baldness to begin with, and despite the fair number of punch grafts received, they were far from adequate in adding a significant coverage of hair to the scalp. Patients with very severe baldness present a difficult problem for the surgeon in determining whether it is wise to initiate a series of hair-transplant procedures. Because of the limits of the donor hair, it is impossible to give a dense coverage to most of these patients. However, a large number of them will be quite happy and delighted with a modest growth of hair on their bare pates and will frequently be pleased simply because that sense of total baldness has been partially eliminated.

Of the 198 questionnaires that were returned completed, 76 patients indicated that they were partially satisfied with the results of the hair-transplant procedures. Of these 76 patients, 32, or 42 percent, stated that they had not completed the series of procedures proposed by the doctor. The reasons for not completing the procedures were varied (Table 19-3).

Of the 76 patients, 10 indicated that the appearance of the frontal hairline was unnatural, 15 stated that they had obvious scars in the

TABLE 19-3. *Reasons for Not Completing the Series of Procedures*

Reasons	Number of Patients
Too costly	9
Too long	6
Too painful	5
Planning additional transplants in the future	5
Did not have enough time	3
Satisfied with results and did not need any more	3
Became ill	1
Travel distance too far	1
Inconvenience of postoperative period	1

front of the scalp, and 8 claimed that they had obvious scars in the back of the scalp. Of the 76 patients, 15 felt that they had difficulty in styling their hair. The most common complaint was that the hair was too thin. Twenty-one indicated this in the questionnaire.

Of the 76 patients, 25 stated that they had minimal loss of hair, whereas 2 alleged that they had considerable loss and 1 complained that he had as much as 50 percent loss of the transplanted hair.

Of the problems with the scalp, the biggest complaint was the persistence of numbness. Four stated that the numbness was transient, lasting only a few months. Three claimed that the scalp was numb for at least 1 year. One had numbness for 18 months. Three indicated that it was still present after several years.

The great majority stated that they had no problems with their scalps since having the transplants. A very small number had redness, dandruff, and scaling in the scalp after the transplants, although these eventually disappeared.

It was also very interesting to examine answers to the overall effect of the hair-transplant procedure on their jobs, their attitudes, and their friends and families. The overwhelming majority answered that the overall effect was good. There was a total of 47 out of 76 patients in this group. Some even stated that the overall effect was very good or "super." Of the 76 patients, 24 said that there was no effect of the hair-transplant procedure on their jobs, attitudes, or friends and families. Two patients did not answer this question.

Of note also was the fact that three patients, although claiming partial satisfaction, asserted that the overall effect of the transplants on their attitude was negative. One claimed that his attitude was bad because not enough of the transplants took and the hair was too thin after a large number of transplants. Another stated that there was very little improvement, and that the procedures were too costly, too slow and painful, and the transplants were too obvious. The third patient declared that he had been coerced by his wife and family

to have the transplant procedures, and he considers hair transplants to be unnecessary and vain. He further announced that he has since removed himself from that family, and he stated that having begun the transplants, he found himself in a seemingly self-perpetuating cycle of further transplants.

Of interest also is how many of the partially satisfied patients would recommend this procedure to their friends or would undergo more transplants if needed. A total of 66 of the 76 partially satisfied patients answered this in the affirmative. Of the 76, 10 stated that they would not recommend the procedure to their friends, although 6 of the 10 felt that they were committed to the operations and would undergo more transplants if needed. Four of the ten stated that they would not undergo any more transplant procedures. The reasons given were that they were not worth the time, money, or inconvenience, and one patient felt that he could never get enough transplants to completely satisfy himself.

Of the 76 partially satisfied patients, a total of 21 had the combination of strip and punch grafts, whereas 55 had only the punch-graft procedures, indicating that roughly 27 percent of the partially satisfied patients had strip grafts as well as the punch grafts.

The questionnaires in which the patients indicated that they were completely satisfied with the hair-transplant procedures were the easiest to tabulate and by far the most pleasant. There were a total of 105 questionnaires that were marked completely satisfied. Of these 105 patients, 41 stated that they did not complete the series of procedures proposed by the doctor. The most common reason for this was that they were planning to have more procedures in the future. Several stated that they were quite satisfied with the results thus far and did not desire to have any more. A very small number (five) felt that the procedure was too painful. Four claimed that it was too long, and one believed that it was too costly.

Two patients mentioned that they had some redness, itching, and scaling, but that they also had these problems previously. A total of 18 patients alleged that they had minimal loss of hair in the transplants. Some stated that they had considerable loss of hair. A small number had some numbness after the transplants. A total of seven patients had numbness that lasted for 4 to 6 months. One patient had numbness for 1 year, and four claimed that it was still present.

None indicated that it had a bad effect on their attitudes, their work, or their families. Every one of them felt that the overall effect was good. In fact, several of the patients actually used superlatives when they described the overall effect of the hair-transplant procedure on their attitudes. They used such words as *excellent, super,* and *very good.* One assured me that it was exactly what he wanted. The hair growth was gradual, and the effects of the operation were unnoticeable. Every one of these patients would recommend this operation to their friends and would undergo more transplants if needed.

Of the 105 patients who were completely satisfied, a total of 25, or 23.9 percent, had a combination of strip and punch grafts.

The overwhelming majority of the completely satisfied patients had no suggestions as to how the procedure could be improved. Of the 105 patients, 90 had no suggestions, and 15 had some interesting suggestions with regard to improving the procedure. One felt that more transplants per session should be done; 40 were too few. He also suggested that the total cost of the operations be reduced, and he highly recommended the strip grafts in the frontal hairline.

Another patient believed that a more efficient way would be to remove a corresponding strip in the frontal scalp before the transplanted strip is inserted. Another stated that the only part of the operation which he found uncomfortable was in the beginning when the injections of anesthetic were given. He felt that if this pain could be eliminated, the patients would have less fear of being operated on. Another recommended that a superficial application of a liquid or other substance which would cause a numbing effect should be used to

help relieve the discomfort caused by the needle at the onset of the procedure. Another suggested that a way should be devised to replace the injection of the anesthetic with some other form of anesthesia.

Another patient thought that the punch grafts were not very productive. He believed that they result in sparse hair growth, and he found that the strips were more satisfactory. He felt that strategic placement of strips throughout the scalp would be preferable to the punch grafts. Another asserted that he would prefer to have double strips in the front and the plugs much closer together. He believed that he could then achieve a full head of hair. Another wanted the total program speeded up, so that he would not have to take so much time off from work.

Of the 76 patients who were partially satisfied with the procedure, 50 had no suggestions as to how the procedure could be improved, and 26 made various suggestions concerning improvements. Eight would have liked to have had more transplants at a sitting. One would have preferred to be hospitalized to get it over with in one operative procedure instead of going through several recovery periods. One suggested that possibly larger plugs could be used. These plugs would contain more hair, thereby minimizing the number of procedures and the follow-up care needed after each transplant procedure.

Three patients hoped that some form of medication could be discovered that would produce hair growth and eliminate surgery. Another felt that including a hair stylist as a consultant to determine a natural hairline before surgery would be helpful.

Two patients who had punch grafts elsewhere, where the donor sites were not sutured, strongly felt that suturing causes much less scarring in the donor sites. Another sent me an article from a lay magazine describing the electric-powered punch graft. This article favored a method employing a motorized unit that rotates a manual punch with a circular cutting head $\frac{1}{4}$ in. in diameter. The surgeon was able to transplant 900 to 1,000 punch grafts in seven to eight weekly sessions. This doctor also recommended the use of the Dermajet to inject the local anesthetic in the donor and recipient areas to minimize the pain.

One patient who had 100 punch grafts done by me and subsequently had 700 additional transplants done by a dermatologist in the New York area made some interesting remarks:

1. The physician should initially state what results could realistically be expected by the patient.
2. The physician should give an estimate of the potential number of transplants needed to complete the procedure.
3. The physician should resist the patient's choice of what may be an unnatural appearing hairline.
4. Suturing appears to produce better results against scarring.
5. A smaller number of transplants at one sitting (25 to 35) appears to produce a better result than 60, 75, or 100 transplants at one time.

Of the 18 patients who were not satisfied, none had any suggestions as to how the operation could be improved. However, one did make a very interesting observation. He believed that the procedure itself was performed satisfactorily, but the patients should know and understand exactly what the results of this procedure really are—that they will still have to cover up significantly. In this patient's opinion, this procedure is clearly not indicated for patients with overall severe baldness.

Final Thoughts

It was obvious from the questionnaires that the most common complaint was that the hair was too thin and that the hair could not be styled satisfactorily. Some claimed that there was obvious scarring in the front and back. A large number of the dissatisfied patients did not complete the series of procedures proposed by the doctor. The most important lesson learned

from these questionnaries was that certain points should be stressed carefully in the preoperative consultation with the patients. All patients should be told that hair transplantation involves a long series of tedious, costly, and sometimes painful procedures. In addition, a realistic description of the possible appearance of the transplanted hair after the series has been completed should be given to each patient. Each patient should be told that no matter how many operative procedures they undergo, they will never achieve a full growth of hair. It should be stressed that the resulting hair may not be quite as thick and dense as they would desire, and that there will be some scarring in the recipient and donor sites.

In addition, it should be emphasized that it is very difficult to determine exactly how many transplants each patient will require. It has been my experience that although a certain number of procedures can be recommended to produce a significant amount of hair, each patient's definition of a significant amount of hair varies. Some patients are quite satisfied with a moderately thin covering of hair which eliminates the sense of baldness, while others will not be satisfied until a dense growth of hair can be achieved by as many hair transplants as the donor sites will allow.

The larger punch grafts (4.25 and 4.5 mm) are much more efficient than the smaller ones (3.5 and 4.0 mm), which are more commonly used. The smaller grafts are useful as fill-ins between the larger grafts after the third or fourth procedure. A total of fifty or sixty 4.5-mm punch grafts done in one procedure will produce as much hair as one hundred and twenty 3.5-mm grafts. The larger punch is also more efficient in causing less scarring in the recipient and donor sites. Suturing the donor wounds has also proven to be important in lessening the morbidity and scarring in these areas. Most dermatologists do not suture the donor wounds. The small size of the punch grafts they use may obviate the necessity of suturing. Any wound in the donor area measuring 4 mm or more should be sutured.

The strip graft continues to be very helpful

in improving the hairline in those patients in whom the punch grafts have not produced adequate density. The placement of strips in other areas of the scalp besides the frontal area, e.g., parietal and occipital, has proven helpful.

There were many complaints of excessive costs and that the procedure took too long. The cost and time can be reduced by using larger punches which produce more hair, thereby cutting down on the total number of grafts and procedures.

Reducing the pain, postoperative numbness, and other symptoms that accompany any series of operations presents a more difficult problem. The use of the Dermajet* helps in reducing the superficial pain of needle penetration but not the expansion pain of injection of the local anesthetic in the subcutaneous tissue.

Farber [2] suggests the injection of a single-dose repository corticosteroid intramuscularly (Celestone Soluspan Suspension)† which he feels considerably reduces edema, pain, residual numbness, and possibly scarring and does not appear to interfere with healing. I have not used systemic steroids, but I have routinely used as preoperative sedation 10 mg diazepam orally, and in some highly nervous patients I have used 100 mg sodium pentobarbital by mouth in addition to the diazepam. This has decreased syncope and has lessened the pain of the injections.

This survey has revealed that the great majority of patients (91.4 percent) that had hair transplants were satisfied with the results. The hair-transplant procedures, when done in carefully selected patients, have been successful for adequate replacement of hair in bald areas of the scalp.

*Robbins Instrument Co., Chatham, N.J. 07928.
†Schering Corporation, Galloping Hill Road, Kenilworth, N.J. 07033.

References

1. Correa-Iturraspe, M., and Arufe, H.N. La cirugia plastica en las alopecias parciales definitivas del cuero cabelludo. *Semana Med.* 111:937, 1957.
2. Farber, G.A., Burks, J.W., and Salinger, C. Hair transplants for male pattern baldness: Long-term subjective evaluation. *South. Med. J.* 65:1380, 1972.
3. Lamont, E.S. A plastic surgical transformation: Report of a case. *West. J. Surg.* 65:164, 1957.
4. Montagna, W., and Ellis, R.A. (Eds.). *The Biology of Hair Growth.* New York: Academic Press, 1958.
5. Okuda, S. Klinische und experimentelle Untersuchungen über die Transplantation von lebenden Haaren. *Jpn. J. Dermatol. Urol.* 46:135, 1939.
6. Orentreich, N. Autografts in alopecias and other selected dermatological conditions. *Ann. N.Y. Acad. Sci.* 83:463, 1969.
7. Orentreich, N. Over the fence: Medical treatment of baldness. *Ann. Plast. Surg.* 1:116, 1978.
8. Szasz, T.S., and Robertson, A.M. A theory of the pathogenesis of ordinary human baldness. *Arch. Dermatol. Syphilol.* 61:34, 1950.
9. Vallis, C.P. Surgical treatment of the receding hairline. *Plast. Reconstr. Surg.* 33:247, 1964.
10. Vallis, C.P. Surgical treatment of the receding hairline. *Plast. Reconstr. Surg.* 44:271, 1969.
11. Vallis, C.P. The Strip Graft Method in Hair Transplantation. In E. Epstein and E. Epstein, Jr. (Eds.), *Skin Surgery* (4th Ed.). Springfield, Ill.: Thomas, 1977.

Robert M. Goldwyn

COMMENTS ON CHAPTER 19

DR. VALLIS, who has been a major innovator in hair-transplant surgery, gives us the benefit of an extensive experience in this remarkably exhaustive analysis of his long-term results. Of interest at the outset are his remarks about the 357 patients who did not have operations. Favorable outcomes of surgery depend obviously on wise patient selection. No good hitter goes after every pitch. It is not unexpected that of 628 patients, only 22 were women—more evidence of man's burden in trying to keep pace with baldness. This is one of the few areas of cosmetic surgery in which males vastly outnumber females.

The key to the operation for male pattern baldness and its results is the fact that transplanted hair grows and flourishes as it would in its original location. If the donor hair assumed the characteristics of the recipient site, the operation would be a useless adventure.

Of the 333 patients having hair transplants, 258 were younger than 41. In response to a questionnaire sent to 563 patients, 181 (91.4 percent) of the 198 who responded stated that they were satisfied with the results. Canvasing former patients to determine their opinion of their treatment takes not only effort, but courage. Few of us like a negative reaction to our surgery, and fewer of us still would put ourselves on the line to elicit dissatisfaction. And even fewer would do what Dr. Vallis did: pursue the nonrespondents on the assumption that they were dissatisfied (a supposition which was not always true, as Dr. Vallis explains).

Some were unhappy with what they considered an unnatural frontal hairline and also with the sparseness of growth of the transplanted hair. In analyzing these patients, Dr. Vallis observed that, in retrospect, they were poor candidates since the donor hair was too scanty from the start. Dr. Vallis makes the further point that too often surgeons mistakenly believe that if the initial transplant shows sparse growth, additional ones will necessarily increase the density of hair. More likely, other sets of transplanted hair will be no more successful. Dr. Vallis's suggestion of doing 10 punch grafts as a test is a good one. If they show growth at the rate of 10 hairs per 4-mm graft, and if the hair is of good quality, additional transplants can then be done with more assurance for the patient and the surgeon. This preliminary operation should eliminate what could have been unfavorable long-term results.

Of interest also in Dr. Vallis's series were those who did not complete their treatment. Their expressed reasons concerned the cost of the procedure, the time, and the pain involved. Although most patients had no complaints referable to their scalp, a few were distressed by persistent numbness, a possibility which should be discussed with the prospective patient.

From Dr. Vallis's 17-year experience, one must conclude that hair transplantation, in the correct patient, is justified because of its satisfactory long-term results.

20

GENERAL skepticism exists regarding the results of excision of xanthelasma palpebrarum—to the extent that some surgeons are reluctant to advocate any treatment. This pessimism may be due partly to limited and disappointing personal experiences, as well as to the clinical misconception that all patients who are treated have the same prognosis. Until recently, the literature has not provided data to refute these attitudes [4, 5], but the results obtained from follow-up on a large series of cases [3] have enabled the physician to better predict the results of treatment and accordingly aid in patient selection.

The controversy surrounding the clinical significance of xanthelasma is relevant to the plastic surgeon because of the frequency with which he sees this type of patient. In addition, the relationship to disorders of lipid metabolism is of current interest. Although xanthelasma is usually considered to be a manifestation of hypercholesterolemia, only one-third of patients with xanthelasma have abnormal serum lipid levels; most of these abnormal levels are of uncertain significance and do not predispose the patient to a higher recurrence rate. The familial and acquired hyperlipidemias (including bilary cirrhosis, myxedema, and diabetes mellitus), while accounting for less than 5 percent of patients, are significant predisposing factors in that there is a marked tendency for xanthelasma recurrence after xanthelasma removal.

Xanthelasma also may be associated with other cutaneous xanthomas (and xanthoma tendinosa) as part of a systemic xanthomatous disorder [1]. Fortunately, this is rare, and the result of excisions of these xanthelasmas is usually a recurrence. Ninety-eight percent of pa-

Bryan C. Mendelson
James K. Masson

RESULTS OF TREATMENT OF XANTHELASMA

tients with xanthomas have the lesion located on the eyelids.

Thus in more than 90 percent of patients, xanthelasma is a localized collection of xanthomatous plaques occurring without any known predisposing condition, even though one-third of the patients have elevated serum lipid levels.

Treatment

Once established, xanthelasma plaques either remain unchanged in size or increase in size and number; they do not decrease. The lesions, of themselves, are harmless and rarely become large enough to obstruct vision. Occasionally, however, they become symptomatic (itchy during perspiration). The usual indication for treatment is for cosmetic correction, since the lesions are prominently located and conspicuously colored (Fig. 20-1). In the absence of a known cause, a rational basis for definitive treatment does not exist, and although local excision is often successful, it can hardly be considered curative.

Nonsurgical techniques such as topical applications of trichloroacetic acid (50 to 75% solution) [2], cautery, carbon dioxide snow, and cryosurgery are practiced, generally by nonsurgeons, and usually more than one application is required for complete removal. For the plastic surgeon, surgical excision is just as easy and more precise.

Results

The results of excision of xanthelasma plaques should be assessed in light of the natural history of the condition, particularly because the results reflect more the underlying diathesis than the adequacy of excision. Typically, the condition commences with one or more round to oval plaques located medially in the skin of the upper eyelids. There is a tendency not only for the plaques to enlarge, but also for further nodules to develop; these may remain discrete or may coalesce. If the condition worsens, multiple, small, or large plaques may become evident on the upper and lower lids.

Recurrent xanthelasma includes not only the recurrence of lesions that had previously been completely excised, but also the later appearance of xanthelasma plaques on the same or different eyelids. It is unusual for a new lesion to develop on the same or different lid without a recurrence at the site of the original excision. This situation tends to be seen in patients with multiple bilateral lesions. One-fifth of patients with "recurrences" have new lesions on the other eyelid.

Forty percent of patients who are treated for the first time will have recurrences. This rate increases to 60 percent for patients being treated for recurrent xanthelasma. If the lesions have been treated only once before, there is a reasonable chance of successful reexcision (recurrence rate of about 50 percent), whereas if previous treatment has failed many times, the chance of success is slight.

When the time elapsed between excision and recurrence is less than 1 year, the proportion of recurrences is highest. The recurrence rate diminishes each year thereafter, and recurrence after 10 years is rare.

Although there is no statistical relationship between the probability of recurrence and the patient's age at which xanthelasma first ap-

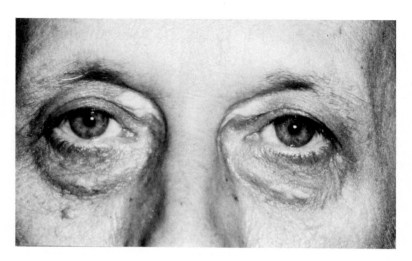

FIGURE 20-1. *Typical appearance of xanthelasma. When all four eyelids are involved, the chance of recurrence is high.*

peared, the younger patients with recurrence seem to have the recurrence sooner after excision than do the older patients.

If all four eyelids have plaques, irrespective of the size of the plaques, the recurrence rate is more than 80 percent, whereas the recurrence rate is 40 percent when one, two, or three eyelids only are involved.

Two factors that are not clearly related to recurrence are a positive family history and elevated serum lipid levels (usually cholesterol). Although one-third of patients have family histories of xanthelasma, the recurrence rate after initial excision is about the same as for those with negative family histories, although the treatment of recurrent xanthelasma in patients with positive family histories is usually unsuccessful. With the exception of the previously mentioned hyperlipidemia syndromes, the presence of elevated serum lipids bears no relationship to the recurrence rate.

Of patients with recurrence after excision, 75 percent believed that the surgery had been worthwhile, in that the recurrent lesions were fewer or smaller than the original lesions or the

time interval before recurrence was satisfactory. However, all patients who had a recurrence within 12 months believed that the treatment was not worthwhile. These were patients who had multiple bilateral plaques and who had recurrences that were usually as pronounced as or greater than the original lesions.

Final Thoughts

Because surgery for the treatment of xanthelasma is simple, safe, and cosmetically satisfying, there are no inherent contraindications to excision, provided the risks of ectropion from excessive skin resection are appreciated. The need to use a skin graft after excision is rare. There is nothing to suggest that the treatment of xanthelasma is otherwise detrimental or specifically increases the likelihood of further deposits.

All patients may be considered in one of three categories in relation to the probability of a successful excision:

1. When the xanthelasma is associated with systemic xanthomas or with an underlying hyperlipidemic syndrome, recurrence is ex-

pected and excision is not generally advocated.

2. When the xanthelasma is typical and the patient is presenting for initial excision, provided all four eyelids are not involved, excision is worthwhile, with a success rate of about 60 percent.

3. When the patient has had a recurrence after a previous excision, the chance of success after another excision is 40 percent. However, if the patient is young and has a rapid development of the recurrence, multiple previous recurrences, or a positive family history, the diathesis toward depositing xanthelasma plaques appears to be greater than the ability of the surgeon to successfully treat the condition.

References

1. Duke-Elder, W.S.   The Lids in Systemic Disease: Xanthomatosis. In W.S. Duke-Elder (Ed.), *System of Ophthalmology* (2nd ed.). St. Louis: Mosby, 1974. Vol. 13, part 1, p. 297.
2. Lussier, M., and Grenier, M.   Traitement du xanthélasma palpébral par méthode chimique. *Union Med. Can.* 96:885, 1967.
3. Mendelson, B.C., and Masson, J.K.   Xanthelasma: Follow-up on results after surgical excision. *Plast. Reconstr. Surg.* 58:535, 1976.
4. Paletta, F.X.   Tumors of the Skin: Xanthomatoses. In J.M. Converse (Ed.), *Reconstructive Plastic Surgery*. Philadelphia: Saunders, 1964. Vol. 1, pp. 342–343.
5. Zarem, H.A., and Lorincz, A.L.   Benign Growths and Generalized Skin Disorders. In W.C. Grabb and J.W. Smith (Eds.), *Plastic Surgery* (2nd ed.). Boston: Little, Brown, 1973. P. 719.

Robert M. Goldwyn

COMMENTS ON CHAPTER 20

THIS well-done study by Drs. Mendelson and Masson emphasizes the value of long-term evaluation. Some may consider xanthelasma a trivial condition, but not so for the patient who has it or the doctor who treats it. That a third of all people with xanthelasma have elevated serum lipids creates concern about their general health. For many patients, these deposits are not only unsightly, but are stigmata of cardiovascular disease—a reminder to themselves and others of their vulnerability to premature death.

Anyone who has tried to eradicate xanthelasma locally must have wondered how much the patient would ultimately benefit. In this excellent study, the authors have given us some of the answers. With more certainty, we can talk to a patient about the probability of success or recurrence following excision. As Drs. Mendelson and Masson state, although there are alternative methods of management, excision is "just as easy and more precise." Often the plaque involves more than the skin, extending through the muscle. Magnification lenses are helpful to avoid incomplete local excision that would soon give rise to the impression of an early recurrence.

The data presented in this chapter do not permit us to attempt a correlation between depth of involvement of the xanthelasma and the rate of its recurrence.

Another fact we should like to know is the incidence of recurrence in grafts usually employed to avoid ectropion. Why the xanthelasma appears most often medially on the lids has never been explained. If the local conditions were altered by grafting, would this proclivity for the inner canthi remain the same? Would the donor site of the graft be a critical factor? Probably not, but without data, one can only conjecture.

21

THERE is a striking scarcity in the literature of long-term follow-up of patients with fibrous dysplasia. This review of patients with craniofacial fibrous dysplasia, seen over a period of 30 years, was undertaken to evaluate the results of various kinds of treatment. Secondarily, it has yielded observations which may contribute to a better understanding of the disease.

Fibrous Dysplasia

Fibrous dysplasia may affect any bone of the skeleton and thus is of interest to a number of medical specialists. The orthopedic surgeon encounters it in the long bones; the thoracic surgeon, in the ribs. The otolaryngologist must consider it in differential diagnosis of tumors of the sinuses and maxilla, and the neurosurgeon in tumors of the skull. It is of concern to the plastic surgeon, who deals with it in the facial skeleton. Because it may be associated with endocrine abnormalities, it is of interest to the endocrinologist and internist. The oral surgeon is familiar with a variety of lesions in the jaw with the same fibro-osseous structure but with a different clinical course and prognosis. Finally, it is a problem to the pathologist, who finds its etiology obscure and its proper classification difficult. References to this disease can be found in the literature of each of these specialties.

Changing Concepts of Fibrous Dysplasia

The variety of names given to fibrous dysplasia in the literature reflects the changing concepts of its nature. It has been referred to variously as ossifying fibroma, osteofibroma, osteitis fibrosa,

378

Michael L. Lewin

CRANIOFACIAL FIBROUS DYSPLASIA

osteitis fibrous deformans, osteodystrophy, hypertrophic osteitis, and many others [16]. Cases of fibrous dysplasia also can be found in the literature under various descriptive terms such as *leontiasis ossea* [31] or *fibrous swelling of the jaws* [2].

In the early part of the nineteenth century, only those cases with large tumefactions attracted medical attention, and they were considered sarcomas. However, many clinicians were aware of their relatively benign nature, recognizing that they differed from the true sarcomas in their slow and noninvasive growth and in their excellent prognosis after resection.

In 1828, James Syme resected two-thirds of the mandible of a 24-year-old man with a huge tumor [21]. He reported this case as an osteosarcoma. Judging from Syme's description and from the Edinburgh Museum specimen, this was a case of fibrous dysplasia. The long-term success of the operation can be attested by the portrait of the patient 30 years later (Fig. 21-1).

Fibrous dysplasia does not conform strictly to the criteria of a neoplasm because of its multifocal origin, polyostotic distribution, self-limiting growth, and possible regression. Although some pathologists consider it a reparative granuloma, in the present prevailing opinion it is classified as a tumor-like lesion [11,18].

Since fibrous dysplasia originates in childhood, the prevalent concept is that it develops from a congenital tissue defect, single or multiple, and is classified as hamartoma. A familiar form of this disease, which occurs in the jaws multifocally and laterally, is known as cherubism [2,12]. It is usually self-limiting and regressive.

Fibrous dysplasia can be compared with cutaneous hemangioma, which, in rare instances, exhibits unrestrained destructive growth but is generally self-limiting and regressive. However, in hemangioma, the changes occur during the first few years of life, while in fibrous dysplasia, the lesion persists over many decades, or a lifetime, and its spontaneous regression is limited.

Distribution

Fibrous dysplasia may be monostotic or polyostotic. In either form it has a predilection for the craniofacial skeleton. The monostotic lesion is most frequently localized in the mandible or maxilla. The polyostotic form is limited to the craniofacial skeleton in three out of four cases. It will usually involve the mandible, maxilla, orbits, cranial base, and vault.

Fibrous dysplasia, in either monostotic or polyostotic form, affects other parts of the skeleton, such as the femur, tibia, humerus, pelvis, and ribs. In about half the cases of generalized polyostotic distribution the craniofacial skeleton is affected in some measure [6,23,31].

If the lesion is monostotic, it is unlikely that other bones will become involved during the course of the disease. Generalized or craniofacial polyostotic fibrous dysplasia frequently follows a certain pattern, either unilateral or symmetrically bilateral.

Morphology

It is characteristic of fibrous dysplasia that the normal osseous structure of the spongiosa, or

379

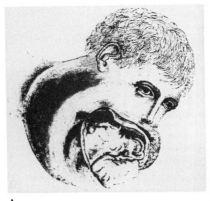

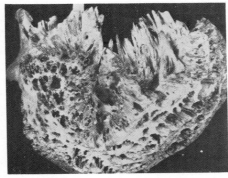

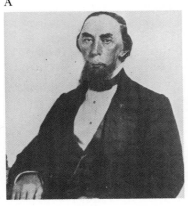

FIGURE 21-1. *(A) Drawing of James Syme's case of mandibular tumor. Specimen weight, 4 1/2 pounds. (B) Macerated specimen preserved in Anatomic Museum, University of Edinburgh. (C) Portrait of patient 30 years after operation. (Reproduced from J.M. Graham, James Syme,* Br. J. Plast. Surg. *7:1, 1954.)*

medulla, is replaced by fibrous tissue with osteogenic proclivities. This manifests itself in the formation of immature, nonlamellar, woven, or fibrous bone. Fibrous or osseous tissue may predominate; a more correct term for this condition might be *fibro-osseous dysplasia.*

The connective tissue may be highly cellular and vascular, with multiple giant cells and hemorrhagic foci, or it may be predominantly collagenous. Degeneration of the collagenous substance results in cyst formation. Osteoblasts and osteoclasts are present in various quantities and distribution. The immature bone may calcify, forming round bodies, the substance of which resembles osteocementum. Many of these variations can coexist side by side within a single specimen [10,11,18].*

*Histological documentation of the reported cases was omitted in this chapter to avoid a large number of additional illustrations.

The lesion begins centrally, distending the cortex as it grows and eventually eroding it. Single or multiple hump-like nodules may appear on its surface. The affected bone contains white or brown areas of firm, rubbery, fleshy tissue which may vary in size from small specks to huge nodules. Interspersed osseous elements give the tissue a gritty consistency. In some instances the lesional tissue may have a soft, chalky character. The prevalence of osseous elements, thickening of the trabeculae, and intense calcification give the lesion a hard, rocklike quality.

Radiological Appearance

The histological makeup of the tumor determines its radiological appearance. This can be visualized best in the mandible. If fibrous elements predominate, a radiolucent, cyst-like shadow is cast, while osseous elements make the lesion more radiopaque [25]. The cortex may be attenuated or eroded. When there is a mixture of fibrous and osseous elements, the radiological shadow acquires a ground-glass texture ("smoke pattern"). Spotty areas of calcification may appear within this outline, or the entire lesion may be of mottled, irregular density.

Radiological details are difficult to visualize in the midface and cranial bones. In the maxilla, ethmoids, and the base of the cranium, fibrous dysplasia has a uniform sclerotic density, either localized as a nodule or diffuse. In the cranial vault, the involved bones appear sclerotic and enlarged, with areas of rarefaction and radiolucency [14].

Monostotic Fibrous Dysplasia

Fibrous dysplasia is a disease of children and adolescents which may persist into later life. The main and frequently only symptom in the craniofacial skeleton is swelling which causes facial deformity. The lesion usually is detected between the ages of 6 and 9.

In a typical history, an asymptomatic facial swelling or asymmetry is noted or an osseous lesion is found on routine dental x-ray examination. In the jaws it is frequently found next to an unerupted tooth. By the time it is noticed, the size of the lesion suggests that it may have existed for a long time. It probably could have been demonstrable in infancy, but radiological survey of asymptomatic children rarely is done at that age. There is, therefore, little information about the incipient stages of this disease.

The most common manifestation of monostotic fibrous dysplasia in the mandible is an intraosseous nodule, localized at its angle. It is "encapsulated" by the cortices and a zone of condensation or sclerosis. Similar lesions may be found in the maxilla or around the ethmoid region.

The usual pattern in the progression of the disease is a slow, often imperceptible enlargement for a few years, after which the growth

ceases and the lesion remains stationary. In several cases, followed for more than two decades, the osseous lesion remained stationary and asymptomatic. Such changes as condensation, sclerosis, calcification, and thickening of cortices were interpreted as signs of maturation (case 1) [17].

Spontaneous regression does occur occasionally. Spotty or partial replacement by normal-looking bone can be demonstrated (case 4). The belief that the disease is active in childhood and that it is arrested during puberty is partially valid. There are some instances when it was first diagnosed or became active again as late as the sixth decade of life. It has been suggested that the earlier it develops, the more aggressively it grows and the poorer the prognosis [10].

A different course has been observed in a number of cases. The lesion enlarges rapidly to alarming proportions, its growth suggesting a malignant tumor. In rapid sequence, the cortex is attenuated, distended, and eroded (cases 3 and 4).

The complications and functional disturbances created by these tumors are due to their physical enlargement. In the mandible, intra-oral tumefaction results in pressure ulceration, difficulty in mastication and speaking, and finally in interference with respiratory exchange. Elsewhere there may be nasal obstruction, displacement of the eyeball, proptosis, optic atrophy, and compression and infection of the tear sac.

Spontaneous fractures, a common manifestation of fibrous dysplasia in the long bones, do not occur in the facial skeleton.

Sarcomatous degeneration of fibrous dysplasia occurs so rarely that it should not be confused with a rapidly growing lesion. Slow et al. [26] collected 33 cases of osteogenic sarcoma arising from fibrous dysplasia. Thirteen of them were localized in the craniofacial skeleton. Most of them had been exposed to radiation previously, and the sarcoma had developed 20 to 30 years later. The authors calculated the incidence of malignant degeneration in fibrous dysplasia at 0.4 percent, rising to 44 percent when radiation had been given. Schwartz and

Albert [24] claim that such malignant transformation is more frequent even without radiation. There is now universal agreement that radiation is contraindicated as a treatment modality.

Craniofacial Polyostotic Fibrous Dysplasia

The facial deformity in the polyostotic form of fibrous dysplasia is usually more severe, affecting different parts of the face [8]. The progression of the disease is similar to that of the monostotic form in that the enlargement continues for several years, usually during childhood and adolescence, and then remains stationary. The disease, whether limited to the craniofacial skeleton or of a more generalized distribution, may remain in remission for decades, perhaps indefinitely [4, 10]. Many of these patients are asymptomatic, the facial deformity being their only handicap.

There is a certain autonomy of the individual lesion, which may continue to enlarge while other lesions remain stationary. Individual tumors in the mandible or maxilla may behave and appear radiologically like a monostotic tumor (cases 5 and 6).

A complex clinical syndrome, usually designated as McCune-Albright's disease, is associated with various endocrinopathies [1,5,20,30]. Skeletal involvement is similar to that in polyostotic fibrous dysplasia, but more severe. The complications and the sequelae can result in loss of sight, hearing impairment, and other functional impediments. Cutaneous pigmentation may or may not be present.

These cases are of great interest to endocrinologists but are rarely referred for surgical treatment. With advances in endocrinology, a more detailed evaluation can be made of hormonal imbalance, and individual hormones can be quantitated. However, there is as yet neither an explanation of the relation of the endocrinopathy and the skeletal disease nor any endocrinological treatment available. My experience has been with only a few adolescents with

long-standing skeletal disease, grossly elevated growth hormone and prolactin, combined with characteristic giantism. There was no radiological evidence of pituitary enlargement. An autopsy in case 9 was disappointing because it provided no morphological basis in the endocrine glands or the hypothalamus for hormonal dysfunction.

No direct correlation could be found between the disease of the bone and the hormonal dysfunction; no long-term longitudinal data on hormonal secretions are available. The bony process is self-limiting and may be arrested even though the hormonal imbalance persists. However, by the time the disease becomes stationary, the patient may be severely disabled.

Differentiation of Fibro-Osseous Dysplastic Lesions

Paget's disease, which often affects the craniofacial skeleton, is recognized as a different entity. It is a disease of advanced age. The main radiological manifestation is hyperostosis ("cotton wool pattern"). The pathologist finds the mosaic appearance of the bone a characteristic of the disease. Nevertheless, occasionally fibrous dysplasia may have hyperostotic features and is then designated as pagetoid.

In 1925 the association of "brown tumors" with parathyroid adenomas was described and established as an independent clinical entity [16]. Clinically, the differential diagnosis is primarily dependent on the finding of increased calcium and decreased phosphorus in the blood serum and other symptoms of hyperparathyroidism.

Fibro-osseous dysplastic lesions in the jaws, with the same histological makeup as fibrous dysplasia, are quite common. However, their clinical course is different [3,4,13,15,32]. They usually are discovered during middle age, remain small, and are self-limiting. They appear as radiolucent, localized lesions, and they eventually are replaced by normal bone or become a dense, sclerosed, calcified mass, referred to as *cementum*. It is assumed that these lesions develop from dentigerous elements. Since periodontal membrane has an osteogenic potential and cementum is closely related to bone, it is difficult to differentiate between lesions of osseous and dentigerous origin. Calcified, deep-staining bodies, identical with cementum, frequently are found in fibrous dysplasia tumors in other craniofacial locations or in the long bones, hence their designation as *cementifying osteofibroma* [6]. Such fibro-osseous lesions are reported as fibrous dysplasia, periapical, ossifying, or cementifying fibroma, periapical cementifying dysplasia, or cementoma.

Langdon et al. [13], discussing ossifying fibroma of the jaws, posed the question, "Is this one disease or six?" These authors and many others believe that the different findings reflect stages of the spectrum of fibro-osseous dysplasia and that they are part of the evolution of the same disease.

Many clinicians and pathologists insist on differentiation between osteofibroma (or cementifying osteofibroma) [4,6] and fibrous dysplasia. The histological characteristics of the former are the presence of some lamellated bone and rimming of the bony trabeculae with osteoblasts.

Osteofibroma is described as a sharply localized, progressive, monostotic, neoplastic tumor requiring complete resection; fibrous dysplasia is a dysplastic lesion, slow growing and regressive. There is often no correlation between such histological findings and the clinical appearance and course of the disease. Recognized bone pathologists, on examination of the same histological slides, have offered conflicting opinions in identifying them [29]. In polyostotic fibrous dysplasia, individual tumors frequently conform to the description of osteofibroma. Such differentiation between these two entities is questionable at best [3,9,13] and confusing to the surgeon managing these tumors. In a number of instances a radical excision of a fibro-osseous lesion was justified by the diagnosis of an osteofibroma.

In the preparation of this chapter I have reviewed cases of craniofacial fibrous dysplasia where objective data were available (photographs, x-rays, and surgical and pathological reports) for a period of at least 10 years. The length of the follow-up period varied from 10 to 35 years.

Such long-term follow-up is difficult to obtain because the population of metropolitan areas is so highly mobile; patients change their residences frequently. There are a large number of institutions and surgeons from whom to choose, and such institutions often change surgeons as well. It is particularly difficult to obtain long-term follow-up on patients who are not under active treatment, are not disabled, and are symptom free.

Case Reports

Out of twenty-odd cases where such information was available, I have selected nine to illustrate the different forms of this disease, its variations, symptomatology, and long-term behavior. Only abbreviated case reports and pertinent findings are presented. None of these patients had either hereditary or familial history or trauma as a plausible causative factor. Five were monostotic, three in the mandible, one in the maxilla, and one in the ethmoid. Two were polyostotic and two were polyostotic with endocrinopathies.

CASE 1

Asymmetry and mild enlargment of the right side of this girl's face were noted at the age of 10. Four years later, in the course of a dental examination, x-rays showed a large lesion occupying the entire right ascending ramus, posterior to the first molar (Fig. 21-2D). The swelling was not disfiguring (Fig. 21-2A), the patient was asymptomatic, and no operation was indicated.

Radiological follow-up for 11 years showed additional signs of maturation, increased condensation, and sclerosis of the cortex. Two pregnancies had no effect on the tumor.

The growth of the tumor was minimal, but at

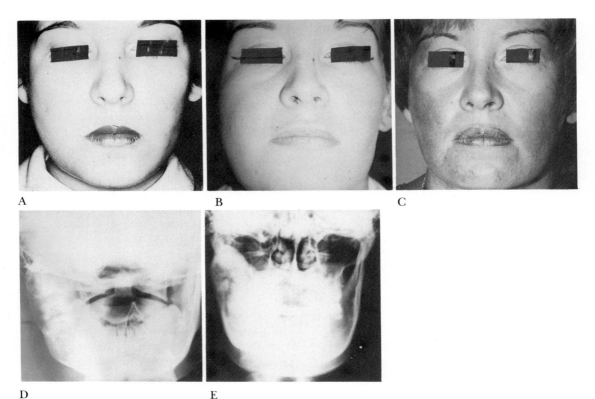

A   B   C

D   E

FIGURE 21-2. *Case 1. (A) Patient at age 14. Note full-*
ness of right side of face. (B) Age 25. Increased swelling of
right side. (C) Age 33, eight years after contouring opera-
tion. Face is symmetrical. (D) Nodule in right mandible
(age 14) with attenuated cortex and mottled opacities. (E)

Nineteen years later (and 6 years after operation), both
cortex and content of nodule are sclerosed. (Reproduced,
with permission, from M.L. Lewin, Fibrous dysplasia of the
mandible in children. Plast. Reconstr. Surg. *25:161–*
173, 1960.)

the age of 25, the patient became aware of fullness in the submandibular area (Fig. 21-2B).
An intraoral contouring operation was performed.

The tumor involved the buccal surface of the
mandible. The cortex was thickened and hard;
the lesional content, gritty, firm, and avascular.
The mandible was contoured to about its normal shape.

Eight years later, the facial contour remained
normal (Fig. 21-2C). Radiologically the nodule
was more opaque and well "encapsulated" by
a sclerotic zone and thickened cortex (Fig.
21-2E). The patient had normal dentition and
was asymptomatic.

Discussion. This is a typical history of fibrous
dysplasia, similar to that of several other pa-

tients followed for 10 to 20 years. The natural
course of the disease was not altered by any
treatment. When the lesion was inactive and
stationary, a contouring operation was performed to correct the asymmetry of the face.

CASE 2

This patient was vaguely aware, throughout his
teens and twenties, of a mild asymmetry and
swelling of the right side of his face. This was
overlooked on induction into the United States
Army (Fig. 21-3A), but was accidentally noticed
later. A hard swelling was found at the angle of
the right mandible. Radiological examination
revealed a fibro-osseous lesion which was
confirmed by biopsy. The patient was discharged from the army because this was considered a preinduction disease.

The swelling enlarged imperceptibly and extended toward the zygoma, but 10 years later it was only mildly disfiguring and asymptomatic (Fig. 21-3B). Radiologically the lesion involved the mandible from the sigmoid notch to the midline (Fig. 21-3F). A contouring operation was advised but declined by the patient.

The tumor progressed slowly for the next 10 years (Fig. 21-3C), but more rapidly during the subsequent 10 years (Fig. 21-3D).

At the age of 65, a resection of the ascending ramus was performed in another institution (Fig. 21-3E and G). The patient died of other causes 4 years later.

Discussion. The lesion had undoubtedly existed in childhood but grew imperceptibly until the seventh decade of life, when it began to progress rapidly. Whether this tumor could have been controlled by a lesser trimming operation is conjectural. The disease was diagnosed by some clinicians as fibrous dysplasia, by others as osteofibroma. Several pathologists, examining the specimen, differed in their opinions. There was no suggestion of malignancy.

CASE 3
Swelling in the right side of the face in this 6-year-old girl was attributed to extraction of a deciduous molar (Fig. 21-4A). X-ray examination showed a radiolucent, cyst-like lesion, occupying the entire ascending ramus of the right mandible (Fig. 21-5A).

By the age of 9, the tumor had progressed to such an extent that the facial deformity was conspicuous and interfered with normal social development. An intraoral trimming operation was performed. The buccal cortex was found to be eroded. A yellow-brown, fleshy tumor the size of a plum was removed. The surrounding diseased bone was curetted.

The tumor continued to grow at a rapid pace, both externally and intraorally. The swelling of the alveolus became so great that the child could not close her mouth. A large pressure ulcer developed over the alveolar crest. The canine and premolar teeth and the sur-

rounding bone were loosened and displaced lingually, crowding the tongue. There was pronounced engorgement and brownish discoloration of the skin over the tumor (Fig. 21-4B). By that time the radiological picture revealed disintegration of the mandible and its replacement by a multiloculated lesion within the septa (Fig. 21-5B).

Since the condition had become life-threatening, a hemimandibulectomy was performed. Mandibular resection extended beyond the midline and included the condyle. The ulcerated mucosa was excised with the specimen. A stainless steel rod was used to stabilize the left mandible (Fig. 21-6A).

A year later, the missing portion of the mandible was replaced with a 6-in.-long fragment of rib. To compensate for future growth, the graft was made long enough so that the mandible was in a prognathic position. A cartilagenous component was included with the rib graft and carved to form the condyle (Fig. 21-6B). Under functional stress, the thin rib graft gradually bent, resulting in its curvature in the submandibular region (Fig. 21-4C). The symphysis receded.

Three years later the convex portion of the reconstructed mandible was excised and replaced with another rib graft overlapping the previous one. Additional pieces of rib were used to reinforce the thin bone graft and to correct the flatness on the right side of the face (Fig. 21-6C and D).

The patient's facial contour at age 34 showed no change from that in Figure 21-4D,E, and F at age 16. The reconstructed condyle was somewhat irregular and small but showed no signs of absorption (Fig. 21-7). Except for a mild flatness in front of the right ear, the patient's facial contour was normal. The deviation of the mandible to the right could be noticed only when the mouth was widely open.

Discussion. This is an example of an aggressively growing fibrous dysplasia. A hemimandibulectomy was performed because the predominantly fibrous pathological tissue had destroyed the mandible, and the bulky intraoral tumor endangered vital functions. Two

386

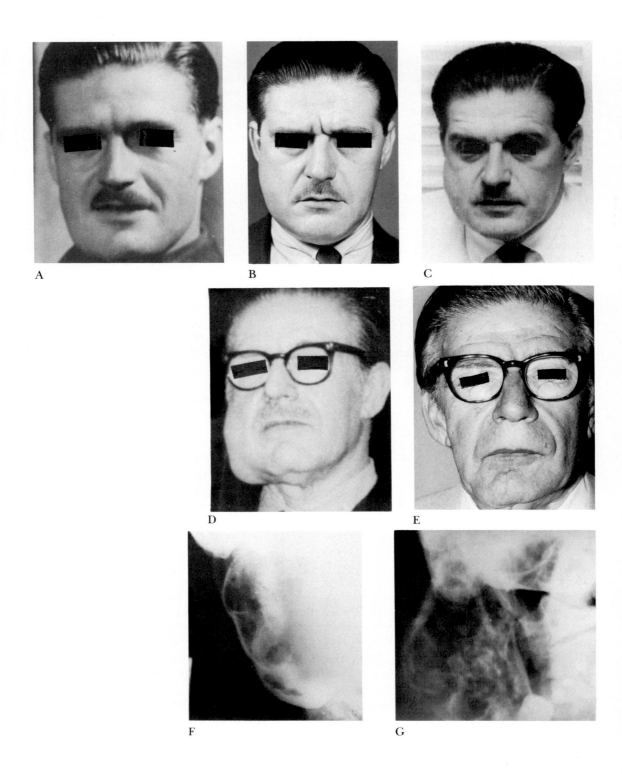

A

B

C

D

E

F

G

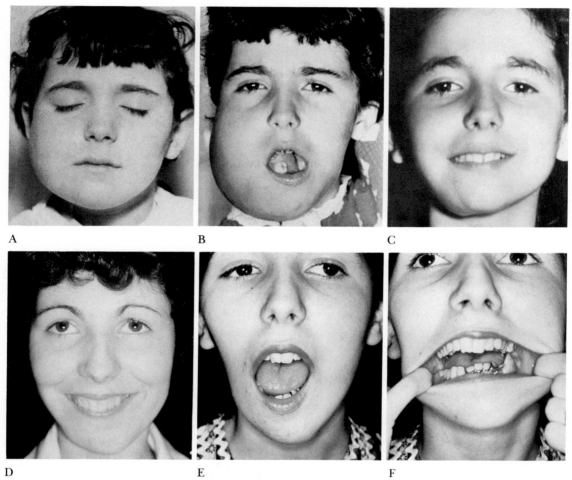

A B C

D E F

FIGURE 21-4. *Case 3. (A) Seven-year-old girl with large cyst-like, mild swelling of right side of face. (B) Fifteen months later, huge intraoral and extraoral tumor. (C) After first bone graft, showing projection of graft into submandibular region. (D,E, and F) Eight years after resection, and 4 years after second bone graft. At age 34, facial* contour remains normal. ([A] and [B] reproduced, with permission, from M.L. Lewin, Fibrous dysplasia of the mandible. Am. J. Surg. 90:951–961, 1955; [C] through [F] from M.L. Lewin, Fibrous dysplasia of the mandible in children. Plast. Reconstr. Surg. 25:161–173, 1960.)

FIGURE 21-3. *Case 2. (A through E) Changes in facial appearance over 35-year period. Note increasing facial asymmetry and swelling of right side. (A) At age 32. (B) At age 46. (C) At age 56. (D) At age 64. (E) At age 69 (4 years after resection). (F) Radiological appearance of lesion at age 46. Cortex attenuated but intact. Lesion is predominantly fibrous with some condensation in center. (G) Eighteen years later (before resection). Atrophic cortex is bulging and seems to be eroded. Lesion still primarily fibrous, with bony septa and condensed core. ([B] reproduced, with permission, from M. L. Lewin, Fibrous dysplasia of the mandible. Am. J. Surg. 90:951–961, 1955.)*

bone-graft procedures were performed to reconstruct the jaw.

CASE 4

This 4-year-old boy developed a swelling of the left side of his face around the upper alveolus in the region of the canine. Within 6 months the swelling increased markedly, extending over the entire maxilla to the orbit and encroaching on the left nasal cavity (Fig. 21-8A).

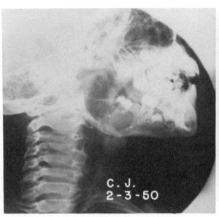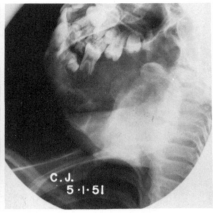

A   B

FIGURE 21-5.   *Case 3. (A) Original x-rays of the right mandible showing a large cyst-like lesion adjacent to an unerupted molar. (B) Fifteen months later, showing a huge tumor with disintegration of osseous mandible and erosion of cortex. Anterior part of tumor predominantly fibrous;* *posterior, fibro-osseous. ([A] reproduced, with permission, from M.L. Lewin, Fibrous dysplasia of the mandible. Am. J. Surg. 90:951–961, 1955; [B] from M.L. Lewin, Fibrous dysplasia of the mandible in children. Plast. Reconstr. Surg. 25:161–173, 1960.)*

The tumefaction of the alveolus and the left side of the palate prevented the child from closing his mouth (Fig. 21-8B). Small ulcerations developed over the alveolus, causing persistent bleeding.

At the operation the maxilla was exposed through a Caldwell-Luc approach. The cortex was eroded and the tumor consisted of gritty, partially rubbery, and partially cystic material. The maxillary sinus was reduced in size and was reamed out. The alveolus, the anterior facial wall, and the pyriform aperture were contoured with osteotomes. Large fragments of bone were removed. Nodules on the hard palate were resected after elevation of mucoperiosteal flaps so that the palate could be reconstituted.

During the subsequent 2 years, the tumor continued to grow slowly, although the external deformity was minimal. Recontouring of the alveolus was performed. Two years later, additional minor trimming was done, and the two impacted teeth were removed.

During the next 6 years, there was no further growth of the tumor; the facial contour, the alveolus, and the palate remained normal (Fig. 21-8D).

Periodic occlusal radiographs revealed that the remaining pathological bone had gradually been replaced by normal bone (Fig. 21-8E).

Discussion.   The aggressive growth of this tumor is similar to the previous case. The operation reduced the tumor substantially, but no attempt was made to resect all the tumor tissue, since this would have resulted in midface mutilation. Subsequent growth of the lesion was limited, slow, and easily controlled by two minor trimming operations. No reconstructive procedure was required. Ten years later there was evidence that the residual tumor had been replaced by normal bone (Fig. 21-8C).

CASE 5

When this boy was about 6 or 7, his parents noticed that his nose was obstructed and that there was a swelling around his right inner canthus. Shortly thereafter, as a result of an accident, his left eye was enucleated.

His parents reported that since the accident the swelling around the right inner canthus had increased rapidly. At the age of 10, he developed an abscess of the right lacrimal sac

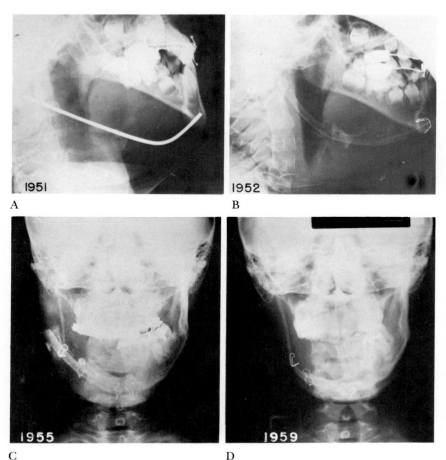

FIGURE 21-6. *Case 3. (A) Postoperative x-rays of mandible with temporary steel rod replacement. (B) Excised mandible replaced with partially decorticated rib. (C) X-rays showing second rib graft after convex portion of first graft was excised. Several on-lay fragments of bone were used to reinforce bone graft. (D) Reconstructed mandible 4 years after last operation. Note contouring of graft which is thin but almost symmetrical with opposite side. Eighteen years later it remained unchanged. (Reproduced, with permission, from M.L. Lewin, Fibrous dysplasia of the mandible in children.* Plast. Reconstr. Surg. *25:161–173, 1960.)*

which required incision, drainage, and repeated irrigation of the canaliculus. His right eye was proptotic and displaced laterally (Fig. 21-9A). The radiological examination showed a large, sclerotic nodule involving the right ethmoid, the orbit, and the nasal cavity (Fig. 21-9C).

Partial resection of the tumor was performed at the age of 11. The tumor was neither sclerotic nor well demarcated, as the radiological findings had suggested. The medial orbital wall had eroded, and two plum-sized nodules were shelled out of the orbit. The tumor replaced the ethmoid cells, the lacrimal bone, and the turbinates with gritty, soft, amorphous bone. It protruded into the pharynx, filling the right nasal cavity and displacing the septum. The nasolacrimal canal was obliterated.

The ethmoid sinuses were curetted. The tumor masses were excised, and the turbinate was amputated. The right canthus was reattached by a transnasal canthopexy.

During the subsequent 5 years, the nasal obstruction gradually recurred. There was a weeks to provide drainage for the lacrimal system. Large nasopharyngeal airways were inserted in both nasal cavities to maintain their patency.

The operation improved the patient's appearance and restored nasal breathing (Fig. 21-9B and D). Tear drainage was sluggish and required occasional irrigation.

Discussion. The pathologist noted the prevalence of cement-like bodies and rendered a diagnosis of cementifying osteofibroma.

Monostotic fibrous dysplasia in the ethmoid area is rather unusual. In this case it encompassed the adjacent bones and intranasal structures so that differentiation from the polyostotic form was blurred. After the first operation, the tumor recurred slowly over a 5-year period. The patient is now an adult and is asymptomatic.

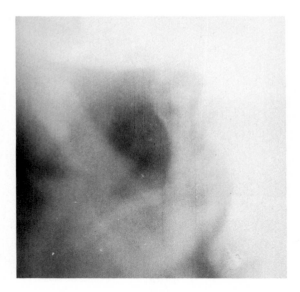

FIGURE 21-7. *Case 3. Reconstructed condyle 25 years later. Cartilaginous component not visible. Some irregular absorption of costal-cartilaginous junction.*

slight fullness at the right inner canthus, and the root of the nose had broadened, giving the nasal bridge a flat appearance. There were intermittent episodes of lacrimal obstruction and infection which required irrigation of the lacrimal sac.

At the age of 16, the operation was repeated, but with more radical resection of the diseased bone. The midline scar on the forehead and dorsum of the nose was reopened. After an osteotomy of the nasal bones, the nasal cavity was entered. The intranasal tumor had spread and flattened the nasal bones and protruded into the right orbit. Extensive resection of the medial orbital wall, the turbinates, the posterior septum, and the adjacent part of the maxilla was performed. The tumor was vascular, but the bleeding was controlled by packing. The displaced septum, which obstructed the opposite airway, was osteotomized and returned to the midline position. Iliac bone grafts were used to reconstruct the medial orbital wall and the nasal bridge. The inner canthi were reattached by a transnasal canthopexy. An angiocatheter was threaded from the lacrimal sac into the nasal cavity and left in place for several

CASE 6

This girl was observed by her pediatrician from the age of 4 because of facial asymmetry and swelling of the left side of the face.

At the age of 10, she was referred to an ophthalmologist who found a 7-mm proptosis and incipient optic atrophy of her left eye. There also was a bone-conduction hearing deficit of the left ear.

By the age of 12, the swelling of the maxilla was moderate, but the swelling of the mandible increased conspicuously (Fig. 21-10A). X-rays showed a diffused opacity of the left maxilla and orbit and thickening and rarefaction of the left cranial vault. In the left mandible there

FIGURE 21-8. *Case 4. (A) Tumor that developed in a 5-year-old boy within a period of 1 year. (B) Main swelling localized in upper alveolus. (C) Serial tangential radiographs during 1 year, showing growth of tumor, which started as a fibrous lesion but developed as a mixture of fibrous and osseous elements ("smoke pattern"). (D) Ten years after operation. (E) Postoperative changes in alveolar bone, followed in occlusal views. (1) Residual pathological bone 1 year after operation. (2) Four years later. (3) Ten years after operation, radiolucency at site of extraction of two unerupted teeth. Remainder of bone has almost normal architecture.*

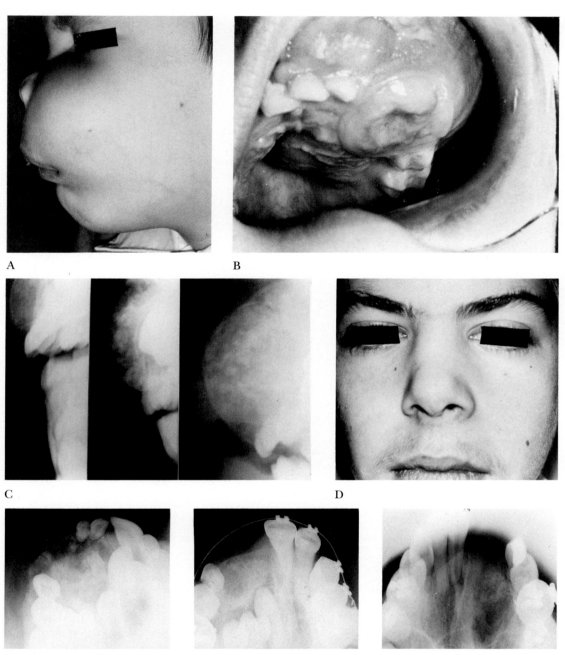

A

B

C

D

E

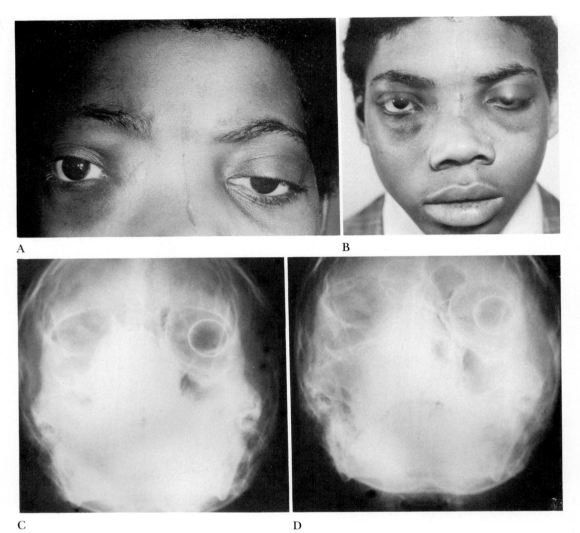

FIGURE 21-9. *Case 5. (A) Fourteen-year-old boy with tumor at right inner canthus, displacing eye. Note spreading of nasal dorsum and complete obliteration of intranasal space. Scar after drainage of abscessed tear sac. Left eye prosthetic. (B) Eight years after first operation. Normal tear drainage and clear nasal passages. (C) Dense sclerotic nodule in right ethmoid area, adjacent maxilla, intranasal and paranasal space, extending into right orbit. (D) After two operations, sclerotic nodule is greatly reduced, both in density and size. Improved aeration of paranasal sinuses.*

was a large nodule with irregular areas of opacities and with a thin cortex. During a year's observation, the lesion did not increase in size and the nodule became more sclerotic.

Since the mandibular tumor was the main aspect of the deformity, a trimming operation was performed. The cortex was of moderate

thickness, and the nodule consisted of gritty material.

Ten years later, the contour of the mandible was normal. The maxillary swelling had decreased. The proptosis of the left eye still measured at 7 mm (Fig. 21-10B). The optic atrophy was more pronounced, but visual acuity re-

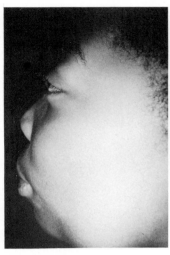
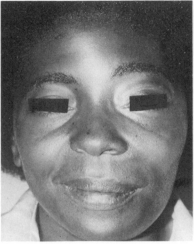
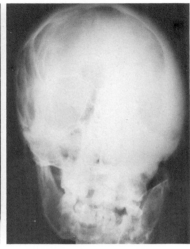

A   B   C

FIGURE 21-10.   Case 6. (A) Thirteen-year-old girl with polyostotic fibrous dysplasia nodule at mandibular angle. Also note swelling of maxilla and proptosis. (B) Patient at age 24, nine years after contouring of mandible. Facial deformity is mild: swelling in malar region and proptosis of left eye. (C) Radiograph at age 24. Nodule in left mandible is sharply outlined and more sclerotic than 10 years earlier. Appearance is typical of monostotic lesion (cases 1 and 2). Diffused sclerosis of left periorbital area, ethmoids, and temporal bone. Density has increased in last 10 years.

mained normal. Radiologically the mandibular lesion was more condensed and sclerosed (Fig. 21-10C). In addition, the calvarium, in the left frontal and parietal region, was uniformly thickened and sclerosed.

Discussion. This is a typical case of a slow-growing, polyostotic fibrous dysplasia involving several bones on the left side of the craniofacial skeleton. The individual lesions seemed to develop and progress independently of each other. The mandibular nodule was identical radiologically, histologically, and in its clinical course with the monostotic lesion in case 1.

Optic atrophy was attributed to the compression of the nerve along the base of the cranium, and the proptosis to the reduction of orbital space. This may have been the result of tumefaction in the orbital surface of the frontal bone or of the sphenoid. Both the proptosis and optical atrophy had progressed slightly during the 13-year period of observation. Up to the present time, this patient's vision has not been affected.

While the cranial component has progressed, the facial tumors have remained stationary over the past 10 years, and the patient has remained asymptomatic.

CASE 7

At the age of 5, a hard growth, the size of a plum, appeared over this boy's left mandible, gradually increasing in size. Within the next 2 or 3 years, a swelling appeared over the left eye, causing a forward and downward displacement of the eyeball. Small, irregular nodules appeared on the left forehead and skull.

By the time the boy was 9, he had a huge swelling of the left mandible which extended down the neck. However, intraorally, the alveolus was not affected, and he had a normal complement of teeth in good occlusion (Fig. 21-11A). Biopsy of the mandibular tumor confirmed the diagnosis of fibrous dysplasia. It was treated by external radiation of 4000 R with no effect.

X-ray examination showed a mottled, dense

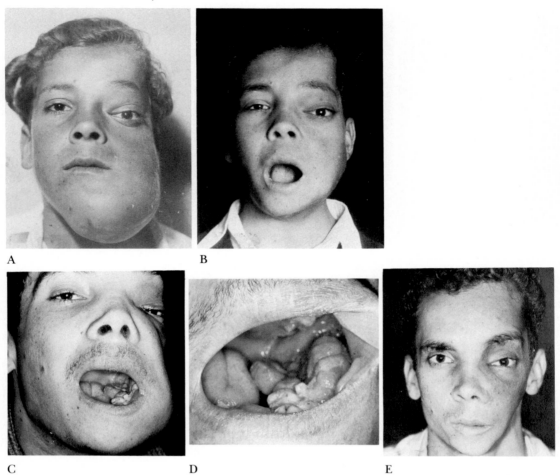

A   B

C   D   E

FIGURE 21-11. *Case 7. (A) Fourteen-year-old boy with mandibular tumor of about 10 years' duration. Note downward displacement of left eye and tumefaction of left forehead. (B) Patient after first operation. (C) Seven years later. Note recurrence of tumor in mandible and new swelling over maxilla and nose. Displacement of left eye has increased, and nodules on forehead and parietal region have grown in size. (D) Enlargement of left alveolus.* *Groove corresponds to imprint of upper teeth. (E) Postoperative appearance of patient after several operations on mandible, maxilla, and cranium. ([A] and [B] reproduced, with permission, from M.L. Lewin, Fibrous dysplasia of the mandible. Am. J. Surg. 90:951–961, 1955; [C] through [E] from M.L. Lewin, Fibrous dysplasia of the mandible in children. Plast. Reconstr. Surg. 25:161–173, 1960.)*

enlargement of the entire left mandible with irregularly calcified septa and fuzzy outline (Fig. 21-12A). The entire half of the left cranial vault was replaced with areas of rarefaction, alternating with areas of condensation. The bone had an irregular, honeycomb appearance. There was marked sclerosis of the floor of the anterior cranial fossa involving the roof of the orbit. A sclerotic nodule occupied the right maxilla and ethmoid region.

An operation was performed at the age of 14 to reduce the huge tumor of the mandible. The cortex was thin and fragmented, and the lesion was of firm, gritty consistency and included

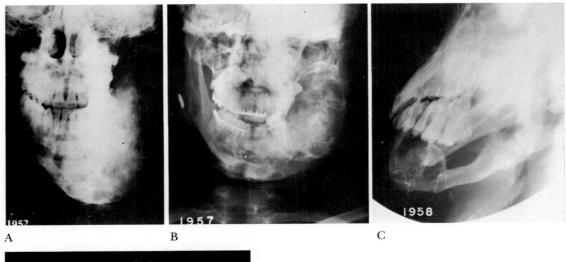

A   B   C

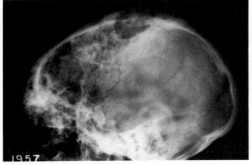

D

FIGURE 21-12.   *Case 7. (A) Exophytic tumor of the mandible with irregular sclerosis. calcification, and fuzzy outline. Diffuse sclerosis of maxilla and ethmoid on left. (B) Recurrent tumor 5 years after extensive trimming of original one. Note "encapsulated" fibro-osseous nodule. Radiological and operative findings are identical to monostotic tumor. Increased sclerosis of left forehead. (C) One year after removal of bulk of tumor in mandible. Because of disintegration of osseous mandible, bone graft was used for reinforcement. Residual tumor still present in mental and subcondylar region. (D) Cranial vault with large areas of rarefaction. Hyperostosis of frontal bone and sclerosis of base of skull. ([A] reproduced, with permission, from M.L. Lewin, Fibrous dysplasia of the mandible. Am. J. Surg. 90:951–961, 1955; [B] through [D] from M.L. Lewin, Fibrous dysplasia of the mandible in children. Plast. Reconstr. Surg. 25:161–173, 1960.)*

white and yellow nodules and cysts of various sizes. Large fragments of bone were removed, and the mandible was recontoured.

The improvement was not only in the patient's appearance but in his attitude. He was no longer depressed and could resume normal social activities (Fig. 21-11B). The condition remained stationary for 3 years, after which both the mandible and maxilla began to enlarge again.

Figure 21-11C shows the patient 5 years after the first operation. There was a diffuse, hard swelling over the left maxilla, extending toward the inner canthus. The left side of the forehead, at the supraorbital ridge, was enlarged, accentuating the effect of the downward displacement of the eye. The tumefaction over the mandible differed from the original condition. It also involved the alveolus, which was greatly enlarged. A deep groove in its

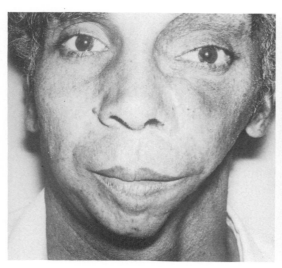

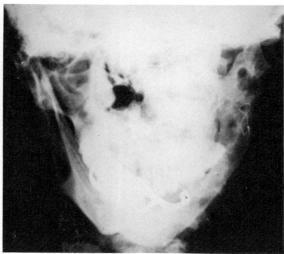

A   B

FIGURE 21-13. *Case 7. (A) Eighteen years later, at age 40. Forehead of normal contour, but left eye depressed. (B) Cyst-like lesion in residual mandible, proximal to old bone graft.*

center, caused by the pressure of the upper teeth, divided the alveolus into two parts (Fig. 21-11D). The lingual side was loosened, tilted inward, and crowded the tongue. Radiologically there was a large "encapsulated" nodule in the left mandible, with intense opacity in the center and radiolucency along the periphery (Fig. 21-12B) The lesions in the maxilla and cranium increased in density and size.

At the operation, the lesion in the ascending ramus was found to be a fleshy, encapsulated nodule, the size of an egg, located within a thin, bony shelf, through which it eroded in several places. A large, encapsulated nodule was enucleated. The loosened and displaced alveolar portion of the mandible was removed. Although no attempt was made to remove all diseased structures, not enough bony element remained in the mandible to maintain its continuity. A few months later, the mandible was reinforced with an iliac bone graft. The graft was joined at both ends to the remaining fibrodysplastic bone and consolidated normally (Fig. 21-12C).

In a separate operation, the maxilla was recontoured, and large fragments of zygoma were excised through an intraoral approach in the upper buccal sulcus. The nodules on the left side of the forehead and in the ethmoid region and the overgrowth of the supraorbital ridge were reduced (Fig. 21-12D). The excised bone was soft and gritty, with multiple cysts and fibrous nodules (Fig. 21-12C).

The patient, now 40 years old and married, has been fully employed for the last 15 years (Fig. 21-13A). Facial contour is almost normal, except for a mild downward displacement of the left eye. Consecutive radiographs show increased thickening of the calvarium, and fibrodysplastic bone is still present in the subcondylar area (Fig. 21-13B).

Discussion. The unilateral polyostotic fibrous dysplasia of the craniofacial skeleton in this patient began at an early age and seemed to become inactive at the beginning of the second decade, by which time there was an enormous external swelling of the mandible. The disease remained inactive for about 5 or 6 years, after which the tumors in the mandible and maxilla enlarged rapidly. The new mandibular lesion resembled, in course and appearance, that of case 3.

Disintegration and fragmentation of the mandible required bone grafting for its reinforcement. Although the graft was inserted into a gap in the fibrodysplastic bone, the consolidation was rapid and uneventful.

During the past 17 years there has been no noticeable activity in any part of the involved craniofacial skeleton, although on radiological examination, the pathological changes persist.

CASE 8

The parents of this boy noticed enlargement and asymmetry of his face and lumps on his skull at the age of 6 or 7. Enlargement of the right side of the face continued at a moderate rate. Around 9 years of age, reduced vision in the right eye was noted.

Between the ages of 10 and 12, several operations were performed in another institution. A partial maxillectomy and trimming of the zygomatic and malar areas was performed through a Fergusson approach. Neurosurgical decompression of the right optic nerve had not improved the existing optic atrophy, and the boy's vision deteriorated further. Fragments of the right frontal bone were excised.

The patient stated that there had been no enlargement of his face or skull after the age of 12, and that his vertical growth had ceased around the age of 18. He had been gainfully employed but was extremely sensitive about his appearance. He also reported mild discomfort in the right hip. Sexual development was normal.

At the age of 22 the patient was 6 ft 6 in. tall and weighed 193 pounds (Fig. 21-14A). There were large areas of dark brown pigmentation on his chest and right upper arm (Fig. 21-14B).

X-rays of his right femur and tibia showed the bone to be of normal configuration but containing large, cyst-like lesions (Fig. 21-14C). Similar lesions were found in the right pelvis.

The upper part of his face and skull were greatly enlarged, particularly in the right malar region, but the lower third was normal in contour. There was a protrusion at the right inner canthus which caused a displacement of the right eye laterally and a broadening of the root of the nose.

Most of the facial enlargement involved the forehead and parietal region. The contour was irregular, with areas of depression and protrusion. The patient had no vision in the right eye, as a result of optic atrophy. There was distortion of the eye fissure, attributable to the earlier operative intervention.

Radiological examination revealed a severe bony overgrowth of the supraorbital ridges and massive thickening of the frontal and parietal areas. The occipital bone was normal. The right ethmoid region was sclerotic, extending into the orbit and broadening the intraorbital distance. The base of the cranium, the right maxilla, and the zygoma were diffusely sclerosed (Fig. 21-14E and F). The mandible was not involved.

Endocrinological workup showed normal levels of gonadotropin, TSH, and thyroid hormone. Random growth hormones varied from 9.4 to 14 ng/ml (normal values 1.5 ng/ml). Prolactin was 38 ng/ml (normal values up to 15 ng/ml).

An operation was performed to reduce the bulk and improve the contour of the midface and forehead. The existing scars on the face were excised, exposing the entire enterofacial wall from the frontal process of the maxilla to the zygoma. The maxilla was recontoured, removing a large fragment from the malar region.

The bony mass protruding into the orbit was reduced, leaving some of the medial wall. The ethmoid cells were thoroughly curetted. The bone was soft, of cancellous consistency. The inner canthus was reattached by a transnasal canthopexy.

The forehead was exposed through a coronal incision. Then, to avoid penetrating the cranial space, multiple drill holes were made to a depth of 3 cm in the frontal area. None of them reached the dura. The frontal bone was extremely vascular and of rock-like consistency. A power saw was ineffective, and osteotomes required a great deal of force. To avoid further trauma to the skull and additional blood loss,

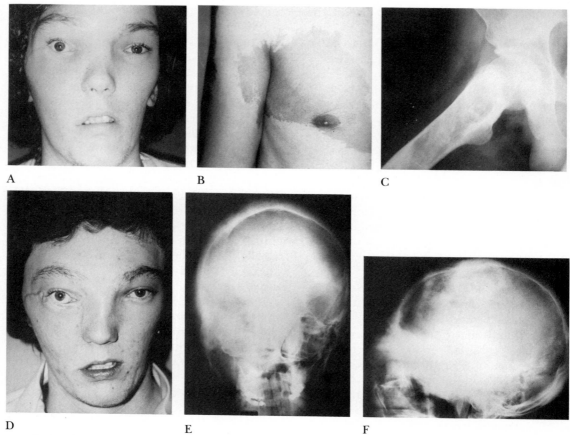

FIGURE 21-14. *Case 8. (A) Patient at age 22. Note deformity of forehead with bulging supraorbital ridges and left frontal parietal region. Depression of right frontal bone. Swelling of right maxilla and zygoma and in right inner canthus. Lateral displacement of right eye (blind). (B) One of pigmented "café au lait" patches. (C) Cyst-like, well-demarcated lesion in right femur remained unchanged for more than 12 years. (D) After operation. Ethmoid mass removed and zygoma trimmed. Contour of forehead normal. (E) Diffuse sclerosis of right midface and cranial skeleton extending over left ethmoid and frontal region. Thickening and fuzzy outline of cranial bones. Mandible not involved. (F) Lateral view of cranial skeleton showing fuzzy hyperostosis of forehead, areas of rarefaction, and sclerosis of anterior cranial vault.*

the contouring was limited to the forehead, particularly to the supraorbital ridges. A total of 350 g of bone was removed. A moderate improvement in the facial appearance was obtained (Fig. 21-14D).

Discussion. This is a classic example of generalized fibrous dysplasia associated with endocrinopathy and skin pigmentation, involving growth hormone and prolactin, both products of the pituitary. Since there was no evidence of enlargement of the sella turcica or of pituitary adenoma, it was assumed that the hypothalamic dysfunction had stimulated the hormonal secretion.

The effect of increased growth hormone in childhood, before the closure of the epiphyses, is giantism, involving the entire vertical growth. Subsequently, one might expect signs of acromegaly, such as enlargement of the acral parts of the body, but there were none.

Comparative x-rays of the long bones and

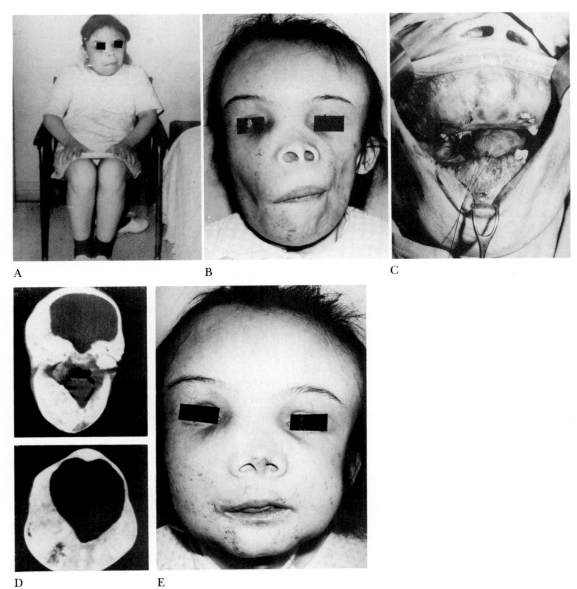

A   B   C

D   E

FIGURE 21-15.   *Case 9. (A) At age 10. (B) Age 18. Patient blind, with severe hearing impairment. (C) Intraoral view. Note enlargement of alveolus and upward displacement of tongue by mass on floor of mouth. (D) CAT scan, coronal and horizontal cuts. Note enlargement of frontal bones, particularly on right side, and crowding of intracranial space. Enlargement of mandible. (E) After first operation on mandible and maxilla.*

pelvis from the age of 7 to 21 showed the lesions to be stationary, with no distortion of the bone. In this respect the patient was asymptomatic.

The craniofacial bones were diffusely involved, particularly the cranial component and the right side of the midface. The mandibles were spared. Optic atrophy was noted early and was attributed to the narrowing of the optic canal. The patient lost the sight of his eye despite decompression of the optic canal.

The skeletal process has been dormant for years, and the patient has been functioning well. While it was important to minimize the facial deformity, an attempt to reduce the size of the calvarium had to be compromised because of the marble-like consistency of the bone and its vascularity.

CASE 9

A Hispanic family noticed that their 3-year-old daughter's head was much larger than that of other children her age. Enlargement continued at a rapid pace, so that at the age of 6 she had to be withdrawn from school because of her grotesque appearance and her failing vision (Fig. 21-15A).

At the age of 9, the circumference of her head was 60 cm. Although she was not menstruating and her secondary sex characteristics were undeveloped, estrogenized vaginal cells were found, suggesting sexual maturity. By the age of 13, her head circumference was 64 cm. She had difficulty in eating and swallowing and was almost totally blind. She also had conductive hearing loss, mostly on the right side.

Because of her monstrous appearance [19], she was isolated at home and cared for by her parents. At the age of 18, she was an unusually tall (6 feet), emaciated girl, weighing 104 pounds, with a head circumference of 73 cm (Fig. 21-15B). Her mandible was tremendously expanded, the tongue pushed upward by a large, bony mass lying on the floor of the mouth in continuity with the mandible. The upper alveolus was equally expanded, and

there were masses on the palate which together with the elevation of the tongue reduced the size of the mouth cavity and the mobility of the tongue (Fig. 21-15C).

The intercanthal distance was about 70 mm. The nose was flat and almost at the level of the cheeks. The forehead and skull were tremendously enlarged.

Radiological examination failed to show any skeletal details, because the x-rays could not penetrate the cranial and facial bones. The disease involved the mandibles, maxillae, and malar frontal bones bilaterally, as well as the base of the cranium. Bone age corresponded to chronological age.

Endocrinological evaluation revealed extreme elevation of the levels of growth hormone and prolactin. The former was 100 times normal, and the nocturnal peak was 800 times normal. The prolactin was 120 ng/ml (normal value 15 ng/ml).

The endocrinologist considered the possibility of pituitary adenoma, pituitary hyperplasia, or hypothalamic dysfunction. The sella turcica could not be visualized.

A comparison of the patient's measurements and photographs at various ages showed the head size had reached its peak around the age of 15.

The patient was hospitalized for several weeks for observation and treatment of her anemia and nutritional state. An operation was planned primarily to improve her oral functions of swallowing and eating.

The mandible was exposed externally and intraorally and completely skeletonized. It was greatly enlarged, extending for about 5 cm below the level of the mental foramina. Bony masses extended along the floor of the mouth and underneath the tongue. The cortex was thickened, hard, and pebbly. Using a Strycker oscillating saw, osteotomes, and bone-biting forceps, the mandible was reduced in size, and all the bone on the floor of the mouth was removed. The bone was extremely hard, resembling cortex, with layers of a chalk-like substance encased within it. The specimen weighed

480 g. The maxillary alveolus was exposed intraorally and reshaped, with removal of an additional 270 g of bone. The bone was very vascular.

The patient made a slow but good recovery. Improvement in appearance of the lower face is shown in Figure 21-15E. She was able to eat, and her nutritional status improved. Efforts were made to construct dentures.

Encouraged by this modest success, 3 months later the surgeon attempted to reduce the size of the forehead, zygomatic, and maxillary regions. Large bony fragments were removed from the zygoma and lateral maxilla. A neurosurgeon made numerous drill holes to estimate the thickness of the frontal bone. The drill penetrated for a distance of 5 cm without reaching the dura. The frontal bone proved to be extremely hard and rock-like. It was impossible to cut through with a saw, and osteotomes met with great resistance. There was profuse bleeding from the cut surface of the bone which was difficult to control by pressure, coagulation, and waxing. The operation was terminated because of a hypotensive episode which was controlled by a massive transfusion. A total of more than 1000 g of bone was removed.

Twelve hours after the operation, the patient developed convulsions and other central nervous system symptoms and died.

At the autopsy, the calvarium was removed with great difficulty. The frontal bone was found to be 9-cm thick, completely obliterating the anterior cranial fossa. The pituitary, the optical chiasma, and the brain stem were embedded in the bone. The brain was compressed into the posterior and middle fossae. The wings of the sphenoid and the petrous pyramids were involved in the disease process. There was evidence of cerebral edema.

A detailed pathological examination showed no abnormalities in the pituitary, other endocrine glands, or the hypothalamus.

The cause of death was assumed to be edema of the brain caused by the surgical trauma. The intracranial space had been greatly reduced by the pathological process, and there was none left to accommodate cerebral swelling.

Discussion. In this case, the endocrinopathy was combined with fibro-osseous dysplasia of unusual severity and rapid progression. There was no evidence of involvement of the remaining skeleton.

The hormonal disturbance involving the growth hormone and prolactin also was unusually severe. Unfortunately, the autopsy did not provide any morphological basis for the endocrinopathy.

The disease process involved the entire craniofacial skeleton, except for the occipital bone. Evidently, compression of the optic chiasma in the early stages led to blindness.

One of the most striking features of this case was the intracranial progression of the disease, involving both the vault and the base of the skull. The 9-cm-thick frontal and parietal bones were not only responsible for the enormous enlargement of the head, but they fused with the sphenoid and petrous bones into an impenetrable mass, reducing the intracranial space by about 50 percent. Neither the middle cranial fossa nor any other cranial nerve was affected.

Surgical Treatment

JAWS

The most frequent operation for patients with fibrous dysplasia was contouring of the mandible. Most mandibular tumors grew outward and downward. They could be reached through an intraoral approach by skeletonizing the buccal and undersurface of the jaw. The tumor was usually located posterior to the mental foramen, but the nerve was exposed and protected.

In most of the cases, the operation was performed when the lesion was mature and stationary. The cortex was expanded, thickened, and sclerosed. The content of the nodule was gritty, with islands of soft tissue, cyst-like structures, and amorphous material.

Sharp osteotomes or a power drill was needed to penetrate the cortex. The bulk of the tumor was removed with osteotomes and curettes, but enough tissue was left behind to maintain the continuity and strength of the mandible.

Often the teeth could be preserved. However, if the entire alveolus was grossly enlarged, it was contoured on the lingual and buccal sides and the teeth were extracted. Only if the enlargement of the mandible was extensive or there was a previous scar, was an external approach utilized. Bleeding was usually profuse but temporary.

When the same operation was performed on an immature, active, predominantly fibrous lesion, the cortex was attenuated, with areas of erosion from which a rubbery, fleshy tumor protruded. Firm, encapsulated nodules of various sizes were often found and were enucleated (cases 3 and 7). They were surrounded by soft lesional tissue of varied fibro-osseous consistency. The lesion was never clearly encapsulated as the radiological picture suggested. The pathological bone was extensively curetted, limited only by the need to maintain the stability of the mandible.

Fractures occurred on several occasions. Arch bars were routinely applied before the operation. When a fracture occurred, the fragments were wired together, but the softness and thinness of the remaining bone made the osseous wiring unreliable. The immobilization was accomplished by intermaxillary fixation. Rapid bone union took place in all instances.

Resection of a segment of the mandible was done in only four cases. In earlier years I attempted resection of all abnormal bone. This entailed sacrificing a large portion of the mandible, as in case 3, where more than half was resected. However, the same "cure" could be effected if only the grossly involved bone was excised. The pathological residual bone, adjacent to the excisional defect, either became sclerotic or seemed eventually to be replaced by normal bone.

When there was mucosal ulceration and inflammation, large fragments of the mucosa were excised. The mandible was stabilized with a Kirschner wire, and the bone graft was delayed.

In retrospect, a primary bone graft could have been used in most cases. In a few instances, when the mandibular bone was disintegrated, bone grafts, both blocks and chips, were used to reinforce the remaining abnormal bone. This is the conventional treatment of fibrous dysplasia lesions in the long bones where stability is essential. Such a procedure proved effective and is indicated in most cases in lieu of complete resection. Invasion of the bone graft by the disease was never demonstrated.

In case 3 a single rib graft was used to replace a hemimandible. In this 9-year-old child the rib was too thin and lacked sufficient rigidity to withstand the functional stresses; it also lacked sufficient bulk to form a well-delineated mandibular angle. The rib graft had the advantage of including the cartilaginous component, which substituted for the missing condyle. Figure 21-7 shows the reconstructed condyle 25 years later, considerably smaller, but functioning normally.

In the fifties I was reluctant to procure large iliac bone grafts in children for fear of interfering in the growth of the pelvic girdle. In the last decade, with the advances in craniofacial surgery for congenital deformities, I have routinely taken a large bone graft from the ilium and osteotomized and reflected the cartilaginous crest, leaving it attached to the gluteal musculature [28]. A large bone graft was removed from the wing of the ilium and the crest returned to its original position. Such iliac grafts, with an ample cancellous component, are preferable for restoration of good contour to the mandible.

In children the bone graft served as scaffolding for the development of the soft tissue. Despite the thinness of the reconstructed mandible, the facial contour in case 3 remained normal, except for a slight flatness in front of the ear.

In none of my cases was a total maxillectomy performed. An external Fergusson approach was avoided, and all contouring operations were done intraorally through the buccal sulcus. An additional subciliary incision was sometimes used for better exposure of the upper part of the maxilla. When massive trimming of the bone was necessary, the lid incision facilitated the visualization and protection of the infraorbital nerve.

The upper alveolus was most frequently involved. The tumor masses sometimes extended inside the pyriform aperture, distorting and obstructing the nose. They were resected after the nasal lining had been reflected and preserved.

The tumor of the facial wall was shaved off with osteotomes. The maxillary sinus was usually obliterated, its mucosa sacrificed with the bone. The rimmed out cavity was drained through an intranasal antrotomy. The epithelialization of the sinus proceeded rapidly. Tumors on the hard palate were resected subperiosteally, preserving the mucoperiosteal flaps.

The lateral part of the maxilla and the malozygomatic complex could be exposed best together with the lateral orbital wall.

In the last decade the extended forehead flap (the coronal incision carried down to the root of the zygoma) has been used to provide exposure of the subtemporal fossa, the orbit, and zygoma without leaving visible facial scars.

ETHMOIDS AND ORBIT

Tumefaction around the inner canthus is a frequent finding in polyostotic craniofacial fibrous dysplasia. It is part of the diffuse involvement of the cranial skeleton, both of its vault and base.

This location is infrequent in monostotic fibrous dysplasia. The monostotic tumor may originate in the ethmoids but involves the medial orbital wall, the lacrimal bone, and the adjacent maxilla. The inner canthus is displaced laterally. The lacrimal sac is dislodged from the lacrimal fossa, and the nasolacrimal duct becomes obstructed. This causes recurrent dacryocystitis. The tumor may extend into the nasal cavity, replacing the turbinates and protruding into the nasopharynx.

With the septum crowded into the opposite side, the nose is totally obstructed. The nasal bones are spread apart and flattened. Extension of the tumor into the orbit leads to proptosis.

Case 5 illustrates such a condition. Although complete resection of the involved tissue was not feasible, an extensive operation was necessary to correct the functional complications and restore facial contour.

The techniques of craniofacial surgery, introduced more than a decade ago, are applicable in such a situation. Reflecting a forehead flap and splitting it in the middle over the bridge of the nose afforded a good exposure to the frontal, orbital, and ethmoid areas and the nasal cavities. After subperiosteal dissection of the orbit, the medial orbital wall was resected. Rhinotomy through the nasal bones exposed the nasal cavity so that the intranasal and nasopharyngeal tumor could be excised or curetted.

Iliac bone grafts were used to reconstruct the nasal bridge and to replace the medial orbital wall. The canthus was reattached by a transnasal canthopexy.

The nasolacrimal duct was reconstructed by threading an angiocatheter through the punctum into the sac and the nasal cavity. After several weeks, an epithelial channel was established which provided drainage of the tear sac.

The most disastrous complication in cases of polyostotic fibrous dysplasia is optic atrophy leading to blindness. It is attributed to compression of the nerve within the optic canal. In case 9 the entire optic chiasma was compressed by the tumor.

Curiously, I have encountered no involvement of any other cranial nerve in fibrous dysplasia. The hearing impairment in two cases was of a conductive type, attributable to changes in the middle ear and mastoid.

Proptosis, or downward displacement of the eye (case 7), can be corrected by resection of the orbital roof and replacement with bone grafts. To retract and protect the anterior cerebral lobe, a frontal craniotomy must be done, an approach frequently used today for reconstruction of congenital or traumatic deformities [27]. However, 20 years ago such a procedure was not considered appropriate for a non-malignant lesion.

Neurosurgical experience with decompression of the nerve in the canal has been poor [7]. In case 8, optic atrophy progressed to complete blindness in 3 to 4 years after such an operation. On the other hand, in case 6, a progressive optic atrophy had been observed for 14 years and the patient still has full vision.

The discouraging results of surgical decompression of the nerve can be attributed to the recurrence of the compression either inside the canal or in another location in the orbit or cranium.

CRANIUM

In four cases of polyostotic fibrous dysplasia, contouring of the frontal and parietal bone was performed. In all the cases the disease involved the anterior part of the cranium, decreasing in intensity toward the occipital bone. The main purpose of the intervention was to reduce the overgrowth of the supraorbital ridges. Visible nodules and irregularities of the frontal, and sometimes of the parietal, bones were shaved.

In two of these cases the supraorbital ridges were of moderate thickness, and some of the nodules consisted of fibro-osseous material with small cysts.

The most severe cranial enlargement was encountered in cases of McCune-Albright disease. The dramatic autopsy findings showed the bony enlargement to be not only external but intracranial as well. The brain was displaced and compressed. The bone was of rock-like hardness and vascular. The operation in this type of case is difficult, intracranial complications and blood loss making it hazardous.

Management of Fibrous Dysplasia

The management of fibrous dysplasia is guided by the following considerations:

1. The tumor is benign. The surrounding tissues are not invaded but may undergo pressure atrophy.
2. It is self-limiting, although its rate of growth and point of arrest are unpredictable.
3. The enlargement of the lesion can be monitored easily, since its main manifestation is a visible enlargement.
4. Clinical observation with repeated x-rays is the best modality to assess the aggressiveness of the disease.
5. Biopsy of the tumor may be important to confirm the diagnosis, exclude malignancy, and reassure the patient. However, it is of limited value in predicting the course of the disease, since different parts of the tumors are in different stages of evolutionary growth.
6. The operation does not influence the biological course of the tumor. If it is actively growing, it will continue after the operation. However, the "debulking" operations may prevent complications and minimize the deformity in anticipation of spontaneous arrest of its growth.
7. The operation should be performed during the inactive phase of the lesion. During the active phase, it should be delayed as long as possible and is indicated only when the tumefaction is disabling or there is the threat of complications.

Final Thoughts

Fibrous dysplasia is one of the most perplexing diseases of the skeletal system. Its etiology is unknown, its pathogenesis uncertain, and its histology diverse. Classified as a tumor, it does not fulfill the customary criteria of a neoplasm.

Clinically the disease has many guises, and its course is unpredictable. It can appear within the craniofacial skeleton as a single or multiple lesion; it can have a generalized distribution throughout the body; and its growth can be slow and benign or rapid and unrestrained.

A treatment plan must be based on the natural history of the disease and requires fine surgical judgment of when to operate and what operation to perform.

Most of my patients were treated in their inactive stage by a conservative operation to reduce the bulk and contour the bone. Resection of all pathological tissues was not feasible because it would have resulted in a mutilating disability. These patients were rehabilitated and remained symptom free for decades. However, there is a chance of a future flare-up of the disease which should be dealt with as conservatively as possible.

In general, monostotic fibrous dysplasia is overtreated [9, 22]; polyostotic fibrous dysplasia is undertreated. Because the surgeon is uncomfortable with leaving a tumor in place, and often alarmed by its rapid growth, there is an inclination to resect whenever feasible. However, when there are multiple lesions, the limitation of surgical treatment is apparent, and few such patients are referred to the surgeon.

Recent developments in craniofacial surgery for congenital deformities have contributed to the management of craniofacial tumors. Most surgeons are now better prepared to treat lesions in the cranium, orbit, and ethmoids, and to handle the subsequent reconstruction.

Acknowledgment

My appreciation to Dr. John Li, Director of Pathology and Laboratories, North Central Bronx Hospital, for his review of histologic slides. His interpretation and assistance were invaluable.

References

1. Albright, F. Polyostotic fibrous dysplasia: A defense of the entity. *J. Clin. Endocrinol.* 7:307, 1947.
2. Caffey, J., and Williams, J.L. Familial fibrous swelling of the jaws. *Radiology* 56:1, 1951.
3. Cooke, B.E.D. Benign fibro-osseous enlargements of the jaws. *Br. Dent. J.* 102:1, 1957.
4. Dehner, L.P. Tumors of the mandible and maxilla in children: I. Clinicopathologic study of 46 histologically benign lesions. *Cancer* 31:364, 1973.
5. DiGeorge, A.M. Albright syndrome: Is it coming of age? *J. Pediatr.* 87:1018, 1975.
6. Eversole, L.R., Sabes, W.R., and Rovin, S. Fibrous dysplasia: A nosologic problem in the diagnosis of fibro-osseous lesion of the jaws. *J. Oral Pathol.* 1:189, 1972.
7. Feiring, W., Feiring, E.H., and Davidoff, L.M. Fibrous dysplasia of the skull. *J. Neurosurg.* 8:377, 1951.
8. Furst, N.J., and Shapiro, R. Polyostotic fibrous dysplasia: Review of the literature with two additional cases. *Radiology* 40:501, 1943.
9. Georgiade, N., Masters, F., Horton, C., and Pickrell, K. Ossifying fibromas (fibrous dysplasia) of the facial bones in children and adolescents. *J. Pediatr.* 46:36, 1955.
10. Harris, W.H., Dudley, H.R., and Barry, R.J. The natural history of fibrous dysplasia: An orthopaedic, pathological, and roentgenographic study. *J. Bone Joint Surg.* [Br.] 44A:207, 1962.
11. Jaffe, H.L. Fibrous Dysplasia. In *Tumors and Tumorous Conditions of the Bones and Joints.* Philadelphia: Lea & Febiger, 1958. P. 117.
12. Jones, W.A., Gerrie, J., and Pritchard, J. Cherubism: A familial fibrous dysplasia of the jaws. *J. Bone Joint Surg.* [Br.] 32B:334, 1950.
13. Langdon, J.D., Rapidis, A.D., and Patel, M.F. Ossifying fibroma—one disease or six? An analysis of 39 fibro-osseous lesions of the jaws. *Br. J. Oral Surg.* 14:1, 1976.
14. Leeds, N., and Seaman, W.B. Fibrous dysplasia of the skull and its differential diagnosis: A clinical and roentgenographic study of 46 cases. *Radiology* 78:570, 1962.
15. Lewin, M.L. Fibrous dysplasia of the mandible. *Am. J. Surg.* 90:951, 1955.
16. Lewin, M.L. Fibrous dysplasia of the mandible in children. *Plast. Reconstr. Surg.* 25:161, 1960.
17. Lewin, M.L. Nonmalignant maxillofacial tumors in children. *Plast. Reconstr. Surg.* 38:186, 1966.
18. Lichtenstein, L. *Bone Tumors.* St. Louis: Mosby, 1952.
19. Markowicz, H., and Shanon, E. Fibrous dysplasia with monster-like deformity. *Laryngoscope* 70:147, 1960.
20. McCune, D.J., and Bruch, H. Osteodystrophia fibrosa. *Am. J. Dis. Child.* 54:806, 1937.
21. Paterson, R. Memorials on the life of James Syme. Edinburgh:Edmonston & Douglas, 1874.
22. Ramsey, H.E., Strong, E.W., and Frazell, E.L. Fibrous dysplasia of craniofacial bones. *Am. J. Surg.* 116:542, 1968.
23. Schlumberger, H.G. Fibrous dysplasia of single bones (monostotic fibrous dysplasia). *Milit. Surg.* 99:504, 1946.
24. Schwartz, D.T., and Alpert, M. The malignant

transformation of fibrous dysplasia. *Am. J. Med. Sci.* 247:1, 1964.

25. Sherman, R.S., and Glauser, O.J. Radiological identification of fibrous dysplasia of the jaws. *Radiology* 71:553, 1958.

26. Slow, I.N., Stern, D., and Friedman, E.W. Osteogenic sarcoma arising in a preexisting fibrous dysplasia: Report of case. *J. Oral Surg.* 29:126, 1971.

27. Tessier, P. Experiences in the treatment of orbital hypertelorism. *Plast. Reconstr. Surg.* 53:1, 1974.

28. Tessier, P. Personal communications, 1978.

29. Waldron, C.A. Fibro-osseous lesions of the jaws. *J. Oral Surg.* 28:58, 1970.

30. Warwick, C.K. Some aspects of polyostotic fibrous dysplasia: Possible hypothesis to account for the associated endocrinological changes. *Chir. Radiol.* 24:125, 1973.

31. Windholz, F. Cranial manifestations of fibrous dysplasia of bone: Their relation to leontiasis ossea and to simple bone cysts of the vault. *Am. J. Roentgenol.* 58:51, 1947.

32. Zimmerman, D.C., Dahlin, D.C., and Stafne, E.C. Fibrous dysplasia of the maxilla and mandible. *Oral Surg.* 11:55, 1958.

Joseph E. Murray

COMMENTS ON CHAPTER 21

DR. LEWIN has prepared a comprehensive study of the interesting pathological process of fibrous dysplasia. He has provided a follow-up of 9 of approximately 20 patients with whom he has had experience. In addition, he includes analysis of the pathological process. The disease transcends specialty designations and is seen by orthopedists, plastic surgeons, endocrinologists, oral surgeons, and pathologists. Etiology is obscure, classification difficult, with a variety names given to this condition. Craniofacial fibrous dysplasia is seldom confused with malignant sarcomas, but may require treatment because the developing mass is impinging on adjacent structures. Rarely, obstruction to the optic nerve may cause incipient blindness unless decompression is performed. Spontaneous regression is limited, although cessation of growth occurs often and is the usual pattern. Dr. Lewin's comparison to the growth of hemangiomas is apt, with his reservation that there is a certain degree of unpredictability in both instances.

Case 7 has an excellent 18-year follow-up, showing the changes in some aspects of the condition along with the persistence of the changes themselves. The functional matrix theory of Moss seems to be confirmed by the observations in cases 3 and 4, where we have excellent remodeling of the bone grafts which had been placed many years before.

Dr. Lewin gives a balanced presentation to this baffling condition, and particularly valuable is his description of the morphology, microscopic appearance, and radiological changes. The differential diagnoses discussed under Craniofacial Polyostotic Fibrous Dysplasia are enlightening and show the importance of a multidiscipled approach to the diagnosis of these patients.

These observations of a few patients over several decades provide a basis for the current concepts of treatment, namely, avoidance of surgery except where the mass itself is producing an unacceptable cosmetic defect or is encroaching upon vital structures such as the optic nerve.

22

THE results of the curative and supportive treatments for facial paralysis in one surgeon's hands over a period of 35 years have been reviewed to estimate the types and progressive variants of the procedures and the quality and longevity of the results [1-7]. The frequency and timing of adjustments and complications and the timing and type of supplemental procedures necessary to retain a relatively reasonable level of competence over a prolonged period of observation were also recorded. To establish the initial and late degree of deformity, quality of amelioration, and rate of attenuation, as well as the improvement by supplemental or complemental procedures in the child, the healthy young adult, the middle-aged, and the aged required an adherence to a standard of examination and a rigidity of operative technique that has not always been maintained. Nonetheless, multiple examinations of the majority of patients over the years have yielded the reasons for the progressive technical changes and timing of procedures. Viewing the results over a perspective of three decades may help establish reasonable goals to which the average surgeon could aspire without developing guilt over an inability to accomplish perfection in every patient.

Sources

During the past 30 years, reconstructive measures for patients with facial paralysis have included nerve reattachments, transfers, grafts, and bypasses, including cranial-nerve transfers, ipsilateral facial-nerve transfers, and of late, cross-face nerve grafts. Dynamic masseter and temporalis muscle transfers of varying types

Bromley S. Freeman

CORRECTION OF FACIAL-NERVE PARALYSIS

have been tested, as has static suspension reconstruction with the use of preserved and autogenous fascia and polypropylene mesh and dermis. Muting or camouflaging of the spastic normal side has been treated by weakening of the opposing antagonists by myotomy, myomectomy, and neurectomy. In addition, multiple mechanical devices for closure of the orbital sphincter and innumerable aesthetic maneuvers of varying extent have been applied in an effort to improve the function and features.

Attempts to discuss the value of the varying techniques, their expectations and drawbacks, and to establish specific indications will be made. Practically all the patients are from my private files, most followed for at least 5 years, some for 25 years. The months of review have provided me with an opportunity to observe the effects of time on the changing attitudes of both patients and surgeon and to become acquainted with the limitations of both.

After an initial presentation in 1961, a second unpublished review of the results of cranial-nerve crossovers was made with James Greenwood in 1968. A study of facial-nerve grafts was published in 1972 [2]. A series of 100 patients operated on for facial paralysis by supportive techniques was reported in 1975 [5] and exposed the shortcomings in recording, examining, and testing. The results of a personal series of patients treated by immediate or early facial-nerve reapproximation, direct neurorrhaphy, direct nerve grafts, and nerve reroutings after tumor surgery were compared. It was obvious that the findings after reestablishing neural continuity could not be used for norms against which to plot the results of the supportive measures. Despite occasional and early

mass movements and spasm, which usually disappeared with training and time, early return of facial-nerve function by neural reapproximation resulted in feature control and balance that were unobtainable in the supportive group, no matter which technique or group of techniques was used (Fig. 22-1).

If neural continuity could not be restored, the basic objectives of surgery on the palsied patient would have to be more realistic. Not only did the surgeon mature, but the patients followed for a longer term than the average 1 or 2 years had matured sufficiently to offer a reasonable subjective guide as to the relative importance of the problems encountered and of the value of additional help proffered. Preferences now led to improvement of speech, chewing, and other functional necessities of the oral sphincter and protection of the eye rather than mere improvement of appearance. Study of an accumulation of rough notes, sketches, photographs, and, rarely, moving pictures of procedures and patients delineated an interesting evolution of technical changes by the author throughout the years. Although the photographs and sketches showed progressive alteration, there was noted an occasional return to simplistic techniques discarded for more modish designs. These designs, again in turn, had been cast aside when, in my hands, they did not live up to their published expectations.

Review entailed rereading office chart histories, referring physicians' notes, multiple electrical studies, hospital charts, and records of brief periodic follow-up reexaminations. There were obvious and sometimes appalling disparities between histories and examinations, both physical and electrical, carried out by the various physicians, residents, technicians, etc. at

409

410

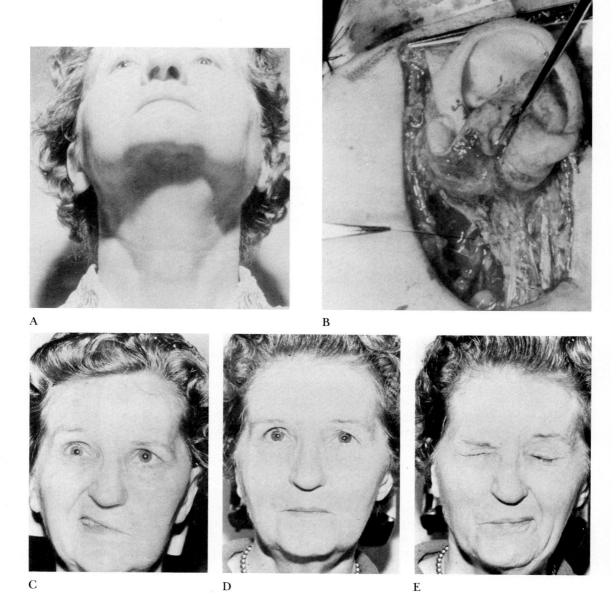

FIGURE 22-1. K.L.P. *(A) Fixed, recurrent, deep lobe and retromandibular mixed tumor. (B) Direct nerve anastomosis after resection of a 1½-cm section of the main trunk of the facial nerve from foraminal exit at time of removal. Laxity of the distal nerves after removal of the total* *gland allowed anastomosis in 1963 with 6-0 nylon (without use of a microscope). (C) Two weeks postoperative. Palsy evident. (D and E) Appearance 8 years later; control and balance.*

the *same* time. This has led to the use by all examiners of standardized forms. It is difficult in a busy practice to allocate sufficient time to digest a detailed history, but in these patients the history and reports of the internists, otologists, neurosurgeons, obstetricians, pediatricians, neurologists, and not infrequently, the previous plastic surgeon must be at hand and digested. Although neurological examination may not be the forte of the general plastic surgeon, it is an essential tool in the armamentarium of those plastic surgeons who would treat facial paralysis. Associated problems caused by damage or alteration of other cranial nerves not infrequently have been disregarded and left untreated by the neurosurgeons or neurologists responsible for primary care.

To evaluate the type and degree of facial paralysis for a permanent base on which to work, the two standard forms mentioned are used. After going over almost 200 charts one realizes that even the experienced surgeon needs a formal routine to detail objective signs of facial paralysis, not only for primary analysis of the defect to be treated, but also for reference in the follow-up. Table 22-1 is one such formal report. The second, a stylized sketch of the facial muscles (Table 22-2), is used by the examiner not only to mark weakness and spasticity of the various muscles, but also to request electromyographic studies of particular muscles. The electrodiagnostician in turn annotates a similar sketch, in addition to his formal report. Although this may be called petrification of examination, it is most essential for true evaluation of a patient.

Electrodiagnostic Testing

Since the chances for technical error in electrodiagnosis include not only needle position and depth, but also the type and size of the needle, it required the greatest care to standardize and quantify results. Although we established a standard form with each laboratory, it was difficult to place reliance on many of our electromyographic examinations. Moreover,

patients who have subtotally recovered from Bell's palsy, bulbar poliomyelitis, and other vascular, inflammatory, and allergic disturbances of the facial nerve characteristically heal with a certain amount of cross-innervation, since the regenerating axons find different pathways to the muscles and often produce associated muscular action in different portions of the face upon stimulation.

The presently available EMG, "computerized" or not, is still imperfect. Despite expensive and advanced equipment and built-in software, EMG interpretations are still based on individual technique, and the interpretation must be correlated with nerve conductivity by a knowledgeable technician and coordinated with the previous examinations by the neurophysiologist and surgeon. Serial examinations and reports of previous examinations must include the electrical changes noted after any surgery or intercurrent disorders. A combination of interested surgeon and diagnostician should assay the problem before the surgeon decides on the type of repair, assists, or modifications to be tried. After rereading some early reports, it is the author's impression that electromyographers must have adequate time and interest and be properly directed by the surgeon to render anything other than an imperfect appraisal of the problem.

Spontaneous Postparalytic Neural Reinnervation: An Etiological and Diagnostic Problem

The results after therapy for facial paralysis, whether surgical, medical, or electrical, must be reviewed against the natural history of the particular disorder causing the disturbance. Neurological reviews have shown that at least three-fourths of the patients who have had Bell's palsy have recovered either completely or with some insignificant but partial residual paralysis of the facial musculature. Spontaneous return of function after surgical excision of the seventh cranial nerve has been described as

TABLE 22-1. *Facial Palsy Examination Form*

Patient name _____ Date _____

Patient number _____

	Right	Left
Forehead .... Furrows		
Movement		
Spasm		
Temporal .... Fossa		
Skin		
Brow .... Level		
Frown		
Spasm		
Redundancy		
Upper lid .... Texture		
Blink		
Close with effort, to—mm		
Synchronous		
Conjunctiva		
Cornea		
Palpebral fissure		
Stare—at rest		
—emotion		
—speech		
Hooded		
Canthal bowing		
Lower lid .... Sag		
Ectropion		
Texture		
Redundancy		
Punctum		
Scars		
Speech .... Slaver		
Drool		
Spit		
Slurred		
Dysarthria		
Mucosal protrusion		

Mastication . . . . Slobber _____ | _____

Noise _____ | _____

Buccal impaction _____ | _____

Suck—liquids _____ | _____

Kiss _____ | _____

Mucosal biting _____ | _____

Nasal . . . . Septum _____ | _____

Sneer _____ | _____

Ala _____ | _____

Block _____ | _____

Mouth . . . . Position of angle _____ | _____

Eversion _____ | _____

Buccal fold _____ | _____

Tongue atrophy _____ | _____

Air leak _____ | _____

Midface . . . . _____ | _____

Nasolabial fold . . . . Type _____ | _____

Sag _____ | _____

Mentolabial groove . . . . _____ | _____

Skin texture . . . . _____ | _____

Skin redundancy . . . . _____ | _____

Platysma . . . . _____ | _____

Bromley S. Freeman, M.D.

infrequent; yet the frequency increases as the time interval lengthens. Omitting the ravages of bulbar poliomyelitis in children, the largest number of patients operated on were those who had loss of the facial nerve because of neoplasm intracranially, intratemporally, or peripherally or those for whom sacrifice of the facial nerve was necessary during the surgical removal of a tumor. Despite the operators' descriptions of deliberate sacrifice of the seventh nerve intracranially, intratemporally, and extratemporally without reconstruction, careful reexaminations over the years showed evidence that a small percentage of the surviving patients had spontaneous, gradual, and partial regrowth of neural fibers from the same side. Minimal reinnervation has occurred, and not necessarily from the fifth or the opposite seventh nerve. Although particularly noted in children after resections involving the parotid gland, this creeping reinnervation has been found several years after the surgical removal of acoustic neuromas in adults in whom total disruption of the nerve was accurately described by the surgeon. This phenomenon makes a decision difficult concerning early neural replacement. Moreover, one wonders about the accuracy of attributing the final re-

TABLE 22–2. *Diagram of Facial Muscles to Record Findings*

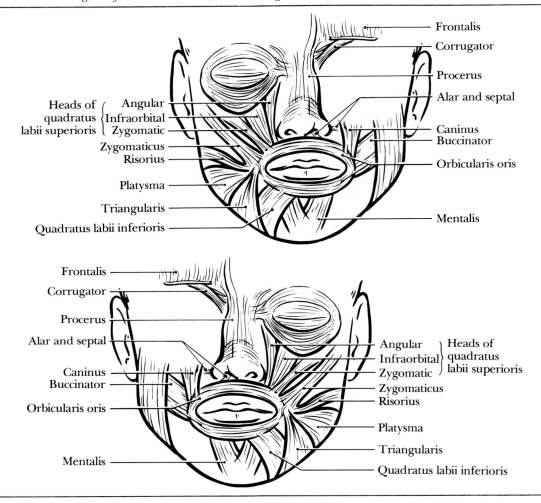

sults, especially after a lapse of several years, to any specific technique of repair. Despite the possibility of unrecognized creeping reinnervation in a small percentage of patients and the occasionally slow (18 months to 3 years) return of neural innervation in fractures of the skull (Fig. 22-2), we cannot leave the patient with a totally paralyzed face which requires alleviation, nor can we close the door to reinnervation by permanently blocking the peripheral branches of the facial nerve.

A classic example is the patient in Figure 22-3, who, at the age of 3 months, had a radical resection of a "malignant hemangioma." Together with the parotid gland and tumor, the major trunk of the facial nerve was accurately described as "removed" by the surgeon and this was confirmed by the pathologist. The patient had a clinically complete palsy of the central and lower two-thirds of the right facial nerve for 15 years. At 16 years of age she was referred for a supportive procedure. Complete denervation of the middle and lower facial muscles was found, and the conduction and electromyographic studies carried out in two separate neurophysiological laboratories reported "complete loss of the lower two-thirds of the nerve with no evidence of viable muscle innervation of the lower face." Preliminary to a temporalis muscle transfer, dissection of the facial nerve through the usual face-lift incision revealed grossly intact facial-nerve branches, although irregular in position and extremely fine, to these same midfacial muscles regarded electronically as denervated as well as by physical examination by experienced examiners, including the author. When these nerves were stimulated, the muscles moved. Instead of a temporalis muscle transfer, an elastic-mesh sling support of the lower two-thirds of the face elevated the side. Six months of assiduous training in a highly motivated adolescent resulted in complete, if weakened, recovery.

In muscles diagnosed electronically as "total muscular denervation" for 15 and even 20 years, biopsies of the facial nerve by electron microscopy of the "atrophic neural branches" have shown histologically normal axons. These occasional findings have been corroborated by Conley (personal communication) and show the amazing potential for regeneration of the facial nerve, which when partial, might well be aided by supplemental procedures.

Neural Rehabilitation

Facial-muscle reinnervation was and is part of the surgical technique in many neurosurgical clinics after extirpation of tumors of the head and neck to ensure early recovery and maintenance of the oral sphincteric tone and to protect the eyes. The procedures carried out through the years have included direct approximation of peripheral facial-nerve segments, loosened sufficiently by parotidectomy for anastomosis to the terminal branches either directly or by nerve grafts. Occasionally, ipsilateral buccal and platysmal branches were rerouted to the branches to the lip. When the lesion was cerebral, temporal, facial-hypoglossal, or facial-accessory, nerve crossovers were done with various modifications over the three decades. The majority of these patients developed and maintained muscle tone.

Although improvement was found in 90 percent of the twelfth- and eleventh-nerve reroutings, over 30 percent had lagophthalmos. All the "hypoglossals" had dysarthria to some degree and a modest amount of mass movement. Only a few had sufficiently good emotional facial reactions to record a level of anything better than "satisfactory" or "fair." Some degree of atrophy of the tongue was present in all the office patients and most patients so treated seen in consultation. Although the majority, having been forewarned, did not complain, not a few requested cosmetic and functional improvement. However, the oral sphincter had sufficient tone to control chewing, eating, and drinking. In the early 1940s, six patients had the descending branch of the hypoglossal nerve attached to the lower peripheral branches of the cut facial nerve. In none was there evidence of restoration of tone. All six were lost to follow-up after 1 year. In the late 1950s, only one-half of the twelfth nerve was employed for anastomosis after the manner of Love, who used this technique until he retired. Although atrophy of the tongue was minimal, those few who responded to questionnaires stated that improvement was fair.

The use of the eleventh or accessory nerve was a simpler procedure for the author and resulted in less of a deformity. However, the use of the sternomastoid branches of the accessory nerve, anastomosed to the lower half of the peripheral branches of the facial nerve, as pioneered by Bragden, produced even less of a deformity, although resurgence of tone in the reinnervated muscles was slow, possibly because of the fine branches. Out of eight sternomastoid transfers, I have had two failures, which presumably must be attributed to technical errors.

Since the majority of these patients were middle-aged and older males, the usual deformities that attend total sections of the twelfth and eleventh nerves were woefully present. The shoulder drop was apparent, especially in workers, but could be compensated for by

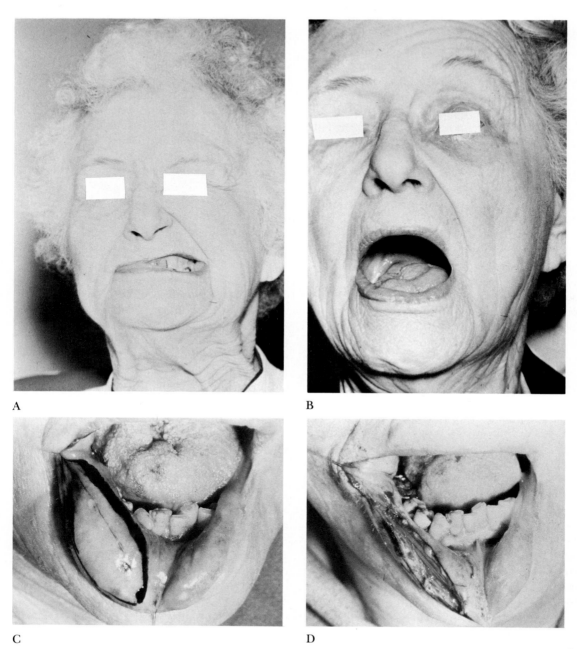

C

D

FIGURE 22-2.   M.R. *Ancillary procedure: labial vermilion excision. (A) Seven years postcraniectomy, facial paralysis after "total removal of facial nerve." (B) Three years later (10 years after paralysis), creeping reinnervation gave control of muscle slowly, but redundant mucosa and evi-* *dent aging on the right, previously paralyzed, side. (C and D) Excision of redundant buccal and labial mucosa. (E and F) After mucosa excisions and blepharoplasty for hooded lid and browlift (no face lift), she is a happy woman. Still well, 1977.*

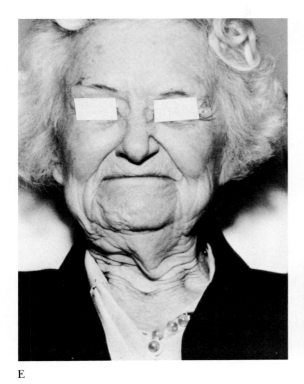

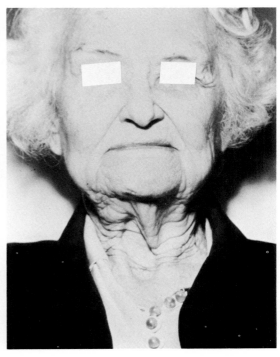

E

F

physical exercise. Not infrequently, typical facial hyperkinesia, which could be considered iatrogenic (especially around the lid), was persistent in several for decades. All the cranial reroutings required auxiliary operative procedures.

Rerouting of ipsilateral peripheral branches to the platysmal muscle to replace the fine nerves of the lower lip has been carried out since 1946, and with excellent and rapid results, despite the relatively large needle, the 6-0 nylon sutures, and the adhesive micropore tape [2, 7]. Two patients explored several years after the neural anastomosis during the course of a later neck dissection showed a small neuroma around the sole suture, but function was excellent. In three patients, function was restored to the lip in less than 3 months. Moreover, no platysmal deficit has been noted, possibly, however, because I neglected to examine for one specifically.

Muscle Transfers

The muscle transfers reviewed (since 1946) include varying techniques in the use of the temporalis and masseter muscles only. Personal attempts to rotate other muscles of the neck have met with early and frank failure and will have to be reviewed by those surgeons who have accomplished working sternocleidomastoid, digastric, and omohyoid motors to the face.

MASSETER TRANSPLANTS

Masseter transplants, the major muscle transfers first used in this series and considered as interpositional insertions of cut masseter muscle for both neurotization and motor, include

1. Subtotal masseter rotation and implantation into the stripped facial muscles with permanent fixation to the nasolabial dermis.
2. Subtotal masseter transfers to a previously

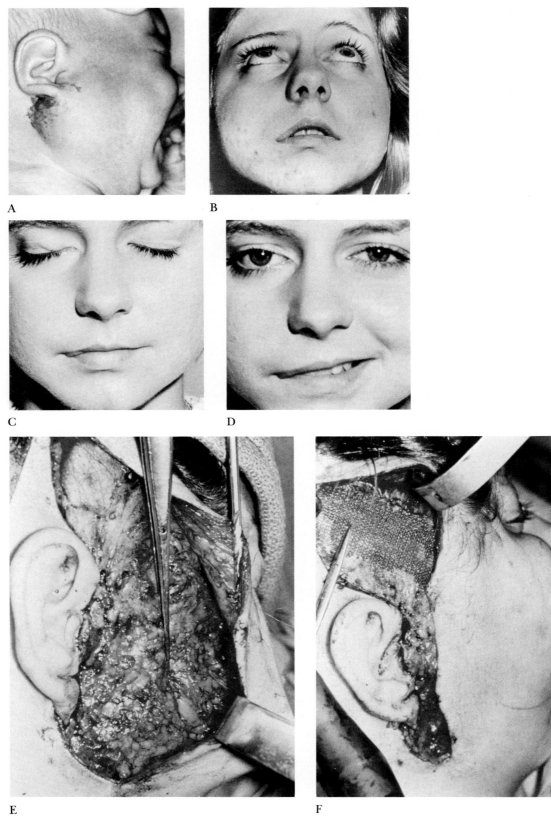

A

B

C

D

E

F

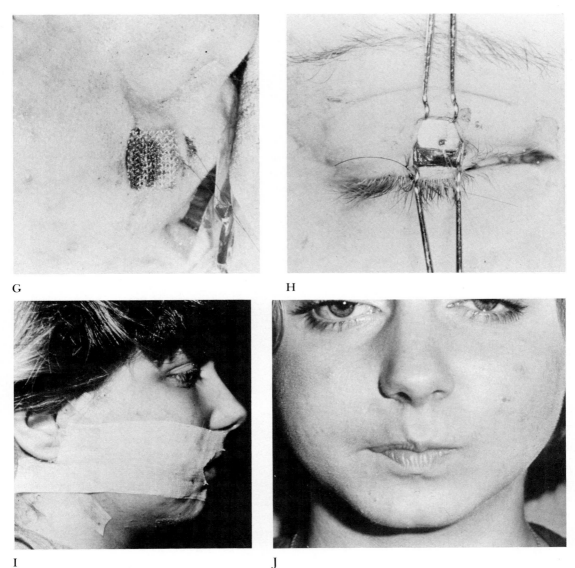

G

H

I

J

FIGURE 22-3.   L.P. *Unrecognized subliminal return treated by neurolysis, mesh elastic lift, and persevering gymnastics. (A) Dissection and removal of "entire" facial nerve with ulcerating hemangioma, age 3 months (confirmed by pathologists' review), by expert plastic surgeon. (B, C, and D) Sixteen years later "complete unilateral right facial paralysis" clinically and electrodiagnostically (camouflaged by plumpness). (E) Preliminary to planned temporalis transfer, exploration of nerve revealed muscle response by stimulation of peripheral branches of the facial nerve (temporal to mentalis). (F and G) Instead,* internal assist by Marlex mesh support to orbicularis oris and to nasolabial fold and (H) temporary gold weight to the upper lid. (I) Postoperative collodion splint. (J) After 6 months of mimetic gymnastics. Patient is improving under mimetic gymnastics. The weight and the Marlex support can be removed if and when the muscles regain adequate strength. Patient's emotional stability has improved remarkably. A classic "creeping reinnervation" was masked and required neurolysis, mechanical assists, and training for restoration.*

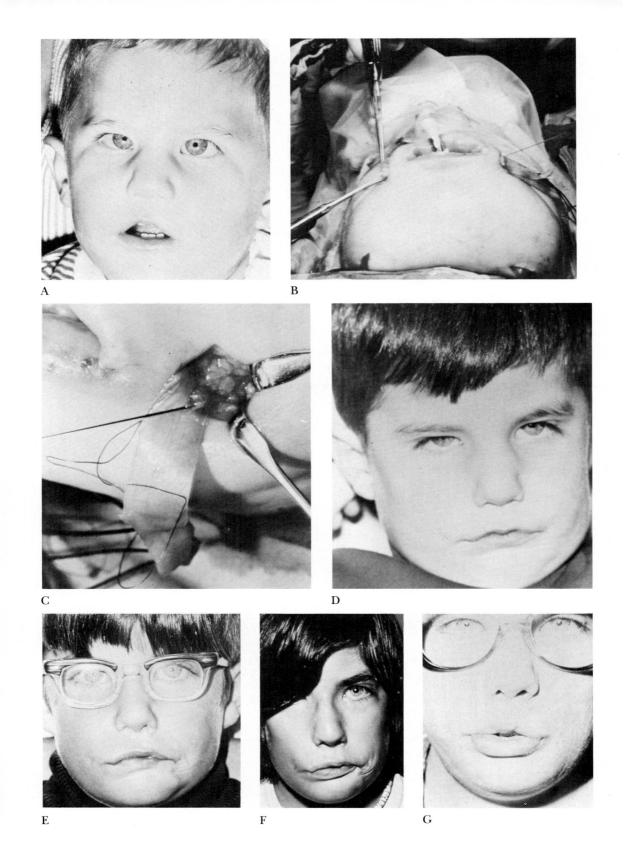

A

B

C

D

E

F

G

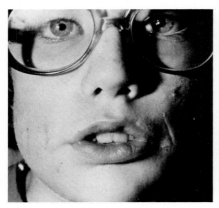
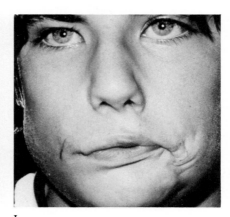

H   I

FIGURE 22-4.   D.C. *Möbius syndrome with bilateral lower facial palsy, accompanied by eye and extremity deformities. (A) 1965, preoperative. (B) Intraoperative, first stage, large fascial bands forming oral sphincter. (C) Second stage, 5 weeks later; attachment of the anterior half of each masseter muscle to the band, 1966. (D) 1968, good control of the lips; eye straightened by muscle surgery. (E) 1970,* *good control, but the right side showing slippage. (F) 1977, increased slippage. Patient requests help. (G and H) 1977, after dissections and reattachment of the masseter to original fascial embouchure. Control of the lips, but a symmetrical dynamic pull. (I) Right tenses well, the left overcorrects. Has improved by exercises.*

constructed circumoral fascial sphincter (Fig. 22-4).
3. Transfers plus directional fascial support from commissure to malar bone or temporal fascia.
4. Transfers with a segmental temporalis muscle lift to the masseter-orbicularis junction (conjoint muscle attachment).

All transfers proved of some value for both immediate and late stabilization. Although occasional evidence of slight neurotization of facial muscles was found by "careful EMG studies," because of the presence of a gross muscle and the prolonged facial muscle training, these findings are felt to be "indecisive" by the author. All offered late and continued fixation and support of the oral sphincter and definite voluntary motion. Twenty percent required later tightening or release because of contracture, foreign-body reaction in implanted fascia after 5 to 15 years (around a nidus of the heavy, braided, nonabsorbable suture material used in securing the muscle under tension), or late but progressive attenuation and fracture of a join that had lasted for years. Excursion on voluntary motion was minimal with the few who maintained prolonged and continuous mimetic gymnastics, and emotional control was relatively negligible but present.

Nonetheless, active, tight sphincters were present 10 to 20 years later in bilateral paralysis of the lower face. In unilateral palsies, certain complemental procedures were frequently necessary. These included (1) release of spasticity of the contralateral muscles by myomectomy or, occasionally, neurectomy; (2) additional transfers of a temporalis muscle segment to the insertion at the commissure; or (3) support, static or elastic, by a broad fascial or polypropylene mesh band fixed securely to the temporalis aponeurosis after proper adjustment. These latter procedures counterbalanced the residual lowering of the angle of the mouth prevalent in maturing children in whom the masseter was inserted with a circumoral band. In adults, the nasolabial fold flattened, disappeared, and required reconstruction by a cosmetic procedure, a dermal sling, a Marlex or fascial uplift, or preferably the dynamic segmental temporalis muscle lift mentioned (see Fig. 22-5).

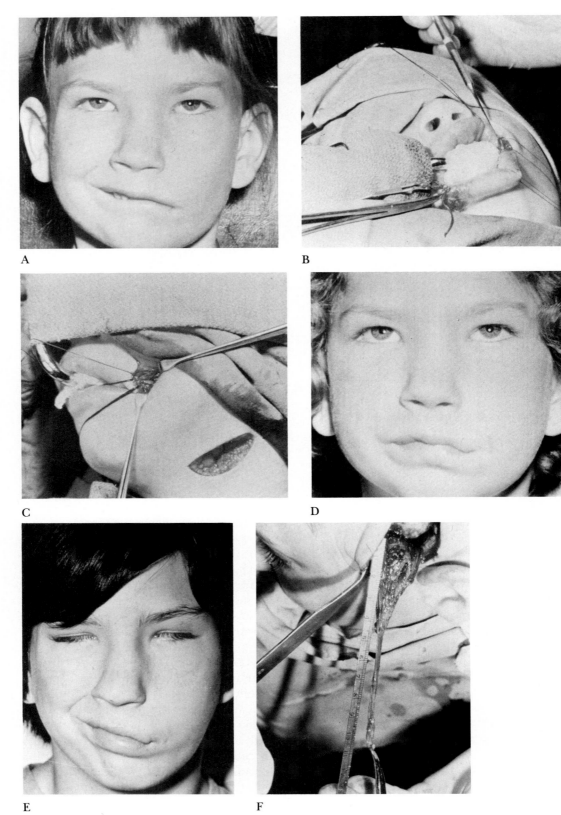

A

B

C

D

E

F

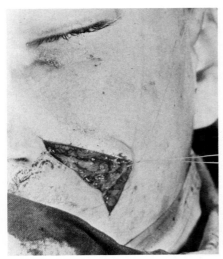
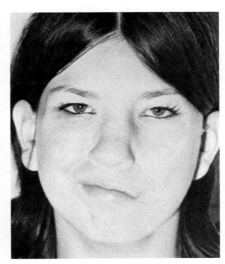

G   H

FIGURE 22-5. B.H. *The necessity of multiple operative procedures, and the difficulty of "titration" of muscle pull. Left facial paralysis; Möbius variant (note eyes). Illustrates downward pull of masseter over the years, requiring stabilization superiorly by temporalis muscle. (A) Preoperative. (B) Insertion of circumorbital sling. (C) Subtotal masseter transfer, 6 weeks later. (D) Immediate postopera-* *tive control. (E) Six years later, control of the lower lip, but none of the upper, and absent nasolabial folds. Lids close almost completely without assist. (F and G) Temporalis muscle transfer to angle (insertion at masseter-circumorbital join). (H) Postoperative, 6 weeks; needs excision of skin and adjustment for further elevation of angle. Nine years later, patient and parents still do not wish further surgery.*

Bilateral masseter muscle transfer was extremely useful in several patients with Möbius's syndrome who have maintained their bilateral muscular activity during chewing and speaking. In these patients there has been no emotional distortion, since they rarely showed facial evidence of emotion except with their eyes. Asynchronism or imbalance was an operative or mechanical pulley imbalance or complication. When a masseter motor was used in unilateral lower facial palsies, distortion with even slight emotional response contrasted with the opposite or spastic side unless extensive and sometimes repeated resection of the antagonist muscles was carried out and the patient was mirror-trained to maintain an unusual, tranquil composure. This was possible in two young adults, but the underlying mental stress must be considerable, since both have developed peculiarly stoic personalities. Expectations for sphincteric control are fair; buccinator replacement, excellent; emotional or nonvoluntary control, poor.

Among the complications found in masseter transfer were late partial tears in the growing adolescent, stretching of the attachment (Fig. 22-4), and late acute but complete dehiscence of the motor insertions of the commissure or lips. Three "pullouts" were corrected after 5, 7, and 12 years, respectively, by secondary dissections and elevation and rotation of the residual masseter muscle, reattaching it to the preexisting scar mass at the angle of the mouth [3]. In two patients, these were aided by the simultaneous creation of a nasolabial fold and tailored balancing of the upper lip by skin as well as mucosa excisions. Skin tethering, noted in one patient at a recall examination 12 years after sphincter construction, was corrected by freeing of the skin from the attachment and immediate mobilization. In another patient, after skin adherence to the internal scar was released, a small piece of Teflon film was temporarily inserted between the "tendon" and the skin and mimetic gymnastic gum chewing was started, which relieved the adherence permanently. The slight but frequent depression of the affected commissure as the patient grew—the majority of masseter transplants were in children or adolescents—accentuated the necessity for carrying out a triangulation of forces by the temporalis muscle lift procedures described as part of the initial operation (Fig. 22-6).

TEMPORALIS MUSCLE

Rotation of temporalis muscle and aponeurosis motor units was the most frequent dynamic procedure in all ages during the past 18 years. Temporalis transfers can be divided into the following:

1. Segmental muscle and aponeurosis for re-creating an orbicularis oculi sphincter.
2. Isolated segmental muscle transfers to an existing attached masseter or fascial transplant to the upper lip and commissure, as well as to replace segmental or partial facial palsies.
3. Subtotal transfers of the posterior or central two-thirds of the temporalis muscle to the middle and lower face.
4. Total muscle and aponeurosis (many-tailed) transfers encompassing orbital, nasal, and oral sphincteric attachments (Fig. 22-7).

All temporalis muscle transfers worked well eventually and were unsurpassed for the prevention and permanent repair of buccinator pseudohernia because of the broad, bony origin, the wide mechanical block of the soft cheek hiatus, and *reconstruction of the sphincter by multiple insertions across to the normal side by the aponeurosis expansion,* which made voluntary action superb. In those patients able to be guided sufficiently long to develop and sustain continued mimetic gymnastics, the large, coarse muscles worked fairly well in subdued emotional expressive changes. However, although no bilateral synchronous, symmetrical, truly emotional reaction could be obtained, the effects on mild but restrained smiling and laughter were *not* grotesque. Several completely rigid

individuals, similar to the two patients mentioned earlier, had sufficient mental and facial control that even with pain, shock, or mirth, little difference could be told from the immobile face of the patient with parkinsonism, except that the mouth was controlled, did not drool, and the eyes closed well and tightly.

During the past 18 years, all the temporalis muscle transfers have been carried out with simultaneous antagonist myomectomies and at least unilateral face lifts. Although much time was spent in facial gymnastic mirror training and reiterated abjurations for constant training, it was most difficult to maintain motivation in the majority of patients. Practically all required creation of a nasolabial fold and permanent brow elevation by dermal attachment to the pericranium, especially after a face lift, both static cosmetic procedures, but they have lasted a decade or more (Fig. 22-8). Several of the nasolabial fold reconstructions had to be repeated when the patient aged, and not a few had early temporary healing problems at the nasolabial fold. Yet brow lifts, possibly because of the bony attachment, have never needed revision and have given excellent results.

It was not until 6 years ago that extensive total temporalis muscle transfers were carried out in individuals over 60. These patients have maintained control at least as well as, and frequently better than, the younger adults for whom it had originally been retained. It has not been considered advisable or necessary to do concomitant cross-face nerve grafts to the muscle for synchronous balance. A few free-muscle transplants in the manner of Thompson have failed, due either to a lack of surgical dexterity or to a lack of understanding of the technique. Fur-

FIGURE 22-6. A.F. *"Congenital facial paralysis" on the left with central third weakness and spasm of the right eye, 1962. (A) During speech. (B) During forced closure. (C) Temporalis muscle strip to aid masseter direction. (D and E) 1971, after masseter muscle transfer to previously placed circumoral fascial reconstruction of embouchure, and resection of antagonist muscles. (F) 1972, ten years postoperative masseter transplant and 8 years postoperative, "needs no surgery and is extremely happy."*

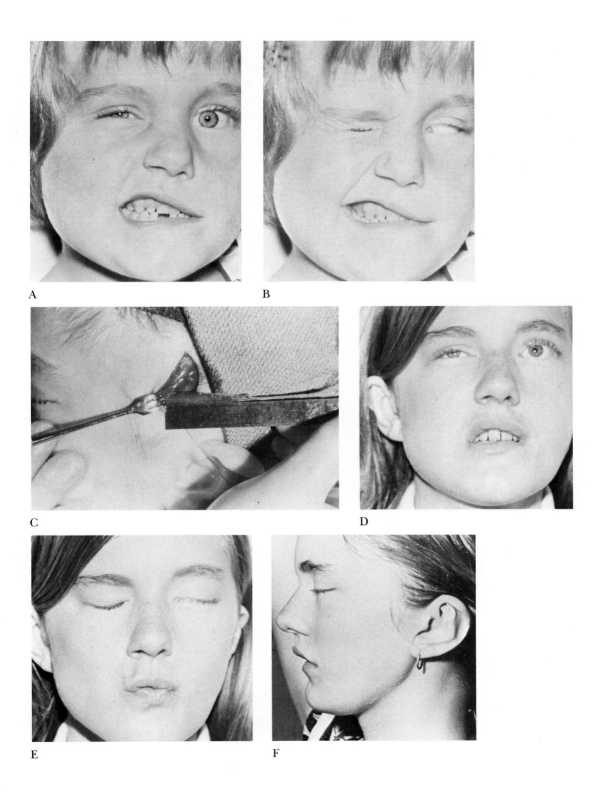

A

B

C

D

E

F

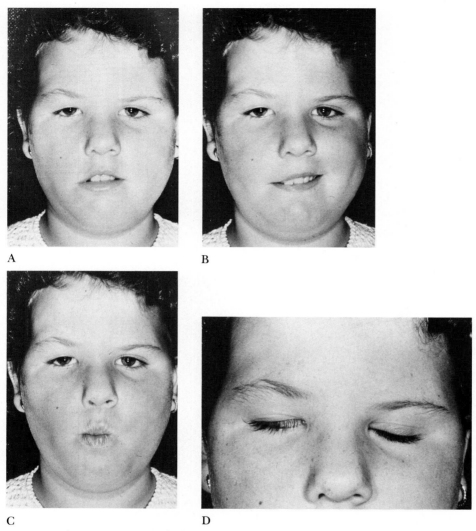

A

B

C   D

FIGURE 22-7.   M.J. *Postoperative temporalis transfer and muscle (contralateral) section. (A through D) Six years after five-tailed temporalis transfer to all sphincters,* *with fair control. Patient is still maintaining mimetic gymnastics. What will she need in 10 years?*

ther reconstruction permitted direct biopsy of the residual scar graft.

Although reports by Thompson and Hekelius are optimistic, free-muscle grafts presently are not equivalent to the transplant of vascularized, neuroticized muscle with a bony attachment and firm insertion into either the nasal periosteum or an anatomically completed oral sphincter continuous with the normal side. The average temporalis transfer allowed ex-

FIGURE 22-8.   G.O. *Temporalis transfer plus need for "aesthetic" ancillary procedures. Classic facial-nerve paralysis with partial loss of the fifth and ninth nerves. Total temporalis transfer to reconstruct orbicularis oculi and oris. (A) Preoperative. (B) Elevation of temporal muscle and aponeurosis. (C) Speaking. (D) Pursing. (E) Relaxed. (F) She needs a face lift.*

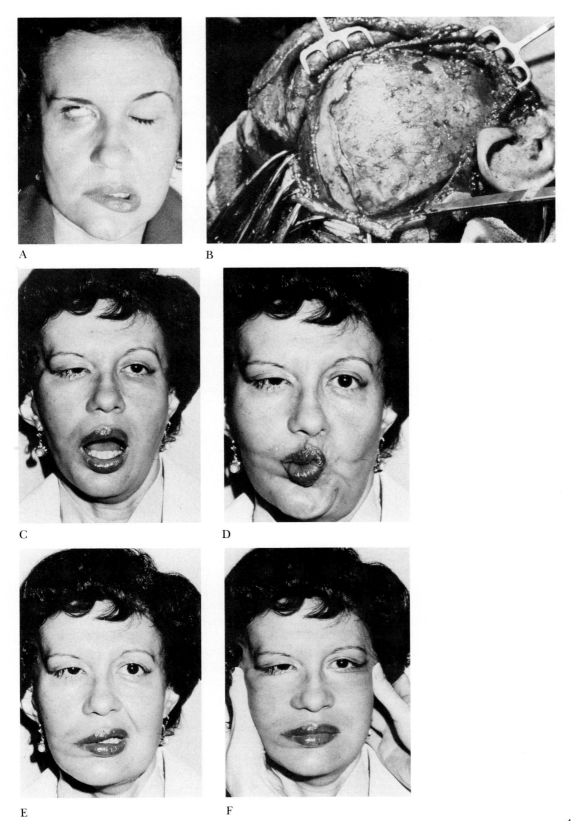

A

B

C

D

E

F

cellent closing of the eyes, with occasional tenting of the lateral commissure away from the globe and a bulge at the lateral border unless either the orbit was fenestrated or the lateral rim grooved. As aging progressed and the tissues thinned, the lid stretched, sagged, and was not as efficient, requiring revision. The angle of the mouth when stabilized was rarely elevated. The abnormality in excessive smiling or with emotional change was an oblique elevation of the contralateral side and an occasional baring of the teeth, preferred by the patient to resection of antagonistic muscles so radically that no emotion could be exhibited. Partial but secure control of both sphincters has been good and has lasted as long as the patient has been followed, some for 20 years. When readjustments were necessary, they were done with as much deliberate delicacy as a tendon operation, and they were guarded against excessive pull for weeks. They can loosen early.

Masseter transfer stabilized the labial angle, but the slight drag downward with growth contrasted with the normal level at rest and with the rapid, if modified, elevation of the usually slightly spastic opposite commissure and nasal levators with motion. Although the temporalis muscle was the preferred dynamic transfer, in a few cases it was not complete, or even available. When the upper two-thirds of the face was normal or balanced in the patient with bilateral lower facial paralysis, bilateral transfer of the anterior two-thirds of the masseter, attached snugly into a well-organized, wide, circumorbital band (inserted in a previous stage) on both sides simultaneously, has proved to be of lasting value when followed from childhood to the adult stage.

Suspension: Elastic and Static

Between 1939 and 1949, unilateral facial paralyses were reconstructed by thin autogenous fascial stripping, as popularized by Blair. Late follow-ups, several as long as 20 years, by mail and in person described a gradual attenuation of the thin facial skin overlying the narrow bands (and in a few cases, palmaris tendons). Frequently, the tense bands compressed the softer, somewhat edematous subcutaneous tissue and were easily seen. After several years, most bands loosened at their medial or peripheral attachments (i.e., the insertions at the inner canthus, filtrum, angle, and center portion of the lower lip), and in a few, reattachment of the still-viable fascia was attempted. This was quite difficult, and replacement by sheets of fascia, freeze-dried or autogenous, were used. Apparently the attachment to the dermis and the now completely denervated and atrophic muscles had weakened at the site of insertion. It was obvious that fascial support required attachment to the normal side for sustained fixation. It was then that I recognized that the oral sphincter had to be reconstructed anatomically by fascial support with continuous attachment to the contralateral motor unit. Deterioration of fascial strips which did not reach the opposite side occurred in 3 years, although a few lasted 5. When augmented by malnutrition and cachexia in terminal patients, dissolution of the suspension seemed to occur in months.

From the fifties to the present time, progressively broad fascial supports, many-tailed and securely fixed to the ala and across both the upper and the lower lips to the normal side, formed a complete anatomical sphincter. These maintained sphincteric action and restored appearance at rest and, occasionally, with voluntary motion (Fig. 22-9). The points of attachments were changed from merely temporal to zygomatic and temporal, as well as to the sternocleidomastoid fascia (to show motion on opening the mouth). (True bony attachment, i.e., mandibular, has been used in two patients.) These broad fascial reconstructive suspensions form a large part of my series of middle-aged patients and have stood the test of time, although the end results have but little semblance of emotion and require occasional adjustments over a period of years [4]. Homografts or freeze-dried irradiated fascia required adjustment at the end of a year or two. Homograft biopsies show little difference from the autografts studied, yet they tear through sooner and require adjustment more frequently, possibly because they are used in the elderly.

Marlex mesh or polypropylene elastic netting was substituted for fascia in the older patients and for temporary suspension. A broad, many-tailed band that reconstructed the embouchure and attached to the temporal region through the face-lift incision by nonabsorbable sutures has worked well. The sutures have been removed easily when necessary. The cephalad end of a few extruded because of poor wound healing in the temporal space, and a few cut through the buccal mucosa when pulled too tightly. Adjustment was easy. The upper limb was stripped from the underlying fascia; the firm insertion, secured on the opposite side, allowed the entire band to be elevated and reattached snugly (Fig. 22-10). Although overcorrection has never been a handicap, the mesh can tear out of tissues if the tension is too great. None of the Marlex *had* to be removed. Some was removed to be replaced by muscle, and some was left in place even after neural reinnervation had taken place. The majority of these patients had little difficulty. Transmucosal insertions of the mesh to the ascending ramus of the mandible worked well and were never pulled out of the bone. Several placed too superficially protruded through the buccal mucosa and were exposed by the pressure of projecting teeth. Not a few patients complained of the mesh being too tight.

Of the seven intraoral insertions, there were no infections. Yet this approach has been discarded because of the possibility of infection and because of the facility with which the external approach lent itself to exact placement. Those placed through the external approach did not have a direct attachment to the mandible. Neither these nor the two fascial strips to the mandible have been reexplored. Those exposed required a patch for continuity and to prevent buccinator hernia. Healing has always been uneventful, despite the age of the patient and the attenuated mucosa.

Temporary and partial suspensions or, as they are called, "assists" were carried out in a number of patients to guide an already working motor to a more desired angle or for a temporary suspension while awaiting neural growth. None of these have been removed, at least by the author.

The Orbicularis Oculi Sphincter

Loss of function of the nerve branches to the eyelids results not only in lagophthalmus and epiphora, but also in spasticity of the ipsilateral levator palpebralis and of the opposite orbicularis muscles. If loss of the sensory branch of the fifth nerve should be included, even if only temporary, the defects may be compounded by potential corneal ulceration. When the denervation of the muscle is prolonged, especially in those past 40, muscle atrophy, gravitational stretching of the nonelastic skin, upper-lid hooding despite lagophthalmus, and lower-lid sagging and eversion are added to the prevalent ectropion. These late changes are most evident in those lids tethered for years by tarsorrhaphies as the sole method of corneal protection.

However, even with the sophisticated canthoplasties involving tarsal resection, with the exception of several patients who had a cranial nerve bypass, later blepharoplasties were necessary if the patients were followed sufficiently long. It appeared that the neural return from some nerve transfers was insufficient to keep the eyelid muscles from atrophy. With the exception of 2 patients, of the 18 that were followed, actual voluntary motor function after cranial nerve transfer was, at best, minimal and usually required some assist. Generally, after a period of 5 or more years, because of relaxation, stretching, and ectropion, further surgical reconstruction was necessary. An occasional patient with the palpebral fissure tightened by both a lateral and medial canthoplasty maintained support and comfort for close to a decade, but the majority of the patients required dynamic reconstructive procedures from 2 to 10 years later.

Of the dynamic procedures reviewed, segmental temporalis myoplasties proved to be tol-

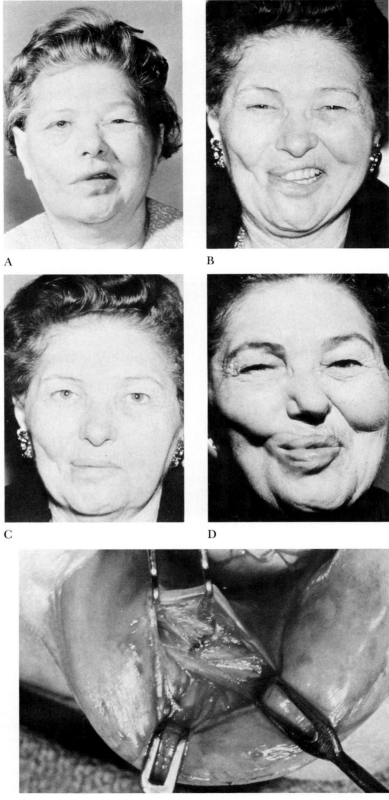

A

B

C

D

E

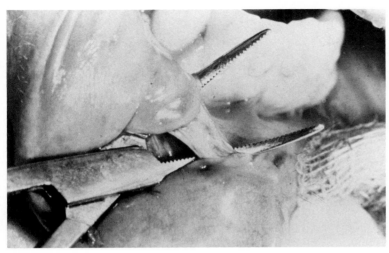

F

FIGURE 22-9.   E.O.B. *Reinnervation after fascial support. Planned permanent fascial support and antagonist release aided and did not impede return of some neural regrowth. Patient referred by a neurosurgeon for "total ablation of the facial nerve" at removal of acoustic neuroma. (A) Many-tailed fascial support to both sphincters, 10 days after surgery. (B and C) Review in 1962 showed control by mimetic gymnastics. (D) 1963, it is obvious she had regained slight control of the orbicularis muscle and a few of the midfacial muscles. No release is needed around the orbicularis. (E) Exposure of tight orbicularis oris allowed freeing of the broad but rounded fascial band to the lower lip, and a step tenoplasty allowed a centimeter release. (F) In 1967 further contracture in the lower lip was released by an open tenotomy. Although the patient died of recurrence of tumor some years later, she had been given 8 years of social and emotional stabilization.*

erated best and often showed functional improvement over a long period. These were not without complication; 4 of 20 cases required some modification, release, tightening, and rerouting; others may have been treated elsewhere. In addition, several had skin tethering. Most, unless the lateral wall was fenestrated or grooved, showed a temporal bulge and a slightly lateralized outer canthus, as well as bowstringing of the rim away from the globe. Eversion occurred in only one patient, and this was repaired with difficulty. None eroded. The myoplasty used was that which Anderson and Schmid have popularized. Two were complete failures and were lost to follow-up. During the last few years, wider ribbons of aponeurosis were used in both upper and lower lids, in an attempt to give structure to the lid sphincter to compensate for the later attenuation and atrophy of the broad, if thin, orbicularis muscular support of the tarsi and soft tissues of the lids, deformed by descent of the atonic brow.

Lid dynamism by various mechanical appliances has been attempted, but with the exception of lid weights, all have been replaced. Because of chronic edema and extrusion, the upper-lid wire springs have been removed (seven out of seven, but Morel-Fatio has an enviable record of permanence). Buried weights of tantalum or gold have been my mainstay for almost three decades and are still the choice for a temporary appliance to close the upper lid. At least 30 such weights have served their purpose and have been removed without injury or scarring. Nor have they prevented later reconstructive procedures when advisable or a normal graceful motion when the muscle has been reinnervated (Fig. 22-11). Minor complications have been positional change, discoloration, and exaggerated skin folds in the atonic lid. Nonetheless the assistance of weights has been invaluable, particularly in patients with some return of tonus, as a temporary measure for the very weak and in the immediate postoperative

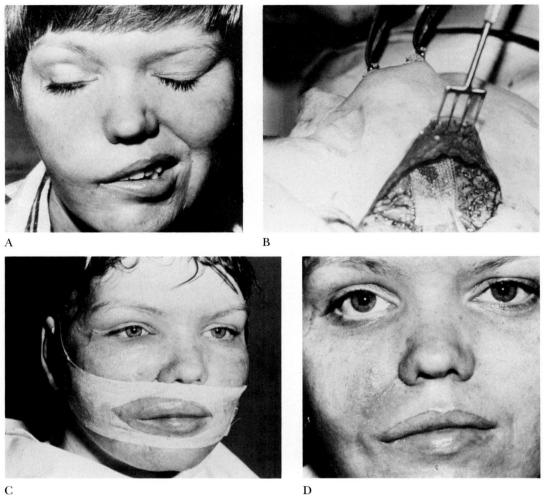

C

D

FIGURE 22-10.   J.M. *Mesh support. (A) Loosening of the temporal attachment of Marlex support 8 years after surgery. (B) Exploration and advancement of Marlex and creation of nasolabial fold. (C) Postauricular splinting maintained for 6 weeks. (D) Ten years after initial Marlex insertion, after nasolabial fold construction and Marlex reattachment. Could use lower lid support.*

period prior to a temporalis repair or a nerve graft. The elastic sphincteric construction of Arion, as modified by Wood-Smith, offers immediate and excellent construction of a sphincter. However, out of 17 immediate, spectacular results, all have had the Silastic loop removed because of thread breakage, stretching, loosening, and in three instances, conjunctival exposure of the band. To avoid disappointment of both patient and surgeon, it should be relegated to temporary use.

Full-thickness graft of the skin to the upper lid has been of value in two patients, but caused an obvious cosmetic blemish. Both had 3 years of fair lid closure until they died. It does offer closure without a foreign body, but with cosmetic impairment. Lower-lid stabilization by fascial and thin cartilage implants has done well. Silastic, Teflon, and Proplast should never be placed under the thin skin and atrophic muscle of the lid. Teflon and Silastic will extrude eventually; black Proplast will discolor the

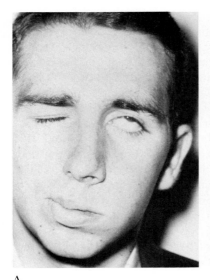
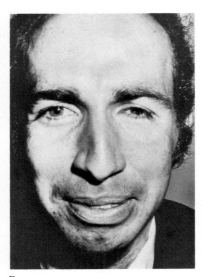

A   B

FIGURE 22-11.   W.H. *Lid weight, removable. Traumatic intracerebral section of nerve. (A) Reconstruction of maxilla, orbit, nose, etc. Refused all aid for palsy except gravity assist; tantalum weight for lid. (B) Eight years after trauma, complete control. Weight adequate to close the eye until regrowth of the nerve 3 years later.*

dermis, and contracture of the pseudocapsule will necessitate removal. Even smooth, prefabricated Silastic bands for support without tension have required removal despite an initial report. Aesthetic blepharoplasty becomes essential as age increases, but no attempt has been made to give a tight, snug upper lid for fear of impairing closure.

It would seem that we must accept asynchronous, asymmetrical lid motion either with myoplasty from the temporalis or with ipsilateral nerve transfer from the masseteric nerve to the upper facial trunk (as proposed by Escat in 1924 and carried out superbly to the lower face by Spira in 1977). It may be that cross-face nerve grafts from the opposite side will give revitalized muscle synchronization and symmetry in a sufficient percentage of attempts to warrant their increased use [7].

Alloplastic Suspension, Assists, and Insertions

Twenty-five years ago, attempts to use stainless steel and tantalum wire and mesh met with failure. A trial of Silastic slings, preliminary to a temporalis muscle transfer, or as a temporary elastic lift, was tried in children and adults. Although the immediate results of several were "good," none lasted over 2 years, after which they had pulled loose or slipped. All have been removed and not replaced. The pseudosheaths resulting after removal of the rods were usually too constricting for the upper portion of the transposed muscle belly and even for the aponeurotic slip. Little difference could be noticed between those few muscle transpositions through a prepared passage and those by direct transfer of the muscle-aponeurosis unit.

In 11 patients the preliminary insertion of a thin sheet of Teflon to prepare a lined cavity for later insertion of either fascia, mesh, or muscle, or inserted temporarily to release skin fixation to adherent muscle or tendon, usually at the angle of the mouth, was done. It has proved unnecessary prior to the insertion of dermis-fat-fascia grafts to obliterate a temporal hollow. The use of a pad of polyurethane or Silastic foam to obliterate the temporal defect has been discarded, although a few may still be in place. Because of the later rigidity and peri-implant capsular changes, preference now would be for a fat-fascia-dermis pad. Usually the cosmetic deformity seems insufficient to warrant its use. A few attempts to use Proplast plaques to attach tendons or alloplastic elastic support in the muscle have been disappointing. Fixation, even in a relatively tranquil face, despite a 3-month delay before applying tension, has been poor. Fortunately, these have been removed rather easily.

Removal of Antagonist Pull

Presently we have not been able to show by electrodiagnostic tests that opposing contralateral muscles are spastic, yet the clinical evidence is sufficient to warrant surgical modification

even in those palsies that are "temporary," or in patients awaiting neural regrowth. Neurectomy, used infrequently, has not been a method of choice during the past 6 years, except coincidentally during the recent use of cross-face nerve grafts when selective nerves are sectioned as a source of axon growth to the paralyzed side. The dissection of the varying multiplicity of the fine branches, especially around the mouth during this procedure, reveals the reason for the relative evanescence of the results of "selective neurectomy" (Fig. 22-12).

Complications of muscle resection, aside from those of wound healing and hematoma, were relatively few and had to do with the return of hyperactivity of sectioned muscle that required further myectomy. The degree of motion loss after surgery varied with the indi-

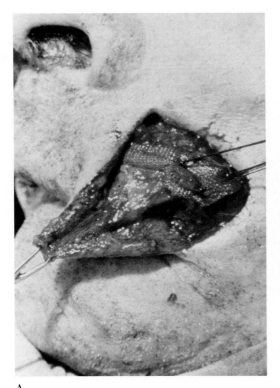
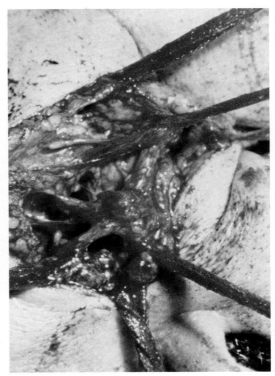

A B

FIGURE 22-12. L.F. *Technique of myectomy for contralateral spasm. (A) Exposure of upper-lip contralateral muscles. (B) Dissection prior to resection. Note multiple fine nerve branches.*

vidual muscles sectioned, the amount removed, and comparatively, with the degree of return in the paralyzed side. Titration of motion is difficult, but mirror training does help. Secondary resections can be difficult. Patients who had myectomy and had considerable nerve recovery to the paralyzed side over the years have neither required nor even inquired as to the advisability of reattachment of the contralateral muscles sectioned. Of those patients, 20 percent could have used further muscle resection, but did not; 10 percent had release of a late postoperative fusion or deep scar. Another 20 percent had additional muscles resected at a second procedure. Temporary weakening (simple myotomy) was included in the series, and in the majority, full muscular action has returned, some as early as 3 months (Fig. 22-13).

Since I have considered myectomy as part of practically every lower and middle face supportive procedure, whether muscle, fascia, or mesh, since 1960, it must be recognized that I am prejudiced toward a procedure that has worked well for so long. Transection of the spastic upper-lid levator has not been carried out, nor have the flaccid muscles been plicated (Nikilson) after impressive failures in a small series.

Physical Gymnastics

Mimetic gymnastics has been offered postoperatively to every patient operated on for relief of facial paralysis. Unfortunately, it has been extremely time-consuming for the physician and his aides, since it is quite difficult to establish sustained interest in the family, and even in the patient, to obtain results sufficiently obvious to the patient to increase motivation. However, in the years 1958 through 1962, a number of patients continued training for more than the usual desultory month or two. A dedicated nurse coaxed and cajoled the patients into continuing their training by sending frequent postcard reminders. Upon her retirement, this ceased. In 1970 a book on face saving

exercises by Marjorie Craig* came to my attention. Here, with judicious elisions, was a training manual needed to stimulate the patient, guide the family, and remind the physician. Patients were told to disregard the conclusions and merely follow the exercises. Since that date, all patients with facial paralysis, temporary or permanent, partial, total, unilateral, or diffuse, have been offered the book and have had the opportunity to train the muscles. Our best results, either in spite of or because of the exercises, have come from that patient group which has maintained facial gymnastics.

Physical reconditioning of the weakened facial muscles, as well as mental adjustments to the realities of appearance and facial function, provides the best means of effecting emotional balance and social rehabilitation of the patient postoperatively. Physical reconditioning has been utilized preoperatively in etiologically obscure and diffuse irregular palsies. With the proper training, physical effects can be obtained with limited yet sufficient success to give the patient a sense of accomplishment against odds and, in addition, some restoration of confidence, even if minor. Preliminary exercises have proven of value diagnostically in several children, and when possible, mimetic gymnastics has been an integral portion of the convalescent treatment of these patients. The surgeon writes the prescription for exercises for specific muscle weaknesses or loss. A graduated series of the exercises depicted in the book is outlined. Although the slim volume gives the patient a ready reference to both the anatomy of the muscles involved and the exercises to be carried out, actual medical supervision of the program with a maximum of effective control by the physician has been necessary. When left solely to the physical therapy aides, it has failed, possibly because of the infrequency with which they see this problem. Like all physical reconditioning, there must be a progressive exercise increase based on the "overload" principle used in training gross body muscles.

*M. Craig. *Face Saving Exercises.* New York: Random House, 1970.

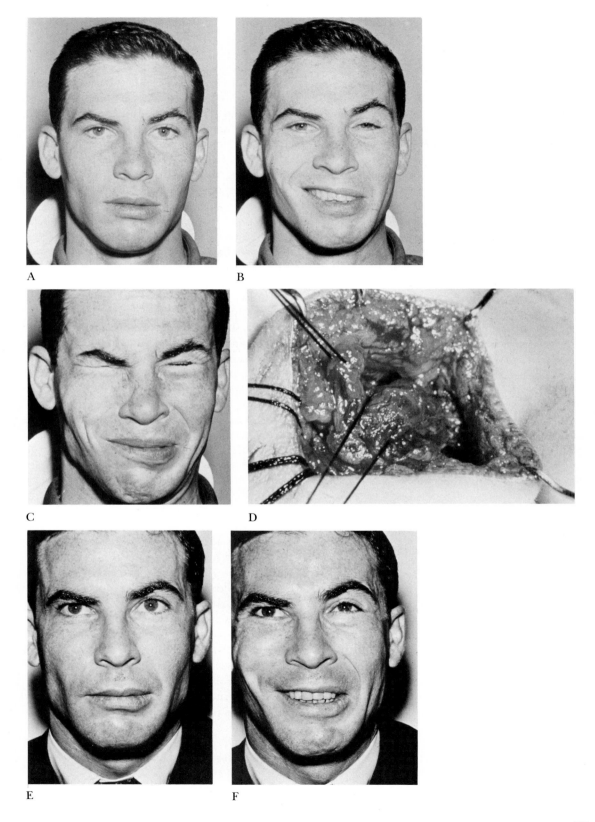

The variations of the postoperative residual require individualization of the program. The immediate full cooperation of the patient shocked by the emotional and physical trauma of brain and/or head and neck surgery is difficult to obtain, and as one would anticipate, this difficulty has been most marked in children. It has been necessary for the physician and family to take an active role in attempting to motivate children years after the surgery has supplied the apparatus. The patients who have done best were examined at least once a month, at which time the slightest evidence of improvement was acclaimed and deviation from the set program corrected. Problems and further expectations are openly discussed. A yearly reanalysis of results and, when requested, a possible prognosis as to a realistic end result can be offered. Obviously, success of surgical treatment improves motivation, but it has been influenced also by the amount of interest that the surgeon and his aide maintained. Surgical failures have not been improved by mimetics, but good results seem to have been enhanced. The immobile faces of some politicians, lawyers, and actors make excellent models for the patient to study. The mirror and the television should cultivate a more socially acceptable result.

Final Thoughts

The surgeon who wishes to engage in the surgical treatment of facial paralysis must take into account the following:

1. Repeated examinations are necessary.
2. There are limitations and a considerable margin of error in the present electrodiagnostic testing methods.
3. Ten percent of patients with "total destruction of the nerve" experience late, spontaneous return of innervation.
4. Normal attrition of facial tissues by abuse and aging is accelerated by loss of neural tone of the muscles.
5. One should reserve the use of the simpler operative procedures for patients needing only partial or temporary assists and for those with a short life expectancy. The remainder of the patients should have as much done as is physiologically proper and possible, at one or two early operative sessions.

References

1. Freeman, B.S. Facial Palsy. In J.M. Converse (Ed.), *Reconstructive Plastic Surgery*. Philadelphia: Saunders, 1964. Vol. 3, pp. 1124–1174.
2. Freeman, B.S. Non-suture Techniques in Facial Nerve Anastomosis. In J. Conley and J.T. Dickinson (Eds.), *Plastic and Reconstructive Surgery of the Face and Neck*. Stuttgart: Thieme, 1972. Vol. 2, pp. 92–95.
3. Freeman, B.S. Techniques for Sphincteric Control in Facial Paralysis. In J. Conley and J.T. Dickinson (Eds.), *Plastic and Reconstructive Surgery of the Face and Neck*. Stuttgart: Thieme, 1972. Vol. 2, pp. 103–106.
4. Freeman, B.S. Late reconstruction of the lax oral sphincter in facial paralysis. *Plast. Reconstr. Surg.* 51:144, 1973.
5. Freeman, B.S. Long-term Results Following Varying Techniques for Facial Palsy. In D. Marshac and J.T. Hueston (Eds.), *Transactions of the Sixth International Congress of Plastic and Reconstructive Surgery*. Paris: Masson, 1976. Pp. 348–350.
6. Freeman, B.S. Synthetic Materials in Orbital and Surrounding Tissue. In D.B. Soll (Ed.), *Management of Complications in Ophthalmic Plastic Surgery*. Birmingham: Aesecularius, 1976. Pp. 45–57.
7. Freeman, B.S. Facial Palsy. In J.M. Converse (Ed.), *Reconstructive Plastic Surgery* (2nd ed.). Philadelphia: Saunders, 1977. Vol. 3, pp. 1774–1867.
8. Freeman, B.S. Ancillary Techniques for the Amelioration of Facial Palsy. In S. Fredricks and G.S. Brody (Eds.), *Symposium on the Neurologic Aspects of Plastic Surgery*. St. Louis: Mosby, 1978. Vol. 17, pp. 307–316.
9. Freeman, B.S. Review of long-term results in supportive treatment of facial paralysis. *Plast. Reconstr. Surg.* 63:215, 1979.

FIGURE 22-13. M.C. *Residual palsy with emotion only, 5 years after partial recovery from cerebral injury; treated by antagonist muscle resection. Result 10 years after injury and 5 years after resection of antagonist muscles. (A) Relaxed. (B) Voluntary. (C) Residual palsy on emotion. (D) Dissection of the facial muscles around the left commissure. (E) Five years later, relaxed. (F) With emotion.*

David W. Robinson

COMMENTS ON CHAPTER 22

THE author has made a significant contribution to the care of patients who have had injury to the facial nerve by sharing his clinical experiences with over 200 patients cared for over the past 35-plus years. A studied plan was made for each patient who was checked carefully and often. Practically all the procedures previously described have been tried and evaluated as to their short- and long-range results. Clinical observations and electromyographic determinations were made frequently and recorded. Although he does not espouse solid set recommendations, he draws conclusions which are valid and based on trial and error.

For immediate injury of the facial nerve extracranially, early or late primary suture produced the best, but not perfect, results. If there was a sizable defect, a free-nerve graft or a cranial-nerve transfer, using preferably the hypoglossal and less often the spinal accessory nerve, produced the advantage of regained muscle tone, which must be weighed against the mass action of all facial muscles as well as the neurological deficit produced in tongue and shoulder. The nerve to the platysma was transferred successfully to the perioral muscles. Early and late return of muscle function without any repair or substitution was observed in about 10 percent of patients.

Muscle transfers employing the temporalis and masseter muscles used as muscle slips with attached fascia have produced much better results than static implants of fascia, Marlex mesh, wire, Silastic, etc. The transfers of neck muscles, sternocleidomastoid, digastric, and omohyoid were not successful. All static procedures have a place, but the face sags in 5 to 10 years. Fascial implants should extend to and be secured to the good nonparalyzed side of the oral sphincter. Gold or tantalum implants aid lid closure to help prevent the exposure dangers of lagophthalmus but were not as good as the temporalis transfer operation. Careful and judicious nerve and/or muscle sections serve as antagonists of the muscles of the seemingly hyperactive unimpaired good side and, with studied suppression of emotion, the patient may learn to keep some balance between the two sides. Resection of the redundant tissues, such as the relaxed sagging side (as with a standard rhytidectomy), the skin, tarsus, and mucosa of the paralytic lower lid, forehead skin just above the brow, and the nasolabial fold with fixation to the dermis, is a useful procedure.

The important key to patient and physician satisfaction has been found because of careful observations, willingness to try varied and multiple corrective procedures in the same patient, and the positive psychological support given the patient. Bromley Freeman states that operations should be performed with deliberate delicacy. His experiences are unique, and his recounting of them are well worth study by reconstructive surgeons dealing with this problem.

23

IN 1963, 1965, and 1972, I published articles [2, 3, 4] on the immediate reconstruction of the mandible and temporomandibular joint which had been developed in the Plastic Surgical Unit at Middlemore Hospital, Auckland, New Zealand. They gave details of the technical problems and ended with evidence that, contrary to widespread belief, bone grafts do not die but continue to live in much the same way as does a skin graft.

This contribution is concerned with the long-term results in such cases, but in order to make this comprehensible, a brief account of the basic principles of the method is needed.

It was applied in reconstruction following resection of the hemimandible for such tumors as myxoma, ameloblastoma, and chondrosarcoma. These tumors often extend to the base of the condylar process so that disarticulation at the temporomandibular joint is necessary. However, since they are not aggressively malignant, it is not necessary to remove any great amount of soft tissue. There is, therefore, no need to defer reconstruction.

Because the patients are often young, it is particularly important to achieve the highest possible standards from the point of view of appearance, dental occlusion, and function at the newly reconstructed temporomandibular joint. The resected part, therefore, must be able to carry a partial denture, any remaining teeth must occlude normally, and the reconstructed temporomandibular joint must function well.

W. M. Manchester

THE LONG-TERM RESULTS IN THE IMMEDIATE RECONSTRUCTION OF THE MANDIBLE AND TEMPOROMANDIBULAR JOINT BY FREE BONE GRAFTING

It seemed to me that these exacting standards could best be met by using an autogenous but largely cancellous (in fact, bicortical) bone graft that was as nearly as possible an exact replica of the normal. The details of the exact placing and fixation of the graft have been dealt with elsewhere, but briefly the method is as follows.

A thin aluminum or pewter pattern of the required hemimandible is applied to the outer surface of the ilium, and a graft including its full thickness is cut out exactly to the shape of the pattern (Fig. 23-1). After its removal, further shaping is needed in order to convert it into a replica of the normal (Fig. 23-2). A view from above shows how the curvature of the ilium on the same side is appropriate (Fig. 23-3).

The theory of temporomandibular joint reconstruction was based on the idea that the joint has two synovial cavities separated by a meniscus (Fig. 23-4). The disarticulation is carried out so as to leave the meniscus in place, thus leaving the upper synovial cavity undisturbed (Fig. 23-5). The bone graft has its condylar head placed in this meniscus, but owing to the fact that it has no articular cartilage, this space is obliterated (Fig. 23-6). The joint, however, can function well with the remaining synovial cavity. The jaw is kept immobilized for 1 month, and it is normal to have quite solid union between the graft and the remaining part at the end of that time.

CASE 1

This man presented in 1964 at the age of 42 years with an ameloblastoma affecting the right hemimandible and recurrent after surgery some 3½ years previously (Fig. 23-7). In September 1964, the hemimandible was removed and replaced by a free bone graft replica (Fig. 23-8). He made an uninterrupted recovery, and union was solid in 4 weeks. An x-ray taken 5 years later shows near perfect symmetry between the two halves (Fig. 23-9). An x-ray of the junction between the graft and the remaining hemimandible shows the state of affairs some 11 years later. A very convincing cortex has developed on both sides (Fig. 23-10). The postoperative appearance was indistinguishable from normal 5 years later (Fig. 23-11). His dental occlusion was also normal 5 years later. The graft has carried a partial denture since reconstruction (Fig. 23-12). Five years later, opening at the reconstructed temporomandibular joint was within normal limits (Fig. 23-13). An x-ray taken 1 month postoperatively shows the trabecular pattern of the graft to be that of the donor site, the ilium, and also the absence of a cortex (Fig. 23-14). Six months later an x-ray shows that the trabecular pattern has changed and a cortex is developing under the influence of functional stress (Fig. 23-15). A panoramic tomogram taken 11 years postoperatively shows remarkably normal mandibular architecture (Fig. 23-16).

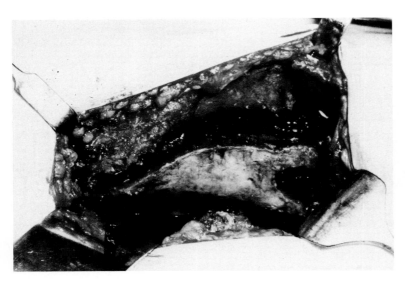

FIGURE 23-1. *The outer surface of the right ilium has been exposed, and a bicortical but largely cancellous bone graft the shape and size of a normal hemimandible is be-* *ginning to emerge. The condylar and coronoid processes are shown at the bottom right of the picture.*

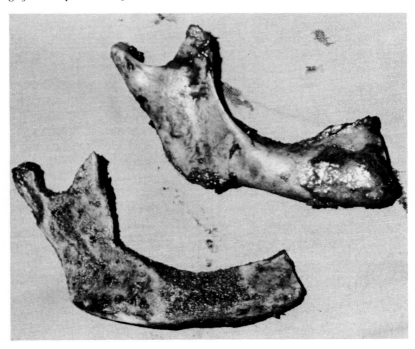

FIGURE 23-2. *The excised and diseased hemimandible above with the bicortical full thickness iliac replica below. (Reproduced, with permission, from W.M. Manchester, Immediate mandibular reconstruction. In Transactions of the Third International Congress of Plastic Surgery. Amsterdam: Excerpta Medica Foundation, 1964.)*

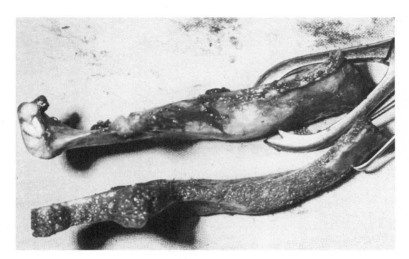

FIGURE 23-3. *The diseased hemimandible and its replica seen from above showing how the curvature of the ilium on the same side is appropriate. (Reproduced, with permission, from W.M. Manchester, Some technical improvements in reconstruction of the mandible and temporomandibular joint. Plast. Reconstr. Surg. 50:249, 1972.)*

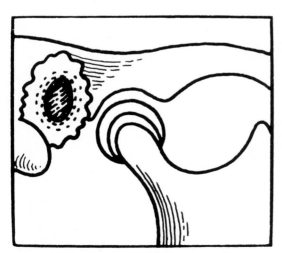

FIGURE 23-4. *The temporomandibular joint has two synovial cavities separated by a meniscus.*

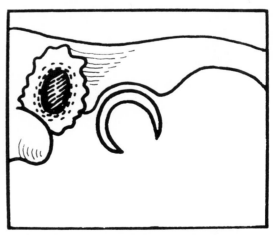

FIGURE 23-5. *The hemimandible has been disarticulated leaving the meniscus in place and thus leaving the upper synovial cavity undisturbed.*

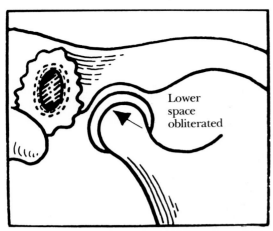

FIGURE 23-6. *The absence of articular cartilage on the condylar process of the graft leads to the obliteration of the lower synovial cavity, but the upper remains and can function well.*

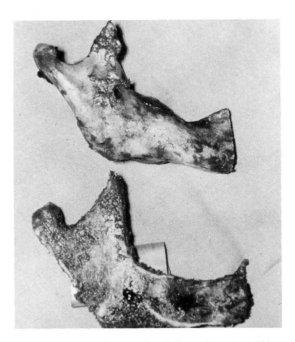

FIGURE 23-8. *The excised and diseased hemimandible and its replica. (Reproduced, with permission, from W.M. Manchester, Some technical improvements in reconstruction of the mandible and temporomandibular joint. Plast. Reconstr. Surg. 50:249, 1972.)*

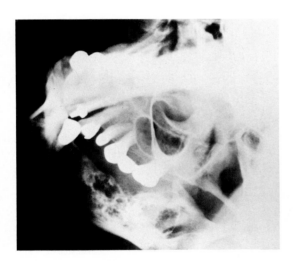

FIGURE 23-7. *This rotated lateral view of the right hemimandible shows a recurrent ameloblastoma extending almost to the base of the condylar process.*

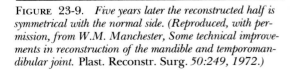

FIGURE 23-9. *Five years later the reconstructed half is symmetrical with the normal side. (Reproduced, with permission, from W.M. Manchester, Some technical improvements in reconstruction of the mandible and temporomandibular joint. Plast. Reconstr. Surg. 50:249, 1972.)*

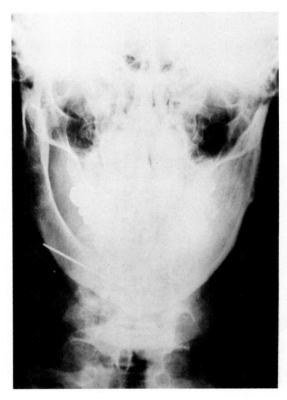

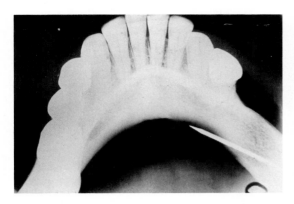

FIGURE 23-10.   *An occlusal x-ray shows the junction of the graft and the remaining mandible 11 years later.*

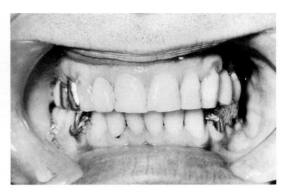

FIGURE 23-12.   *Five years postoperatively there is normal dental occlusion. (Reproduced, with permission, from W.M.Manchester, Some technical improvements in reconstruction of the mandible and temporomandibular joint. Plast. Reconstr. Surg. 50:249, 1972.)*

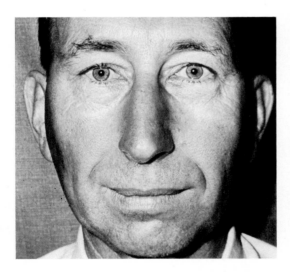

FIGURE 23-11.   *Five years postoperatively the appearance is normal. (Reproduced, with permission, from W.M. Manchester, Some technical improvements in reconstruction of the mandible and temporomandibular joint. Plast. Reconstr. Surg. 50:249, 1972.)*

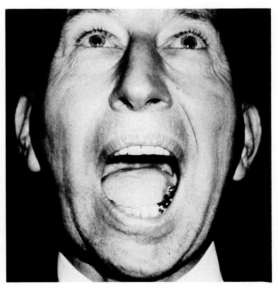

FIGURE 23-13.   *Jaw opening 5 years postoperatively is normal. (Reproduced, with permission, from W.M. Manchester, Some technical improvements in reconstruction of the mandible and temporomandibular joint. Plast. Reconstr. Surg. 50:249, 1972.)*

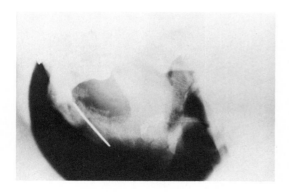

FIGURE 23-14. *This x-ray taken 1 month postoperatively shows the trabecular pattern of the donor site, the ilium.*

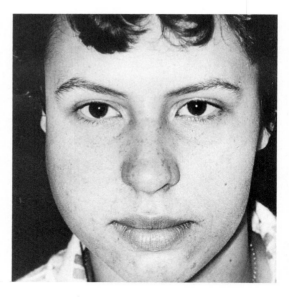

FIGURE 23-17. *Preoperative appearance of a 16-year-old girl with a myxoma of the right hemimandible. (Reproduced, with permission, from W.M. Manchester, Immediate mandibular reconstruction. Transactions of the Third International Congress of Plastic Surgery. Amsterdam: Excerpta Medica Foundation, 1964.)*

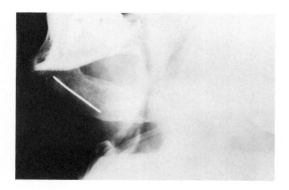

FIGURE 23-15. *Six months later the trabecular pattern has changed and a cortex has developed above and below.*

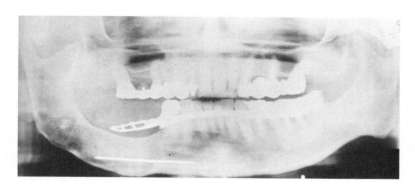

FIGURE 23-16. *Eleven years postoperatively a panoramic tomogram shows this same graft to have developed a cortex and to be surprisingly symmetrical with its fellow of the opposite side.*

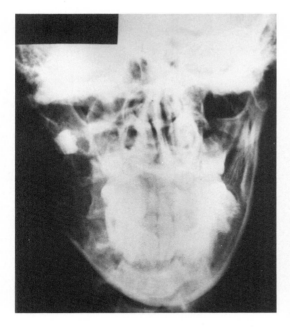

FIGURE 23-18.   *The tumor is expanding and replacing the right hemimandible, and there is an ectopic tooth in the sigmoid notch. (Reproduced, with permission from W.M. Manchester, Immediate mandibular reconstruction. Transactions of the Third International Congress of Plastic Surgery. Amsterdam: Excerpta Medica Foundation, 1964.)*

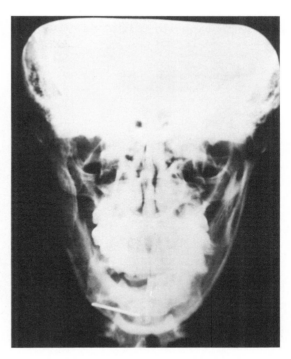

FIGURE 23-19.   *The graft is symmetrical with the normal side. (Reproduced, with permission, from W.M. Manchester, Immediate mandibular reconstruction. Transactions of the Third International Congress of Plastic Surgery. Amsterdam: Excerpta Medica Foundation, 1964.)*

CASE 2

This 16-year-old girl presented in 1959 with a myxoma of the mandible (Fig. 23-17). An x-ray shows a large tumor expanding and replacing the right hemimandible with an ectopic tooth in the region of the sigmoid notch (Fig. 23-18). The hemimandible and temporomandibular joint were reconstructed using a free grafted replica in October of 1959. A postoperative x-ray taken a year later shows a symmetrical mandible (Fig. 23-19). Three and a half years postoperatively, the dental occlusion was normal, and the graft has carried a partial denture ever since (Fig. 23-20). Jaw opening at the reconstructed temporomandibular joint 3½ years postoperatively was normal, the condyle riding up on the eminentia articularis (Fig. 23-21). An x-ray taken 1 month postoperatively shows the trabecular pattern of the donor site, the ilium (Fig. 23-22). Six months later the pattern has changed and a cortex has developed (Fig.

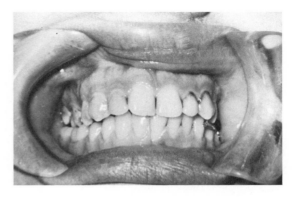

FIGURE 23-20.   *Many years later the dental occlusion is normal and a partial denture is carried on the graft. (Reproduced, with permission, from W.M. Manchester, Immediate reconstruction of the mandible and temporomandibular joint. Br. J. Plast. Surg. 18:291, 1965.)*

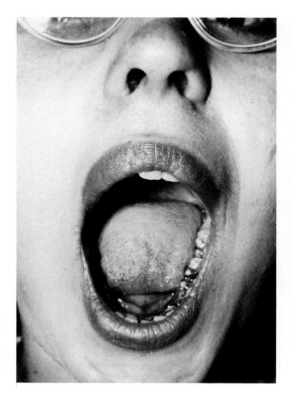

FIGURE 23-21. *Jaw opening is normal in this case. This can only be accomplished if the condyle is riding up on the eminentia articularis. (Reproduced, with permission, from W.M. Manchester, Immediate reconstruction of the mandible and temporomandibular joint.* Br. J. Plast. Surg. *18:291, 1965.)*

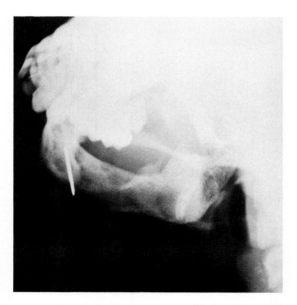

FIGURE 23-23. *Six months postoperatively a cortex has developed.*

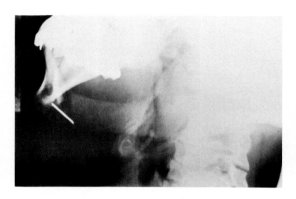

FIGURE 23-22. *One month postoperatively the trabecular pattern is that of the donor site.*

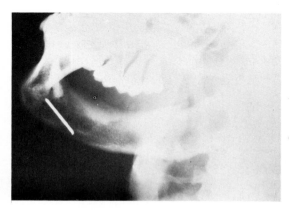

FIGURE 23-24. *Six years postoperatively much more normal mandibular architecture is shown as a result of functional stresses.*

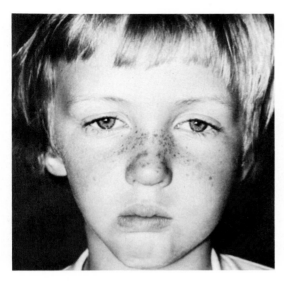

FIGURE 23-25.   *A 6-year-old girl who some 2½ years previously has had the right hemimandible excised for what was thought to be a fibrosarcoma, but what was in fact a myxoma of the mandible.*

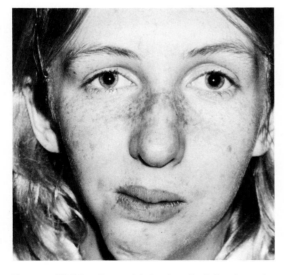

FIGURE 23-26.   *Same girl showing the deformity at the age of 17.*

23-23). Six years later the whole structure is much denser and now resembles normal mandible (Fig. 23-24).

CASE 3

When this patient was 3 years old in 1958, her hemimandible was removed without reconstruction for what at that time was diagnosed as a fibrosarcoma, but which later examination of the original slide showed to be a myxoma of the mandible. When first seen by myself, she was 6 years old (Fig. 23-25). It was decided to put off reconstruction until she was 16 (Fig. 23-26). In September of 1971, the hemimandible and temporomandibular joint were reconstructed, but because the point of resection anteriorly was at the symphysis, the graft needed much more curvature than that naturally provided by the ilium. The graft was therefore given greater curvature by an osteotomy near the symphysis, as seen in Figure 23-27. A K-wire has been used to fix these two fragments at the osteotomy site. When photographed 2 years later, there was a great improvement in her appearance (Fig. 23-28). An x-ray shows the bone graft 3 months later with a K-wire at the symphyseal join and also at the osteotomy site (Fig. 23-29). The important thing is that both the symphyseal junction and the osteotomy site were solidly united in 1 month. This could clearly not have happened if the graft were dead, since the osteotomy site is nowhere in contact with living bony tissue or even periosteum. This fact will be referred to later in the discussion on the fate of the grafted bone.

CASE 4

This 60-year-old patient reported to us with a recurrent ameloblastoma at the angle of the right hemimandible but extending a long way forward in the body, as seen in an x-ray taken in June 1976 (Fig. 23-30). The hemimandible was removed and replaced at an operation performed in July of 1976, and a postoperative x-ray taken about 1 month later shows the typical trabecular pattern of the ilium (Fig. 23-31). A postoperative picture taken about a year later shows that there is no interference with the in-

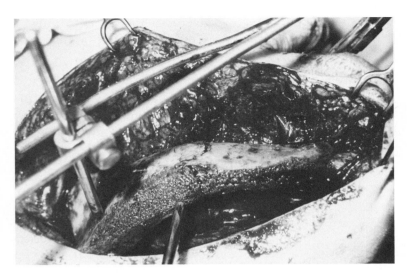

FIGURE 23-27. *Same patient as in Figures 23-25 and 23-26. This photograph shows a bicortical, but largely cancellous, bone graft that has been reshaped by an osteotomy some little distance from the symphysis, which itself is at the right of the incision. A K-wire has immobilized this osteotomy.*

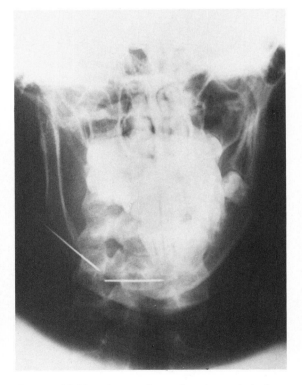

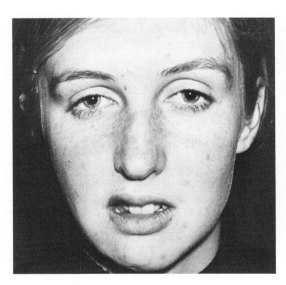

FIGURE 23-28. *Her postoperative appearance 2 years later.*

FIGURE 23-29. *An x-ray 3 months postoperatively shows both the osteotomy site and the point of junction in the symphyseal region. There is good symmetry of the two halves.*

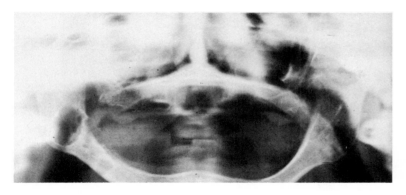

FIGURE 23-30. *A recurrent ameloblastoma at the right angle of the jaw in a 60-year-old woman.*

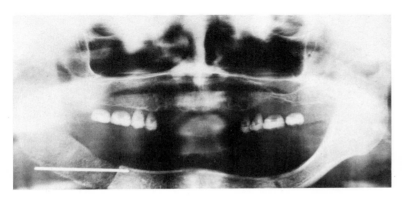

FIGURE 23-31. *The x-ray appearance 1 month post-operatively.*

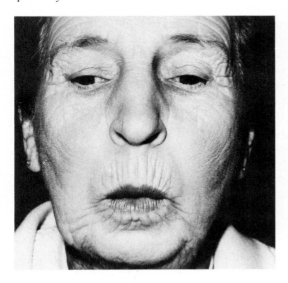

FIGURE 23-32. *The patient is pouting her lips, and there is no interference with the innervation of the lower lip.*

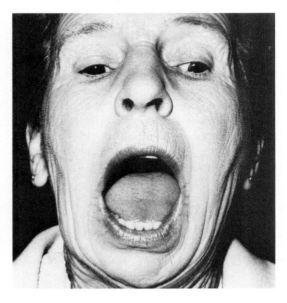

FIGURE 23-33. *Jaw opening is normal at the reconstructed temporomandibular joint.*

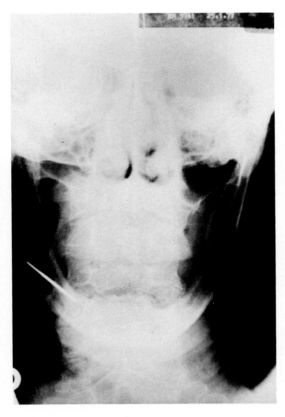

FIGURE 23-34. *Postoperative x-rays show good symmetry between the two halves.*

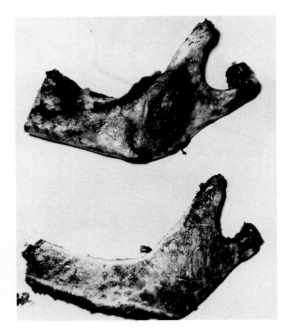

FIGURE 23-35. *The resected hemimandible and its replica.*

nervation of the lower lip (Fig. 23-32). A year later, mandibular opening was normal (Fig. 23-33). It is interesting to note that this patient was able to wear her preoperative denture on her newly reconstructed hemimandible 6 weeks later. Another postoperative x-ray shows the normal symmetry of the mandible (Fig. 23-34).

CASE 5

This man reported in 1976 with an ameloblastoma of the left hemimandible. It was excised and reconstructed using a bicortical cancellous replica (Fig. 23-35). Some 6 weeks postoperatively, a small abscess developed in the stitchline. This was opened, drained, went on discharging for about a month, and then healed completely. A postoperative panoramic tomogram taken afterward shows an area where

some bone absorption has taken place (Fig. 23-36). The important thing about this is that if the bone graft were dead in the immediate postoperative period and therefore a foreign body, infection of this kind would have meant removal of the whole bone graft. In fact, this bone graft has behaved just as a normal bone would have, and this seems to provide clear evidence of its survival from the beginning.

CASE 6

In June 1962 this man was seen, with a history of having had a block dissection of the neck following a melanoma of the lower lip. During that block dissection it was found that melanomatous tissue was entering the mental foramen, and it was impossible to clear this. It was therefore known that the inferior alveolar canal contained melanomatous tissue. The hemimandible was removed and a bicortical cancellous graft was introduced in June of 1962. He made good progress, but after a few months, widespread secondaries developed and he died 11 months postoperatively. His

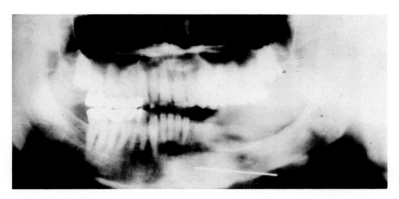

FIGURE 23-36. *This panoramic tomogram shows the symmetry between the two halves, but an area of absorption is seen just in front of the angle at the inferior border. This was the result of a small hematoma that became infected, and some bone loss occurred, but the whole graft was not lost.*

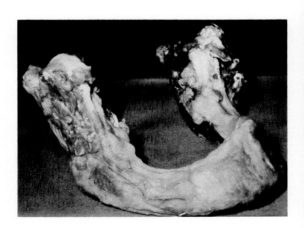

FIGURE 23-37. *This hemimandible was taken from the patient described as case 6. It was reconstructed on the side nearest the camera, 11 months previously. A K-wire can be seen near the inferior border, and the alveolar mucosa upon which he wore a denture is seen on the graft. (Reproduced, with permission, from W.M. Manchester, Immediate reconstruction of the mandible and temporomandibular joint. Br. J. Plast. Surg. 18:291, 1965.)*

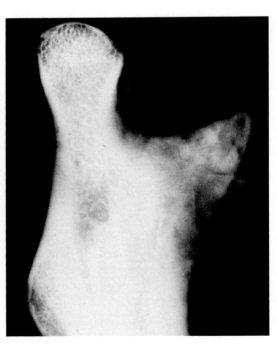

FIGURE 23-38. *A postmortem x-ray of the specimen. This is the normal side and shows the trabecular pattern. (Reproduced, with permission, from W.M. Manchester, Immediate reconstruction of the mandible and temporomandibular joint. Br. J. Plast. Surg. 18:291, 1965.)*

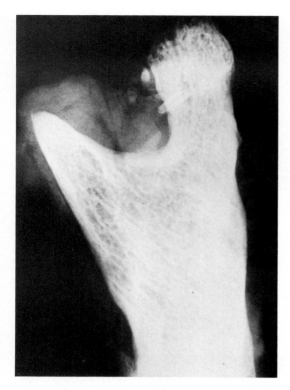

FIGURE 23-39. *This is the reconstructed side 11 months after the bone graft was introduced. The trabecular pattern is that of the mandible and not of the ilium. A cortex has developed where there was no cortex at the time of the transfer. (Reproduced, with permission, from W.M. Manchester, Immediate reconstruction of the mandible and temporomandibular joint.* Br. J. Plast. Surg. *18:291, 1965.)*

wife kindly allowed us to recover the reconstructed hemimandible (Fig. 23-37). This shows the reconstructed part nearest the camera, and it is possible to see the K-wire protruding from the inferior border of the mandible. The muscles of mastication have reattached themselves in convincing fashion, and the alveolar mucosa is seen adherent to the grafted hemimandible. He wore a denture on this until he died.

Postmortem x-rays of this reconstructed hemimandible were taken, and that of the normal side gives an idea of the trabecular pattern (Fig. 23-38). An x-ray of the reconstructed side, 11 months postoperatively,

shows that the bone graft has developed a cortex apart from its own original one, especially in the sigmoid notch region, and the trabecular pattern is that of the mandible (Fig. 23-39). It is inconceivable that if this bone graft were dead it could have been reabsorbed and replaced by bone from the symphyseal region in the short space of 11 months, which it would have to have done if the old theory is correct. This lends further substance to the idea that these bone grafts do not die but continue to live and undergo remodeling to suit them to their new position and function.

The Fate of the Grafted Bone

For many years it has been held, more particularly among the ranks of orthopedic surgeons, that free bone grafts do not survive transplantation but merely form a scaffolding for the ingrowth of new bone from the two ends between which they are placed. It seems inescapable in the light of evidence supplied by the preceding cases that, provided the technical standards which are necessary to ensure the survival of a skin graft are applied to the free transplantation of bone grafts, these too survive in the same way. They then undergo architectural changes to suit them to their new position and functional stresses. Everyone knows that if a skin graft is put onto a hematoma, the blood coagulates in the vascular system of the graft, that part of the graft becomes an infarct, and because it is at the surface, it soon is infected and becomes an ulcer. If, however, it is put onto a vascular bed without the intervention of a hematoma, connections are rapidly established between the vascular system of the bed and that of the graft, and the graft survives. If vascular soft tissues are applied to a largely cancellous bone graft without the intervention of a hematoma, it seems certain that the same thing happens. The following facts seem to provide convincing proof of this.

1. If the bone graft requires further shaping than the curvature of the ilium naturally provides, the bone graft can be fractured and im-

mobilized with a K-wire into some better shape. This fracture or osteotomy unites at the same rate as a fracture of the normal mandible does and is therefore solid in 1 month. This could not possibly happen if the bone graft were dead (case 3).

2. If a cancellous bone graft is exposed by the breaking down of the stitch line or by a small area of infection, only a small part is lost and the rest survives, just as would happen in a normal bone. If it were completely dead, as we are asked to believe, it would be a foreign body, and the whole dead bone graft would have to be removed before healing could be achieved (case 5).

3. The trabecular pattern is remodeled very quickly in response to functional stresses that are applied to it and at a place very remote from the only point of bony contact. This could not happen if the bone graft were dead, and it is inconceivable that in such a short space of time it could have been replaced by bone from the symphyseal region, the only point of bony contact. This happens even when all the periosteum is excised as well (case 6). The only possible explanation for the persistence of the belief that bone grafts die is the fact that many orthopedic surgeons do in fact put their bone grafts into hematomata. In these cases, they are very deep below the surface and do not become infected. The necrosis is therefore aseptic. When this is the case, of course, the earlier theory probably does hold good.

It is hard to believe that the observations made in these cases can have any other explanation than that the bone grafts survive and are vascularized from the beginning. However, this can happen only if the graft is in intimate contact with vascular soft tissue everywhere without the intervention of hematoma.

Final Thoughts

1. The long-term results of a previously published method of immediate reconstruction of the hemimandible and temporomandibular joint have been illustrated in a number of cases.

2. The cosmetic results have been shown to be within normal limits many years later.

3. The dental occlusion has been shown to be normal many years later, as has the ability of the graft to carry a partial or full denture.

4. Function at the temporomandibular joint can be normal or very little short of it.

5. The fate of the grafted bone has been discussed and evidence produced to suggest that if the technical standards are high enough, the grafts are rapidly vascularized and survive as skin grafts do.

6. Free grafting in cases where vascular soft tissues are present has been shown to be the treatment of choice for reconstruction of the mandible and temporomandibular joint. For this type of case it has many advantages over the more elaborate free compound flap transfers that have recently been described. These latter leave more disfigurement of the donor site and are more time consuming. They will certainly have a place in the reconstruction of bony and soft tissue defects created by the excision of, say, squamous cell carcinoma of the floor of the mouth, especially where much of the mucosa and overlying skin have had to be sacrificed, and especially where the soft tissues have been irradiated.

References

1. Jaffe, H.L. *Tumors and Tumerous Conditions of the Bones and Joints.* Philadelphia: Lea & Febiger, 1958. P. 435.

2. Manchester, W.M. Immediate Mandibular Reconstruction. In T.R. Broadbent (Ed.), *Transactions of the Third International Congress of Plastic Surgery.* Amsterdam: Excerpta Medica, 1964. P. 1087.

3. Manchester, W.M. Immediate reconstruction of the mandible and temporomandibular joint. *Br. J. Plast. Surg.* 18: 291, 1965.

4. Manchester, W.M. Some technical improvements in the reconstruction of the mandible and temporomandibular joint. *Plast. Reconstr. Surg.* 50: 249, 1972.

5. Mowlem, R. Bone grafting. *Br. J. Plast. Surg.* 16: 293, 1963.

Joseph E. Murray

COMMENTS ON CHAPTER 23

THIS lucid and concise chapter embodies careful preoperative planning, superb technical skills, and critical follow-up. The type of resection suitable for these repairs is reserved, as the author states, for those tumors of low malignant potential. For more extensive resections, especially those following x-ray treatment, blood-bearing soft tissues in the form of pedicle or revascularized flaps are needed.

In spite of the limited applicability of these elegant techniques, the contributions of Mr. Manchester are monumental not only in the excellence of the functional result, but also because of the extra dividends obtained from his careful physiological observations. The healing of fractures within the autotransplanted iliac graft, the control of localized infection within the graft, the migration of teeth, and the remodeling of the trabeculae from those of the ilium to those of the mandible are striking evidences that these grafts are in fact surviving in toto and not serving merely as a dead scaffold on which host cells regrow.

A few careful observations such as reported in this chapter can be contrasted with the chaos that can result from a review of some of the experimental work on bone graft remodeling. Experimental work has led to conflicting concepts of the differing results because of differences in the animal models and the site and source of the bone grafts.

Mr. Manchester has shown that for the human mandible, remodeling does occur and can almost completely simulate the normal side if sufficient time has elapsed following the grafting. I was most impressed by his observations on the mandibular graft which was removed at death. The striking reattachment of the muscle, and even of the mucosa, to the grafted bone demonstrates the ability of muscle to reattach under normal stimuli. Muscular reattachment following mandibular osteotomy with or without bone graft is a subject of intense interest in this current era of craniofacial surgery. Planning experimental models to test the various hypotheses of muscle reattachment is a difficult chore, and the experiments are expensive to complete, being dependent on long-term follow-up studies of individual, large experimental animals, e.g., the dog or primate. In a study of long-term bone grafts in my own patients, I have found that in children especially remodeling can be so complete as to simulate perfectly the normal mandible. In several patients who have had sequential bone grafting in the treatment of hemifacial microsomia, I have found evidence of the bone graft only by the wires which had been placed several years previously.

Bone grafts do survive intact in the human without undergoing resorption and creeping substitution if solid bony union is obtained in at least one area of the graft to the host. Loss of osteotomized bone can occur even though the blood supply to an osteotomized fragment is unimpaired. This localized resorption of osteotomized bone is presumably due to localized hematoma.

Mr. Manchester's chapter is a model of superb clinical observation, careful surgical technique, and imaginative postoperative evaluation.

24

THE late results of untreated or inadequately treated facial fractures *in adults* are generally obvious. In addition to visible facial asymmetry and deformity (Fig. 24-1), these patients may have symptoms of malocclusion, trismus, diplopia, sinusitis, hearing loss, and diminished nasal airway. Prevention of such morbidity lies with an aggressive approach to prompt diagnosis and definitive treatment. Similarly, the complications of inadequately treated facial fractures in adults require an aggressive reversal or supplementation of static deformities. This is often accomplished through the use of autogenous bone grafts or alloplastic materials. More significant, however, are the sequelae of facial fractures *in children*. The seriousness of fractures in infants and young children is compounded by the effect of the fractures on future facial growth and development.

Repeated analysis of pediatric facial fractures confirms their rarity, particularly during the first 5 years of life. It is not until the midteens that the frequency and pattern of fractures approach those of adulthood. The comparative immunity of children to facial fractures is due to both environmental and anatomical factors. Before the age of 5, most children have a relatively protected existence under parental scrutiny. Falls are common, but weight, height, and distance are usually small and therefore so are the gravitational forces generated. The face is small in relation to overall head size until a child reaches the teens. The face is more flexible, and the large number of resilient growth centers permits a greater degree of distortion to occur before fracture occurs. There is relatively more cancellous and less cortical bone in children, accounting for the increased elasticity and greater incidence of greenstick fractures.

In a review of 2,386 consecutive facial fractures treated in one author's (RCS) private practice over an 11-year period (1961–1972),

Richard Carlton Schultz
Jeffrey Meilman

FACIAL FRACTURES IN CHILDREN

188 cases fell into the age range from 1 to 16 years. Of these, 15 fractures occurred in children less than 5 years of age, accounting for 8 percent of pediatric facial fractures in this series. One hundred and twenty (64 percent) were nasal fractures; 27 (14 percent), mandibular fractures; 15 (8 percent), orbital rim fractures; 14 (7½ percent), zygomatic fractures; and 12 (6½ percent), maxillary fractures. Vehicular trauma accounted for 40 percent of the fractures, while 32 percent were due to falls and athletic injuries. Of even these young children, 36 percent had other associated injuries.

All the pediatric fractures in this series were treated in the hospital. Considerable tact and patience often were required, and most procedures were carried out under either local anesthesia and heavy sedation or general anesthesia. Generally, a one-stage procedure was sufficient. Because of the rapidity of fracture healing in children, early and proper reduction was an essential element to achieve a satisfactory result. Anatomical reduction became difficult after 7 days, and occasionally was not possible after 14 days. Sometimes associated injury delayed treatment, but every effort to overcome treatment delay was made to prevent complications and undesirable results.

Complications such as cerebrospinal fluid rhinorrhea and ophthalmic injuries with late ophthalmological sequelae were not observed more frequently than in adults. Infections were uncommon in promptly reduced facial fractures, even when associated with severe soft tissue injury. Malunion with associated deformity was the major long-term complication—usually from inadequate stabilization or delayed treatment.

Considering the face in thirds, hypertelorism resulting from unreduced or improperly reduced nasoethmoid fractures was the most difficult long-term complication in fractures of the upper third of the face. Persistent nasal deformity resulting from improper or nonreduction of nasal fractures is a major complication in the middle third of the face. Excess bone formation and cartilage distortion can occur with a potential diminution in midfacial growth, although this was not our experience, nor has it been a major noted occurrence in larger series. With maxillary fractures, only severe nasoethmoid or orbital fractures resulted in local residual deformity. We did not find the impairment of facial growth that was emphasized by both McCoy et al. [32] and Rowe [38, 39].

It is in the lower third of the face that condylar fractures damage the articular surfaces and growth centers to produce the most severe deformities in later life. This is due to growth retardation of the affected ramus, together with functional impairment resulting from ankylosis. Because of this concern for growth retardation, there is little indication for surgical interference with a child's condyle or articular surface.

Questionnaires were sent to all 188 pediatric facial fracture patients, who were studied from 5 years to 16 years after treatment. Fifty-nine questionnaires were undeliverable because of change of address; sixty-five questionnaires were answered and returned, covering nasal, mandibular, orbital, zygomatic, and maxillary fractures. The patients and their parents were asked to rate any residual problem relating to their facial fracture from mild to severe and state their concern in their own words. Those patients listing residual long-term complications were contacted by telephone and in person.

The majority of subjective complaints came from the 47 patients who had had nasal fractures. Eight complained of partially obstructed nasal breathing and two of sinus headaches, but

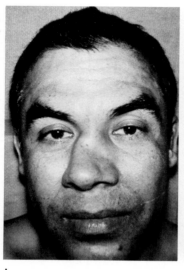
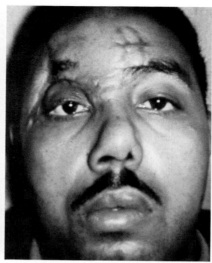
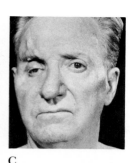
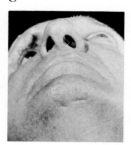

A B

C

D

FIGURE 24-1. *Healed deformities from unreduced facial fractures. (A) Unreduced, healed nasal fracture in a former boxer. (B) Healed, unreduced supraorbital fracture and a nasal fracture from an intentional injury. (C and D) Unreduced, healed, depressed zygoma fracture from an automobile accident. (Reproduced with permission from Schultz, R.C.,* Facial Injuries, *1st edition, Copyright © 1970, and 2nd edition, Copyright © 1977 by Year Book Medical Publishers, Inc., Chicago.)*

only two complained of a residual irregularity on the nasal dorsum. These two children were examined, and both indeed had a minor irregularity of the bony dorsum. In only one instance was there a complaint of retardation of nasal growth (Fig. 24-2).

None of the 10 mandibular fracture returns in this study showed residual complaints of any kind. Review of the 27 pediatric mandibular fractures in this series, however, showed no severe crushing fracture of either the condylar growth center or articular surface.

Only one of the five patients who had follow-up of orbital and zygomatic fractures complained of a supraorbital scar but no bony deformity. The five follow-up reports of maxillary fractures comprising all varieties of Le Fort classifications listed no complications whatsoever. Of the five patients (aged 4 to 11) with maxillary fractures, the two sustained at age 6 showed mild facial elongation and flattening but no evidence of facial growth attenuation.

This limited study, though statistically unimpressive, would seem to bear out our original contention that an aggressive approach to prompt diagnosis and treatment minimizes unfavorable sequelae to facial fractures even in children. However, the numerous considerations and concerns for pediatric facial fractures follow.

Rationale of Treatment

As already pointed out, fractures of the facial bones are far less common in children than in adults. The facial skeleton is less brittle, having a high degree of bone vascularity with high osteogenic potential. The bony structures have not yet calcified and suture lines not yet closed, and the facial skeleton is less prominent than the neurocranium. During the second year of life, the facial bones begin to overtake the cranium in rate of growth, but it is not until the end of the first decade of life, with greater pneumatization of the paranasal sinuses and replacement of deciduous teeth with permanent dentition, that the facial skeleton emerges

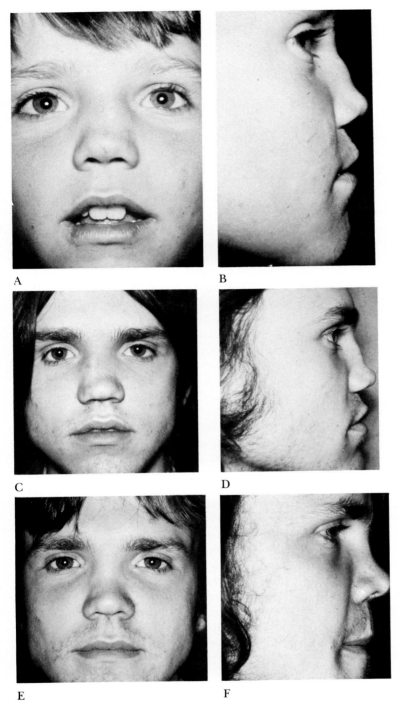

A

B

C

D

E

F

FIGURE 24-2. *Retarded nasal growth, secondary to an unreduced nasal fracture. (A and B) Eight-year-old patient with a healed, unreduced nasal fracture. (C and D) Patient at age 19, showing same deformity and the effect of arrested nasal growth. (E and F) Appearance 1 month after open reduction of the healed nasal deformity and sub-* *mucous resection. Patient refused a recommended bone graft that could further improve the appearance of his nose. (Reproduced with permission from Schultz, R.C., Facial Injuries, 2nd edition. Copyright © 1977 by Year Book Medical Publishers, Inc., Chicago.)*

461

from the cranial base. Supraorbital and glabellar fractures are exceedingly uncommon in small children. When present, they are often associated with frontal or temporal skull fractures. Therefore, they represent serious injury, and the patient should be observed for intracranial complications.

The frontal sinuses develop at varying ages. Although precursors of the frontal sinuses appear as early as the fourth fetal month, rudimentary development of the sinuses does not begin until the end of the first year of life. The rate of pneumatization is then variable, but by age 6 it is generally present to some extent. Visualization of the frontal sinuses by x-ray accordingly can be uncertain, depending on age and rate of development.

Open reduction of supraorbital and glabellar fractures is indicated when a deformity is found by observation, palpation, or x-ray study. Penetration of the posterior wall of the frontal sinuses by fracture connotes injury by powerful forces, and cerebral damage should be suspected. If intracranial aerocele is seen on skull x-rays, dural tear is present and cerebrospinal rhinorrhea will probably occur. Neurosurgical evaluation is indicated in such cases. The operative management of fractures in this area is the same as in adults. Reconstruction of healed depressed deformities with alloplastic materials is usually postponed until the facial bones have reached their growth potential.

Scott and Symonds [46], pointing out that the cranium increases in size fourfold compared with the twelvefold increase in the size of facial bones, stress that the growth of the nasal septum is the primary factor in the downward and forward movement of the facial skeleton. Severe injury to this structure in childhood is liable to lead to a growth failure of the middle third of the facial skeleton and the development of a saddle deformity of the nose (Fig. 24-2). The principal growth of the mandible occurs in an area of hyaline cartilage situated beneath the fibrous tissue covering the articular surface. A severe blow directed along the long axis of the mandible before 3 years of age tends to burst open the thin-walled, highly vascular

condyle, which causes an intracapsular fracture with hemarthrosis and gross disorganization of the growth cartilage, resulting in subsequent deformity.

During birth, mechanical strain and stresses of a prolonged delivery may lead to septal deviation. Similarly, a delivery aided by forceps may cause zygomatic arch or temporomandibular joint fracture, resulting in temporomandibular ankylosis and developmental atresia of the mandible (Fig. 24-3). Because of the superficial position of the facial nerve, paralysis due to injury by forceps pressure is also observed.

Infants and young children fall frequently, fortunately only from places as high as a crib or bed. The relative infrequency of facial bone fracture in children is supported by the recent literature [15, 16, 26, 40], which indicates a less than 1 percent incidence of facial fractures from birth to 5 years of age. In 5,367 cases of facial fractures [15, 16, 32, 37, 40, 43], only 5 percent happened to children up to 12 years old.

As far as the geometry of the face is concerned, protruding areas are more likely to sustain injury. Thus the nasal bones are most commonly traumatized, followed by the mandible and malar bone [35, 45]. The overlying soft tissues of the face absorb energy and spread impact forces over a wide area, thereby reducing the trauma. Since the long-term results of maxillofacial trauma depend on the tolerance of different parts of the face to trauma, it is interesting to realize that the nasal bones have the lowest tolerance levels. The zygomatic arch is the second most fragile facial area. The maxilla is sensitive to localized horizontal impacts, and the mandible is much more sensitive to lateral than to frontal impacts because in the latter there is considerable energy absorption from opening and retrusion of the jaw. The frontal bone is the most resistant to injury, requiring from 10 to 6,400 times the force to produce nasal fracture [35].

In an analysis of 122 fractures in 109 children, Kaban, Mulliken, and Murray [17] found 45 percent nasal fractures, 32 percent mandibular fractures, and 20.5 percent zygo-

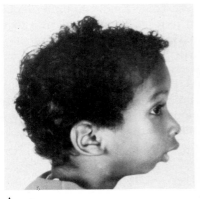
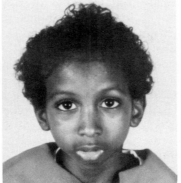
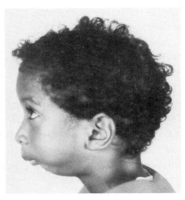

A

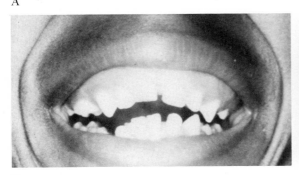
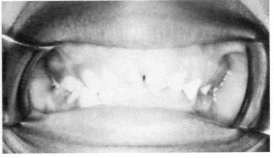

B

FIGURE 24-3. *Temporal mandibular joint ankylosis and developmental atresia of mandible, secondary to birth trauma. (A) Mandibular atresia, age 5. (B) Total mandibular excursion and occlusion, age 5.*

matic-maxillary fractures. McCoy [32], in his analysis of pediatric facial fractures, found the mandible to be the most common site (40 percent), followed by nasal fractures (23.3 percent), and then orbital-malar fractures (16.3 percent). Most series confirmed the higher incidence of facial fractures in male children, probably the result of more physical activity among boys. It should be realized that forces great enough to cause bony facial injury in children often cause injury to other areas of the body in more than half the patients, e.g., skull fracture, central nervous system injuries, long-bone fractures, closed chest injuries, and ocular trauma [32, 45]. These associated injuries, of course, may have significant long-term sequelae.

Knowledge of patterns of facial growth lends insight to the significance of bony injury at certain ages. From birth to age 12, the face undergoes almost continuous growth. However, cephalometric x-ray studies show that this growth can be divided into rapid and slow phases. The first 6 months of life represent a very rapid phase of facial growth, whereas the period from 6 months to 4 years represents a relatively slow growth rate. Growth from age 4 to 7 years is relatively rapid, but is slow from 9 to 15 years. The last period of growth, particularly in the male, is from 15 to 19 years. Bone injuries occurring during periods of rapid growth have a greater potential for deformity than those occurring during periods of slower growth. Repeated observations have shown that condylar injury before the age of 3 will probably result in severe deformity, injuries occurring after age 6 are apt to result in moderate deformity, and injuries after age 12 will result in only slight deformity. Closed reduction techniques tend to minimize additional insult to growing bone.

The general principles of treatment of pediatric maxillofacial injuries are essentially the same as those in the adult, namely, fixation of the fragments in their correct alignment with teeth in occlusion until union has taken place. The degree of precision required in the child is not quite as great as in the adult, since the replacement of deciduous teeth by the permanent teeth and the adaptive potential of alveolar bone can bring about a considerable degree of self-correction if alignment or articulation is not perfect. Furthermore, during childhood a certain amount of residual malocclusion can be corrected by orthodontic treatment. Also, the developing bone predisposes to greenstick fractures [21]. As a result of the high degree of osteogenic activity, union takes place in about half the time taken for an adult, and loose fragments can become quite adherent to one another in 3 or 4 days. Therefore, pediatric facial fractures should be reduced as soon as possible, for delay may result in a difficult reduction. Life-threatening injuries to other parts of the body take precedence in therapy, and delayed treatment in the critically ill patient increases the chances for malunion or nonunion. Swelling, ecchymoses, and hematoma may obscure the true nature of the fracture. Lastly, lack of patient cooperation may significantly delay diagnosis and treatment.

Undue surgical manipulation should be avoided in general, since it may induce additional injury to growth centers of the facial bones. During the period of mixed dentition, open reduction of the mandible or maxilla should be more conservative than in the adult. Drill holes should not be placed through a tooth bud. However, advantage should be taken of existing lacerations for a direct approach to the fracture for wiring of the fragments. Graham and Peltier [14], MacLennan [25], Freid [11], and others conclude that conservative management in children prevents complications with associated vulnerable tooth buds and growth centers. Deciduous teeth have short bulbous crowns and are poor abutments

for wires or arch bars. This makes interdental immobilization more difficult in children than in adults. A major factor in the management of children is patient cooperation; many reductions require general anesthesia [21].

Mathog and Rosenberg [30] state that children with complications from facial fractures can become emotionally depressed. Most complications develop during the period immediately following the trauma.

Nasal Fractures

Since a child's bony nasal pyramid is a proportionally small part of the nose, a nasal fracture may not present as obviously as in an adult, especially in the presence of edema. Radiographs are even less useful in a child than in the adult for demonstrating a nasal fracture. Significant numbers of associated fractures of the facial skeleton are present in a third of nasal fracture patients, and lacerations present in over half of the cases [31]. Nasal fractures should be reduced immediately, prior to the onset of edema, or delayed until after the edema has subsided, usually 4 to 6 days in children. Even minor disfigurements should be reduced, since these may be accentuated by growth (Fig. 24-2).

Bergland and Borchgrevink [3] described four patients with bilateral cleft of the primary palate with a normal secondary palate and no connection between the septum and the secondary palate. They found no evidence of influence of either prenasal or postnasal growth of the maxilla or facial growth. They reviewed the literature and found that in other instances where no hard tissue junction between the nasal septum and secondary palate existed, facial growth and occlusion were unaffected. Indeed, experience in craniofacial surgery also indicates that the septum, when resected, has little or no effect on facial growth.

In severe nasal fractures with collapse of the nasal dorsum, involvement of the frontal process of the maxilla can occur. This may involve injury to the lacrimal bone and to the lacrimal collecting system, with excessive tearing and resultant recurrent infection (dacrocystitis). Detachment of the medial canthal ligaments with widening of the intercanthal distance (hypertelorism) can occur, with resultant loss of the caruncle and prominent epicanthal folds.

In such injuries, open reduction with wire fixation of fragments is desirable. Injuries to the medial canthal ligament should be handled by identifying the ligaments and wiring them to each other or to stable bone fragments. If canthal displacement is not corrected early, hypertelorism may be permanent. Early repair is less difficult than late repair, which is complicated by the adjacent scar tissue.

The dacrocystic component of the naso-orbital fracture presents with swelling and redness of the sac area. Occasionally one can express viscous or purulent fluid from the duct by upward pressure on the sac. Exploration of the puncta and collecting system with a probe or fluorescein dye defines the level of obstruction. Antibiotics, ophthalmic solutions, probing, and irrigation may all be necessary to control infections of the duct system. Patency may develop after several months. If patency cannot be obtained, reconstruction or bypass of the duct system is indicated. Naso-orbital fractures are often associated with fractures of the orbital floor.

Children sustaining severe nasal fractures or comminuted nasal fractures may show developmental deformities years later despite correct initial treatment. A flattened nasal dorsum, varying degrees of nasomaxillary recession, and hypertelorism can occur, but the most frequent long-term complication (50 percent) found by Fry [12], Mayell [31], and Winters [53] is a compromised airway caused by deviation and thickening of the septum. Many of these children become mouth breathers and may suffer from chronic rhinitis and sinusitis. Surgical intervention (submucous septal resection) is required to relieve the obstruction. This treatment should not be postponed until the child has reached adolescence for fear of interfering with nasal growth. Surgical procedures to relieve obstruction should be conservative. They

consist of thinning the septal cartilage, scoring the cartilage, or bone grafting (Fig. 24-4) to relieve the deformity. Further definitive surgery may be indicated during adolescence [12].

The long-term follow-up of a reduced pediatric nasal fracture from the point of view of appearance is of interest. From the standpoint of subjective review, complaints are few, but on objective assessment of the bony cartilaginous dorsum for breathing and straightness, only a fourth were considered satisfactory [31]. The remainder had some broadening, deviation, or depression of the bridge, although in no case was it very marked. The cartilaginous portion of the dorsum was most often deviated. In rare instances, skillful nasal reduction or subsequent open reduction of a healed nasal fracture in the adult can produce a more pleasing nasal form than the nasal silhouette had before injury (Fig. 24-5).

Mandibular Fractures

The long-term results of mandibular fractures are influenced by the treatment, which is determined by the specific location of the fracture, and that, in turn, is related to the age of the child. In the younger child (under 10), two-thirds of the fractures involve the condyle compared with only 40 percent in those 11 to 15 years of age [21]. Fractures of the mandibular body are second in frequency. In the adult population, Bernstein found the body of the mandible followed by the angle to be the most frequently involved sites [5, 6]. There is generally an increase in other associated facial bone fractures in the older age groups.

The general principles of treatment to achieve the best results are essentially the same as with adults, namely, fixation of fragments in their correct alignment, with teeth in occlusion, until union has taken place. In children, the simplest methods that will relieve the symptoms of malocclusion, swelling, tenderness, and pain and also provide adequate reduction and stabilization should be chosen. Small occlusal imperfections in children under 10 years of age

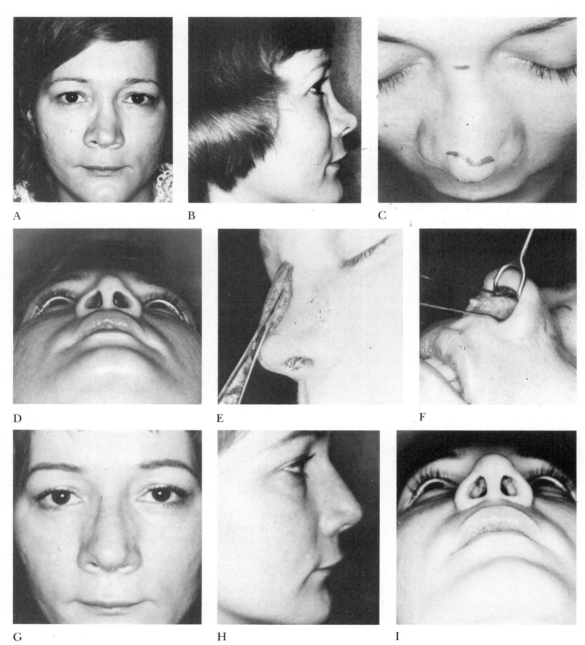

A

B

C

D

E

F

G

H

I

FIGURE 24-4. *Healed nasal fracture deformities with bone resorption are frequently best treated by autogenous bone grafts, ordinarily taken from the iliac crest. (A through D) Appearance of patient with healed nasal fracture deformity, demonstrating angulation and loss of nasal height. (E and F) Size and shape of bone graft and method of insertion through routine intercartilagenous incision. (G, H, and I) Appearance of patient 1 year following bone-grafting procedure. (Reproduced with permission from Schultz, R.C., Facial Injuries, 2nd edition. Copyright © 1977 by Year Book Medical Publishers, Inc., Chicago.)*

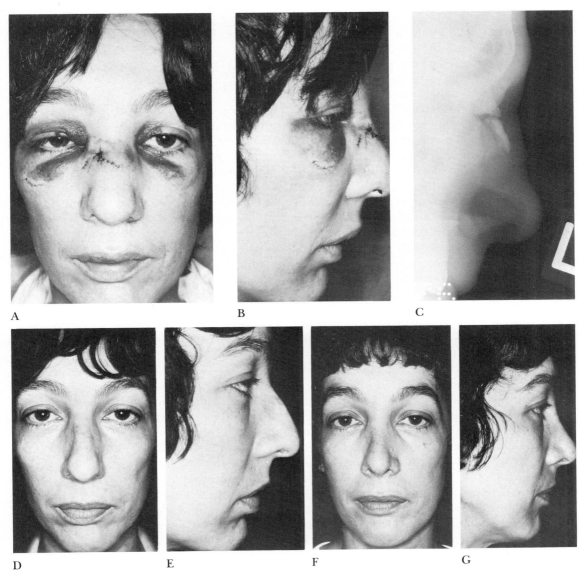

A B C

D E F G

FIGURE 24-5.   *Depressed nasal fracture in adult, treated initially by closed reduction, followed subsequently by open reduction and rhinoplasty for eventual improvement of preinjury appearance. (A, B, and C) Patient sustained open depressed fractures of the nasal bones and laceration of the right cheek from an accident in the home. Closed reduction of the nasal fractures was performed following injury. (D and E) Fractures healed with secondary deformity.*

Open reduction of healed nasal fracture deformity was performed 8 months after injury. Recontouring and shortening of the nose was accomplished at this same time. (F and G) Final appearance 6 months following open reduction and rhinoplasty. (Reproduced with permission from Schultz, R.C., Facial Injuries, 2nd edition. Copyright © 1977 by Year Book Medical Publishers, Inc., Chicago.)

will be overcome in the course of eruption of the permanent teeth by the adaptive potential of alveolar bone with the stress of mastication. Nonetheless, this does not mean that good fixation initially after injury is not required. Indeed, children tend to loosen most types of apparatus more readily than adults, and considerable care and ingenuity are needed in the design and application of methods of jaw fixation. Fortunately, union takes place in about half the time taken for an adult, most fractures being firm in 3 or 4 weeks. In younger children particularly, the demarcation between medullary and cortical bone is not as evident as in adults, and fractures of the jaw tend to be more a distortion of the bony contour or the "greenstick" type of deformity than a sharply defined fracture line. Minor crack fractures of the mandible generally require no immobilization.

In our series of patients, the two major factors influencing the treatment were the site of the fracture and the developmental state of the dentition. Fractures of the angle and body generally require intermaxillary fixation. As in adults, open reduction with direct interosseous wiring is usually indicated only in badly displaced body or angle fractures (Fig. 24-6). Injury to permanent tooth follicles can occur when drill holes are not placed sufficiently close to the inferior border of the mandible. Elaborate head caps and external devices should be avoided in children because of the need for almost continuous adjustment. However, orthodontic bands are highly suitable for fixation when they are in place at the time of injury [21].

Treatment of displaced fractures of the body of the mandible is influenced by the lack of nondental bony substance available for direct interosseous wire fixation. During the period of mixed dentition, deciduous teeth are exfoliating and permanent teeth just erupting. This may interfere with the use of interdental wire and arch bars. Interdental wiring is further complicated because primary teeth are conically shaped and thus hold wire ligatures poorly. When these factors make the conventional methods of open interosseous wiring such as arch bar or Blair-Ivy eyelet loop fixation inap-

propriate, a custom fabricated acrylic trough splint can be used [40] (Fig. 24-7).

Condylar Fractures

More recently, unilateral fractures without gross displacement in children younger than 10 years of age have been treated by encouraging motion. Bilateral condylar fractures with a moderate to major degree of displacement are simply immobilized for 2 to 3 weeks, followed by progressive mandibular motion. As with adults, only fractures of the condyle with gross fragment separation or longitudinal fractures extending obliquely down the ramus of the mandible require open reduction and wiring (Fig. 24-8). The long-term results in our patients have justified this approach. From the serial radiographs of MacGregor and Fordyce [24] and the experimental work on rhesus monkeys by Walker [52] and Boyne [7], condylar fractures with deviation or displacement undergo partial resorption and recontouring. By muscular movement causing gradual repositioning of the fractured fragment, these factors combine to reproduce a comparatively normal condylar articular process in function and appearance. The condylar growth center remains active. Clinically, it has been demonstrated radiographically [18] that the fractured and displaced condyle in children undergoes resorption and reconstruction within 6 to 12 months under the influence of the physiological stress and strains of mastication. The fracture deformity of the condyle is corrected and the reconstituted condyle is frequently relocated in the glenoid fossa.

Complications

Complications of mandibular fractures can be short term, such as nonunion or malunion, or long term, such as ankylosis of the condyle or arrested growth of the condyle. In the younger pediatric age group, nonunion is rarely seen, but in the older age groups, 24 percent of the fracture population, despite adequate treatment, can be expected to develop this complication [29]. Nonunion is characterized by pain and abnormal mobility. Often there is tenderness over the site of nonunion, and occlusion will be abnormal. Several mechanisms may account for this disturbance in bone healing, such as local infection, poor reduction and immobilization, and postoperative trauma. A decreased blood supply can lead to a replacement of osteogenic cells by fibroblasts, with subsequent fibrosis between segments of the fracture. Treatment consists of control of local infection, adequate immobilization, debridement if necessary, and bone grafting when indicated.

Malunion is a common complication following mandibular fracture in children. The healing of bone fragments in poor apposition may affect not only the appearance, but also the occlusion, although the latter is not so important as in adults. Treatment delay while more serious injuries are corrected encourages initial healing that is difficult to correct. Sometimes ecchymoses and swelling camouflage displaced fragments. Malunion results from inadequate reduction and immobilization, especially with unfavorable angle fractures. Resulting premature contact of the teeth requires occlusal adjustments by grinding techniques (equilibration). Occasionally, one or more displaced teeth require orthodontic treatment or removal with prosthetic replacement. Only rarely is surgery necessary to correct the malunion.

Comminuted intracapsular condylar fracture involving severe disorganization of the articular surface in a child prior to the age of 5 or 6 carries an especially poor long-term prognosis because this injury results in an arrest of the cartilaginous growth in the subarticular region. Walker [51] investigated 50 patients with arrest in the development of the condyle and noted that 2 of 14 patients with bilateral injuries were severely affected. MacLennan [25], in his review of 180 condylar fractures, likewise emphasized considerable deformity in later years after crushing injury to the condylar cartilage, especially when the injury occurred before the age of 2½ years. The failure of growth in patients with unilateral injuries results in a deviation toward the affected side with some retrognathia, while in patients with bilateral injuries, a severe degree of retrognathia may occur. The only treatment of value for the intracapsular comminuted fracture is to avoid immobilization, keeping the jaw moving to prevent ankylosis.

Ankylosis is characterized by progressive trismus, which causes difficulty in speech and eating and, therefore, possible malnutrition. The patient is unable to open the jaw more than 5 mm (Fig. 24-3). The true incidence is unknown. Trauma is implicated as the primary cause, but some patients develop this complication without a history of significant injury. It is suspected that minor trauma may go unnoticed and yet cause pressure on the condyle and injury to the joint surfaces. A crushing injury to the relatively soft articular surface, especially at a young age, may result in fragmentation, extravasation of blood, and disruption of the growth center from subsequent avascular necrosis. The most commonly accepted theory suggests that bleeding around the joint stimulates abnormal fibrosis and ankylosis. The meniscus is thereby destroyed, and fibrous bands obliterate the joint space. These fibers become calcified, and the condyle may develop proliferative changes [51]. Bony fragments occurring with fracture dislocations of the condyle may fuse in and around the glenoid fossa. In some cases, infection stimulates the proliferative process. It is uncertain whether the mandibular shift, the micrognathia, or the shortened ramus occurs from growth center disturbance per se or from nonuse of the jaw.

Most surgeons agree that ankylosis should be relieved in childhood, since the problems associated with an inadequate diet, dental disease, and inaccessibility to the oral cavity and pharynx in an emergency far outweigh any theoretical advantage of preserving a viable growth center with damaged osteogenic potential. The preferred treatment is surgery. Mechanical opening of the jaw either under anesthesia or with exercise devices has proven to be ineffective. Condylectomy with excision of the an-

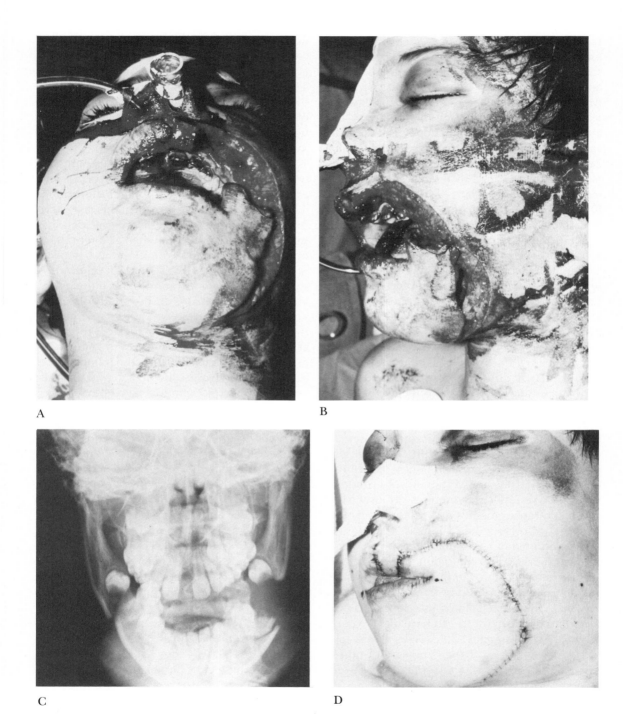

A

B

C

D

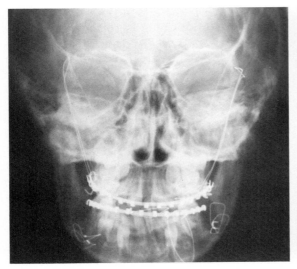

E

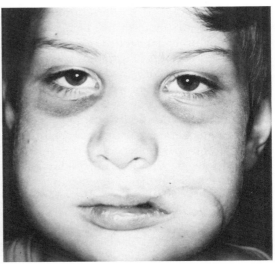

F

FIGURE 24-6. *Open reduction with direct interosseous wiring for badly displaced fractures of the body and angle of the mandible was partially performed through the soft tissue injury. (A and B) Appearance of 9-year-old patient initially, showing massive soft tissue wounds of lower face. (C) Posteroanterior view of mandible, demonstrating gross separation of bilateral mandibular fractures. (D) Appearance of patient immediately following open reduction and wound closure. (E) Posteroanterior x-rays of facial bones,* showing bilateral figure-of-eight interosseous wire fixation of mandibular fractures, circummandibular wire fixation of mandibular arch, and internal suspension of maxilla to frontal bone for concomitant LeFort II maxillary fractures. (F) Appearance of patient 2 months following injury. (Reproduced with permission from Schultz, R.C., Facial Injuries, 2nd edition. Copyright © 1977 by Year Book Medical Publishers, Inc., Chicago.)

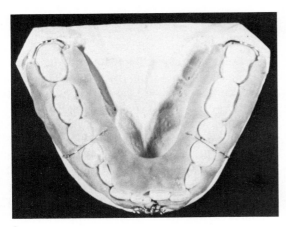

A

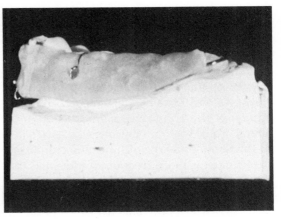

B

FIGURE 24-7. *Custom fabricated acrylic trough splint. (A and B) Acrylic trough splints can provide excellent immobilization of the mandible when a mandibular fracture is undisplaced and stable. The lingual and buccal portions of the splint are joined by malleable wire behind the posterior molar teeth. It is tightened and locked anteriorly with wire* loops. It can also be stabilized further by interdental wires passed through the splint and the gingiva. (Reproduced with permission from Schultz, R.C., Facial Injuries, 2nd edition. Copyright © 1977 by Year Book Medical Publishers, Inc., Chicago.)

kylosed tissue should be done, usually at the time the deciduous teeth are being shed and permanent premolar teeth are erupting. The short ramus may be elongated by osteotomy or a bone graft inserted if necessary at this same time. The opposite normal ramus may sometimes also be sectioned to allow a pivotal point for rotation around the coronal plane.

The pathogenesis of temporomandibular ankylosis is poorly understood. It is suggested that too long a period of immobilization encourages fixation of the joint, whereas too short a period may stimulate inflammation of the joint space. It is logical, therefore, to immobolize condylar fractures for short periods of time when indicated, and although the surgeon hopes for a bony union, a fibrotic nonunion with good motion is acceptable and certainly preferable to even partial ankylosis [30].

Fractures of the Zygoma and Orbital Floor

Far behind the frequency of nasal and mandibular fractures in the pediatric age group are zygomatic fractures and fractures of the maxilla. Zygomatic fractures occur mostly in older children, usually as a result of vehicular trauma. Considerable force is required to fracture the resilient zygoma of a child, and the fracture usually takes the form of a fracture dislocation. Lack of complete closure of the frontozygomatic suture also explains the infrequency of this type of fracture. Orbital fractures are also usually characterized by a separation of this frontozygomatic junction in the lateral orbital wall with downward displacement of the floor. This type of unilateral craniofacial detachment is more frequent in the child than the Le Fort III bilateral craniofacial dysfunction. McCoy et al. [32] found the incidence of pure pediatric zygomatic fractures to be 4.7 percent and zygomatic with orbital fracture to be 16.3 percent. In his pediatric series, Rowe [38, 39] states that the incidence of zygomatic fractures necessitating operative treatment was a mere 0.3 percent. Malar complex fractures with asymmetry and flattening of the eminence

or fractures of the orbital rim with a palpable step-off deformity must be corrected accurately within the first 5 to 7 days to avoid later dysfunction and deformity. Unlike the situation in the adult (Fig. 24-1), after this type of fracture has healed in the child, it is not as amenable to correction by refracturing or by bone grafting.

Depressed malunited zygomatic fractures vary in their severity. Often there is residual hypoesthesia of the cheek or flatness of the cheek, and the lateral canthus may be pulled inferiorly, giving a slanted appearance to the palpebral fissure. In addition, the inferior displacement of the fracture may impinge against the coronoid process resulting in an open bite. Fortunately, malunion of the zygoma is rare. Martin et al. [28] reported a 10 percent incidence in zygomatic fractures. Dingman [10] noted that complications are more common with conservative closed reduction of the original fracture.

Malunited zygomatic fractures occur either because of an unstable reduction or because periorbital and cheek swelling obscured the bony depression and reduction was not attempted. Occasionally the fracture may be adequately reduced but accidental pressure on the face moves the fragments out of position [21].

"Blowout" Fractures

The etiology of orbital "blowout" fractures, unassociated with zygomatic fracture, is similar to that in adults. They are caused by the patient being hit in the orbital region with a ball or another child's fist or by trauma received in automobile accidents (Fig. 24-9). To prevent late problems, these fractures should be corrected as soon as possible, through an infraorbital approach with preservation and realignment of the floor fragments, release of the entrapped orbital contents, and if necessary, placement of an alloplastic implant (Silastic) or a thin bone graft under the periosteum of the floor of the orbit. A Caldwell-Luc approach can be used if the antrum is sufficiently pneumatized. Blowout fractures older than 10 to 14 days should be treated with either an alloplastic implant or a bone graft. Proper repositioning of these structures prevents adhesions between the globe, the periorbital fat, the inferior rectus and inferior oblique muscles, and the orbital floor.

Diplopia and enophthalmus are complications that may follow various types of orbital floor fractures. Although infrequent, diplopia may be a complaint immediately following injury; later, enophthalmos becomes a more obvious sign. Injury to and entrapment of the periorbita may cause subsequent inflammation and fibrosis, with adherence to the orbital walls and impairment of muscle function. Herniated or ecchymotic orbital fat may undergo necrosis. This condition is worsened by fracture expansion of the orbital floor, which permits the globe to sink deeper into the orbit and makes the eye appear small. Complete correction of late enophthalmos caused by a healed, enlarged, and depressed bony orbit can seldom be accomplished by simple procedures such as alloplastic or bone-graft supplementation of the orbital floor and side walls or relocation of the lateral or medial canthal "ligaments." Complete relocation and recontouring of the entire bony orbital cone by excision and supporting bone grafts are usually required to correct such deformities.

Loss of vision can develop from postoperative orbital hemorrhage, trauma to the optic nerve, central artery occlusion, or thrombosis of the optic vein [36]. To prevent this complication following surgery, every effort should be made during reduction to avoid excessive pressure or tension on the globe. Alloplastic material should be kept under the periosteum and notched in the area of the optic nerve when placement far posterior in the orbit is necessary.

Maxillary Fractures

The typical LeFort lines of fracture are rarely seen in children [26, 27, 32, 39]. Transverse maxillary (LeFort I) and pyramidal (LeFort II) fractures are occasionally encountered (Fig. 24-10). Unless gross displacement exists, unilateral maxillary fractures seldom warrant open reduction in children for fear of inflicting further damage on the growing bone and unerupted dentition. Problems with fixation are similar to those encountered in the treatment of mandibular fractures because of the presence of poorly retentive teeth.

Even when properly reduced, midfacial fractures may eventually lead to a scaphoid facial deformity because of injury to the growth centers of the maxilla and nasal septum. With maxillary growth there is not only a forward and downward component, but a constant remodeling of the multiple regional parts. The development includes a displacement away from the cranial base, a posterior enlargement corresponding to lengthening of the dental arch, and an anterior resorption of the malar region. The nasal vaults grow forward and laterally, while the descent of the premaxillary area occurs by resorption on the superior and anterior surface of the nasal spine and by bony deposition on the inferior surface. It is fortunate that this complex scenario is seldom interrupted by maxillary fracture in childhood.

Incomplete reduction and immobilization of maxillary fractures, however, are the most frequent causes of malunion with elongation of the face, flattening, and malocclusion even in the pediatric age group. Fortunately, many cases of malunion are not severe, and camouflage can be achieved with onlay bone grafts [8]. Malunion can best be prevented by deferring surgical repair until most of the swelling has disappeared. More accurate visual evaluation and palpation of the deformity will then facilitate precise reduction of the fractures. Timing of the reduction then becomes critical, however, since bony healing occurs rapidly thereafter. Remobilization of a malunited maxillary fracture in children is extremely difficult after 2 to 3 weeks as opposed to the remobilization of a similar fracture in the adult.

Dental Injuries

Maxillofacial trauma during childhood commonly results in injury to the anterior teeth.

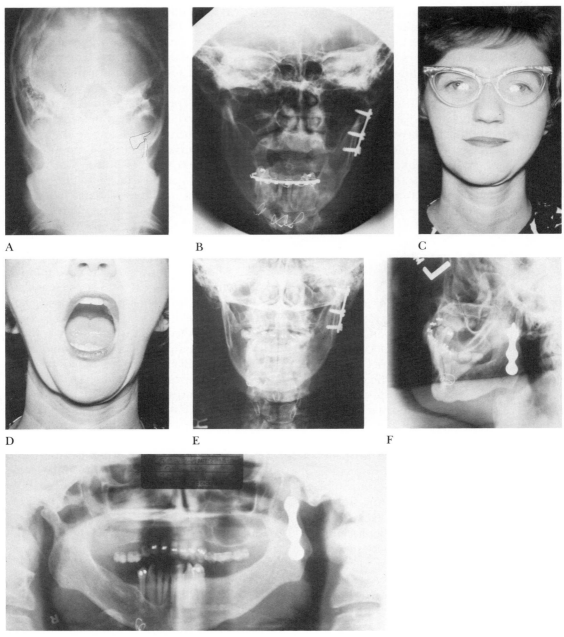

A

B

C

D

E

F

G

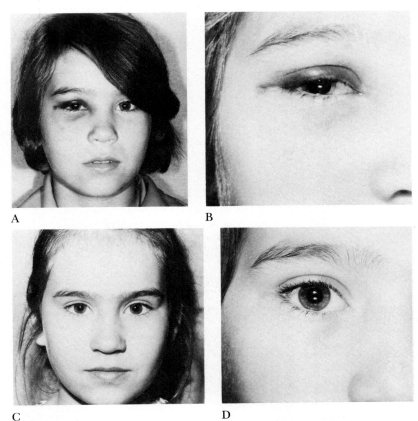

A   B

C   D

FIGURE 24-9.   *True "blowout fractures" of the orbit are rare in children, as in adults. (A and B) Blowout fracture of the orbital floor resulting from being hit with a tennis ball. Note periorbital ecchymosis and dilated pupil. (C and*

D) Appearance of same patient 3 months following open reduction and insertion of Silastic sheet to orbital floor through lower-eyelid incision. The patient had no residual symptomatology.

FIGURE 24-8.   *Indications for open reduction of condylar fractures are rare in adults and even more rare in children. (A) X-ray of patient with gross displacement of condylar neck fracture (in association with multiple fractures of the symphysis), preventing closed reduction. (B) Postoperative x-ray showing reduction and internal fixation of left condyle with metal plate and screws. Also visible are internal fixation of multiple fractures at the symphysis and interdental fixation of anterior mandibular teeth with single arch bar. (C and D) Appearance of the patient 3 months following operation, demonstrating a full range of mandibular motion. (E, F, and G) X-rays of the same patient 11 years following injury and repair, demonstrating healing and good alignment and viable mandibular condyle. (Reproduced with permission from Schultz, R.C.,* Facial Injuries, *1st edition, Copyright © 1970, and 2nd edition, Copyright © 1977 by Year Book Medical Publishers, Inc., Chicago.)*

Traditionally these dental injuries are divided into those which involve deciduous and those which involve permanent dentition. Injuries to deciduous dentition most often occur between the ages of 1 and 2½ years when children are learning to walk. They fall frequently, sometimes injuring the face and anterior teeth. Because of the relative softness of the premaxilla at this age, the most common injury is one of displacement of the upper incisors. This may result either in intrusion of the tooth into the premaxilla, a loosening or partial dislocation with lingual or buccal displacement, or a total tooth avulsion.

Intruded teeth frequently reerupt in subsequent weeks and may reach full eruption in 4

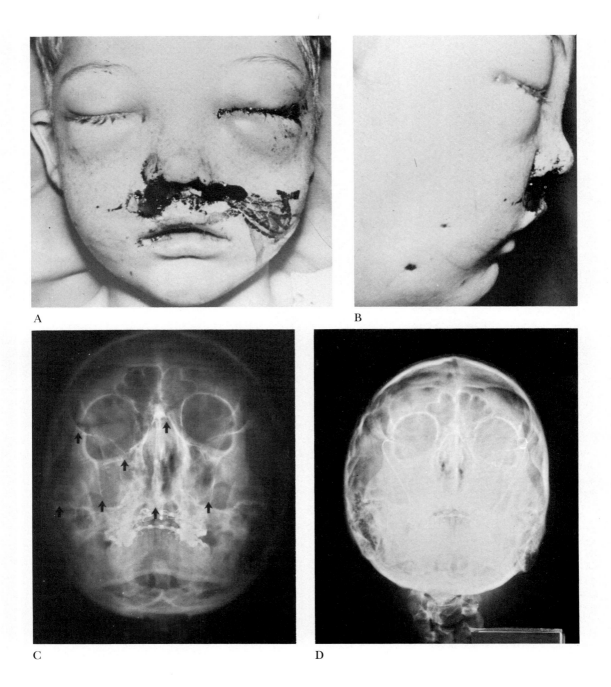

A

B

C

D

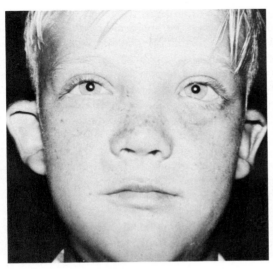

E

FIGURE 24-10. *Asymmetrical LeFort-type fractures, resulting from an automobile accident, in a 6-year-old boy. (A and B) Typical appearance of a "free-floating" maxilla. Bloated, markedly edematous, elongated midface is characteristic. Note bilateral epistaxis. The patient also had cerebrospinal rhinorrhea. (C) Water's x-ray view showing multiple fracture sites. Arch bars are already ligated to upper and lower dental arches in preparation for open reduction. (D) Postoperative Water's view, showing wire suspension of maxilla from temporal bones bilaterally. Suspension arch bars are ligated to upper dental arch. (E) Appearance of patient 6 months following open-reduction procedure. The patient had good occlusion. (Reproduced with permission from Schultz, R.C., Facial Injuries, 1st edition. Copyright © 1970 by Year Book Medical Publishers, Inc., Chicago.)*

to 6 months. In a child younger than 2½ years of age with incomplete root formation, these intruded teeth may retain normal vitality after reeruption. Calcific degeneration and necrosis of the pulp are common sequelae to the reeruption of intruded teeth once root formation is mature, in children older than 2½ or 3 years of age.

Elaborate methods for the fixation of loose deciduous teeth are contraindicated. Generally, partial dislocation of deciduous teeth should be reoriented intraorally when sufficiently stable, otherwise they should be removed, followed in some instances by placement of a space maintainer. The future of partially dislocated teeth is related to the maturity of the dental root at the time of injury. The capacity of teeth, particu-

larly those with an open apex, to retain viability is considerable given immobilization for 3 to 4 weeks and the prevention of infection. Total avulsion of deciduous teeth is less common than other forms of displacement, but it results in the greatest damage to the overlying permanent teeth.

Fracture of the crowns and roots of deciduous teeth is comparatively rare and far less common than in the permanent teeth. Fractured crowns with exposed dentin but without pulpal involvement should be protected until definitive dental restoration can be carried out. An extensive crown fracture will invariably involve the pulp, and the tooth should be extracted. Root fractures, particularly those involving the coronal portions of the root, should be extracted. Simultaneous surgical removal of the apical portions of the fractured root is necessary to prevent later interference in the eruption of permanent teeth. Fractures in the apical portions of the root usually heal uneventfully [41].

Trauma to deciduous teeth such as just described, because of the close anatomical relationship between the apices of primary teeth, may harm developing permanent dentition. According to various studies, the prevalence of such disturbances ranges from 12 to 69 percent.

In Andreasen's and Ravn's [1] review of 103 patients with 213 traumatized permanent teeth, the following disturbances in mineralization and morphology were found: white or yellow-brown discoloration of enamel in 23 percent; discoloration of teeth and enamel associated with circular enamel hypoplasia in 12 percent. Other disturbances in morphology, such as crown dilaceration, later root angulation, and partial or complete arrest of root formation, were found in 6 percent of patients. Disturbances in permanent dentition were found to be less frequent in patients whose injury occurred after 4 years of age.

White or yellow-brown enamel discoloration with a circular enamel hypoplasia occurred especially in younger individuals, whereas enamel discoloration without enamel hypoplasia also was seen in older age groups. This relation seems to indicate that the developing permanent tooth germ is especially sensitive to injuries during its early developmental stages. However, disturbances in mineralization do occur even when radiographic examination at the time of injury reveals complete crown formation, indicating that secondary mineralization of enamel takes place over an extended period of time and is still going on during initial phases of root development. On the contrary, circular enamel hypoplasia will occur only when the injury is sustained during crown formation, possibly a result of localized arrest of enamel matrix formation due to ameloblast injury [1].

Disturbances in permanent dentition seem to be related to the type of injury sustained. The low frequency of disturbances found after subluxation indicates that this type of impact disrupts the thin tissue barrier between the primary tooth and its permanent successor only to a minor degree. On the other hand, in an intrusion injury the alveolar socket is fractured or crushed, and the incidence of permanent tooth disturbance rises. Lastly, comparison of the complication rates of different treatment procedures on primary dentition which effect disturbances in permanent dentition shows no significant differences. Injury to the permanent tooth germ is sustained at the moment of trauma [1].

The prevalence of accidental injuries to permanent anterior teeth in children between the ages of 5 and 15 years varies between 4 and 9 percent and occurs more commonly in boys [13]. Just as with the deciduous teeth, the upper incisors are the most frequently traumatized, and the injuries result from play at home or at school. Approximately 12 percent of the injuries in Gelbier's study of English school children occurred from organized contact sports; the remainder were due to automobile and bicycle accidents. Injuries to enamel only require smoothing of the tooth surface. If the injury exposes a considerable area of dentin, the latter should be covered as quickly as possible for comfort and to obviate irritation to the underlying pulp, including irreversible pulpitis and pulp necrosis. Treatment of traumatic in-

juries to the pulp depends largely on the age of the child and the maturity of the dentition. When root formation is incomplete in patients seen within 3 days of trauma, the usual treatment is vital pulpotomy. In cases in which root formation is complete at the time of injury, a total pulpotomy is usually done. Here the entire pulp is extirpated and the root canal filled with occlusive material [13].

Injury involving the coronal half of the root, either by extensive crown fracture or transverse root fracture, usually requires extirpation of the entire root. With injury involving the apical half of the root, the prognosis is much improved. Treatment usually involves splinting, and the root heals by fibrous union when immobilization is adequate and the fracture site remains free of infection.

Subluxed permanent teeth and their associated aveolar bone should be repositioned and splinted by conventional methods, such as arch bars or cap splints. They frequently become nonvital and require root-canal therapy and root-canal filling at a later date, particularly when the root formation is complete at time of injury. In cases of complete avulsion of a permanent tooth when the root is immature with the apex widely open, the tooth should be reimplanted and stabilized in the socket within a few minutes of injury. In these instances the prognosis for pulp revascularization, reinnervation, and continued root formation is good, although the coronal portions of the pulp will usually undergo calcific degeneration. Reimplantation of a complete avulsion when root formation is mature, especially when the avulsion is over 30 minutes old, will invariably lead to root resorption. This resorption may be an exceedingly slow process, taking 10 years or more. Reimplantation in such cases should include pulp removal, pulp space restoration, and splinting [41].

Final Thoughts

Despite the tragic facial deformities commonly seen in adults following untimely or inadequate treatment of facial fractures, the greatest concern for late sequelae from facial fractures lies with those occurring in children. By a late follow-up study of our own limited series of facial fractures in 188 children, as well as study of numerous other larger series, we have shown the major long-term problems to be anticipated. The prevention of these sequelae lies with an aggressive approach to diagnosis and appropriate timing of definitive treatment. We have attempted to review the principles of management of children's facial fractures by describing the fundamentals of growth and development of the facial bones and the pathophysiology resulting from fracture. Although facial fractures in children are relatively uncommon and serious late sequelae are rare, the possible occurrence and seriousness of these sequelae must be kept in mind, for their consequences involve not only disturbed facial growth and development, but frequently lifetime functional impairment as well.

References

1. Andreasen, J.O., and Ravn, J.J. The effect of traumatic injuries to primary teeth on their permanent successors: II. A clinical and radiographic follow-up study of 213 teeth. *Scand. J. Dent. Res.* 79:284, 1971.
2. Bales, C.R., Randall, P., and Lehr, H.B. Fractures of the facial bones in children. *J. Trauma* 12:56, 1972.
3. Bergland, O., and Borchgrevink, H. The role of the nasal septum in midfacial growth in man elucidated by the maxillary development in certain types of facial clefts: A preliminary report. *Scand. J. Plast. Reconstr. Surg.* 8:42, 1974.
4. Bernstein, L. Maxillofacial injuries in children. *Otolaryngol. Clin. North Am.* 2:397, 1969.
5. Bernstein, L., and McClurg, F.L., Jr. Mandibular fractures: A review of 156 consecutive cases. *Laryngoscope* 87:957, 1977.
6. Blevins, C., and Gores, R.J. Fractures of the mandibular condyloid process: Results of conservative treatment in 140 patients. *J. Oral Surg.* 19:392, 1961.
7. Boyne, P.J. Osseous repair and mandibular growth after subcondylar fractures. *J. Oral Surg.* 25:300, 1967.
8. Converse, J.M., and Campbell, R.M. Bone grafts in surgery of the face. *Surg. Clin. North Am.* 34:375, 1954.
9. Dawson, R.L.G., and Fordyce, G.L. Complex fractures of the middle third of the face and their early treatment. *Br. J. Surg.* 41:254, 1953.
10. Dingman, R.O. Symposium: Malunited fractures of the zygoma. Repair of the deformity. *Trans. Am. Acad. Ophthalmol. Otolaryngol.* 57:889, 1953.
11. Freid, M.G., and Baden, E. Management of fractures in children. *J. Oral Surg.* 12:129, 1954.
12. Fry, H. Nasal skeletal trauma and the interlocked stresses of the nasal septal cartilage. *Br. J. Plast. Surg.* 20:146, 1967.
13. Gelbier, S. Injured anterior teeth in children: A preliminary discussion. *Br. Dent. J.* 123:331, 1967.
14. Graham, G.G., and Peltier, J.R. The management of mandibular fractures in children. *J. Oral Surg.* 18:416, 1960.
15. Hagan, E.H., and Huelke, D.F. An analysis of 319 case reports of mandibular fractures. *J. Oral Surg.* 19:93, 1961.
16. Halazonetis, J.A. The "weak" regions of the mandible. *Br. J. Oral Surg.* 6:37, 1968.
17. Kaban, L.B., Mulliken, J.B., and Murray, J.E. Facial fractures in children: An analysis of 122 fractures in 109 patients. *Plast. Reconstr. Surg.* 59:15, 1977.
18. Kaplan, S.I., and Mark, H.I. Bilateral fractures of the mandibular condyles and fracture of the symphysis menti in an 18-month-old child: Two year preliminary report with a plea for conservative treatment. *Oral Surg.* 15:136, 1962.
19. Khosla, V.M., and Boren, W. Mandibular fractures in children and their management. *J. Oral Surg.* 29:116, 1971.
20. Leake, D., Doykos, J., III, Habal, M.B., and Murray, J.E. Long-term follow-up of fractures of the mandibular condyle in children. *Plast. Reconstr. Surg.* 47:127, 1971.
21. Lehman, J.A., Jr., and Saddawi, N.D. Fractures of the mandible in children. *J. Trauma* 16:773, 1976.
22. Lewin, W. Cerebrospinal fluid rhinorrhoea in closed head injuries. *Br. J. Surg.* 42:1, 1954.
23. Lu, M. Reimplantation of avulsed anterior teeth in patients with jaw fractures. *Plast. Reconstr. Surg.* 51:377, 1973.
24. MacGregor, A.B., and Fordyce, G.L. The treatment of fracture of the neck of the mandibular condyle. *Br. Dent. J.* 102:351, 1957.
25. MacLennan, W.D. Consideration of 180 cases of typical fractures of the mandibular condylar process. *Br. J. Plast. Surg.* 5:122, 1953.
26. MacLennan, W.D. Fractures of the mandible in children under the age of six years. *Br. J. Plast. Surg.* 9:125, 1956.
27. MacLennan, W.D. Injuries involving the teeth and jaws in young children. *Arch. Dis. Child.* 32:492, 1957.

28. Martin, B.C., Trabue, J.C., and Leech, T.R. An analysis of the etiology, treatment and complications of fractures of the malar compound and zygomatic arch. *Am. J. Surg.* 92:920, 1956.

29. Mathog, R.H., and Boies, L.R., Jr. Nonunion of the mandible. *Laryngoscope* 86:908, 1976.

30. Mathog, R.H., and Rosenberg, Z. Complications in the treatment of facial fractures. *Otolaryngol. Clin. North Am.* 9:533, 1976.

31. Mayell, M.J. Nasal fractures: Their occurrence, management and some late results. *J. R. Coll. Surg. Edinb.* 18:31, 1973.

32. McCoy, F.J., Chandler, R.A., and Crow, M.L. Facial fractures in children. *Plast. Reconstr. Surg.* 37:209, 1966.

33. Moss, M.L., Bromberg, B.E., Song, I.C., and Eisenman, G. The passive role of nasal septal cartilage in mid-facial growth. *Plast. Reconstr. Surg.* 41:536, 1968.

34. Mustardé, J.C. Facial Injuries in Children. In J.C. Mustardé (Ed.), *Plastic Surgery in Infancy and Childhood.* Philadelphia: Saunders, 1971. Pp. 178–206.

35. Nahum, A.M. The biomechanics of maxillofacial trauma. *Clin. Plast. Surg.* 2:59, 1975.

36. Nicholson, D.H., and Guzak, S.V., Jr. Visual loss complicating repair of orbital floor fractures. *Arch. Ophthalmol.* 86:369, 1971.

37. Pfeifer, G. Kieferbruche im Kindesalter und ihre Auswirkungen auf das Wachstum. *Fortschr. Kiefer. Gesichtschir.* 11:43, 1966.

38. Rowe, N.L. Fractures of the facial skeleton in children. *J. Oral Surg.* 26:505, 1968.

39. Rowe, N.L. Fractures of the jaws in children. *J. Oral Surg.* 27:497, 1969.

40. Rowe, N.L., and Killey, H.C. *Fractures of the Facial Skeleton* (2nd ed.). Edinburgh, Engl.: Livingstone, 1968.

41. Rowe, N.L., and Winter, G.B. Traumatic Lesions of the Jaws and Teeth. In J.C. Mustardé (Ed.), *Plastic Surgery in Infancy and Childhood.* Philadelphia: Saunders, 1971. Pp. 154–175.

42. Schreiber, C.K. The effect of trauma on the anterior deciduous teeth. *Br. Dent. J.* 106:340, 1959.

43. Schuchardt, K., Brichetti, L.M., and Schwenzer, N. Frakturen des Gesichtsskelettes. *Stoma* 13:159, 1960.

44. Schultz, R.C. One thousand consecutive cases of major facial injury. *Rev. Surg.* 27:394, 1970.

45. Schultz, R.C. *Facial injuries* (2nd ed.). Chicago: Year Book, 1977.

46. Scott, J.H., and Symons, N.B.B. *Introduction to Dental Anatomy* (5th ed.). Edinburgh: Livingstone, 1967.

47. Selliseth, N.E. Traumatisering ay primare incisiver og de folger som kan iakttas ved frambrudd av de permanente tenner. Ph.D. Thesis, Oslo, 1967.

48. Stenstrom, S.J., and Thander, B.L. Effects of nasal septal cartilage resections of young guinea pigs. *Plast. Reconstr. Surg.* 45:160, 1970.

49. Stenstrom, S.J., and Thander, B.L. Healing of surgically created defects in the septal cartilages of young guinea pigs. *Plast. Reconstr. Surg.* 49:194, 1972.

50. Taatz, H. Untersuchungen über Ursachen und Häufigkeit exogener Zahnkeimschaden. *Dtsch. Zahn. Mund. Kieferheilkd.* 37:468, 1962.

51. Walker, D.G. The mandibular condyle: Fifty cases demonstrating arrest in development. *Dent. Pract.* 7:160, 1957.

52. Walker, R.V. Traumatic mandibular condylar fracture dislocations: Effect on growth in the *Macacus* rhesus monkey. *Am. J. Surg.* 100:850, 1960.

53. Winters, H.P.J. Isolated fractures of the nasal bones. *Arch. Chir. Neerl.* 19:159, 1967.

54. Zellner, B. Schnelzmissbildungen am permanenten Gebiss nach Milchzahnluzation. *Zahnaerztl. Prax.* 9:1, 1956.

Joseph E. Murray
Leonard B. Kaban

COMMENTS ON CHAPTER 24

THIS chapter on the long-term results of the treatment of facial fractures correctly emphasizes the principles of repair in an effort to avoid the unsatisfactory sequelae of inadequate or incorrect early surgery. Poor results in adults are secondary to inadequate diagnosis and treatment and consist of asymmetries of the orbits, enophthalmos, diplopia, nasal deformity, nasal obstruction, malocclusion, mandibular hypomobility, and other temporomandibular joint problems. Assessment of the long-term results in children is more difficult because of the additional variable of facial growth.

The data presented by Schultz and Meilman, on 188 pediatric facial fractures, are similar to those reported from the Children's Hospital Medical Center [3]. As in the Children's Hospital series, all patients were treated in the hospital. This may lead to a low estimate of the total incidence of pediatric fractures, since many (especially nasal fractures) are nondisplaced and the patients are treated in the office. Because of the lack of information on nonhospital-treated patients, the incidence of late complications of mildly displaced facial fractures is unknown. For example, how many patients with nasal septal problems later in life actually had unremembered trauma as a child?

The Children's Hospital experience with the relative incidence of facial fractures was similar to this report. We also found that nasal fractures were the most common pediatric fractures, followed by mandibular, zygomatic and orbital, and then maxillary fractures. In our series, falls were the most common etiology of facial fractures, whereas in this report vehicular trauma is first. This, however, usually depends on the location of the reported institution in relation to interstate and other high-speed highways.

The early complications of facial trauma depend on the etiology and location of the injury. Most authors agree that these complications are not observed more frequently in children than in adults. We also found that infection is a rare complication if the fractures are treated promptly. However, especially in mandibular fractures, the infection rate increases dramatically if the patient delays more than 24 hours in seeking treatment. This is especially true when the fracture is compounded into the mouth.

The effect of midface fractures of facial growth is controversial and difficult to evaluate. McCoy et al. [5] and Rowe [7, 8] have emphasized the possibility of growth impairment. It is our experience, and that of this report, that growth abnormalities after trauma are rare. However, the incidence of midfacial fractures in children is quite low, and long-term follow-up of large numbers of patients is impossible. This low incidence of midface injuries is probably secondary to the prominence of the calvarium in relationship to the facial skeleton. In most cases, the calvarium protects the face, and if both areas are injured, a severe skull fracture often results in the death of the patient. Our experience has been that if the occlusion is restored and the function of extraocular muscles, facial muscles, and muscles of mastication is intact, major growth impairment does not occur.

In cases of mandibular fracture, those involving the condyle have the greatest potential for long-term adverse affects on mandibular growth. In our experience, these problems occur after overaggressive treatment of mandibular fractures in children. Schultz and Meilman also emphasize the point that overzealous surgical manipulation should be avoided in children, since it may induce injury to growth centers and may damage permanent tooth buds in the vicinity of drill holes and wires. In the case of condylar fractures in children, one has to be careful not to immobilize the jaw excessively. Intermaxillary fixation for more than 10 days or 2 weeks may result in mandibular hypomobility and ankylosis. This is probably secondary to immobilization in the presence of blood clot, periosteum, and the high degree of osteogenic potential in children. Furthermore, the goal of the treatment of subcondylar fractures is not to obtain a perfect anatomical union, but rather to obtain a functional joint.

The concept of the "condylar growth center" as an anatomical entity has become less important recently. It is now felt that if the jaw functions normally and there is good mandibular movement, the mandible will grow symmetrically and at a normal rate [6, 9]. We therefore treat unilateral or bilateral subcondylar fractures with a short period of immobilization (7 to 14 days) if there is pain, trismus, or malocclusion. If there are no symptoms and no malocclusion, the patient is treated with a liquid diet and heat, without immobilization [3, 4]. The patient is followed closely with midline opening exercises to prevent future malocclusion, deviation on opening, or temporomandibular joint dysfunction. Occasionally, after the initial immobilization, we place the patient in guiding elastics to correct deviation on opening. Surgery is rarely indicated for subcondylar fractures, except in a severely medially displaced and dislocated fracture where the proximal fragment impairs mandibular mobility.

Long-term complaints of breathing problems after nasal fractures are difficult to evaluate for several reasons. A large number of minimally or radiographically nondisplaced nasal fractures are seen by individual practitioners, and no registry of such cases exists. Later in life, if the patient has a complication, the earlier trauma may have been forgotten and the relationship not appreciated. On the other hand, some nasal septal and external anatomical deformities are related to earlier trauma for insurance purposes only. It would be interesting to correlate subjective complaints and objective anatomical findings in a large number of patients with "posttraumatic nasal deformity."

Our results in the treatment of orbital and zygomatic complex fractures in children are similar to those reported by Schultz and Meilman. Early treatment usually leads to good long-term results with few complications. Re-

cently, there has been some controversy over the indications for surgical treatment of blowout fractures [1, 2]. We agree with Schultz and Meilman that early treatment for blowout fractures in the presence of enophthalmos, limitation of ocular movement, and paresthesia provides the best chance to avoid the late complications of enophthalmos and diplopia. We disagree, however, with the statement that a "Caldwell-Luc approach can be used if the antrum is sufficiently pneumatized." We feel that the maxillary sinus is rarely large enough in children to get good visibility of the orbital floor. In addition, it is our experience that when the antrum is used for correction of blowout fractures, it is better to expose the orbital floor from above also. This way one avoids blindly pushing bony fragments toward the globe.

This chapter on the long-term results of facial fractures in children emphasizes principles of repair that are well based on experience. The excellence of the results reflects good judgment and the surgical skills employed. As in most other reports of facial fractures in children, a reference was made to the rarity of these injuries. We should remember that most reports from the literature include only hospitalized patients, and we may be overlooking a large number of children who sustain minor variations of these injuries but are not diagnosed by the examining physician or pediatrician in the office or accident room.

Schultz and Meilman analyze very well the factors of parental protection of children, the position of the facial bones, the small mass of the child, and the usually moderate impact involved. The principles of wound healing and bony repair are also pertinent and emphasized in this chapter. The important principle that adequate repair is essential in achieving significantly improved long-term results also is well stated.

References

1. Converse, J.M.   Orbital and Naso-orbital Fractures. In P. Tessier, A. Callahan, J.C. Mustardé,

and K.E. Salyer (Eds.), *Symposium on Plastic Surgery in the Orbital Region.* Vol. 12. St. Louis: Mosby, 1976, pp. 79–106.

2. Furnas, D.W.   Emergency Diagnosis of the Injured Orbit. In P. Tessier, W. Callahan, J.C. Mustardé, and K.E. Salyer (Eds.), *Symposium on Plastic Surgery in the Orbital Region.* Vol. 12. St. Louis: Mosby, 1976, pp. 67–78.

3. Kaban, L.B., Mulliken, J.B., and Murray, J.E. Facial fractures in children: An analysis of 122 fractures in 109 patients. *Plast. Reconstr. Surg.* 59:15, 1977.

4. Leake, D., Doykos, J., III, Habal, M.B., and Murray, J.E.   Long-term follow-up of fractures of the mandibular condyle in children. *Plast. Reconstr. Surg.* 47:127, 1971.

5. McCoy, F.J., Chandler, R.A., and Crow, M.L. Facial fractures in children. *Plast. Reconstr. Surg.* 37:209, 1966.

6. Moss, M.L., and Rankow, R.   The role of the functional matrix in mandibular growth. *Angle Orthod.* 38:95, 1968.

7. Rowe, N.L.   Fractures of the facial skeleton in children. *J. Oral Surg.* 26:505, 1968.

8. Rowe, N.L.   Fractures of the jaws in children. *J. Oral Surg.* 27:497, 1969.

9. Sørensen, D.C., and Laskin, D.M.   Facial growth after condylectomy or osteotomy in the mandibular ramus. *J. Oral Surg.* 33:746, 1975.

INDEX